MW00843949

Hsu

12/17/2020

Applied Immunohistochemistry
in the Evaluation of Skin Neoplasms

Jose A. Plaza • Victor G. Prieto
Editors

Applied Immunohistochemistry in the Evaluation of Skin Neoplasms

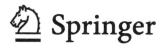 Springer

Editors
Jose A. Plaza
Miraca Life Sciences
Dermatopathology Division
Dallas, TX, USA

Victor G. Prieto
Department of Pathology
University of Texas MD Anderson
Cancer Center
Houston, TX, USA

ISBN 978-3-319-30588-2   ISBN 978-3-319-30590-5   (eBook)
DOI 10.1007/978-3-319-30590-5

Library of Congress Control Number: 2016933774

© Springer International Publishing Switzerland 2016
This work is subject to copyright. All rights are reserved by the Publisher, whether the whole or part of the material is concerned, specifically the rights of translation, reprinting, reuse of illustrations, recitation, broadcasting, reproduction on microfilms or in any other physical way, and transmission or information storage and retrieval, electronic adaptation, computer software, or by similar or dissimilar methodology now known or hereafter developed.
The use of general descriptive names, registered names, trademarks, service marks, etc. in this publication does not imply, even in the absence of a specific statement, that such names are exempt from the relevant protective laws and regulations and therefore free for general use.
The publisher, the authors and the editors are safe to assume that the advice and information in this book are believed to be true and accurate at the date of publication. Neither the publisher nor the authors or the editors give a warranty, express or implied, with respect to the material contained herein or for any errors or omissions that may have been made.

Printed on acid-free paper

This Springer imprint is published by Springer Nature
The registered company is Springer International Publishing AG Switzerland

Contents

Contributors

Rami Al-Rohil, M.D. Section of Dermatopathology, Department of Pathology, University of Texas, M.D. Anderson Cancer Center, Houston, TX, USA

Aurelio Ariza, M.D. Department of Pathology, Hospital Universitari Germans Trias i Pujol, Barcelona, Spain

Phyu P. Aung, M.D., Ph.D. Department of Pathology, The University of Texas M.D. Anderson Cancer Center, Houston, TX, USA

Jonathan L. Curry, M.D. Section of Dermatopathology, Department of Pathology, University of Texas, M.D. Anderson Cancer Center, Houston, TX, USA

Julio A. Diaz-Perez, M.D. Division of Dermatopathology, Department of Pathology, Wake Forest Baptist Medical Center, Winston-Salem, NC, USA

Brendan Craig Dickson, B.A., B.Sc., M.D., M.Sc., F.C.A.P., F.R.C.P(C.) Department of Pathology and Laboratory Medicine, Mount Sinai Hospital, Toronto, ON, Canada

Tammie Ferringer, M.D. Department of Dermatology, Geisinger Medical Center, Danville, PA, USA

Department of Laboratory Medicine, Geisinger Medical Center, Danville, PA, USA

Maria Teresa Fernández Figueras, M.D. Department of Anatomic Pathology, Hospital Universitari Germans Trias i Pujol, Barcelona, Spain

Heather Froehlich, M.D. Dermatopathology Division, Miraca Life Sciences, Irving, TX, USA

Laura Fuertes, M.D. Department of Dermatology, Fundación Jiménez Díaz, Universidad Autónoma, Madrid, Spain

Juan F. García, M.D., Ph.D. Department of Pathology, M.D. Anderson Cancer Center Madrid, Madrid, Spain

Danny Ghazarian, M.B., Ch.B., Ph.D., F.R.C.P.C. Laboratory Medicine Program, University Health Network, Toronto, ON, Canada

Ayman Al Habeeb, M.B.B.S., F.R.C.P.C. Department of Laboratory Medicine and Pathobiology, University Health Network, Toronto, ON, Canada

Doina Ivan, M.D. Department of Pathology, University of Texas, M.D. Anderson Cancer Center, Houston, TX, USA

Department of Dermatology, University of Texas – M.D. Anderson Cancer Center, Houston, TX, USA

Sebastien Labonte, M.D., F.R.C.P(C.) Department of Pathology, CHU-L'Hotel-Dieu de Quebec, Quebec City, QC, Canada

José Luis Mate, M.D. Department of Pathology, Hospital Universitari Germans Trias i Pujol, Barcelona, Spain

Roberto N. Miranda, M.D. Department of Hematopathology, University of Texas, M. D. Anderson Cancer Center, Houston, TX, USA

Ana M. Molina-Ruiz, M.D. Department of Dermatology, Fundación Jiménez Díaz, Universidad Autónoma, Madrid, Spain

Priyadharsini Nagarajan, M.D., Ph.D. Department of Pathology, Section of Dermatopathology, The University of Texas MD Anderson Cancer Center, Houston, TX, USA

Jose A. Plaza, M.D. Miraca Life Sciences, Dermatopathology Division, Dallas, TX, USA

Victor G. Prieto, M.D., Ph.D. Department of Pathology, University of Texas, M. D. Anderson Cancer Center, Houston, TX, USA

Luis Requena, M.D. Department of Dermatology, Fundación Jiménez Díaz, Universidad Autónoma, Madrid, Spain

Sadia Salim, M.D. Department of Dermatopathology, Miraca Life Sciences, Irving, TX, USA

Martin Sangueza, M.D. Department of Pathology, Hospital Obrero Nro 1, La Paz, Bolivia

Omar P. Sangüeza, M.D. Department of Pathology, Wake Forest University School of Medicine, Winston-Salem, NC, USA

Department of Dermatology, Wake Forest University School of Medicine, Winston-Salem, NC, USA

Olayemi Sokumbi, M.D. Section of Dermatopathology, Department of Dermatology, Medical College of Wisconsin, Milwaukee, WI, USA

Gustavo Tapia, M.D. Department of Pathology, Hospital Universitari Germans Trias i Pujol, Barcelona, Spain

Michael T. Tetzlaff, M.D., Ph.D. Department of Pathology, Section of Dermatopathology, The University of Texas MD Anderson Cancer Center, Houston, TX, USA

Department of Translational and Molecular Pathology, The University of Texas MD Anderson Cancer Center, Houston, TX, USA

Carlos A. Torres-Cabala, M.D. Dermatopathology Section, Department of Pathology, University of Texas, M.D. Anderson Cancer Center, Houston, TX, USA

Department of Dermatology, University of Texas, M.D. Anderson Cancer Center, Houston, TX, USA

Danielle M. Wehle, M.D.M.S. Department of Dermatopathology, Miraca Life Sciences, Irving, TX, USA

Part I

Immunohistology of Epithelial Tumors

Immunohistology and Molecular Studies of Epithelial Tumors

Heather Froehlich and Jose A. Plaza

Basal Cell Carcinoma

Basal cell carcinoma (BCC) is the most common cutaneous neoplasm. In one population-based study in Rochester, Minnesota, the annual incidence for BCC was estimated at 146 cases per 100,000 persons [1]. Risk factors include exposure to sunlight and, to a lesser degree, ionizing radiation and arsenic exposure [2].

Histologically, cells of BCC resemble cells of the basal layer of the epidermis; however, the cell of origin for BCC remains unclear and controversial. The varying histologic subtypes may arise from different cellular compartments of the skin, particularly stem cells of the interfollicular epidermis and from the upper infundibulum [3]. Although multiple histologic patterns exist for BCC, the clinical subtypes of BCC can be more broadly classified into indolent-growth and aggressive-growth subtypes [4, 5]. Subtypes with indolent growth include superficial and nodular types. Subtypes with aggressive growth include morpheaform (sclerosing, infiltrative),

micronodular, and basosquamous [4]. Although most BCCs are treated successfully by surgical excision, more aggressive subtypes have the potential to be locally destructive or metastasize. Metastatic BCC is rare, with an incidence reported at 0.03 % [6, 7].

The nevoid basal cell carcinoma syndrome (NBCCS) is an autosomal disorder manifesting as hundreds to thousands of BCCs in a single patient in addition to odontogenic keratocysts, palmar and plantar pits, and increased incidence of other neoplasms including medulloblastomas and rhabdomyosarcomas [8]. Patients with NBCCS have one defective copy of the patched 1 (PTCH1) tumor suppressor gene on chromosome 9q22, which encodes a receptor for the Sonic hedgehog (SHH) pathway [9, 10]. Biallelic inactivation of the PTCH1 gene results in constitutive upregulation of SHH signaling which is required for BCC proliferation and survival [11, 12]. Mutations in PTCH1 gene and subsequent upregulation of HH signaling occurs both in NBCCS and in sporadic BCCs. A minority of sporadic BCCs have mutations in the downstream smoothened (SMO) protein that also leads to SHH upregulation and BCC carcinogenesis [13–16]. Other somatic mutations that contribute to BCC carcinogenesis include p53 mutations, the majority of which are presumably ultraviolet (UV)-induced [17].

On histology, BCC shows nests of basaloid keratinocytes surrounded by stoma, often with peritumoral retraction and peripheral palisading

H. Froehlich, M.D. (✉)
Dermatopathology Division, Miraca Life Sciences,
Irving, TX, USA
e-mail: HFroehlich@MiracaLS.com

J.A. Plaza, M.D.
Miraca Life Sciences, Dermatopathology Division,
6655 MacArthur Boulevard, Dallas, Texas 75039, USA
e-mail: jplaza@miracals.com

© Springer International Publishing Switzerland 2016
J.A. Plaza, V.G. Prieto (eds.), *Applied Immunohistochemistry in the Evaluation of Skin Neoplasms*, DOI 10.1007/978-3-319-30590-5_1

of lesional cells. Mucin is often present. Mitotic and apoptotic cells are frequent. Different subtypes of BCC demonstrate different histologic patterns.

Superficial BCC shows connection to the epidermis with downward buds of basaloid cells, often with peritumoral retraction. Nodular BCC shows nests, often large, that extend into the papillary and reticular dermis. Peritumoral retraction and mucin pooling is frequent. Morpheaform BCC shows infiltrative strands of BCC within a thick, collagenous stroma, that can often extend into the deep dermis and subcutis. Micronodular BCC shows small round nests of BCC with an associated dense stroma that can extend deep into the dermis or subcutis. Basosquamous BCC or metatypical BCC shows a basaloid cell morphology but with areas of keratinization.

The diagnosis of BCC with an adequate sample is often straightforward without any immunohistochemical stain required. Different subtypes of BCC, however, on a superficial shave biopsy, may raise the possibility of other diagnoses that require alternative treatment modalities. In such circumstances, IHC can be applied, in addition to morphologic criteria, to favor one diagnosis over the other.

Infiltrative BCC, microcystic adnexal carcinoma (MAC), and desmoplastic trichoepithelioma (DTE) can show morphologic similarities and immunohistochemistry stains are useful in this differential. BerEP4 shows positivity in BCC and DTE, whereas MAC is typically negative. BerEP4, however, can be negative in the center or surface of BCC and in areas with a more squamoid morphology [18]. BerEP4 positivity is seen not only in basal cell carcinoma but in poromas, porocarcinomas, chondroid syringomas, hidradenomas, and primary mucinous carcinoma [19]. CK15 is positive in 90% of MACs, 100% of DTEs and is negative in BCC and squamous cell carcinomas (SCC) [20]. Androgen receptor (AR) positivity can be seen in superficial, nodular, and most infiltrative basal cell carcinomas and is negative in most desmoplastic trichoepitheliomas; however, AR positivity is reported in classic trichoepithelioma, trichoblastoma, and sebaceous carcinoma, all of which may enter the differential [21–23]. Pleckstrin

homology-like domain, formerly A, member 1 (PHLDA1) is also reportedly useful to differentiate infiltrative BCC from DTE. DTE is positive for PHLDA1 and infiltrative BCC is typically negative; however, other subtypes of BCC, particularly micronodular BCC, can be positive in up to one third of cases [24]. (Fig. 1.1a, b).

BCC with squamous metaplasia versus SCC with basaloid features can be a difficult differential on histologic grounds. BCC shows strong and diffuse staining for both CK17 and CK14, in addition to Ber-EP4 and although SCC can show occasional positivity for each marker individually, it should not show diffuse positivity for all markers [25].

Sebaceous carcinoma (SC) is an aggressive neoplasm that may histologically mimic other malignant tumors, especially BCC and SCC; therefore, its recognition is important for appropriate treatment. In the past, Oil Red O was used to identify intracytoplasmic lipids in sebaceous lesions in fresh frozen tissue; however, standard permanent tissue processing extracts the intracellular lipids and often nonspecifically highlights macrophages and non-lipid laden cells in the background stroma. Many studies have analyzed conventional markers such as EMA, Ber-EP4, androgen receptor, CK7, and P53 [21, 26–28]; but these studies have shown variable results and the markers have mostly been analyzed individually rather than as part of a comprehensive panel. New studies have investigated the utility of lipid droplet proteins as markers of SC. The use of antibodies against the PAT family of lipid droplet-associated proteins perilipin (PLIN1) and adipophilin showed great success within specific diagnostic contexts. Adipophilin is more sensitive than Oil Red O in highlighting cytoplasmic lipid vesicles, and the sensitivity of adipophilin in poorly differentiated SC is approximately 82%. We recently published a large series of SC and compared the immunohistochemical profile with BCC and SCC [29]. In our series, all SCs were EMA positive (100%); however, in a minority of SC cases, EMA was only focally and irregularly positive in cases of poorly differentiated SC. All cases of BCC were negative for EMA but SCC expressed EMA in 72.72% of cases. As reported previously, our study also proved that

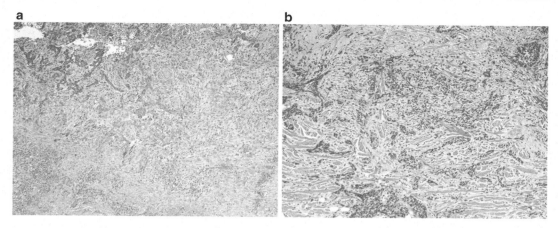

Fig. 1.1 (**a**) This is an example of infiltrative BCC. In small or in limited tissue samples, lesions can show similarities with a desmoplastic trichoepithelioma. (**b**) Infiltrative BCC composed of small cords and fascicles of basaloid cells

immunohistochemical detection of EMA is useful only in differentiating SC from BCC; however, in poorly differentiated cases of SC, EMA can be negative or only focally positive. EMA alone is not useful to differentiate SC from SCC. Some authors evaluated the diagnostic utility of CK 7 to separate SC from both BCC and SCC. Such studies have had variable results with some showing high sensitivity and specificity to separate SC from BCC and SCC. Our experience differs to the previous studies in terms of CK7 expression in both SCC and BCC. Our results also showed that 28.5 % of BCC, 9 % of SCC, and 88.8 % of cases of SC expressed CK7. Most cases of SCC did not express CK7; thus, immunohistochemical detection of CK7 in neoplastic cells may be valuable in differentiating SC from SCC in most instances. CK7 is not a reliable marker to separate SC from BCC. Ber-EP4 is an epithelial marker that has been utilized and studied previously in this context. Up to 25 % of SC can express Ber-EP4; whereas 100 % of BCC cases are positive (diffusely and strongly positive) and 100 % of SCC are negative, suggesting that Ber-EP4 is a reliable marker in differentiating SC (EMA+/Ber-EP4−/+) from BCC (EMA−/Ber-EP4+) and SCC (EMA+/−/Ber-EP4-) when combined with other markers such as EMA or protein lipid markers and it should not be used alone for such a distinction. Adipophilin is a monoclonal antibody raised against a protein on the surface of intracellular lipid droplets, and it has been shown to be expressed in sebocytes and sebaceous lesions. Recent studies have investigated the utility of lipid droplet proteins as markers of SC and has been reported to be a sensitive marker for SC. In some of these studies, adipophilin has been reported to show a nonspecific granular uptake of antibody in the epithelial cells of BCC and SCC creating diagnostic confusion. In addition, it is our experience that in cases of SCC in situ granular cytoplasmic expression of adipophilin can be easily misinterpreted as intraepithelial SC, representing a diagnostic pitfall. The bubbly/vacuolar cytoplasmic expression that corresponds to intracytoplasmic lipid vacuoles would support the diagnosis of SC. In our study, we found adipophilin expression in all cases of SC which was defined as membranous labeling of intracytoplasmic lipid globules [29]. In our view, histology remains the gold standard for diagnosis of SC, and we suggest that the immunohistochemical assessment for epithelial markers and lipid droplet-associated proteins are a helpful diagnostic adjunct in the assessment of such tumors. Immunostaining for epithelial markers should be performed once careful standard microscopic evaluation has taken place. If these results are nonconclusive for SC, the prospective diagnosis can be confirmed by a lipid droplet-associated protein, such as adipophilin (Fig. 1.2a–k).

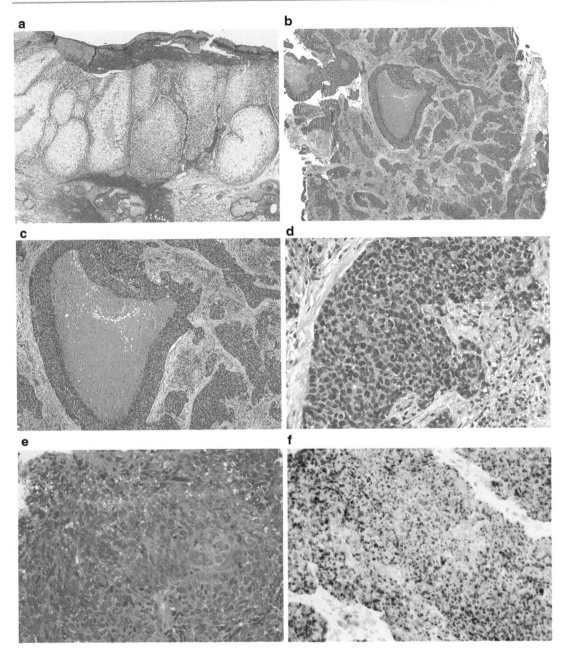

Fig. 1.2 (**a**) This is an example of a low grade sebaceous carcinoma. These neoplasms are usually easily diagnosed on H&E and do not need IHC workup. (**b**) This a poorly differentiated sebaceous carcinoma. Note the basaloid features and the comedo necrosis. These neoplasms can be confused with other malignancies such as basal cell carcinoma and squamous cell carcinoma. (**c**) High power of a poorly differentiated sebaceous carcinoma. Note the lack of sebaceous differentiation requiring IHC to further classify the process. (**d**) Poorly differentiated sebaceous carcinoma. A diagnostic clue is the presence of a subtle vacuolar pattern in the cytoplasm of the neoplastic cells.

(**e**) Another example of poorly differentiated sebaceous carcinoma. Note the subtle cytoplasmic vacuoles in the basaloid cells. (**f**) Cytoplasmic vacuolar pattern with adipophilin. (**g**) Sebaceous carcinoma. EMA is strongly positive. (**h**) This is a example of BCC with clear cell features. This neoplasm was localized in the eyelid of a 56-year-old man. The ddx of this neoplasm is with sebaceous carcinoma. (**i**) BCC with clear cell features. High power of the basaloid cells with clear cell differentiation. (**j**) BCC with clear cell features. Adipophilin stain is negative, but notice the focal granular staining that is classically seen in BCC. (**k**) BCC with clear cell features. EMA is negative

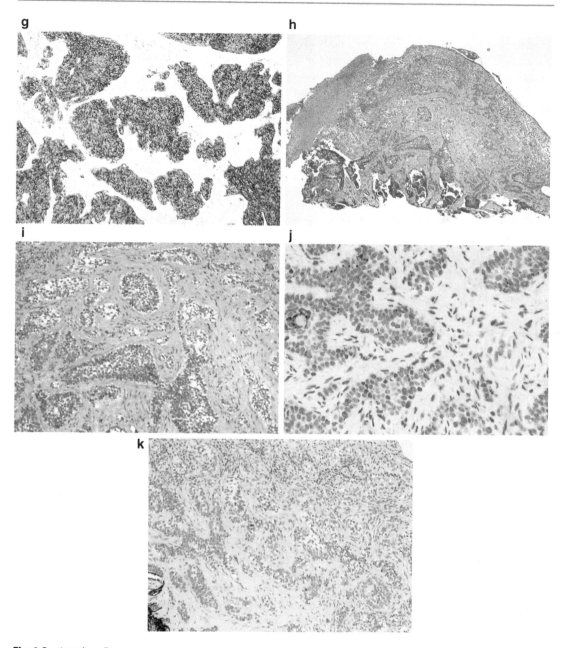

Fig. 1.2 (continued)

Another common problem in dermatopathology is the distinction between trichoepithelioma and BCC. Histomorphologic analysis has become in recent years more difficult because of the use of small shave biopsies, which for the most part deprive the histomorphologist of many architectural clues to the correct diagnosis. Trichoepitheliomas are hamartomatous tumors with follicular differentiation and a mesenchymal response equivalent to that seen in a normal hair follicle. Histopathologic features that favor a diagnosis of trichoepithelioma include a well circumscribed symmetrical lesion with symmetric and smooth margins, mesenchymal body differentiation usually in the form of germs and papillae, a cribriform pattern of neoplastic basaloid cells, clefts within the stroma and between the stroma and adjacent normal dermis, cornification of neoplastic epithelial cells that can be seen in association with foreign body granulomas, and a highly fibrotic stroma resembling that of perifollicular connective tissue. In contrast, histopathologic features that will favor a diagnosis of BCC, include an asymmetrical poorly circumscribed lesion, often with jagged borders, numerous necrotic neoplastic cells often en masse, frequent presence of melanin in germinative cells, frequent presence of acid mucosubstances within aggregations of epithelial cells and in the stroma, clefts between neoplastic cells and stroma, an edematous stroma, infiltrates of inflammatory cells, and frequent ulceration. Due to the major differences in management and prognosis of these two lesions, a correct diagnosis is desirable and expected. A number of studies have evaluated ancillary diagnostic tools, such as the immunohistochemical studies using CD34, CK15, CK14, Ber-Ep4, bcl-2, p53, etc., but have provided only limited support and diagnostic utility in the adjunctive histological separation of BCCs from trichoepitheliomas. Additionally, some studies have expressed the opinion that these two neoplasms may represent different points along the same neoplastic spectrum and are therefore difficult to differentiate on immunohistochemical techniques. We analyzed the expression of podoplanin (D2–40) in this setting. This antibody is a well-known lymphovascular marker that has been shown to react in the basal layer of the outer root sheath of hair follicles, peripheral germinative cells of sebaceous glands, and some cutaneous neoplasms. In our study, we found expression of podoplanin in 22.20 % of BCC's and in 95 % of trichoepitheliomas. Also, podoplanin expression in trichoepitheliomas was noted to be present not only in the basal layer of the tumor cells but also in the suprabasal layer of the tumor cells, as opposed to BCC's in which the positivity was primarily located in the basal layer of the tumor nests. The

overall sensitivity and specificity of podoplanin immunoreactivity to separate primary BCC's from trichoepitheliomas was 95.5 % and 77.8 %, respectively, in this study [30]. The fact that a subset of BCC's can express podoplanin could embrace the premise that these neoplasms may have the potential for multilinear differentiation.

Clear Cell Acanthoma

Clear cell acanthoma (CCA), originally reported by Degos et al., presents as a solitary, circumscribed pink or red papule or nodule, often with a collarette of scale [31]. Although CCA has previously been considered as a benign epidermal neoplasm, more recent findings suggest that CCA represents a localized inflammatory dermatosis akin to psoriasis [32, 33].

Typically, an acanthotic and psoriasiform epidermis is present, sharply demarcated from the surrounding normal epidermis. Lesional keratinocytes demonstrate cytoplasmic clearing with abundant glycogen which can be highlighted with PAS staining. Neutrophils are characteristically present within the lesion and in the overlying stratum corneum.

IHC findings demonstrate positive staining for CKAE1/AE3, CK34BE12, and negative staining for CAM5.2, a staining pattern that parallels the normal epidermis and psoriasis, further lending support to the concept of clear cell acanthoma as a localized inflammatory process [33, 34].

Intraepidermal Epithelioma of Borst–Jadassohn

Whether or not intraepidermal epithelioma of Borst–Jadassohn (IEBJ) represents a histologic pattern or a distinct tumor entity has been a matter of much debate. Many authors prefer to ascribe the term "Borst–Jadassohn phenomenon" (BJP) to a morphologic pattern of nested atypical keratinocytes situated within normal epidermis. The BJP has been described in a variety of lesions such as Bowen's disease, actinic keratoses, hidroacanthoma simplex, and seborrheic keratoses.

Tumors that features the Borst–Jadassohn phenomenon prominently include clonal seborrheic
keratosis and clonal Bowen's disease, which can
be challenging to differentiate on histologic
grounds. Immunohistochemistry can aid the morphologic impression. A study performed by Lora
et al. [35] evaluated the IHC expression of several antibodies and demonstrated that the lesional
cells of BJP are positive for epidermal growth
factor-receptors (EGF-R) in a cell membranous
pattern as well as Ki-67, p63, and p53 in clonal
seborrheic keratosis, clonal Bowen's disease,
hidroacanthoma simplex, and porocarcinoma.
Nests of BJP were negative for CK7 and CK19.
CK5/6 positivity was seen in nests of clonal seborrheic keratosis and hidroacanthoma simplex,
but was negative in clonal Bowen's disease and
porocarcinoma [35]. More recently, lumican
expression has been utilized to differentiate
hidroacanthoma simplex and clonal seborrheic
keratosis. Lumican is expressed in most lesions
of hidroacanthoma simplex, but is negative in
most seborrheic keratoses, with some exceptions
[36]. Lumican positivity can also be seen in
Bowen's disease but is typically negative in normal keratinocytes within the epidermis [36].

Bowenoid Papulosis

Bowenoid papulosis (BP) histologically resembles Bowen's disease (BD) but shows a distinct
clinical presentation as multiple papules that
develop on the penis, vulva, perineum, or perianal regions, generally on a younger population than Bowen's disease. Lesions may rarely
spontaneously regress, but have the potential
for progression into an invasive tumor and,
rarely, metastasis. BP is associated with human
papilloma virus (HPV) [37] and is considered
transmissible through sexual or vertical transmission [38].

BP histologically resembles Bowen's disease
with full-thickness keratinocyte atypia and mitoses. Epidermal acanthosis, hyperkeratosis, and
parakeratosis are also seen. Although lesions
appear nearly identical histologically, the nuclei
in bowenoid papulosis are reportedly smaller

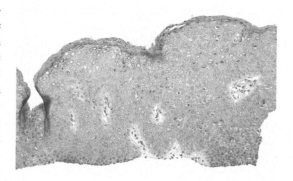

Fig. 1.3 Bowenoid papulosis. Without appropriate clinical history these lesions can be easily mistaken for SCC
in situ

with less pleomorphism than Bowen's disease
[39]. (Fig. 1.3)

Immunohistochemistry is not helpful in distinguishing between BP and BD. Both can
express p16, which classically demonstrates diffuse positive staining [40, 41]. Expression of p16
is also present, however, in condyloma, though
with more focal, scattered positivity compared to
BP [40]. HPV is involved in the pathogenesis of
BP and may disrupt the regulation of cell cycle
related proteins, cyclin D1 and cyclin E [42].
Immunohistochemistry, polymerase chain reaction, and in situ hybridization are all methods
commonly employed to detect and subtype
HPV. Identification of high-risk subtypes in BP is
important for the patient and for their sexual partners who are at risk of HPV transmission.

Clear Cell Papulosis

Clear cell papulosis (CCP) presents as multiple
hypopigmented macules and papules [43, 44].
Histologically, the lesion demonstrates clear cells
along the basal layer of the epidermis. No cytologic atypia or mitotic figures are seen. The histologic differential includes Toker's cell of the
nipple, Paget's disease, extramammary paget's
disease, clear cell squamous cell carcinoma in
situ, melanoma in situ, and sebaceous carcinoma
in situ.

Clear cell papulosis and the lack of overt atypia should readily distinguish CPP from malignant neoplasms. On IHC, lesional cells are positive for CAE1, CEA, EMA, GCDFP-15 [44]. Scattered mucin positivity is also seen, in contrast to Toker cells, which are mucin negative [45]. Clear cells are positive for IKH-4, and negative for lysozyme, which is suggestive of an eccrine secretory origin [46]. Long term follow-up shows CCP to be a benign, asymptomatic entity that often partially regresses and requires no treatment [47].

Pseudoepitheliomatous Hyperplasia

Pseudoepitheliomatous hyperplasia (PEH) is a reactive epidermal proliferation that shows histologic resemblance to SCC. Clinical presentation depends on the underlying process; however, lesions generally present as a scaly or crusted plaque or nodule, often one to several centimeters in size. Histologically, lesions of PEH demonstrate irregular epidermal hyperplasia with downward projections into the reticular dermis. Mild cytologic atypic may be present; however, necrosis or atypical mitotic figures are usually absent. Without a detailed clinical history, and without a systematic approach to exclude a variety of disorders that feature PEH as a secondary lesion, a biopsy could easily be misinterpreted as well-differentiated squamous cell carcinoma.

PEH is classically present in association with numerous disorders, particularly deep fungal infections, conditions with chronic irritation or inflammation, and various neoplastic conditions. Distinguishing between PEH and SCC can be challenging, and although an immunohistochemistry panel utilizing p53, E-cadherin, and MMP-1 can be of use on mucosal biopsies [48], the same stains do not reliably distinguish the two entities in a cutaneous setting. Immunohistochemistry stains for p53 protein have not proven helpful in differentiating PEH from SCC, nor does CD1a staining for Langerhans cells distinguish the entities, despite various proposals that either stain might be of value in the distinction between reactive and neoplastic proliferations [49]. More

recently, matrix metalloproteinase-19 and tumor suppressor protein p16 have been demonstrated to be potential markers distinguishing PEH and SCC. Loss of MMP-19 and p16 may favor malignancy in the particular setting of a chronic wound [50]. Studies examining the role of epidermal growth factor receptor have not demonstrated EGFR to play a pathogenic role for PEH [51, 52].

Molecular studies may hold promise in the future for distinguishing PEH from SCC. One study series examined the molecular pathways and genes involved in SCC and PEH by using gene expression microarrays [53] and then identified two genes, C15orf48 and KRT9, which had distinct gene expression patterns for SCC and PEH [54]. Using a multiplex TaqMan PCR assay, the two conditions could be distinguished with high sensitivity.

Actinic Keratoses

Actinic keratosis clinically present as erythematous, scaly lesions on sun-exposed skin. Lesions arise as a consequence to UV radiation exposure or immune suppression [55, 56]. Histologically, actinic keratoses can display a variety of patterns, but classically demonstrate parakeratosis, acanthosis, and squamous dysplasia involving the basal layer of the interadnexal epidermis. Several histologic variants of actinic keratosis exist including hypertrophic, acantholytic, and pigmented subtypes [57–59]. There can be difficulty distinguishing actinic keratosis from early squamous cell carcinoma in situ and the two entities often form part of a continuum of histologic findings. Histologically, actinic keratosis can resemble superficial basal cell carcinoma. In these instances, Ber-EP4 can be useful. Epidermal buds of superficial basal cell carcinoma are positive for Ber-EP4 staining, whereas basal epidermal cells of actinic keratosis are negative [60].

Squamous Cell Carcinoma In Situ

Squamous cell carcinoma in situ presents as an erythematous plaque, often sharply demarcated from the surrounding skin. Histologically, keratinocyte dysplasia is present in all layers of the epidermis and involves intraepidermal adnexal epithelium with overlying parakeratosis. Keratinocytes often have abundant, pale cytoplasm with numerous mitoses and varying degrees of nuclear atypia and hyperchromasia. Squamous cell carcinoma in situ with prominent clear cell change can raise the histologic differential of Paget's disease, extramammary Paget's disease (EMPD), melanoma in situ, or, rarely, intraepithelial sebaceous carcinoma [61]. Histologic features that support the diagnosis of squamous cell carcinoma in situ include keratinization of cells, intercellular bridges, and keratohyaline granules [62]; however, in difficult cases, immunohistochemical studies are useful to arrive at the correct diagnosis. SCCIS stains positive with p63 [63]. EMPD typically is positive for mucicarmine, carcinoembryonic antigen (CEA), CK7, CAM5.2, and Ber-EP4 [62, 64–67]. There are reports, however, of SCCIS with CK7 and CAM5.2 positivity, and positive staining should be interpreted with caution and within the appropriate clinical context. [64, 68] Intraepithelial sebaceous carcinoma can show positivity for EMA, Ber-EP4, androgen receptor (AR), and adipophilin [21, 69].

Pagetoid SCCIS (PSCCIS) is a well-documented variant of SCCIS that has a tendency to occur on sun-exposed skin, such as the extremities and head/neck area. [70] Squamous cell carcinoma can develop in non-sun exposed areas of the body as well, especially in immunocompromised patients. Some PSCCIS have been described in the genital areas. The main differential diagnosis of PSCCIS in the genital area is with EMPD, specifically primary EMPD, where the neoplastic process arises within epidermis itself, as opposed to secondary involvement from an internal organ. Because of the potential overlap in histological features and anatomic distribution of PSCCIS and EMPD, immunohistochemistry may be helpful in the workup of these cutaneous pagetoid neoplasms. Intraepidermal lesions with pagetoid distribution can cause diagnostic difficulties. While there are some important histologic clues to separate PSCCIS from EMPD, they

may not be sufficient to render a definitive diagnosis. Keratohyaline granules, single cell keratinization, and intercellular bridges in the tumor cells are histologic changes that will favor the diagnosis of PSCCIS. Histochemical and immunohistochemical studies can be of value in distinguishing these lesions; however, caution must be exercised in their interpretation as they can represent diagnostic traps. Positive mucicarmine is of value in diagnosing EMPD in most cases, but not all cases are positive for mucin. CEA expression is generally considered as evidence of glandular differentiation and supports the diagnosis of EMPD; however, rare cases of EMPD can be negative for this marker and some PSCCIS are positive. Paget cells also express GCDFP-15, in line with an apocrine epithelial differentiation, but its expression is only observed in two-thirds of cases. CK7 has been regarded as the immunohistochemical stain of choice in the diagnosis of EMPD, but few cases of PSCCIS have been reported to stain positive for this marker. CAM 5.2 has been reported to be useful in separating these neoplasms, as cases of EMPD tend to express this marker but rare cases of PSCCIS can be positive for this marker. More recently, Ber-EP4 has been reported to be a useful marker for differentiating EMPD from PSCCIS, showing moderate to strong positivity in all cases of EMPD. We reported the use of p63 in this setting. In our series we found that all cases of primary EMPD were negative for p63 and all cases of PSCCIS expressed p63. This lack of expression in EMPD is because these neoplasms arise from the intraepidermal portion of apocrine glands. In the context of pagetoid cutaneous neoplasms, p63 appeared to be a sensitive and specific marker for PSCCIS. Our results confirmed that strong nuclear positivity for p63 in the pagetoid cells is highly specific for PSCCIS. A point of caution is that the rare secondary EMPD from urothelial carcinomas may express p63 (however, most secondary EMPD cases are negative) (Fig. 1.4a–h).

Intraepithelial sebaceous carcinoma can mimic SCC in situ. Intraepithelial sebaceous carcinoma is usually associated with sebaceous carcinoma; however, rare cases can present without the presence of an invasive component. In such

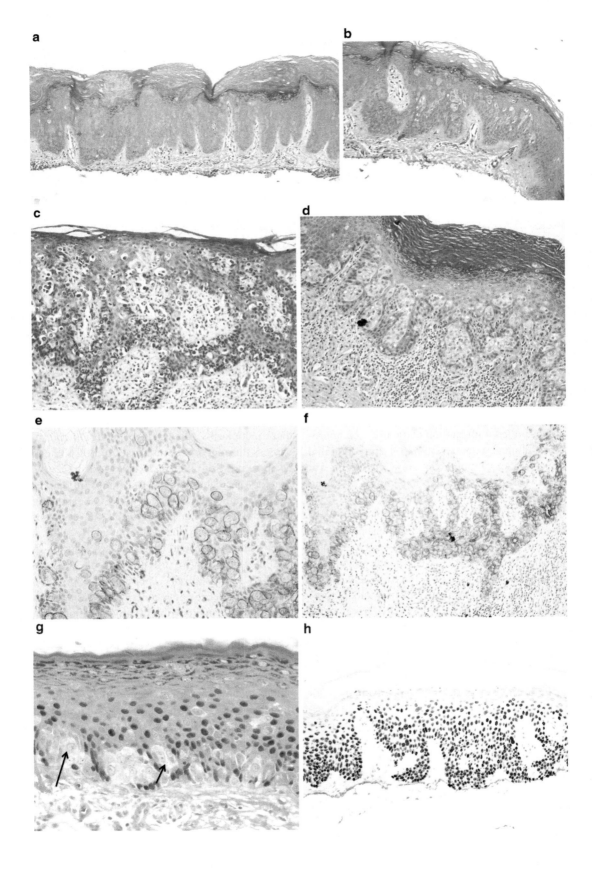

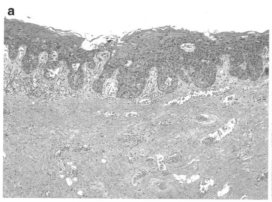
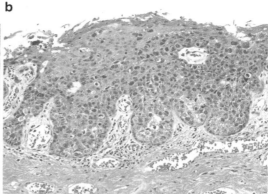

Fig. 1.5 (**a**) Intraepidermal sebaceous carcinoma in situ. This variant of sebaceous carcinoma can be easily mistaken for SCC in situ. (**b**) Intraepidermal sebaceous carci-noma in situ. Diagnostic clue is the presence of scattered large cells with clear/bubbly cytoplasm

cases, it does not extend beyond the epidermal basement membrane and/or lacks any association with preexisting sebaceous glands. In some instances it is very difficult to make an accurate diagnosis given the rarity of intraepithelial disease. Histologic features to consider include a proliferation of intraepidermal atypical basaloid cells with enlarged and hyperchromatic nuclei intermingled with vacuolated cells containing bubbly cytoplasm and scalloped nuclei and disordered cell growth. The constellation of histological findings demonstrating vacuolated cells containing bubbly cytoplasm and scalloped nuclei and adipophilin positivity by immunohistochemistry supports the diagnosis of intraepithelial sebaceous carcinoma [69] (Fig. 1.5a, b).

Rarely, intraepidermal neuroendocrine carcinoma (Merkel cell carcinoma, MCC) enters the histologic differential and immunohistochemistry, particularly MCC positivity for CK20, chromogranin, and synaptophysin, can help confirm the diagnosis [71].

Squamous Cell Carcinoma

The World Health Organization (WHO) classification of cutaneous squamous cell carcinomas (SCC) includes spindle-cell (sarcomatoid) SCC, acantholytic SCC, verrucous SCC, SCC with horn formation, and lymphoepithelial SCC subtypes. Another classification scheme proposed by Cassarino et al. includes several more variants, each stratified by their risk of metastic potential [72, 73]. Low-risk variants (</= 2 % risk) include SCC arising in actinic keratosis, verrucous SCC, spindle cell SCC, and tricholemmal carcinoma. Intermediate malignant potential variants (3–10 % risk) include acantholytic SCC, lymphoepithelioma-like carcinoma, and Jadassohn tumor with invasion. Several squamous cell carcinoma variants are high risk (>10 % risk), including invasive Bowen's disease, adenosquamous carcinoma, desmoplastic SCC, and SCC that arises in chronic conditions or radiation.

Fig. 1.4 (**a**) Pagetoid SCC in situ. Note the full thickness atypia along with scattered pagetoid cells. (**b**) Pagetoid SCC in situ. Note the increased number of pagetoid keratinocytes within epidermis. This variant of SCC can be confused with extramammary Paget's disease. (**c**) Extramammary Paget's disease. Note the similarities with pagetoid SCC in situ. (**d**) Extramammary Paget's disease. Diagnostics clues include the lack of keratohyaline granules and intercellular bridges. (**e**) Extramammary Paget's disease. CAM 5.2 expression. (**f**) Extramammary Paget's disease. CK 7 expression. (**g**) Extramammary Paget's disease. This is a p63 and H&E counterstain and note the neoplastic cells are negative for p63 (*arrow*). (**h**) Pagetoid SCC in situ. The cells are positive for p63 (neoplastic and non-neoplastic keratinocytes)

Verrucous Squamous Cell Carcinoma

Verrucous carcinoma was first described by Ackerman in 1948 [74]. Clinically, verrucous carcinoma involves mucosal surfaces, anogenital sites, and plantar surfaces and present as exophytic warty growths. Lesions on mucosal surfaces and anogenital sites are HPV related; however, a weaker association exists with HPV occurring on cutaneous sites [38]. Verrucous SCC is considered low-grade.

Histologically, lesions demonstrate acanthosis, papillomatosis with overlying parakeratosis. At the base of the tumor, the lesion demonstrates a broad, pushing border with blunt epithelial projections into the dermis. Cytologically, keratinocytes demonstrate minimal cytologic atypia. The differential includes epithelial hyperplasia and verrucous lesions. Immunohistochemical expression of p53 and Ki-67 have been reported to aid in the differential with stronger expression in basal and suprabasal cells in verrucous carcinoma [75–77].

Spindle Cell Squamous Cell Carcinoma

Spindle cell (sarcomatoid) SCC, when associated with radiation exposure, typically follows an aggressive course. Without a prior history of radiation, spindle cell SCC is considered low-risk [72]. On histology, spindle cell SCC is composed of cytologically atypical spindle cells with numerous mitotic figures and often with a lack of overtly squamous morphology. The differential includes spindle cell melanoma, atypical fibroxanthoma/pleomorphic undifferentiated sarcoma and cutaneous leiomyosarcoma/atypical smooth muscle neoplasm. Immunohistochemistry can confirm the diagnosis with positive cytokeratin staining; however, not all spindle cell SCC demonstrate positivity with all cytokeratins. High molecular weight cytokeratins, such as CK34BE12 and CK5/6 are the most sensitive in this variant of SCC [72, 78–82] compared to low molecular weight cytokeratins (CAM5.2, CK8/18) or pan-cytokeratins (CKAE1/AE3) [83, 84]. Immunostaining for p63 is also useful, but

can occasionally show focal positivity in AFX [82, 84]. The p40 isoform of p63 demonstrates higher sensitivity and may be a better marker in select cases [82]. (Fig. 1.6a–f)

The distinction of AFX from sarcomatoid carcinomas, may be difficult despite the use of immunohistochemistry, given that a subset of sarcomatoid carcinomas may lack cytokeratin expression (1). Many immunohistochemical markers have been regarded as reliable for AFX including CD10, CD99, CD163, and CD68 [80, 85]; however, they have not shown sufficient sensitivity and specificity to replace the more common approach which is a diagnosis of exclusion. Several studies have examined the use of p63 in AFX, showing that p63 is negative while consistently positive in sarcomatoid carcinoma. Conflicting results have been observed in other studies showing the lack of sensitivity of p63 in squamous cell carcinomas as well as the positivity of p63 in non-epithelial malignancies including AFX and melanoma. We reported that poorly differentiated squamous cell carcinomas (sarcomatoid carcinomas) can be negative for p63, as we found expression in only 6/10 cases, with one case showing only focal expression [86]. This finding represents a potential diagnostic pitfall, especially when only a limited panel of immunohistochemical stains is performed. AFX represents a relatively indolent lesion when compared to sarcomatoid carcinoma and due to the major differences in management and prognosis, a correct diagnosis is desirable and expected. Awareness of this phenomenon is critical when evaluating sarcomatoid carcinomas and sometimes a battery of immunostains can help to demonstrate epithelial differentiation. Also, cases of sarcomatoid carcinoma may entirely lose immunohistochemical markers of epithelial differentiation, which then may be confirmed by ancillary studies, such as ultrastructural analysis.

Acantholytic Squamous Cell Carcinoma (Adenoid)

Acantholytic, or adenoid SCC, first described by Lever, demonstrates areas of gland-like, or pseudoglandular proliferation, a phenomenon secondary

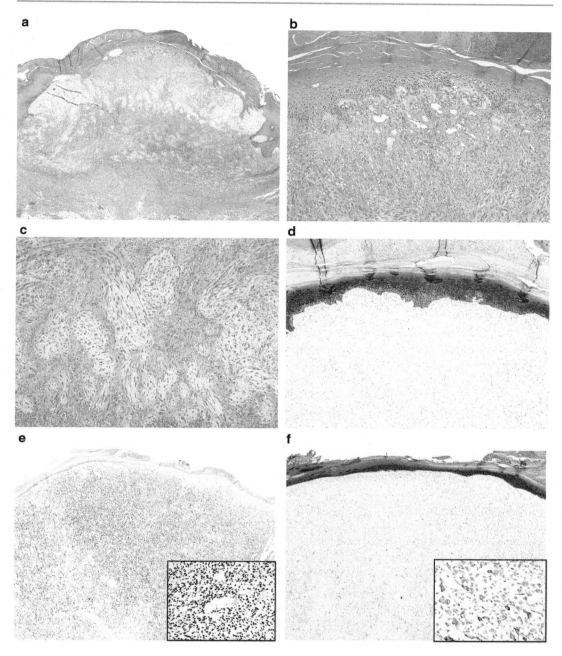

Fig. 1.6 (**a**) Sarcomatoid carcinoma. Note a poorly differentiated neoplasm in dermis. These neoplasms require IHC stains to arrive to the correct diagnosis. (**b**) Sarcomatoid carcinoma. In some cases a clear cut in situ component cannot be identified as depicted in this example. (**c**) Sarcomatoid carcinoma. Note the presence of malignant spindle cells in dermis with a fascicular pattern. (**d**) Sarcomatoid carcinoma. It is very important to order the correct battery of immunostains when analyzing these tumors. Cytokeratin stains are usually positive but can be negative in some cases (as depicted in this image with wide spectrum keratin). (**e**) Sarcomatoid carcinoma. P63 is often positive (but in rare occasions can be negative; thus, multiple epithelial marker need to be ordered). (**f**) Sarcomatoid carcinoma. These neoplasms are often positive for high molecular weight cytokeratin (34bE12)

to loss of cohesion, or acantholysis. Metastatic risk has been reported as high as 19% [87]. Altered desmosomal cadherins most likely contribute to the acantholytic phenomenon and formation of gland-like structures in adenoid SCC and may promote invasion and more aggressive behavior [88–91]. Adenoid SCC is positive for CKs, EMA, and negative for PAS-d, mucicarmine, and CEA. [87] (McKee, pg 1128), which helps distinguish adenoid SCC from metastatic adenocarcinomas and eccrine carcinomas.

Lymphoepithelioma-Like Carcinoma

Lymphoepithelioma-like carcinoma (LELC) of the skin, first described by Swanson et al. is a rare malignant neoplasm that resembles nasopharyngeal carcinoma [92]. Similar lesions have been reported at other sites, including salivary gland, thymus, tonsil, and uterine cervix [92]. Unlike its counterpart in the nasopharynx, LELC of skin is typically not associated with Epstein-Barr virus [68, 93–96], with rare exception [97].

Histologically, LELC is comprised of islands of cytologically atypical epithelial cells with abundant cytoplasm and vesicular nuclei surrounded by a dense lymphocytic infiltrate, often with an uninvolved overlying epidermis. On low power, aggregates of epithelioid cells may suggest germinal centers. If the subtle cohesion between the epithelial cells is overlooked, the lesion can be misinterpreted as lymphocytoma cutis, cutaneous lymphadenoma, or a B-cell lymphoma [98]. Other carcinomas can mimic LELC such as BCC, spiradenocarcinoma, and carcinoma with thymus-like differentiation (CASTLE) [99–101]. Of the above entities, CASTLE, which demonstrates Hassall's corpuscles, can be excluded on histologic grounds. Given the broad differential, immunohistochemical stains are routinely performed in the diagnosis of LELC of skin.

Epithelial cells demonstrate cytokeratin and EMA positivity, and are CK7, CD20 negative [93, 102]. LELC is often considered a variant of SCC and therefore distinguishing between inflamed SCC and LELC may be impossible.

BCC should be EMA negative and Ber-EP4 positive in contrast to LELC. Merkel cell carcinoma with lymphoepithelioma-like pattern has been described and immunostains for CK20 and synaptophysin can be useful in this setting [103]. Melanocytic markers are negative in LELC; however, scattered S100 positive cells have been described in the inflammatory infiltrate [93]. (Fig. 1.7a–d)

Adenosquamous Carcinoma

Adenosquamous carcinoma (ASC) of the skin is a rare tumor that is considered to have aggressive clinical behavior. The differential includes metastatic adenocarcinoma, secondary involvement of the skin by an underlying salivary gland tumor, and other cutaneous neoplasms such as primary mucoepidermoid carcinoma. Clinical history is essential when an adenosquamous carcinoma is encountered and should include a review of any potential metastases or primary salivary gland neoplasms.

Adenosquamous carcinoma displays areas of squamous differentiation consisting of islands and infiltrative nests of atypical keratinocytes, often with keratocysts, in addition to areas with glandular differentiation [104]. Mucoepidermoid carcinoma (MEC) of the skin, which also demonstrates glandular and squamous areas, has caused some confusion in the literature with ASC despite reportedly different biologic behaviors [105]. Histologically, MEC demonstrates more obvious goblet cells interspersed with squamous cells and lacks the stromal desmoplasia often associated with adenosquamous SCC [106, 107]. Invasive Bowen's disease can show glandular differentiation, but also shows Bowen's disease in the overlying epidermis [108–110]. Acantholytic squamous cell carcinoma, in contrast to ASC, does not show true gland formation. Desmoplastic SCC, which otherwise may show similar features to the squamous areas of ASC, does not have glandular differentiation. Some authors consider ASC to be a high risk subtype of SCC, on a spectrum with desmoplastic SCC [104, 110]. ASC shows diffuse positivity for p63 and CK5/6 [110].

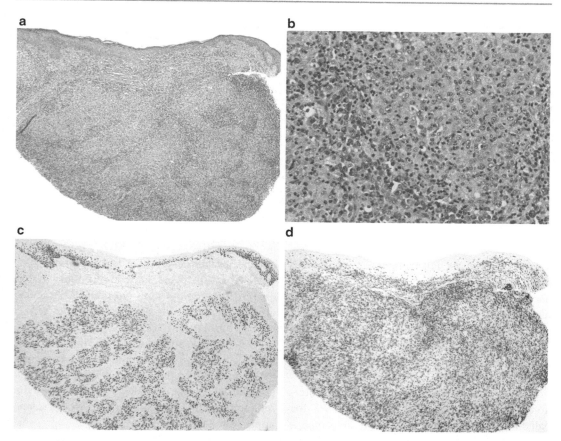

Fig. 1.7 (**a**) Lymphoepithelioma-like carcinoma. Note the high number of lymphocytic cells obscuring the atypical epithelial cells. (**b**) Lymphoepithelioma-like carcinoma. High power image showing the cell with abundant cytoplasm and vesicular nuclei surrounded by a dense lymphocytic infiltrate. (**c**) Lymphoepithelioma-like carcinoma. P63 highlights the neoplastic population of epithelial cells in dermis. (**d**) Lymphoepithelioma-like carcinoma. CD3 highlights the dense population of T-cells in the background

Glandular differentiation in ASC can be highlighted by CEA,CK7, mucicarmine, or alcian blue staining [104, 106, 110].

Desmoplastic Squamous Cell Carcinoma

Squamous cell carcinoma that demonstrates more bland cytology with a prominent component of desmoplasia, the lesion is classified as a spindle cell/desmoplastic SCC, which is categorized as high risk [111–113]. Desmoplastic growth in SCC confers an increased risk for local recurrence and metastasis [114]. The differential includes desmoplastic melanoma, atypical fibroxanthoma, infiltrative neoplasms such as sclerosing basal cell carcinoma, microcystic adnexal carcinoma, in addition to non-epithelial entities such as scar, dermatofibroma, and dermatofibrosarcoma protuberans. In a case series by Velazquez et al., a panel of cytokeratins, particularly pankeratin, CK34BetaE12, and p63 demonstrated diffuse positivity in lesional spindle cells [115]. Desmoplastic melanoma, a histologic mimic of desmoplastic SCC, is often MART1 and HMB45 negative and can raise diagnostic challenges; however, SOX10 expression helps distinguish desmoplastic melanoma from other entities, including spindle cell carcinoma [116].

Merkel Cell Carcinoma

Merkel cell carcinoma is associated with risk factors such as UV exposure and immune suppression, including patients with CLL [117–119]. Clinically, lesions present as violaceous papules or nodules on the head and neck, upper or lower extremities, and less often on sun-protected sites.

On low power, the initial impression is of a "blue-cell tumor". The lesion is usually circumscribed, but may have an infiltrative periphery. Cytologically, cells have minimal cytoplasm and a finely granular "salt and pepper" chromatin pattern. Frequent mitoses are present and lymphovascular invasion is often found at the periphery. The differential includes basal cell carcinoma, metastatic small cell carcinoma, either pulmonary or extrapulmonary, Ewing's sarcoma, and metastatic neuroendocrine carcinoma from other organ systems. In a small biopsy sample, intraepidermal spread can be prominent and cutaneous T-cell lymphoma and melanoma may enter the histologic differential diagnosis.

The diagnostic workup for Merkel cell carcinoma should begin with knowledge of the patient's clinical history and any previous malignancies. On immunohistochemistry, MCC is positive for CAM5.2, CKAE1/3, CK20, CK34BE12, synaptophysin, chromogranin, neuron-specific enolase, and EMA in addition to neural markers CD56 and neurofilament (NF) protein. CK20 most often displays a characteristic paranuclear dot-like pattern, but can also demonstrate a mixed membranous, diffuse, or cytoplasmic expression pattern. Negative markers include S100, LCA, and CK7, with rare reports of CK7 positivity [120–123]. (Fig. 1.8a–g)

The main differential for MCC includes metastatic small cell carcinoma of the lung. A panel including CK20, p63, CK7, and TTF1 is helpful; MCC is typically negative for CK7 and TTF1; however, both CK7 positive tumors [120–123] and TTF-1 positive tumors [124, 125] have been reported. CD99 and Fli-1 are also positive in MCC, making distinction between MCC and Ewing's sarcoma difficult. Fluorescence in situ hybridization (FISH) analysis for a reciprocal translocation of the ESWR1 gene can aid in this differential [126].

Merkel cell carcinoma expresses both PAX-5 and Tdt [127, 128] similar to small cell lung carcinoma, but the expression of these markers does not imply a B-cell origin to MCC [129]. DEK, a nuclear protein chromatin architectural factor that is overexpressed in retinoblastoma, colon cancer, melanomas, and high-grade neuroendocrine carcinoma, also shows strong and diffuse nuclear positivity in MCC [130]. Although DEK expression may not be useful in distinguishing MCC from its histologic mimics, its expression may be a result of the Merkel cell polyomavirus genome integration and down regulation of the retinoblastoma protein during Merkel cell carcinoma pathogenesis [130].

Merkel cell carcinoma has clonal integration of a polyomavirus [131]. When McPyV is integrated, the large T antigen domain is truncated, which has a higher binding affinity to the Rb protein [132]. When the large T antigen protein binds to phosphorylated Rb protein, pRB no longer suppresses E2F, a transcription factor critical for transition from G1 to S phase [132]. Viral integration and subsequent expression of large T antigen is thought to cause cell cycle dysregulation by binding and inactivation of the Rb tumor sup-

Fig. 1.8 (**a**) Merkel cell carcinoma. Note the tumor cells with neuroendocrine features including minimal cytoplasm with salt and pepper nuclei. (**b**) Merkel cell carcinoma. CK 20 showing the classic dot-like cytoplasmic staining. (**c**) Merkel cell carcinoma. It is not unusual for Merkel cell carcinoma to show CK20 expression with membranous staining. (**d**) Merkel cell carcinoma. Rarely, Merkel cell carcinoma can show expression with CK7 and be negative for CK20. (**e**) Intraepidermal Merkel cell car-cinoma. This variant can be difficult to recognize, especially in superficial biopsies in which only minimal dermis is available for inspection. (**f**) Intraepidermal Merkel cell carcinoma. Note the single cells within epidermis with pagetoid upward migration. The differential diagnosis of this variant includes melanoma and lymphoma. (**g**) Intraepidermal Merkel cell carcinoma. CK20 stain shows nice dot-like cytoplasmic staining within the epidermis and dermis

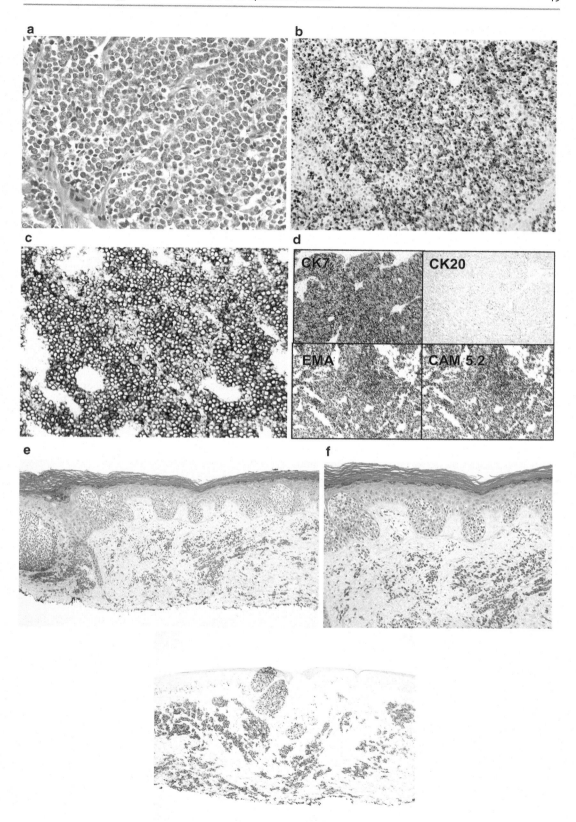

pressor protein, which is the key step in the development of Merkel cell carcinoma [133]. In McPyV negative tumors, several tumors have demonstrated truncating mutations in the Rb1 gene, providing further evidence for the retinoblastoma protein pathway involvement in Merkel cell carcinomas [133].

Although the majority of MCC are exclusively dermal, involvement of the epidermis has been reported in less than 10% of cases. Most reported cases of MCC with epidermotropism have an underlying dermal component; however, rare cases of only epidermal MCC have been reported. Histologically, the tumor cells confined to the epidermis can appear lentiginous with single cells along or just above the basal layer, and/or form compact nests or aggregates like Pautrier's microabscesses. Cellular aggregates may be confined to the base of rete, associate with acrosyringia, or more frequently spread through the epidermis in a pagetoid fashion. The epidermis may be hyperplastic, attenuated, or ulcerated. The neoplasms that likely simulate pagetoid MCC are melanoma in situ and cutaneous T-cell lymphoma; however, other important diagnostic considerations include pagetoid squamous cell carcinoma in situ, extramammary Paget's disease, porocarcinoma, sebaceous carcinoma, and metastatic small cell carcinoma. Cytokeratin 20 has been shown to be particularly useful in distinguishing MCC from many other neoplasms (as explained above), when used in conjunction with other relevant immunohistochemistry stains.

References

1. Chuang TY, et al. Basal cell carcinoma. A population-based incidence study in Rochester, Minnesota. J Am Acad Dermatol. 1990;22(3):413–7.
2. Guo HR, et al. Arsenic in drinking water and skin cancers: cell-type specificity (Taiwan, ROC). Cancer Causes Control. 2001;12(10):909–16.
3. Grachtchouk M, et al. Basal cell carcinomas in mice arise from hair follicle stem cells and multiple epithelial progenitor populations. J Clin Invest. 2011;121(5):1768–81.
4. Sexton M, Jones DB, Maloney ME. Histologic pattern analysis of basal cell carcinoma. Study of a series of 1039 consecutive neoplasms. J Am Acad Dermatol. 1990;23(6 Pt 1):1118–26.

5. Crowson AN. Basal cell carcinoma: biology, morphology and clinical implications. Mod Pathol. 2006;19 Suppl 2:S127–47.
6. Lo JS, et al. Metastatic basal cell carcinoma: report of twelve cases with a review of the literature. J Am Acad Dermatol. 1991;24(5 Pt 1):715–9.
7. Uzquiano MC, et al. Metastatic basal cell carcinoma exhibits reduced actin expression. Mod Pathol. 2008;21(5):540–3.
8. Gorlin RJ. Nevoid basal-cell carcinoma syndrome. Medicine (Baltimore). 1987;66(2):98–113.
9. Stone DM, et al. The tumour-suppressor gene patched encodes a candidate receptor for Sonic hedgehog. Nature. 1996;384(6605):129–34.
10. Gailani MR, et al. Developmental defects in Gorlin syndrome related to a putative tumor suppressor gene on chromosome 9. Cell. 1992;69(1):111–7.
11. Hutchin ME, et al. Sustained Hedgehog signaling is required for basal cell carcinoma proliferation and survival: conditional skin tumorigenesis recapitulates the hair growth cycle. Genes Dev. 2005;19(2):214–23.
12. Adolphe C, et al. Patched1 functions as a gatekeeper by promoting cell cycle progression. Cancer Res. 2006;66(4):2081–8.
13. Gailani MR, et al. The role of the human homologue of Drosophila patched in sporadic basal cell carcinomas. Nat Genet. 1996;14(1):78–81.
14. Aszterbaum M, et al. Identification of mutations in the human PATCHED gene in sporadic basal cell carcinomas and in patients with the basal cell nevus syndrome. J Invest Dermatol. 1998;110(6):885–8.
15. Xie J, et al. Activating Smoothened mutations in sporadic basal-cell carcinoma. Nature. 1998;391(6662):90–2.
16. Reifenberger J, et al. Missense mutations in SMOH in sporadic basal cell carcinomas of the skin and primitive neuroectodermal tumors of the central nervous system. Cancer Res. 1998;58(9):1798–803.
17. Reifenberger J, et al. Somatic mutations in the PTCH, SMOH, SUFUH and TP53 genes in sporadic basal cell carcinomas. Br J Dermatol. 2005;152(1):43–51.
18. Yu L, Galan A, McNiff JM. Caveats in BerEP4 staining to differentiate basal and squamous cell carcinoma. J Cutan Pathol. 2009;36(10):1074–176.
19. Sellheyer K, et al. The immunohistochemical differential diagnosis of microcystic adnexal carcinoma, desmoplastic trichoepithelioma and morpheaform basal cell carcinoma using BerEP4 and stem cell markers. J Cutan Pathol. 2013;40(4):363–70.
20. Hoang MP, et al. Microcystic adnexal carcinoma: an immunohistochemical reappraisal. Mod Pathol. 2008;21(2):178–85.
21. Ansai S, et al. Sebaceous carcinoma: an immunohistochemical reappraisal. Am J Dermatopathol. 2011;33(6):579–87.
22. Arits AH, et al. Differentiation between basal cell carcinoma and trichoepithelioma by immunohistochemical staining of the androgen receptor: an overview. Eur J Dermatol. 2011;21(6):870–3.

23. Izikson L, Bhan A, Zembowicz A. Androgen receptor expression helps to differentiate basal cell carcinoma from benign trichoblastic tumors. Am J Dermatopathol. 2005;27(2):91–5.

24. Yeh I, McCalmont TH, LeBoit PE. Differential expression of PHLDA1 (TDAG51) in basal cell carcinoma and trichoepithelioma. Br J Dermatol. 2012;167(5):1106–10.

25. Linskey KR, et al. BerEp4, cytokeratin 14, and cytokeratin 17 immunohistochemical staining aid in differentiation of basaloid squamous cell carcinoma from basal cell carcinoma with squamous metaplasia. Arch Pathol Lab Med. 2013;137(11):1591–8.

26. Jakobiec FA, Mendoza PR. Eyelid sebaceous carcinoma: clinicopathologic and multiparametric immunohistochemical analysis that includes adipophilin. Am J Ophthalmol. 2014;157(1):186–208. e2.

27. Fan YS, et al. Characteristic Ber-EP4 and EMA expression in sebaceoma is immunohistochemically distinct from basal cell carcinoma. Histopathology. 2007;51(1):80–6.

28. Bayer-Garner IB, Givens V, Smoller B. Immunohistochemical staining for androgen receptors: a sensitive marker of sebaceous differentiation. Am J Dermatopathol. 1999;21(5):426–31.

29. Plaza JA, et al. Role of Immunohistochemistry in the Diagnosis of Sebaceous Carcinoma: A Clinicopathologic and Immunohistochemical Study. Am J Dermatopathol. 2015;37(11):809–21.

30. Plaza JA, et al. Immunolabeling pattern of podoplanin (d2-40) may distinguish basal cell carcinomas from trichoepitheliomas: a clinicopathologic and immunohistochemical study of 49 cases. Am J Dermatopathol. 2010;32(7):683–7.

31. Degos R, et al. Epidermal tumor with an unusual appearance: clear cell acanthoma. Ann Dermatol Syphiligr (Paris). 1962;89:361–71.

32. Finch TM, Tan CY. Clear cell acanthoma developing on a psoriatic plaque: further evidence of an inflammatory aetiology? Br J Dermatol. 2000;142(4):842–4.

33. Zedek DC, Langel DJ, White WL. Clear-cell acanthoma versus acanthosis: a psoriasiform reaction pattern lacking tricholemmal differentiation. Am J Dermatopathol. 2007;29(4):378–84.

34. Ohnishi T, Watanabe S. Immunohistochemical characterization of keratin expression in clear cell acanthoma. Br J Dermatol. 1995;133(2):186–93.

35. Lora V, Chouvet B, Kanitakis J. The "intraepidermal epithelioma" revisited: immunohistochemical study of the Borst-Jadassohn phenomenon. Am J Dermatopathol. 2011;33(5):492–7.

36. Takayama R, et al. Expression of lumican in hidroacanthoma simplex and clonal-type seborrheic keratosis as a potent differential diagnostic marker. Am J Dermatopathol. 2014;36(8):655–60.

37. Wade TR, Kopf AW, Ackerman AB. Bowenoid papulosis of the penis. Cancer. 1978;42(4):1890–903.

38. Dubina M, Goldenberg G. Viral-associated nonmelanoma skin cancers: a review. Am J Dermatopathol. 2009;31(6):561–73.

39. Yu DS, et al. Morphometric assessment of nuclei in Bowen's disease and bowenoid papulosis. Skin Res Technol. 2004;10(1):67–70.

40. Kazlouskaya V, et al. Expression of p16 protein in lesional and perilesional condyloma acuminata and bowenoid papulosis: clinical significance and diagnostic implications. J Am Acad Dermatol. 2013;69(3):444–9.

41. Harvey NT, Leecy T, Wood BA. Immunohistochemical staining for p16 is a useful adjunctive test in the diagnosis of Bowen's disease. Pathology. 2013;45(4):402–7.

42. Zhou L, et al. Expression of cyclin D1 and cyclin E significantly associates with human papillomavirus subtypes in Bowenoid papulosis. Acta Histochem. 2013;115(4):339–43.

43. Kuo TT, Chan HL, Hsueh S. Clear cell papulosis of the skin. A new entity with histogenetic implications for cutaneous Paget's disease. Am J Surg Pathol. 1987;11(11):827–34.

44. Kuo TT, et al. Clear cell papulosis: report of three cases of a newly recognized disease. J Am Acad Dermatol. 1995;33(2 Pt 1):230–3.

45. Kohler S, Rouse RV, Smoller BR. The differential diagnosis of pagetoid cells in the epidermis. Mod Pathol. 1998;11(1):79–92.

46. Kim YC, Mehregan DA, Bang D. Clear cell papulosis: an immunohistochemical study to determine histogenesis. J Cutan Pathol. 2002;29(1):11–4.

47. Tseng FW, et al. Long-term follow-up study of clear cell papulosis. J Am Acad Dermatol. 2010;63(2):266–73.

48. Zarovnaya E, Black C. Distinguishing pseudoepitheliomatous hyperplasia from squamous cell carcinoma in mucosal biopsy specimens from the head and neck. Arch Pathol Lab Med. 2005;129(8):1032–6.

49. Galan A, Ko CJ. Langerhans cells in squamous cell carcinoma vs. pseudoepitheliomatous hyperplasia of the skin. J Cutan Pathol. 2007;34(12):950–2.

50. Zayour M, Lazova R. Pseudoepitheliomatous hyperplasia: a review. Am J Dermatopathol. 2011;33(2):112–22. quiz 123-6.

51. Mott RT, et al. Melanoma associated with pseudoepitheliomatous hyperplasia: a case series and investigation into the role of epidermal growth factor receptor. J Cutan Pathol. 2002;29(8):490–7.

52. Barkan GA, Paulino AF. Are epidermal growth factor and transforming growth factor responsible for pseudoepitheliomatous hyperplasia associated with granular cell tumors? Ann Diagn Pathol. 2003;7(2):73–7.

53. Ra SH, et al. Molecularly enriched pathways and differentially expressed genes distinguishing cutaneous squamous cell carcinoma from pseudoepitheliomatous hyperplasia. Diagn Mol Pathol. 2013;22(1):41–7.

54. Su A, et al. Differentiating cutaneous squamous cell carcinoma and pseudoepitheliomatous hyperplasia by multiplex qRT-PCR. Mod Pathol. 2013;26(11):1433–7.

55. Sober AJ, Burstein JM. Precursors to skin cancer. Cancer. 1995;75(2 Suppl):645–50.

56. Alam M, Ratner D. Cutaneous squamous-cell carcinoma. N Engl J Med. 2001;344(13):975–83.

57. Billano RA, Little WP. Hypertrophic actinic keratosis. J Am Acad Dermatol. 1982;7(4):484–9.

58. Carapeto FJ, Garcia-Perez A. Acantholytic keratosis. Dermatologica. 1974;148(4):233–9.

59. James MP, Wells GC, Whimster IW. Spreading pigmented actinic keratoses. Br J Dermatol. 1978;98(4): 373–9.

60. Tope WD, Nowfar-Rad M, Kist DA. Ber-EP4-positive phenotype differentiates actinic keratosis from superficial basal cell carcinoma. Dermatol Surg. 2000;26(5):415–8.

61. Al-Arashi MY, Byers HR. Cutaneous clear cell squamous cell carcinoma in situ : clinical, histological and immunohistochemical characterization. J Cutan Pathol. 2007;34(3):226–33.

62. Chang J, et al. Diagnostic utility of p63 expression in the differential diagnosis of pagetoid squamous cell carcinoma in situ and extramammary Paget disease: a histopathologic study of 70 cases. Am J Dermatopathol. 2014;36(1):49–53.

63. Reis-Filho JS, et al. p63 expression in normal skin and usual cutaneous carcinomas. J Cutan Pathol. 2002;29(9):517–23.

64. Williamson JD, et al. Pagetoid Bowen disease: a report of 2 cases that express cytokeratin 7. Arch Pathol Lab Med. 2000;124(3):427–30.

65. Mai KT, et al. Pagetoid variant of actinic keratosis with or without squamous cell carcinoma of sun-exposed skin: a lesion simulating extramammary Paget's disease. Histopathology. 2002;41(4):331–6.

66. Lau J, Kohler S. Keratin profile of intraepidermal cells in Paget's disease, extramammary Paget's disease, and pagetoid squamous cell carcinoma in situ. J Cutan Pathol. 2003;30(7):449–54.

67. Sellheyer K, Krahl D. Ber-EP4 enhances the differential diagnostic accuracy of cytokeratin 7 in pagetoid cutaneous neoplasms. J Cutan Pathol. 2008;35(4): 366–72.

68. Clarke LE, et al. Expression of CK7, Cam 5.2 and Ber-Ep4 in cutaneous squamous cell carcinoma. J Cutan Pathol. 2013;40(7):646–50.

69. Currie GP, Plaza JA, Harris GJ. Intraepithelial sebaceous carcinoma: a case report of an unusual occurrence. Am J Dermatopathol. 2014;36(8):673–6.

70. Raju RR, Goldblum JR, Hart WR. Pagetoid squamous cell carcinoma in situ (pagetoid Bowen's disease) of the external genitalia. Int J Gynecol Pathol. 2003;22(2):127–35.

71. Tan BH, Busam KJ, Pulitzer MP. Combined intraepidermal neuroendocrine (Merkel cell) and squamous cell carcinoma in situ with CM2B4 negativity and p53 overexpression(*). J Cutan Pathol. 2012;39(6): 626–30.

72. Cassarino DS, Derienzo DP, Barr RJ. Cutaneous squamous cell carcinoma: a comprehensive clinicopathologic classification—Part one. J Cutan Pathol. 2006;33(3):191–206.

73. Cassarino DS, Derienzo DP, Barr RJ. Cutaneous squamous cell carcinoma: a comprehensive clinicopathologic classification--part two. J Cutan Pathol. 2006;33(4):261–79.

74. Ackerman LV. Verrucous carcinoma of the oral cavity. Surgery. 1948;23(4):670–8.

75. Nakamura Y, et al. Verrucous carcinoma of the foot diagnosed using p53 and Ki-67 immunostaining in a patient with diabetic neuropathy. Am J Dermatopathol. 2015;37(3):257–9.

76. Adegboyega PA, Boromound N, Freeman DH. Diagnostic utility of cell cycle and apoptosis regulatory proteins in verrucous squamous carcinoma. Appl Immunohistochem Mol Morphol. 2005;13(2):171–7.

77. Ashida A, et al. Low p53 positivity in verrucous skin lesion in diabetic neuropathy occurring on the dorsum of the foot. Int J Dermatol. 2013;52(3):378–80.

78. Sigel JE, et al. The utility of cytokeratin 5/6 in the recognition of cutaneous spindle cell squamous cell carcinoma. J Cutan Pathol. 2001;28(10):520–4.

79. Gray Y, et al. Squamous cell carcinoma detected by high-molecular-weight cytokeratin immunostaining mimicking atypical fibroxanthoma. Arch Pathol Lab Med. 2001;125(6):799–802.

80. Heintz PW, White Jr CR. Diagnosis: atypical fibroxanthoma or not? Evaluating spindle cell malignancies on sun damaged skin: a practical approach. Semin Cutan Med Surg. 1999;18(1):78–83.

81. Winfield HL, et al. Monophasic sarcomatoid carcinoma of the scalp: a case mimicking inflammatory myofibroblastic tumor and a review of cutaneous spindle cell tumors with myofibroblastic differentiation. J Cutan Pathol. 2003;30(6):393–400.

82. Morgan MB, Purohit C, Anglin TR. Immunohistochemical distinction of cutaneous spindle cell carcinoma. Am J Dermatopathol. 2008;30(3): 228–32.

83. Folpe AL, Cooper K. Best practices in diagnostic immunohistochemistry: pleomorphic cutaneous spindle cell tumors. Arch Pathol Lab Med. 2007; 131(10):1517–24.

84. Dotto J, Glusac E. Best practices in diagnostic immunohistochemistry: pleomorphic cutaneous spindle cell tumors. Arch Pathol Lab Med. 2008;132(5):732.

85. Hartel PH, et al. CD99 immunoreactivity in atypical fibroxanthoma and pleomorphic malignant fibrous histiocytoma: a useful diagnostic marker. J Cutan Pathol. 2006;33 Suppl 2:24–8.

86. Buonaccorsi JN, Plaza JA. Role of CD10, wide-spectrum keratin, p63, and podoplanin in the distinction of epithelioid and spindle cell tumors of the skin: an immunohistochemical study of 81 cases. Am J Dermatopathol. 2012;34(4):404–11.

87. Nappi O, Pettinato G, Wick MR. Adenoid (acantholytic) squamous cell carcinoma of the skin. J Cutan Pathol. 1989;16(3):114–21.

88. Jurcic V, Kukovic J, Zidar N. Expression of desmosomal proteins in acantholytic squamous cell carcinoma of the skin. Histol Histopathol. 2015;30(8): 945–53.

89. Bayer-Garner IB, Sanderson RD, Smoller BR. Syndecan-1 expression is diminished in acantholytic cutaneous squamous cell carcinoma. J Cutan Pathol. 1999;26(8):386–90.

90. Bayer-Garner IB, Smoller BR. The expression of syndecan-1 is preferentially reduced compared with that of E-cadherin in acantholytic squamous cell carcinoma. J Cutan Pathol. 2001;28(2):83–9.

91. Griffin JR, et al. Decreased expression of intercellular adhesion molecules in acantholytic squamous cell carcinoma compared with invasive well-differentiated squamous cell carcinoma of the skin. Am J Clin Pathol. 2013;139(4):442–7.

92. Swanson SA, et al. Lymphoepithelioma-like carcinoma of the skin. Mod Pathol. 1988;1(5):359–65.

93. Requena L, et al. Lymphoepithelioma-like carcinoma of the skin: a light-microscopic and immunohistochemical study. J Cutan Pathol. 1994;21(6):541–8.

94. Ferlicot S, et al. Lymphoepithelioma-like carcinoma of the skin: a report of 3 Epstein-Barr virus (EBV)-negative additional cases. Immunohistochemical study of the stroma reaction. J Cutan Pathol. 2000;27(6):306–11.

95. Fenniche S, et al. Lymphoepithelioma-like carcinoma of the skin in a Tunisian patient. Am J Dermatopathol. 2006;28(1):40–4.

96. Lyle P, Nakamura K, Togerson S. Lymphoepithelioma-like carcinoma arising in the scar from a previously excised basal cell carcinoma. J Cutan Pathol. 2008;35(6):594–8.

97. Aoki R, et al. A case of lymphoepithelioma-like carcinoma of the skin associated with Epstein-Barr virus infection. J Am Acad Dermatol. 2010;62(4):681–4.

98. Sagatys E, Kirk JF, Morgan MB. Lymphoid lost and found. Am J Dermatopathol. 2003;25(2):159–61.

99. Hinz T, et al. Lymphoepithelioma-like carcinoma of the skin mimicking a basal cell carcinoma. Eur J Dermatol. 2009;19(2):179–80.

100. Chetty R, et al. Spiradenocarcinoma arising from a spiradenocylindroma: unusual case with lymphoepithelioma-like areas. J Cutan Med Surg. 2009;13(4):215–20.

101. Bayer-Garner IB, et al. Carcinoma with thymus-like differentiation arising in the dermis of the head and neck. J Cutan Pathol. 2004;31(9):625–9.

102. Hall G, et al. Lymphoepithelioma-like carcinoma of the skin: a case with lymph node metastases at presentation. Am J Dermatopathol. 2006;28(3):211–5.

103. Ben Abdelkrim S, et al. Merkel cell carcinoma with lymphoepithelioma-like pattern: a case report of an exceedingly rare variant of Merkel cell carcinoma with lymph node metastases at presentation. Case Rep Pathol. 2011;2011:840575.

104. Fu JM, McCalmont T, Yu SS. Adenosquamous carcinoma of the skin: a case series. Arch Dermatol. 2009;145(10):1152–8.

105. Riedlinger WF, et al. Mucoepidermoid carcinoma of the skin: a distinct entity from adenosquamous carcinoma: a case study with a review of the literature. Am J Surg Pathol. 2005;29(1):131–5.

106. Patel V, et al. Cutaneous adenosquamous carcinoma: a rare neoplasm with biphasic differentiation. Cutis. 2014;94(5):231–3.

107. Suarez-Penaranda JM, et al. Primary mucoepidermoid carcinoma of the skin expressing p63. Am J Dermatopathol. 2010;32(1):61–4.

108. Saida T, Okabe Y, Uhara H. Bowen's disease with invasive carcinoma showing sweat gland differentiation. J Cutan Pathol. 1989;16(4):222–6.

109. Fulling KH, Strayer DS, Santa Cruz DJ. Adnexal metaplasia in carcinoma in situ of the skin. J Cutan Pathol. 1981;8(2):79–88.

110. Ko CJ, Leffell DJ, McNiff JM. Adenosquamous carcinoma: a report of nine cases with p63 and cytokeratin 5/6 staining. J Cutan Pathol. 2009;36(4):448–52.

111. Petter G, Haustein UF. Squamous cell carcinoma of the skin--histopathological features and their significance for the clinical outcome. J Eur Acad Dermatol Venereol. 1998;11(1):37–44.

112. Petter G, Haustein UF. Histologic subtyping and malignancy assessment of cutaneous squamous cell carcinoma. Dermatol Surg. 2000;26(6):521–30.

113. Breuninger H, et al. Desmoplastic squamous epithelial carcinoma of the skin and lower lip. A morphologic entity with great risk of metastasis and recurrence. Hautarzt. 1998;49(2):104–8.

114. Brantsch KD, et al. Analysis of risk factors determining prognosis of cutaneous squamous-cell carcinoma: a prospective study. Lancet Oncol. 2008;9(8):713–20.

115. Velazquez EF, Werchniack AE, Granter SR. Desmoplastic/spindle cell squamous cell carcinoma of the skin. A diagnostically challenging tumor mimicking a scar: clinicopathologic and immunohistochemical study of 6 cases. Am J Dermatopathol. 2010;32(4):333–9.

116. Palla B, et al. SOX10 expression distinguishes desmoplastic melanoma from its histologic mimics. Am J Dermatopathol. 2013;35(5):576–81.

117. Robak E, et al. Merkel cell carcinoma in a patient with B-cell chronic lymphocytic leukemia treated with cladribine and rituximab. Leuk Lymphoma. 2005;46(6):909–14.

118. Tadmor T, et al. Increased incidence of chronic lymphocytic leukaemia and lymphomas in patients with Merkel cell carcinoma—a population based study of 335 cases with neuroendocrine skin tumour. Br J Haematol. 2012;157(4):457–62.

119. Engels EA, et al. Merkel cell carcinoma and HIV infection. Lancet. 2002;359(9305):497–8.

120. Tsai YY, et al. CK7+/CK20- Merkel cell carcinoma presenting as inguinal subcutaneous nodules with subsequent epidermotropic metastasis. Acta Derm Venereol. 2010;90(4):438–9.

121. Pilloni L, et al. Merkel cell carcinoma with an unusual immunohistochemical profile. Eur J Histochem. 2009;53(4), e33.

122. Beer TW. Merkel cell carcinomas with CK20 negative and CK7 positive immunostaining. J Cutan Pathol. 2009;36(3):385–6. author reply 387.

123. Calder KB, et al. A case series and immunophenotypic analysis of CK20-/CK7+ primary neuroendocrine carcinoma of the skin. J Cutan Pathol. 2007;34(12):918–23.

124. Ishida M, Okabe H. Merkel cell carcinoma concurrent with Bowen's disease: two cases, one with an unusual immunophenotype. J Cutan Pathol. 2013;40(9):839–43.

125. Koba S, et al. Merkel cell carcinoma with cytokeratin 20-negative and thyroid transcription factor-1-positive immunostaining admixed with squamous cell carcinoma. J Dermatol Sci. 2011;64(1):77–9.

126. Funakoshi T, et al. Application of electron microscopic analysis and fluorescent in situ hybridization technique for the successful diagnosis of extraskeletal Ewing's sarcoma. J Dermatol. 2015;42(9):893–6.

127. Mhawech-Fauceglia P, et al. Pax-5 immunoexpression in various types of benign and malignant tumours: a high-throughput tissue microarray analysis. J Clin Pathol. 2007;60(6):709–14.

128. Zur Hausen A, et al. Early B-cell differentiation in Merkel cell carcinomas: clues to cellular ancestry. Cancer Res. 2013;73(16):4982–7.

129. Murakami I, et al. Immunoglobulin expressions are only associated with MCPyV-positive Merkel cell carcinomas but not with MCPyV-negative ones: comparison of prognosis. Am J Surg Pathol. 2014; 38(12):1627–35.

130. Patel RM, et al. DEK expression in Merkel cell carcinoma and small cell carcinoma. J Cutan Pathol. 2012;39(8):753–7.

131. Feng H, et al. Clonal integration of a polyomavirus in human Merkel cell carcinoma. Science. 2008;319(5866):1096–100.

132. Houben R, et al. An intact retinoblastoma protein-binding site in Merkel cell polyomavirus large T antigen is required for promoting growth of Merkel cell carcinoma cells. Int J Cancer. 2012;130(4): 847–56.

133. Cimino PJ, et al. Retinoblastoma gene mutations detected by whole exome sequencing of Merkel cell carcinoma. Mod Pathol. 2014;27(8):1073–87.

Part II

Adnexal Neoplasms

Immunohistology and Molecular Studies of Sweat Gland Tumors

2

Ana M. Molina-Ruiz, Laura Fuertes, and Luis Requena

Introduction

Adnexal tumors are generally classified according to two principles: (1) benign versus malignant, and (2) line of differentiation: that is, which normal cutaneous structure the lesion most resembles: hair follicle, apocrine/eccrine gland, or sebaceous gland. Although such a classification scheme seems simple at first glance, the reality is that there is still considerable controversy on how to catalog many lesions [1]. Furthermore, tumors of cutaneous sweat glands are uncommon, with a wide histopathological spectrum, complex classification, and many different terms often used to describe the same neoplasm [2].

It is important to understand the basic structure and the physiological function of human sweat glands in order to study the neoplasms that originate from them. Moreover, expression of individual cytokeratins and other markers in normal eccrine and apocrine glands is outlined in Table 2.1. The human body has $3–4 \times 10^6$ sweat glands, two types of which are generally recognized, namely, eccrine and apocrine sweat glands [3]. The average density of eccrine and apocrine sweat glands varies according to the person and anatomic site. The sites of maximum distribution of eccrine glands are the palms, soles, axillae, and forehead, while apocrine glands are most numerous in the axilla and anogenital area [4]. In addition to the eccrine and apocrine glands, two other skin sweat glands have recently been described: the apoeccrine and the mammary-like glands of the anogenital area [5, 6].

Normal Apocrine Glands

Apocrine sweat glands, which are derived from the folliculo-sebaceous-apocrine germ, are restricted to the axillae, anogenital and inguinal regions, the periumbilical and periareolar areas, and, rarely, the face and scalp. Apocrine glands become active at puberty and secrete a proteinaceous viscous sweat which has a unique odor. Specialized apocrine glands are found on the eyelids (Moll's glands) and in the auditory canal (ceruminous glands). The breast is sometimes regarded as a modified apocrine gland [7]. Apocrine glands are composed of a secretory glandular portion in the lower dermis and subcutis, a straight ductal component which is indistinguishable from the eccrine duct, and a terminal intra-infundibular duct which opens

A.M. Molina-Ruiz • L. Fuertes • L. Requena (✉)
Department of Dermatology, Fundación Jiménez Díaz, Universidad Autónoma, Madrid, Spain
e-mail: amolinar@fjd.es; lfuertes@fjd.es; lrequena@fjd.es

© Springer International Publishing Switzerland 2016
J.A. Plaza, V.G. Prieto (eds.), *Applied Immunohistochemistry in the Evaluation of Skin Neoplasms*, DOI 10.1007/978-3-319-30590-5_2

Table 2.1 Expression of cytokeratins and other markers in normal eccrine and apocrine glands (Data from [4])

Markers	Eccrine gland				Apocrine gland			
	Dermal duct		Secretory coil		Dermal duct		Secretory coil	
	Luminal cells	Basal cells	Secretory cells	Myoepithelial cells	Luminal cells	Basal cells	Secretory cells	Myoepithelial cells
CK4	−	−	−	−	NA	NA	NA	NA
CK7	−	−	+	−/+	+	−	+	+
CK8	−	−	+	−	−	−	+	−
CK10	+	−	−	−	+	−	−	−
CK13	−	−	−	−	NA	NA	NA	NA
CK14	+	+	−	+	NA	+	NA	+
CK15	NA	NA	NA	NA	−	NA	+	NA
CK18	−	−	+	−	−	−	+	−
CK19	+	−	+	−	+	NA	+	NA
CK 20	−	−	−	−	NA	NA	NA	NA
CAM 5.2	−	−	+	+	NA	NA	+	+
CK 1/5/10/14	+	+	−	−	+	+	NA	+
S100 protein	−	−	+	+	−	−	−	+

into the follicular infundibulum. The secretory part consists of large tubules with large, round to oval lumina, sometimes containing homogenous eosinophilic or pale basophilic material, the product of apocrine secretion. The luminal cells show an ample, eosinophilic, and finely granular cytoplasm, and are immunoreactive to low molecular weight keratin (LMWK), epithelial membrane antigen (EMA), and carcinoembryonic antigen (CEA). A conspicuous feature of apocrine secretory cells is their "decapitation" mode of secretion whereby an apical cap, formed at the luminal border of the apocrine cells, separates off from the cell and is discharged into the lumen. Another typical feature of these cells is the presence of intracytoplasmic small, brightly eosinophilic granules (zymogen granules) in a supranuclear location. Zymogen granules are PAS-positive and diastase resistant, and represent lysosomes that contain sialomucin, lipid, and iron. The cells in the secretory part are surrounded by a layer of spindled myoepithelial cells that express S-100 protein, p63, smooth muscle actin (SMA), and calponin [4]. Their contraction aids in the delivery of their secretory products. Peripheral to the myoepithelial cell layer lies a distinct basement membrane. The ductal component of the apocrine glands is composed of an inner luminal layer of small cells with scant cytoplasm and a peripheral layer of small cuboidal basophilic cells with round nuclei that expresses p63. A deeply eosinophilic homogeneous cuticle is recognized. Finally, the glandular epithelium of the apocrine glands often expresses gross cystic disease fluid protein 15 (GCDFP-15) and androgen receptors, which may be useful in the assessment of lesions suspicious of apocrine carcinoma [2].

Normal Eccrine Glands

Eccrine sweat glands, smaller than apocrine sweat glands in size, are distributed all over the body surface but not on the lips, external ear canal, clitoris, or labia minora. Eccrine glands secrete hypotonic sweat consisting mostly of water and electrolytes. Their main function is the control of body temperature [3]. The eccrine unit is composed of a secretory portion and a ductal component. The secretory coil lies in the lower reticular dermis and is composed of two populations of epithelial cells: clear cells, which contain glycogen in their cytoplasm, and dark cells, which contain vacuoles filled with mucin. Both types of luminal cells are surrounded by a discontinuous myoepithelial cell layer that stains for S-100 protein, SMA, calponin, and p63. S-100 protein also stains the luminal epithelial cells [4]. The transition from the distal portion of the secretory coil to the proximal fragment of the duct is abrupt and is known as the ampulla. The ductal component, indistinguishable from an apocrine duct, is composed of two parts: the intradermal duct and the intraepidermal component (acrosyringium). The intradermal duct is composed of two layers of small cuboidal basophilic cells with round nuclei and there is an eosinophilic homogeneous cuticle lining the luminal aspect of the inner cell layer. The cells in the excretory coil express positivity for LMWK, EMA, and CEA, as well as S100 protein and p63 in the basal layer only. The intraepidermal duct (acrosyringium) has a characteristic spiraling course, is composed of a single layer of luminal cells, and has an acelular eosinophilic cuticle. This intraepidermal duct is surrounded in the lower part by two or three layers of outer cells. In the middle squamous layer, ductal cells comprising the acrosyringium start to keratinize, demonstrating keratohyaline granules, and the cuticle is no longer visible. Acrosyringeal cells stain for high molecular weight keratin (HMWK) and cytokeratin (CK) 14. Finally, skin tumors with eccrine differentiation often express positive immunohistochemical staining for estrogen and progesterone receptors [8], this has important clinical implications, as affected patients may be partially treated with hormonal therapy [9].

Apoeccrine Glands

Apoeccrine sweat glands have been proposed to represent a third, separate category of human sweat glands [10], although this is still controversial and requires further study. It has been suggested that these glands develop during puberty from the eccrine sweat glands (transformation or transgression of eccrine glands into apocrine glands) or from eccrine-like precursor sweat glands. Apoeccrine glands are mostly found in the axillary region, and within lesions of nevus sebaceus of Jadassohn (NSJ) [5]. Their presence would explain the existence of some adnexal lesions that have both eccrine and apocrine differentiation, as has been proposed in some examples of syringocystadenoma papilliferum (SCAP) or Fox–Fordyce disease [11].

Mammary-Like Glands

Cutaneous mammary-like glands (MLG) are now recognized to be a normal component of the skin in the anogenital region, including the perianal skin. MLG are unique in having features of apocrine, eccrine and mammary glands, and the previous assumption that these glands represent ectopic/accessory breast tissue lying along the milk line (mammary ridge) is now believed to be incorrect. Many adnexal lesions of the anogenital area are now recognized to be of MLG origin, and a helpful feature in attributing MLG origin to an adnexal tumor is the presence of normal MLG in the deep dermis and subcutaneous fatty tissue, in the vicinity of the lesion of interest, with a transition zone between benign and lesional areas [12, 13].

In this chapter a detailed practical approach to the most important general features of benign and malignant sweat glands tumors of the skin is intended, striving to maintain a common and acceptable terminology in this complex subject. For this purpose, we will follow the classification scheme outlined in Table 2.2. Furthermore, a comprehensive and functional approach to the use of immunohistochemistry in the diagnosis of sweat gland neoplasms is also described. The most relevant monoclonal antibodies, for use with immunoperoxidase techniques, in the diagnosis and classification of sweat gland tumors are listed in Table 2.3. Finally, molecular studies will be discussed where appropriate.

Table 2.2 Classification of sweat gland tumors

Differentiation	Benign	Malignant
Apocrine	Hidradenoma Spiradenoma/Cylindroma Syringocystadenoma papilliferum Adenoma of the nipple Ceruminous gland adenomas Moll's gland adenomas Hidradenoma papilliferum Myoepithelioma	Hidradenocarcinoma Spiradenocarcinoma/Cylindrocarcinoma Syringocystadenocarcinoma papilliferum Apocrine carcinoma Extramammary Paget's disease Mucinous carcinoma Endocrine mucin-producing sweat gland carcinoma Hidradenocarcinoma papilliferum Aggressive digital papillary adenocarcinoma
Eccrine	Poroma Syringoma Syringofibroadenoma	Porocarcinoma
Eccrine and apocrine	Apocrine/eccrine hidrocystoma Apocrine/eccrine nevus Tubular adenoma Benign mixed tumor	Syringoid carcinoma Microcystic adnexal carcinoma Adenoid cystic carcinoma Malignant mixed tumor of the skin

Table 2.3 Most relevant antibodies in the diagnosis of sweat gland tumors

Antibody	Role in the diagnosis of sweat gland tumors
Carcinoembryonic antigen (CEA)	Indicates ductal differentiation of both apocrine and eccrine type. It is expressed in the secretory and excretory portions of the eccrine gland. In apocrine glands is positive at the luminal edge of the excretory duct, but in negative the secretory portion
Epithelial membrane antigen (EMA)	Expressed in both the secretory portion and the excretory duct of eccrine and apocrine glands
CAM5.2	Reacts with the apocrine gland and supposedly the duct, and the eccrine secretory coils, but not the eccrine duct
MNF116	Detects the low and intermediate molecular weight keratins (5, 6, 8, 17, and 19), stains the basal cells of the epidermis and adnexae. It is found in all epithelial tumors, including adnexal ones
34βE12/CK903	It recognizes CK1, CK10, and CK14, which are expressed in ductal and squamous epithelia, basal cells, and myoepithelial cells. Reacts with basal cells from normal eccrine ducts and some apocrine gland tumors
Antibodies to individual keratins	Not of much assistance in routine diagnosis, but they have given a valuable insight into the possible derivation and/or differentiation of various eccrine tumors
Gross cystic disease fluid protein 15 (GCDFP-15)	Intense immunoreactivity in the luminal edges of the secretory tubules and the excretory ducts of the eccrine and apocrine glands
Human milk fat globulin 1 and 2 (HMFG-1, HMFG-2)	Expressed in the normal apocrine glands and tumors with apocrine differentiation
Vimentin, α-smooth muscle actin, s-100 protein, p63, calponin	Markers of myoepithelial cells which are seen in most sweat gland tumors considered to differentiate toward the secretory coil of sweat glands, and in most of the traditional apocrine tumors
Estrogen, progesterone and androgen receptors	Usually expressed in the apocrine sweat glands and tumors with apocrine differentiation
p53	Present in some sweat gland carcinomas; rarely present in benign tumors
Ki-67	The mitotic rate is an important indicator of malignancy
CD44	Strongly expressed in the eccrine coil secretory cells, it has not proved a useful marker of sweat gland differentiation in tumors
Ferritin	Demonstrates ferritin in the outermost layer of the eccrine and apocrine ducts
IgA and secretory component	Detect antigen in the lumen and on the surface of the epithelium of sweat glands
IKH-4, EKH-5, and EKH-6	Stain the secretory coil of the eccrine glands
SKH1	Reacts with the secretory portion and coiled duct of the eccrine gland and the secretory portion of apocrine glands

Cysts and Hamartomas

Apocrine Hidrocystoma, Eccrine Hidrocystoma, and Apocrine Cystadenoma

According to the latest WHO classification of cutaneous tumors, apocrine hidrocystomas are cystic adenomas that arise from the apocrine secretory coil, whereas eccrine hidrocystomas represent retention cysts of the eccrine duct [14]. It can be difficult to distinguishing between apocrine hidrocystoma and eccrine hidrocystoma in cases with compression of the epithelial lining of the apocrine hidrocystoma due to cyst distension by excessive secretions.

Apocrine hidrocystoma is a cystic lesion that despite its apocrine derivation it is rare at sites rich in normal apocrine glands. It is usually found as a solitary lesion on the head and neck area of middle aged patients, although multiple lesions have also been documented sporadically or as a feature of ectodermal dysplasia (Schöpf-Schulz-Passarge syndrome) and focal dermal hypoplasia (Goltz syndrome) [15–17]. Similar lesions on the eyelids are also known as Moll's gland cysts [18], and penile variants are now thought at least in part to represent median raphe cysts rather than true apocrine cysts. Apocrine hidrocystoma presents as an intradermal, dome-shaped, translucent, bluish-black cystic nodule measuring up to about 1 cm. Some patients report worsening in summer months or with excessive heat that decreases during the winter months [19].

Microscopically, apocrine hidrocystoma consists of a large unilocular or multilocular cystic space situated within the dermis. The cystic spaces are usually lined by a double layer of epithelial cells: an outer layer of flattened vacuolated myoepithelial cells and an inner layer of tall columnar cells with eosinophilic cytoplasm and basally located, round or oval vesicular nuclei. Decapitation secretion is usually present, and papillary projections of epithelium into the lumen are found in about one-half of cases. Occasionally, the cyst cavity is partially replaced by a papillary or adenomatous proliferation, and the term "apocrine cystadenoma" is used to refer to these lesions [20].

Immunohistochemistry reveals that apocrine hidrocystoma is a complex tumor, and that lesions with a proliferative component (apocrine cystadenoma) are different from the pure cystic form and have increased Ki-67 staining, especially in areas with a genuine papillary growth pattern. EMA and CEA are demonstrable in the luminal aspects of the epithelial cells, which themselves express various cytokeratins, including 34β E12 (CK1/5/10/14), CK7, CK8, CK18, CK19, and others [21]. It is said that simple epithelial cytokeratins are not expressed in the eccrine retention variant of hidrocystoma. Differentiation between eccrine and apocrine lesions is also said to be achieved by using human milk fat globulin 1 (HMFG-1) and GCDFP-15, which are usually only expressed by the apocrine sweat gland [22]. Finally, the myoepithelial layer can be highlighted with SMA, calponin, and p63. Staining with S-100 protein is variable.

Apocrine and Eccrine Nevi

Eccrine nevus (nevus sudoriferous, sudoriferous hamartoma) is a rare hamartoma of the eccrine unit which typically presents in childhood or adolescence and has a predilection for the upper extremities. Apocrine nevus is a congenital, benign, and persistent adnexal cutaneous hamartoma composed of ostensibly normal apocrine glands and ductal structures within a fibrous stroma. It is not uncommon to find an apocrine nevus component in lesions of nevus sebaceus of Jadassohn or SCAP.

Histologically, eccrine nevi have localized increased number and size of eccrine glands. The variant called eccrine angiomatous hamartoma has, in addition to the eccrine glands, adipose tissue and small capillaries. In apocrine nevi the apocrine glands are more numerous than in other areas of mature skin and display a disordered architecture. The overlying epidermis may be slightly hyperplastic with papillomatosis, and it may contain buds of basaloid cells, occasionally forming similar aggregates to basal-cell carcinoma (BCC). The apocrine glands proliferate in the reticular dermis and may extend into the subcutaneous fat in a circumscribed but unencapsulated fashion, where they present within a delicate fibrous stroma [23, 24].

Immunohistochemical studies of apocrine nevi show similar features to those of normal apocrine sweat glands, thus being positive for EMA and

CEA, LMWKs, such as CK7, and GCDFP-15,while negative for HMWKs and S-100 protein [25]. Moreover, p63 can be expressed by basal cells of excretory ducts and by myoepithelial cells of the secretory coils [24, 26]. Ki-67 demonstrates that apocrine nevi show a low proliferation potential, which is consistent with the clinically benign and stable nature of these hamartomas [24].

Syringocystadenoma Papilliferum

SCAP is a benign lesion that occurs most commonly on the scalp or forehead. About 30 % of cases are associated with a congenital lesion, usually a nevus sebaceous of Jadassohn, and for this reason it is not always possible to be certain at what age the SCAP component developed [27]. Probably half are present at birth or develop in childhood [28]. It usually presents as one or several yellowish papules, sometimes arranged linearly, and with reduced or absent hair growth. The lesions increase in size at puberty, becoming papillomatous and often crusted.

Microscopically, SCAP is composed of ducts and papillary projections lined by two layers of epithelial cells: cuboidal at the periphery and columnar cells with abundant, basophilic cytoplasm in the luminal layer. A connection to the preexisting follicular infundibula may usually be found. The stroma of the papillary processes characteristically contains numerous plasma cells. There may be a background of features of nevus sebaceus of Jadassohn. The main diagnostic issues are the distinction from SCAP hidradenoma papilliferum and to detect features of associated nevus sebaceus of Jadassohn, because such lesions, although very rarely, may give raise to secondary malignant neoplasms

SCAP expresses AE1/AE3, CAM 5.2, EMA, and CEA (Fig. 2.1). The inner layer is

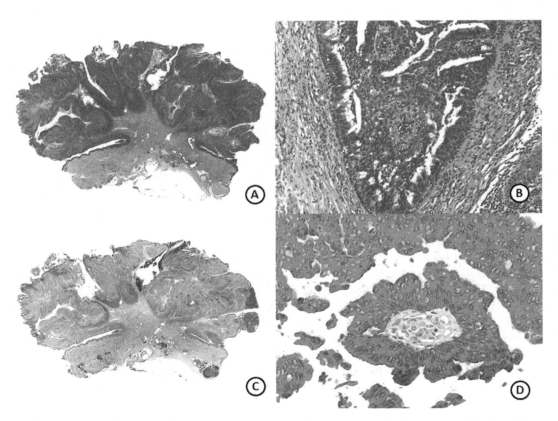

Fig. 2.1 (**a**): Syringocystadenoma papilliferum with prominent epidermal hyperplasia. (**b**) Papillary structures lined by two layers of epithelial cells and plasma cells in the stroma. (**c**) The same case immunohistochemically studied for CEA. (**d**) The epithelium lining the papillae exhibit CEA immunoexpression

positive for SMA. The results of markers of apocrine differentiation are variable. Some authors have found GCDFP-15 and HMFG-1 negative, while others have found GCDFP-15 and/or HMFG-2 present [29, 30]. The luminal cells constantly express CK7 and often CK19, whereas expression of other markers such as CK1/5/10/14, CK14, and CK5/8 is variable. The plasma cells secrete IgA and IgG and they are polyclonal.

Finally, genetic analysis using polymorphic markers at 9q22 (locus for the *PTCH1* gene) and markers at 9p21 flanking the tumor suppressor gene p16, showed LOH at 9q22 in 2 of 10 cases of SCAP, whereas 3 of 7 cases manifested allelic deletions at 9p21 [31].

Benign Tumors

Tubular Adenoma

According to the latest WHO classification of cutaneous tumors, "tubular adenoma" is the term used to encompass a spectrum of tumors including tubular apocrine adenoma and papillary eccrine adenoma, amongst others. Tubular adenomas are slowly growing, circumscribed nodules situated in the dermis or subcutaneous tissue, and have been described at a variety of sites including the scalp, face, eyelid, axilla, leg, and genitalia [32]. The last, however, may represent an adenoma of the anogenital MLG [33]. Those that present on the scalp often arise in a background of nevus sebaceus of Jadassohn and are sometimes associated with SCAP.

Histologically, tubular adenoma usually presents as circumscribed intradermal lobules of well-differentiated tubular structures that sometimes extend into the subcutis. Occasionally, the neoplastic tubules communicate with the overlying epidermis through duct-like structures or dilated follicular infundibula. The tubules exhibit apocrine features with an inner layer of cylindrical cells, often showing "decapitation" secretion, and a connective tissue stroma in which only small numbers of chronic inflammatory cells are present, in contrast to SCAP in which numerous plasma cells are usually found. However, cases of

tubular adenoma have been reported with features of SCAP in the upper part of the lesion and probably these two lesions are more related than previously was thought [34, 35].

Immunohistochemical studies have shown that the luminal epithelial cells are positive for CEA, EMA, and various cytokeratins, including CK7 [36, 37]. The myoepithelial cells can be highlighted with SMA or S-100 protein. However, myoepithelial cell markers are often not expressed in the peripheral layer of atrophic distended tubules or in solid areas of immature squamous metaplasia. HMFG-1 and GCDFP-15 may also be expressed [36–38].

Hidradenoma Papilliferum

Hidradenoma papilliferum is a benign neoplasm that occurs almost exclusively in females, with predilection to the vulva and perianal region. Rare cases of hidradenoma papilliferum have been reported in males, and in extra-anogenital locations, particularly the head and neck area [39], but probably they represent examples of other adenomas with a prominent papillary component. It usually presents as a solitary, small and asymptomatic lesion. Human papilloma virus (HPV) has been suggested as having a potential role in the histogenesis of this neoplasm [40], although this observation needs further study.

Histopathologically, hidradenoma papilliferum arises from apocrine glands or possibly the anogenital MLG. It usually presents as a well-circumscribed solid or cystic dermal nodular lesion, not connected to the epidermis. It is formed of frond-like papillae or tubulopapillary structures that are lined by a two-cell layer: luminal cuboidal or low columnar epithelial cells with apical secretions, resting on an outer myoepithelial cell layer.

Immunohistochemically, the tumor cells often express LMWKs, EMA, CEA, HMFG, and GCDFP-15 [41, 42]. Furthermore, estrogen, progesterone, and androgen receptors are commonly expressed in hidradenoma papilliferum [43]. This and the presence of histomorphological features analogous to benign breast diseases gives further evidence to a possible origin of hidradenoma papilliferum from MLG. The myoepithelial cells express S-100 protein and SMA.

Ceruminous Gland and Moll's Gland Adenomas

A ceruminous adenoma, also known as adenoma of the ceruminous gland and ceruminoma, is a benign neoplasm that arises from the ceruminous glands located in the external auditory canal. These tumors develop in a very specific location, as these glands are found within the outer one third to one half of the external auditory canal, more commonly along the posterior surface [44]. On the other hand, Moll's glands are presumed to be the origin of the few lesions with apocrine differentiation that occur on the eyelids. The most common is apocrine hidrocystoma, which has already been described above. But Moll's glands are also the origin of much rarer benign tumors grouped under the term "Moll's gland adenoma" [4].

Ceruminous adenomas usually present as uncapsulated, but well circumscribed tumors. Connection to the epidermis is not usually seen unless the surface is ulcerated [44]. The tumor shows a dual or biphasic appearance, with glandular or cystic spaces showing inner luminal secretory cells with abundant granular, eosinophilic cytoplasm subtended by basal, myoepithelial cells at the periphery, adjacent to the basement membrane. The luminal cells often show decapitation secretion and yellow-brown, lipofuscin-like pigment granules (cerumen) in their cytoplasms [44]. Moll's gland adenomas usually show benign architectural and cytologic features with solid, solid-cystic, cribriform, or tubular-papillary patterns of growth. Remnants of Moll's glands can sometimes be seen in the vicinity of the neoplasm.

In ceruminomas, immunohistochemistry confirms the biphasic nature of the tumor. All cells are positive with pancytokeratin and EMA. The luminal cells are positive with CK7, while basal/myoepithelial cells are positive with CK5/6, p63, S100 protein, and SMA [44, 45]. CD117 can also be expressed in both populations. Finally, the tumor cells are negative with chromogranin, synaptophysin, and CK20 [44].

Nipple Adenoma

Nipple adenoma is a benign neoplasm that is often misdiagnosed as Paget's disease of the breast clinically or as ductal breast carcinoma histopathologically. It usually occurs in women around 50 years of age as a nodule under the areola or nipple. There is often erythema, erosion or ulceration of the epidermal surface, and sometimes, patients refer pain or discharge of a liquid material related to the menstrual cycle.

Microscopically, nipple adenoma presents as an endophytic, wedge shaped lesion, which usually opens to the epidermal surface or the follicular infundibulum. It consists of tubular elements lined by a double layer of epithelial cells, separated by fibrous septa. Inside the tubules, there is often an eosinophilic and homogeneous material that seems to correspond to apocrine secretion, and decapitation secretion can also be observed in the luminal cells lining the tubules.

Immunohistochemical studies have demonstrated that nipple adenoma does not express estrogen, progesterone, or androgen receptors, and the HercepTest is negative. SMA and p63 are expressed in the basal layer of the neoplastic tubules, supporting the benign nature of the lesion [46].

Apocrine Hidradenoma

Apocrine hidradenoma is a relatively common benign adnexal neoplasm which can have variable histomorphological patterns, reflected by the various terms that have been used to describe this entity: nodular hidradenoma, clear cell hidradenoma, eccrine acrospiroma, clear cell myoepithelioma, clear cell papillary carcinoma, solid-cystic hidradenoma, and apocrine hidradenoma. Apocrine hidradenomas usually present as solitary, skin-colored or reddish papules and/or nodules. They may be large, measuring up to 2 cm or more in diameter, and can occur at any anatomic location and any age.

Microscopically, the predominant growth patterns are solid and/or solid-cystic, seen together in about 90 % of cases, with variation in the ratio of the solid and cystic areas from case to case [4]. It is usually centered in the dermis and well circumscribed, but large tumors may involve the subcutis. It is composed of lobules of uniform eosinophilic or clear, glycogen-rich cells. Ducts can be seen throughout the lesion, some of them dilated and forming cystic areas and "decapitation" secretion is usually seen in some areas of the luminal border. In some cases, mucinous cells are also seen in that luminal border. Some areas may also show squamous differentiation (keratin pearls) or clear cell changes. The stroma is fibrous and may show extensive hyalinization or even keloidal appearance.

Ancillary studies are rarely needed for diagnosis, but immunostains may be helpful on occasions to highlight Glands and ducts when they are sparse, which helps in the distinction of hidradenoma from other clear cell tumors, such as tricholemmoma or cutaneous metastasis from renal cell carcinoma. Apocrine hidradenoma is a heterogeneous tumor with different staining profiles within the main cellular subtypes and architectural regions of the neoplasm. Immunohistochemistry usually demonstrates variability in the expression of the various keratin subtypes in different parts of the tumor, however, CK7, CAM5.2 (Fig. 2.2), and EMA/CEA (luminal border) are expressed in most tumors [47, 48]. Tumor cells are usually negative for S-100 protein (which reveals only Langerhans cells) [49].

Recent molecular studies have documented the presence of a chromosomal translocation $t(11;19)$ in hidradenomas, that results in fusion of the mucoepidermoid carcinoma translocated 1

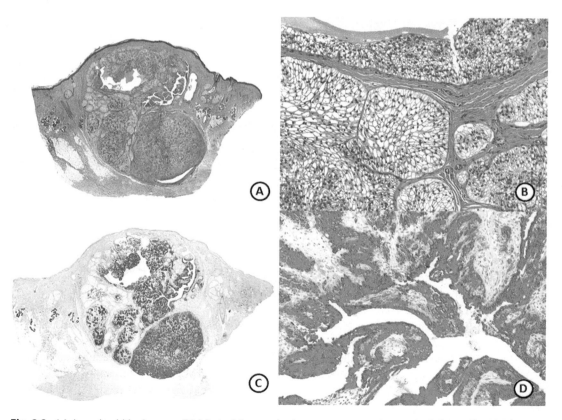

Fig. 2.2 (**a**) Apocrine hidradenoma. (**b**) Most of the neoplastic aggregates are composed of clear cells. (**c**) The same case immunohistochemically studied for CAM 5.2. (**d**) Strong expression for CAM 5.2 in the neoplastic epithelial cells

(*MECT1*) gene on chromosome 19p13 with the mastermind-like 2 (*MAML2*) gene on chromosome 11q21 [50, 51]. This translocation is said to be more common in cases with predominant clear cell differentiation, although it has also been observed in tumors with a mixed cell population, including cases completely devoid of clear cells. This translocation is not restricted to hidradenomas, and has also been described in salivary gland tumors, such as mucoepidermoid carcinoma and Warthin's tumor, as well as mucoepidermoid carcinoma of the cervix [50–52].

Cutaneous Mixed Tumor

Cutaneous mixed tumor is a rare, benign adnexal tumor of sweat gland origin, which is most commonly seen in the head and neck region of patients in the sixth and seventh decades. These tumors usually present as asymptomatic, slow growing masses, mostly affecting the nose, cheek and upper lip [53, 54]. Because of the presence of cartilage, mixed tumor of the skin has also been called "chondroid syringoma," but this term is best avoided as the neoplasm bears no resemblance to a syringoma and cartilage is not a constant feature. The etiopathogenesis of these tumors is unknown, and both an epithelial and a mesenchymal origin have been proposed [55].

Microscopically, cutaneous mixed tumors show both an epithelial and a mesenchymal component, similar to benign mixed tumors of the salivary glands, the so-called pleomorphic adenomas. They usually present as circumscribed nodules composed of bland epithelial cells, arranged in cords, ducts, or tubules. The stromal component is most often myxoid-cartilaginous, but can also be hyaline/fibrous, fatty, osteoid, or be minimal or absent. Cutaneous mixed tumors are classified into apocrine and eccrine types based on the histopathological appearance of the neoplastic tubules, because the eccrine variant shows round ducts lined by a single layer of epithelial cells, while apocrine variant exhibits elongated tubules lined by two layers of epithelial cells. Areas of follicular and/or sebaceous differentiation have only been described in the apocrine variant.

In the eccrine type of mixed tumor the cells express CEA, pancytokeratins, CK7, and S-100 protein [56], while in apocrine mixed tumor, hyaline cells are an accepted feature of myoepithelial differentiation and express actins, S-100 protein (Fig. 2.3), p63, and calponin [57]. Calponin, actins and p63 are negative in the eccrine variant of mixed tumor [57]. Gonzalez Guerra et al. [58] found that the neoplastic epithelium of the tubular structures of eccrine mixed tumor expressed strong immunoreactivity for calretinin, supporting a differentiation towards the secretory portion of the eccrine glands, while apocrine mixed tumor expressed calretinin only in the most keratinized areas of the ductal structures, which may represent areas of either ductal sebaceous differentiation or tricholemmal differentiation.

It has recently been demonstrated that rearrangement of pleomorphic adenoma gene 1 (*PLAG1*) leads to aberrant expression of its protein and is pathogenically relevant in the development of salivary pleomorphic adenomas. A genetic link between salivary pleomorphic adenoma and cutaneous mixed tumor has been subsequently established because most cutaneous mixed tumors express distinct nuclear immunostaining for PLAG1, with moderate or strong intensity in a significant number of neoplastic cells and positive gene rearrangement for *PLAG1* [59] and for EWSR1 [60] have been detected in cutaneous mixed tumors and cutaneous myoepitheliomas. These findings support the notion that salivary pleomorphic adenomas, cutaneous myoepitheliomas, and cutaneous mixed tumors are myoepithelial neoplasms, which are genetically related.

Syringoma

Syringomas usually present as multiple small, skin-colored papules around the eyelids, mostly in young women. Other locations are axilla, abdomen, and vulva. Histologically, they present as symmetrical and well-circumscribed lesions, confined to the upper dermis with no connection, with the overlying epidermis. They are composed of monomorphous cuboidal cells with small

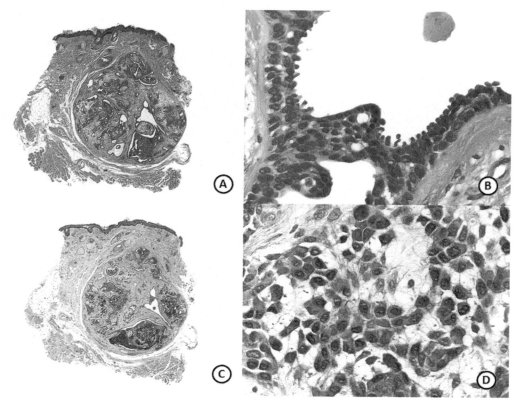

Fig. 2.3 (**a**) Apocrine mixed tumor. (**b**) Elongated tubular structures lined by two layers of epithelial cells with evidence of "decapitation" secretion in the luminal border. (**c**) The same case immunohistochemically studied for S100 protein. (**d**) Strong S100 protein immunoexpression in neoplastic myoepithelial cells

nuclei and inconspicuous nucleoli. Similar cells line ductal structures with small lumina, which may be empty or contain secretions. Calcification and granulomatous inflammation are sometimes observed [61, 62].

Syringomas express CK6 and CK10, both are said to stain the straight duct, with CK6 being a marker for the inner ductal cells and CK10 being a marker for the middle tumor cells. Other cytokeratins variably expressed include CK1, CK5, CK11, CK19, and CK14 [63, 64]. Studies on expression of progesterone and estrogen receptors in syringoma, including those located on the vulva, show conflicting results. Progesterone receptors are expressed in most syringomas, supporting the view that they are under hormonal control, but the expression seems to be less frequent in cases on the vulva. Syringomas usually express CEA and EMA (Fig. 2.4) in the lumina

of the ducts, and are usually negative for GCDFP-15 [65]. The expression of S100 protein family members has been also studied showing that syringomas are positive for S100A2, S1007, and S100P [66].

Spiradenoma, Cylindroma, and Spiradenocylindroma

Although originally considered to represent separate entities, the close relationship between spiradenoma and cylindroma became obvious after identification of lesions with hybrid features of both neoplasms, for which the term spiradenocylindroma was proposed, and nowadays, spiradenoma, cylindroma, and spiradenocylindroma are viewed as a morphologic continuum [4]. Although traditionally thought to be eccrine neoplasms, apocrine and

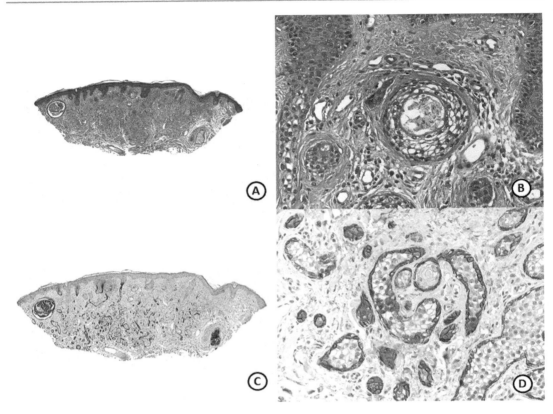

Fig. 2.4 (**a**) Clear-cell syringoma. (**b**) Ductal structures are lined by clear-cells. (**c**) The same case immunohistochemically studied for EMA. (**d**) The outer layer of some neoplastic epithelial aggregates express EMA

follicular differentiation has subsequently been shown in these three neoplasms suggesting that they differentiate along the lines of the folliculo-sebaceous-apocrine unit. All three neoplasms occur either sporadically or as a part of the Brooke–Spiegler syndrome in which they manifest as multiple lesions in various combinations with other adnexal neoplasms, mostly trichoblastoma [67–69]. They usually present as solitary, skin-colored or violaceous, small, asymptomatic nodules affecting adult to elderly patients in the head and neck area.

Microscopically, spiradenomas usually show one or several dermal circumscribed lobules of basaloid cells, with no connection to the epidermis. The nests are composed of two types of epithelial cells; one with a small, dark nucleus, mainly at the periphery of the cellular aggregates, and a second type with large and pale nuclei, sometimes located around small lumina with eosinophilic, PAS-positive, and diastase-resistant material.

Spiradenomas tend to be more vascular and show more likely edematous and cystic stromal changes than cylindromas. Cylindromas typically show multiple small aggregates of basaloid cells surrounded by pink hyaline basement membrane material. Cylinders of hyaline membrane are often seen in the center of such aggregates. Two types of epithelial cells are usually found: a peripheral cell with a large basophilic nucleus and a tendency for palisading, and a larger centrally located paler cell with a vesicular chromatin pattern.

Spiradenomas and cylindromas express identical cytokeratin patterns. Neoplastic cells express CK5/6. In areas with ductal differentiation, luminal cells mainly express ductal markers (CK6, CK14, and CK19) and, less prominently, CK7 [70–74]. When immunostained for myoepithelial markers, these three tumors usually reveal patchy reactivity, with areas showing positivity for some of these markers alternating with completely negative areas (Fig. 2.5) [74]. Basement membrane material seen around the nodules as well as intratumoral droplets stain for collagen IV [72, 73]. Staining for S-100 protein and CD1a reveals intratumoral dendritic cells thought to represent Langerhans cells [70]. Rare benign neoplasms manifest focal positivity for p53, limiting the use of this marker in the differential diagnosis from malignant lesions evolving from benign spiradenoma, cylindroma, and spiradenocylindroma [75].

Lesions occurring in the context of Brooke–Spiegler syndrome are associated with germ line and somatic mutations in the *CYLD* gene located on chromosome 16q [76]. Somatic mutations detected in neoplastic tissue in syndrome-associated lesions include both a sequence mutation and LOH at the gene locus. LOH at 16q has also been demonstrated in rare sporadic cylindromas and spiradenomas.

Poroma Group

These tumors usually originate from the outer cells of the intraepidermal (acrosyringeal) excretory ducts of eccrine the sweat gland. However, there are reports of poromas showing sebaceous, follicular and apocrine differentiation, and the term "apocrine" poromas has been used for those tumors [77]. Poromas usually occur in adults, with predilection to palms and soles, and less frequently the head and neck, and trunk regions. They are usually solitary and rarely multiple, and may present as superficial plaques or dermal nodules, with tendency to ulceration and bleeding.

Histopathologically, four main variants of poromas are recognized and distinguished according to their location in relation to the epidermis and the size of the neoplastic aggregates:(1) hidroacanthoma simplex, also known as intraepidermal poroma, composed of round nests

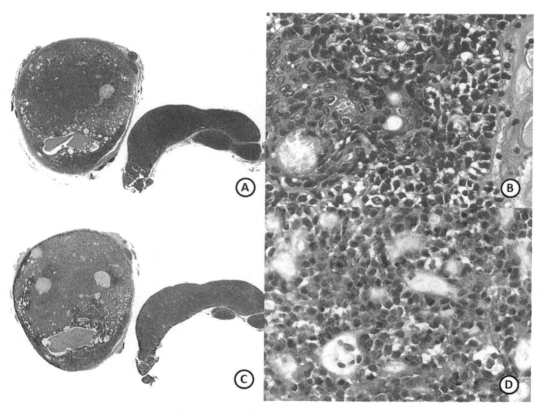

Fig. 2.5 (**a**) Spiradenoma. (**b**) Small ductal structures within the neoplastic aggregates. (**c**) The same case immunohistochemically studied for calponin. (**d**) Strong calponin immunoreactivity for neoplastic cells

of neoplastic cells confined within the epidermis; (2) classic poroma, composed of lobules of neoplastic cells involving both the epidermis and the dermis; (3) dermal duct tumor, characterized by small aggregates of neoplastic cells limited to the dermis, with few or no epidermal connection; and (4) poroid hidradenoma, characterized by single or few large solid neoplastic aggregates involving the dermis with cystic areas inside [78]. All poromas usually consist of solid sheets and nodules composed of two types of neoplastic cells: (1) Poroid cells, which are small basaloid cells, monomorphous and cuboidal, with a well-defined cell membrane, round nuclei and scant cytoplasm; and (2) Cuticular cells, which are larger than poroid cells, with ample eosinophilic cytoplasm, vesicular nuclei and evidence of primitive ductal differentiation in the form of small cytoplasm vacuoles. Well-formed ductal structures are also lined by cuticular cells. Areas of necrosis *en masse* are also frequently found. In intraepidermal lesions, neoplastic aggregates are sharply delineated from adjacent keratinocytes. Foci of squamous differentiation and clear cell change are sometimes seen. The intervening stroma shows abundant vascularization.

Immunohistochemical studies in poromas demonstrate positivity of ductal structures for EMA, CEA, and GCDFP-15. The neoplastic cells are immunoreactive for MNF116 and AE1/AE3 cytokeratins, but not for CAM5.2. Staining for CK7 is variable (Fig. 2.6). Poroid cells are positive for CK14 and are negative for CK10. In contrast, cuticular cells are positive for CK10, CK6, CK1 and /5/10/14, CK10/11, simple epithelial keratins (CK7, CK8/18, and CK19), and "basal" keratins (CK5/8 and CK14) [79]. The cuticular cells have been shown to have similar keratin expression patterns in "eccrine" and "apocrine" poromas. Cuticular cells are often positive for p53, but this feature alone should not be interpreted as a sign of malignant transformation [80].

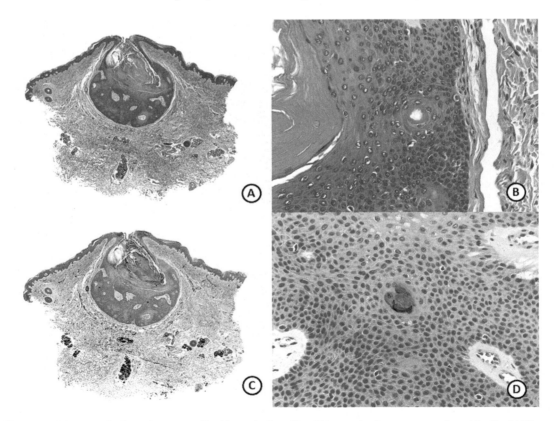

Fig. 2.6 (**a**) Poroma. (**b**) Ductal structures lined by cuticular cells within neoplastic aggregates of poroid cells. (**c**) The same case immunohistochemically studied for CK7. (**d**) Ductal structures show CK7 immunoreactivity

Three of seven studied poromas showed loss of heterozygosity in the *APC* gene, but the meaning of this genetic anomaly remains uncertain [81].

Myoepithelioma

Myoepitheliomas are exceedingly rare cutaneous tumors that arise in the dermis, subcutaneous fat or soft tissues. They are derived from myoepithelial cells which are found in the skin as a discontinuous peripheral layer around eccrine and apocrine glands. Analogous to salivary gland tumors, cutaneous myoepitheliomas are composed of myoepithelial and stromal components of mixed tumors, but lack the ductal epithelial component. Cutaneous myoepitheliomas usually present as firm, well-circumscribed, skin-colored or violaceous nodules ranging in size from 0.5 cm to 2.5 cm [82], although tumors located within

deeper soft tissue may present as larger masses measuring up to 12 cm. [83].

Microscopically, cutaneous myoepitheliomas present as unencapsulated, circumscribed nodules consisting of a pure population of myoepithelial cells with no evidence of glandular or ductal differentiation as is seen in the more commonly encountered mixed tumor. They are situated in the dermis or subcutis, and composed of a variety of cell types, including spindle-shaped, epithelioid, histiocytoid, and plasmacytoid (hyaline) cells [84]. The cells usually have pale eosinophilic cytoplasm and relatively monomorphous ovoid nuclei with inconspicuous nucleoli. Some tumors have very little stroma, while others have a myxoid or collagenous hyalinized stroma.

Immunohistochemistry shows that the tumoral cells often express vimentin, EMA, S100 protein, and a wide spectrum of cytokeratins, although keratin staining is quite variable [85]. Myoid differentiation markers such as SMA (Fig. 2.7),

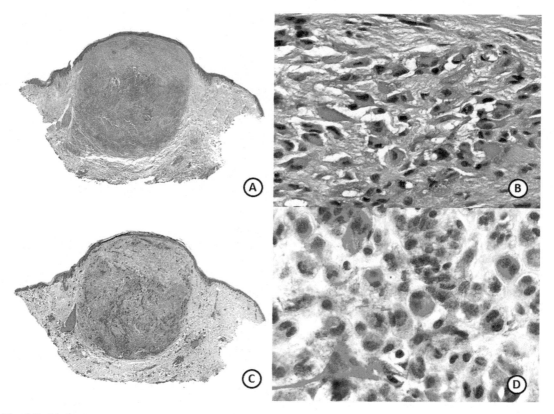

Fig. 2.7 (a) Cutaneous myoepithelioma. (b) Neoplastic cells showing eosinophilic cytoplasm and eccentric nuclei. (c) The same case immunohistochemically studied for SMA. (d) Strong immunoreactivity of neoplastic cells for SMA

muscle specific actin and calponin, as well as other markers like (HHF35) and glial fibrillary acid protein (GFAP) are seen inconsistently [86]. Desmin, synaptophysin, and chromogranin are usually negative [4].

Malignant Tumors

Syringocystadenocarcinoma Papilliferum

Syringocystadenocarcinoma papilliferum (SCACP) is an extremely rare cutaneous adnexal neoplasm representing the malignant counterpart of SCAP from which it usually evolves [1]. To date, less than 30 cases have been reported, and of those, only three had locoregional metastases [87–89]. The majority of cases reported were located in the head and neck region, or less commonly the perineal area and extremities of middle aged to elderly individuals. Clinically, SCACP presents as an enlarging flesh-colored to hyperpigmented exophytic nodule ranging in size from 0.5 to 13 cm [90].

SCACP is characterized histologically by disorderly arranged papillary projections, cytologic atypia and loss of the double layered epithelium [2]. Most tumors have been associated with nevus sebaceus of Jadassohn.

Although there is no definitive immunohistochemical profile for SCACP, this tumor is often positive for CEA and GCDFP-15. The in situ component may be positive with calponin, SMA and p63, which stain the peripheral myoepithelial cell layer. Moreover, p63 expression favors a primary sweat gland neoplasm of the skin rather than a cutaneous metastasis from a visceral adenocarcinoma [91, 92]. The epithelial cells stain with CK7 which may also be used to identify intraepithelial pagetoid spread [93]. An increased Ki-67 staining has been reported [4].

Cribriform Carcinoma

Cribriform carcinoma is a rare but distinctive histopathologic variant of cutaneous apocrine carcinoma that was originally described by Requena et al. in 1998 in a series of five cases [23, 94]. This neoplasm appears in adults and seems to be more common in females. The preferred sites of cribriform carcinoma are the lower and upper limbs.

On histopathology, the neoplasm usually shows no connection with the epidermis or adnexal structures and appears as a relatively symmetric, well-circumscribed dermal nodule, which involves the full thickness of the dermis and sometimes extends to the subcutaneous fat. The tumor is composed of multiple interconnected solid aggregations of epithelial cells that are punctuated by small round spaces in the fashion of a sieve. The cells show round or oval, hyperchromatic, slightly pleomorphic nuclei, inconspicuous or absent nucleoli, granular chromatin, and scant eosinophilic cytoplasm [23, 94].

The neoplastic cells are positive for different cytokeratins including MNF116, AE1/AE3, CAM5.2, and CK7as well as for CEA and EMA (Fig. 2.8), the last two staining the ductal component more intensely. However they are negative for CK20, GCDFP-15, and S-100 protein. Smooth muscle markers as SMA, muscle-specific actin, and calponin can be detected in the spindle cells of the stroma, which probably correspond to myofibroblasts, but not in the neoplastic cells [94].

Cutaneous Mucinous Carcinoma

Primary cutaneous mucinous apocrine carcinoma with neuroendocrine differentiation usually presents as a solitary papule, nodule, or plaque, typically affecting middle-aged or elderly individuals. It may occur anywhere, but has a predilection to involve the head and neck region, in particular the eyelids and scalp. The tumors are usually slow growing.

Hematoxylin and eosin-stained sections of this tumor show a nodular tumor involving the dermis with no connection to the epidermis. The tumor consists of solid, cystic or cribriform nests "floating" in pools of mucin, separated by thin fibrous septa. Neoplastic cells can show a low degree of atypia but mitotic figures are uncommon [95, 96].

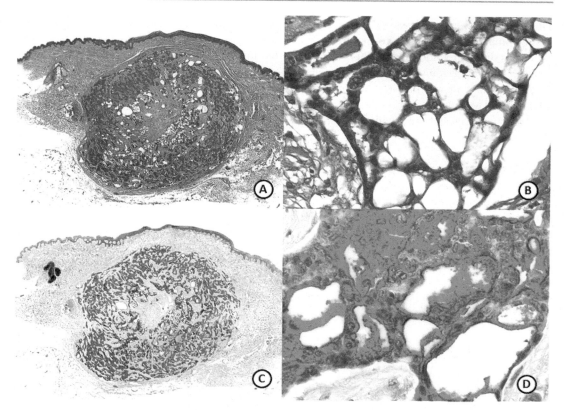

Fig. 2.8 (**a**) Primary cutaneous cribriform carcinoma. (**b**) Small ductal structures within solid aggregates resulting in a cribriform pattern. (**c**) The same case immunohistochemically studied for EMA. (**d**) EMA shows stronger expression in neoplastic cells lining ductal structures

On immunohistochemistry, neoplastic cells show positive expression of CK7, EMA, estrogen and progesterone receptors, and are negative for CK20 [97, 98]. Neuroendocrine markers such as chromogranin, synaptophysin, or neuron-specific enolase, show variable and sometimes focal expression [99–101]. The differential diagnosis with metastatic mucinous carcinoma, especially with metastatic mucinous breast carcinoma, may be extremely difficult, even with immunohistochemistry. Both tumors express CK7, hormone receptors, and some neuroendocrine markers. Some authors have suggested that the presence of an in situ component surrounded by myoepithelial cells highlighted by p63 and CK5/6 at the periphery of the tumor may be an additional criterion in favor of a primary carcinoma [97, 102, 103].

Endocrine Mucin-Producing Sweat Gland Carcinoma

Endocrine mucin-producing sweat gland carcinoma (EMPS) is an uncommon low-grade sweat gland carcinoma with an infiltrating growth pattern. It develops mostly in women and shows a predilection for the periorbital region [104–113]. Histopathologically, the neoplasm shows analogous features to endocrine ductal carcinoma/solid papillary carcinoma of the breast. EMPS shares some clinical and morphological similarities to primary mucinous carcinoma of the skin. The tumor is characterized by large monomorphous epithelial cells with little nuclear pleomorphism and only a few mitotic figures. In some areas, neoplastic cells are arranged in a rossete-like pattern.

This solid- cystic tumor shows mucin within cystic small spaces, cribriform areas and expresses the neuroendocrine markers synaptophysin, chromogranin (Fig. 2.9) and neuron specific enolase in varying staining intensities [104–113]. The tumor cells are also positive for estrogen and progesterone receptors.

Hidradenocarcinoma Papilliferum

Hidradenocarcinoma papilliferum is an extremely rare neoplasm, with very few reported cases in the literature [114–116]. Owing to the paucity of observations, the clinical features of hidradenocarcinoma papilliferum are not well established, but there do not appear to be obvious differences from long-standing hidradenoma

papilliferum in which focal areas of ductal carcinoma in situ (DCIS) may be an incidental finding.

Histologically, DCIS ex-hidradenoma papilliferum appears as a typical hidradenoma papilliferum in which 1 or more foci of crowded epithelial cells may be found, showing pleomorphic hyperchromatic nuclei and abnormal mitotic figures. Retention of myoepithelial cells around such areas is indicative of DCIS.

Immunohistochemically, demonstration of a preserved peripheral myoepithelial layer around the dysplastic epithelium is a prerequisite for the diagnosis of DCIS. The proliferating index (Ki-67) is higher in the areas of DCIS compared with the benign portions of the neoplasm, but there has been no p53 expression in the few cases examined [117].

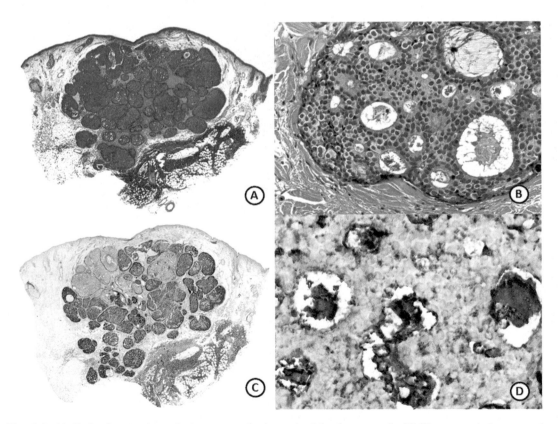

Fig. 2.9 (a) Endocrine mucin-producing sweat gland carcinoma. (b) Neoplastic aggregates showing ductal structures some of them containing mucin within the lumina. (c) The same case immunohistochemically stained for chromogranin. (d) Chromogranin is expressed in the cytoplasm of neoplastic cells and in a stronger way within the lumina

Digital Papillary Adenocarcinoma

Digital papillary adenocarcinoma (DPA) is an uncommon cutaneous malignancy first described by Helwig in 1979 with the term "aggressive digital papillary adenoma" [118, 119]. Because of the lack of histopathologic criteria to allow the distinction between adenoma and adenocarcinoma and predict the clinical behavior of these tumors, the term "aggressive digital papillary adenoma" was later abandoned and the lesion was considered a carcinoma. However, the aggressive course of the neoplasm has also been questioned recently [120, 121]. It often occurs as a single, mildly painful mass and almost exclusively occurs on the volar site of the fingers and toes and on the adjacent skin of the palms and soles [120].

Microscopically, the tumor usually involves both the dermis and the and/or subcutis, and the silhouette of the lesion may be nodular and/or infiltrative. There is usually a combination of solid, solid cystic, cribriform, and tubular growth patterns. Papillary projections into luminal spaces are common, but may on occasion be rare or absent. The stroma may be variably fibrotic. The spectrum of histologic appearances ranges from obvious carcinoma to adenoma-like well-differentiated tumors.

Immunohistochemical studies have shown positivity for S100 protein, CEA, and cytokeratins [119], and may be useful in the differential diagnosis of DPA from metastatic adenocarcinoma. A recent immunohistochemical study of a series of 31 cases of papillary carcinoma demonstrated diffuse positivity for MNF116 pan-cytokeratin, whereas CEA and EMA highlight the luminal border of the tubules. SMA and calponin highlight a myoepithelial layer around tubular/glandular structures, as did p63 and podoplanin [122]. One approach is to investigate the expression of basal epithelial markers such as 34βE12 and p63, which may serve as a good indicator for primary cutaneous origin as well as in situ growth of this neoplasm. Proliferation index with Ki-67 is usually high (Fig. 2.10).

Ceruminous and Moll's Gland Carcinomas

Ceruminous carcinomas are rare malignancies usually presenting with a mass or pain in the outer ear canal of middle aged patients. Tumors are large for the anatomic site [123]. Histopathologically, the tumors are classified as ceruminous adenocarcinoma, NOS, ceruminous adenoid cystic carcinoma, and ceruminous mucoepidermoid carcinoma. The ceruminous adenocarcinoma may be difficult to distinguish from ceruminous adenoma. They usually demonstrate an infiltrative pattern with moderate to severe nuclear pleomorphism, increased mitotic index and rarely necrosis.

Reported examples of Moll's gland adenocarcinomas have shown variable features. Some have been predominantly solid, whereas others have displayed mostly tubular or ductal growth, but all have malignant architectural features. With respect to cytologic appearances, both low-grade and high-grade lesions have been described. In rare examples, evolution from a preexisting benign Moll's gland lesion has been suggested [4].

Malignant Mixed Tumor

Malignant apocrine mixed tumor is a rare tumor of the skin, most often found on the trunk and extremities, which are not the usual sites of the benign variant. Approximately 50 cases have been described to date. Although the majority of tumors have developed de novo, there are some documented examples which appear to have arisen within a preexistent benign mixed tumor. Clinically, the tumor is not distinctive and presents as a flesh-colored or erythematous nodule, predominantly affecting the distal extremities (the foot being the commonest site) [124]. Malignant mixed tumor is an extremely high-grade neoplasm with a metastatic rate of approximately 60 % and a mortality of roughly 25 % [124, 125]. The existence of a malignant counterpart of eccrine mixed tumor is controversial. Some of the reported malignant eccrine

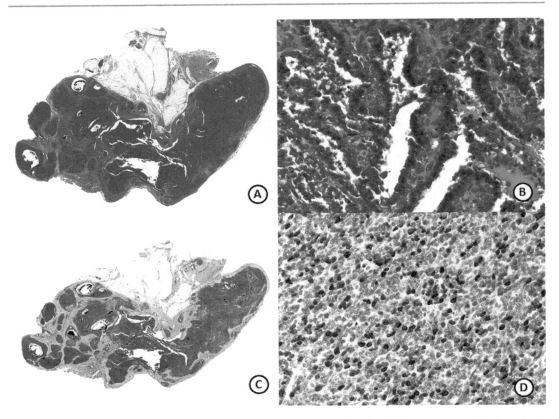

Fig. 2.10 (**a**) Digital papillary adenocarcinoma. (**b**) Papillary structures lined by atypical cells with hyperchromatic nuclei. (**c**) The same case immunohistochemically stained for Ki-67. (**d**) Numerous nuclei of neoplastic cells express Ki-67

mixed tumors of the skin have been found to represent malignant mixed tumors of the salivary glands involving the skin, and further studies are needed to clarify this issue [4].

Histopathologically, the tumors are composed of an epithelial and a mesenchymal component, the latter consisting of myxomatous and cartilaginous areas. The epithelial component predominates at the periphery of the tumor, where there are cords and nests of cuboidal or polygonal cells with some glandular structures. There is variable pleomorphism and scattered mitoses. Mesenchymal elements are progressively more abundant towards the center. Ossification is occasionally present. The histological appearance may be a poor indicator of the biological behavior of a particular tumor in this category, and the identification of a benign precursor lesion has only rarely been histologically documented [126, 127].

Immunohistochemically, the epithelial cells express pancytokeratin, AE1/AE3, CAM 5.2, EMA, CEA, and variably S-100 protein [128–130]. Intracytoplasmic lumina may be outlined with CEA. The luminal epithelial cells also show binding to the lectin *Ulex europaeus* [128–130]. The stromal cells are S-100 protein positive and variably express keratin. SMA and GFAP positivity has been variably reported as present or absent, while androgen receptors have not been detected.

Apocrine Adenocarcinoma

The term "primary cutaneous apocrine carcinoma" is a generic term that encompasses a wide spectrum of primary cutaneous carcinomas showing apocrine differentiation. Due to the complex nosology of apocrine carcinoma, in this chapter, the term cutaneous apocrine adenocarcinoma will be restricted to malignant epithelial neoplasms that manifest unequivocal signs of apocrine secretion, but lack the defining microscopic features of the above mentioned well-defined lesions, such as digital papillary adenocarcinoma, mucinous carcinoma, syringocystadenocarcinoma papilliferum, and malignant apocrine mixed tumor. Also, the term will not be used to refer to other well-defined carcinomas associated with a specific glandular origin (Moll's glands, ceruminous glands, or anogenital mammary-like glands). The clinical features of this tumor are not distinctive, and lesions have been reported to occur in several areas with the axilla appearing to be the most commonly involved site.

Microscopically, the majority of the reported examples are characterized by a glandular, tubular, papillary, tubulopapillary, diffuse, or solid growth pattern centered on the dermis and subcutaneous tissue. In contrast to apocrine adenoma, the tumor is usually poorly circumscribed and frequently presents an infiltrating border. The epithelial cells have abundant eosinophilic cytoplasm, and decapitation secretion is invariably present. Pleomorphism and mitotic activity are variable features, but become more prominent in poorly differentiated variants. The tumor is commonly accompanied by a dense hyaline stroma.

Immunohistochemically, the tumor cells consistently express cytokeratins, including CAM 5.2, CK7, CK15, AE1/AE3, usually GCDFP-15 and variably CEA [131]. Controversial information has been published on the expression of S-100 protein, EMA, lysozyme, α_1-antitrypsin, and α_1-antichymotrypsin. In a significant subset of tumors expression of estrogen, progesterone, or androgen receptors is seen [131]. An in situ component is best identified by an intact peripheral basal/myoepithelial cell layer reactive for calponin, p63, and actin; however, this myoepithelial layer is lost in some cases [4, 32].

Porocarcinoma

Porocarcinomas are aggressive tumors with potential for local recurrence, and nodal and distant metastases [132]. They usually arise within preexisting benign poroid tumors, frequently located in the lower extremities. Histologically they are characterized by an asymmetrical, solid, and nodular growth pattern, with infiltrative or pushing borders. The neoplasm is composed of poroid and cuticular cells, similar to those of poroma, but with varying degrees of nuclear atypia, hyperchromatic nuclei, and prominent nucleoli. Both in situ and invasive forms have been described [2].

Immunohistochemistry shows that poroid cells are positive for CK7. EMA and CEA (Fig. 2.11) have been reported to be positive in the lumina of ductal structures [133, 134], however, poorly differentiated porocarcinomas with no luminal differentiation did not express CEA [132, 134]. The presence of scattered dendritic melanocytes, positive for S-100 protein and HMB-45, has been reported in both poromas and porocarcinomas [135]. Some authors have proposed that CK19 can be useful in the distinction of porocarcinoma from squamous cell carcinoma (SCC), as it is expressed in 67 % of porocarcinomas versus 18 % of SCC. S-100 protein is another useful marker in the differential diagnosis of this neoplasm from tumors with more prominent myoepithelial differentiation such as spiradenoma, apocrine hidradenoma, and cutaneous mixed tumors. In these tumors neoplastic aggregates of myoepithelial cells are positive with S-100 protein, whereas in porocarcinoma the positive cells are scattered dendritic cells [136]. The diagnostic role of other markers (p16, RB protein, beta-2-microglobulin) has been investigated, but they seem to have no relevance in routine practice [137, 138].

Extramammary Paget's Disease

Extramammary Paget's disease (EMPD) is an uncommon cutaneous malignant neoplasm arising in areas with high density of apocrine glands, most commonly in the vulvar and perianal region of middle-aged females, and less commonly the axilla. It has also been reported in areas with modified apocrine glands, such as the eyelids and external auditory canal. Apocrine gland origin or

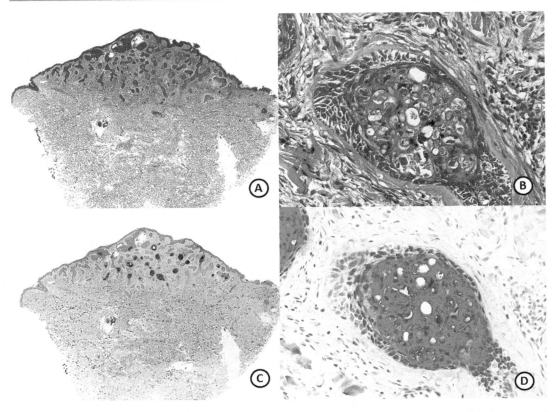

Fig. 2.11 (**a**) Porocarcinoma. (**b**) Some of the neoplastic aggregates show necrosis en masse, pleomorphic nuclei and small ductal structures. (**c**) The same case immuno-histochemically studied for CEA. (**d**) CEA is expressed by most of neoplastic cells

apocrine differentiation of cells in EMPD has been generally accepted [2]. Lesions usually present as erythematous eczematoid slowly spreading plaques and erosive ulceration in older individuals. The size of the lesion usually correlates with its duration.

Histologically, there is a proliferation of single and small clusters of large cells within the epidermis, which have less defined intercellular bridges and exhibit glandular differentiation, occasionally showing intracytoplasmic luminal and ductal formation. The tumor cells in Paget's disease have abundant pale cytoplasm and large pleomorphic nuclei. Mitoses are usually present [7]. The epidermis is usually hyperplastic and there is often overlying hyperkeratosis and parakeratosis. A chronic inflammatory cell infiltrate is found in the upper dermis [8]. An underlying in situ or invasive adnexal carcinoma may be

present. This may show apocrine differentiation, but in other cases it is not possible to determine the cell of origin.

With immunoperoxidase techniques Paget's cells stain for AE1/AE3, LMWK, and CK 7 (Fig. 2.12), with variable positivity seen for EMA and CEA. GCDFP-15, androgen receptors, and Her2/neu are also commonly expressed in EMPD, whereas estrogen and progesterone receptors are not [139–141]. Variable staining of cells has been reported for HMFG [142]. HER-2 protein is expressed in some cases. Prostate-specific antigen (PSA) is expressed in the pagetoid cells of many cases associated with an underlying adenocarcinoma of the prostate, but it may also be expressed in cases without an associated carcinoma [143]. Matrix metalloproteinases (MMP-7, MMP-19) are often expressed in cases with an underlying carcinoma [144]. Other

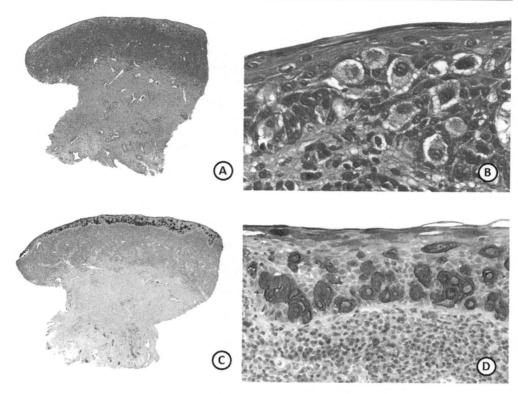

Fig. 2.12 (**a**) Extramammary Paget disease involving the glans penis. (**b**) Paget cells in pagetoid pattern involving the epithelium. (**c**) The same case immunohistochemically studied for CK7. (**d**) CK7 is expressed by Paget cells

proteins that can be expressed in Paget's disease include insulin-like growth factor-1 receptor, p-AKT, p-ERK1/2, Stat3, Stat5a, E-cadherin, cyclin D_1, and Bcl-xL [145–147]. Overexpression of p53 is correlated with stromal invasion. Ber-EP4 can aid in the differential diagnosis from Bowen's disease as it labels all cases of extramammary Paget's disease but none of the other pagetoid neoplasms [148].

Immunohistochemical expression of apomucin MUC1, MUC2, MUC5AC has been proposed as a helpful tool for histopathologic differential diagnosis among mammary Paget disease, extramammary Paget disease, and epidermotropic metastasis in the anogenital skin from adjacent visceral adenocarcinomas [149]. MUC1 is commonly expressed in most cases of mammary Paget disease. In contrast, MUC5AC is a unique mucin that is expressed in most cases of extramammary Paget disease, but not in mammary Paget disease. In cases of mammary Paget disease

associated breast ductal carcinoma, both Paget cells and underlying ductal carcinoma exhibit the phenotype MUC1+MUC2−MUC5AC−. This mucin phenotype is also expressed by Toker cells. In patients with perianal Paget disease associated with rectal adenocarcinoma, Paget's cells express MUC2 constantly, but the expression of MUC1 and MUC5AC is variable. Cases of vulvar and scrotal intraepidermal extramammary Paget disease with no identifiable underlying malignancy express a uniform phenotype of mucin MUC1+MUC2−MUC5AC+, whereas cases of extramammary Paget disease associated with underlying apocrine carcinoma have a phenotype characterized by MUC1+MUC2−MUC5AC−, identical to that of normal apocrine glands. Bartholin's glands express a mucin phenotype identical to that of intraepidermal extramammary Paget disease. These results support that: (1) Mammary Paget disease may arise from either mammary glands or epidermal Toker cells;

(2) Intraepidermal extramammary Paget disease in the anogenital areas may arise from ectopic MUC5AC+ cells originating from Bartholin's or some other unidentified glands; and (3). Unique expression of MUC2 in perianal extramammary Paget disease indicates its origin from colorectal mucosa. In conclusion, the study of mucin gene expression is useful in the histopathologic differential diagnosis among mammary Paget disease, extramammary Paget disease and epidermotropic metastasis in anogenital skin from an adjacent colon adenocarcinoma.

Spiradenocarcinoma and Cylindrocarcinoma

Malignant neoplasms arising in preexisting benign spiradenoma and cylindroma, are rare, and approximately 100 cases having been reported to date [4]. The most common benign neoplasm giving rise to a malignant tumor is spiradenoma, followed by cylindroma. The microscopic appearances of these malignant tumors are heterogeneous, as is the terminology used by different authors. The lesions mostly occur as sporadic solitary neoplasms, or as a component of Brooke–Spiegler syndrome. Sporadic tumors occur mainly in elderly patients and usually involve the back, neck, and scalp, where they present as solitary tumors ranging in size from 2 to 17.5 cm. In Brooke–Spiegler syndrome patients, malignant lesions develop as large, rapidly growing, bleeding, or ulcerated tumors in a background of multiple, smaller, either grouped or confluent papules or nodules, which represent preexisting benign neoplasms [150, 151].

Histopathologically, features suggesting possible malignant potential include an infiltrating growth pattern and loss of mosaic appearance, hyaline sheaths, and biphasic cellular distribution. Nuclear pleomorphism, prominent nucleoli, and frequent or abnormal mitoses are also features seen in these malignant neoplasms.

Immunohistochemistry may be of help in highlighting ductal differentiation, the latter expressing EMA and CEA. The background population of tumor cells express CAM5.2, S-100

protein and GCDFP-15 expression with variable intensity [152]. Although immunostaining for p53 has been suggested to differentiate benign spiradenoma and cylindroma from their malignant counterparts, its utility is limited by its heterogeneous pattern of expression, especially the occasional lack of staining in clearly malignant areas and the occurrence, of focal weak positivity in the benign residual tumor or in unequivocally benign neoplasms [76].

Finally, cases associated with Brooke–Spiegler syndrome usually show a germ-line mutation of the *CYLD* gene. There appears to be no correlation between the germ-line mutation type and the clinical phenotype that would suggest malignant transformation [4]. Despite relatively frequent immunopositivity for p53, mutations of the *TP53* gene are rare in malignant lesions [76].

Microcystic Adnexal Carcinoma

Microcystic adnexal carcinoma (MAC), also called sclerosing syringomatous carcinoma or sclerosing sweat duct carcinoma is an uncommon malignant neoplasm, which is widely believed to be of eccrine origin. However, the presence of infundibular keratinous cysts and the description of apocrine and sebaceous differentiation has been described in many cases [2, 153]. This may suggest that both eccrine and apocrine variants of this neoplasm do exist. It typically develops on the mid-face of young, middle-aged, or elderly woman, and has a tendency toward persistent and local recurrence (approximately 50 %) [154], but not to metastatic potential [155, 156]. In particular, the upper lip and the glabella are the commonest locations.

Histopathologically, MAC is composed of a poorly circumscribed proliferation of non-atypical epithelial neoplastic cells infiltrating the dermis and subcutaneous tissue, with prominent perineural and intraneural invasion. The neoplastic cells are small, uniform, and basaloid, and show no or minimal cytological atypia and mitotic activity. Keratin-filled microcysts are often present in the superficial dermis. Tubular and ductal structures lined by a single layer of neoplastic cells dominate the deeper parts of the lesion. The tumor stroma is characteristically sclerotic.

With immunohistochemistry, the tumor cells express AE1/AE3, and the ductal differentiation and intracytoplasmic lumen formation are positive for EMA and CEA [157]. LeuM1 is usually positive as wells as CD15, while Ber-EP4 (Fig. 2.13) and S100 protein show variable expression [158, 159]. The proliferation rate, as determined by Ki-67, is usually low [160].

Adenoid Cystic Carcinoma

Primary cutaneous adenoid cystic carcinoma (ACC) is a very rare malignant neoplasm affecting older adults, with a female predominance. It can occur in different anatomical sites, most commonly in the scalp [161]. The tumor has a 50 %

local recurrence rate, but metastasis to regional lymph nodes and distant organs is rare [162].

Histopathologically, ACC is indistinguishable from its salivary gland counterpart, and it usually presents as a dermal tumor that forms tubuloalveolar structures lined by atypical basaloid epithelia and associated with the formation of basophilic "cylinders" of myxoid matrix substance. Globules and cylinders of brightly eosinophilic basement membrane-like material complete the picture [163, 164]. Mitoses are typically inconspicuous. An important criterion in ACC in any anatomical location is the striking propensity of these tumors to manifest perineural infiltration.

Immunohistochemically, the tumor cells express low and high molecular weight keratin and broad-spectrum keratins. The presence of ductal differentiation can be confirmed with EMA and CEA, which are frequently expressed in the

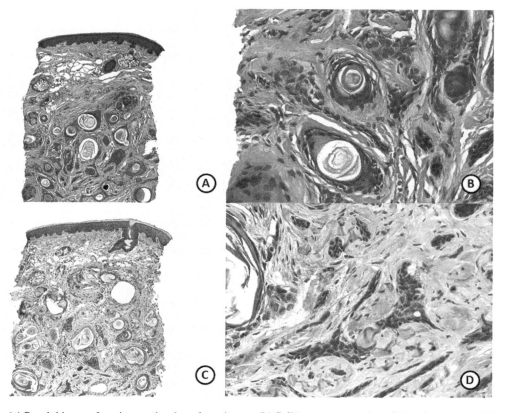

Fig. 2.13 (**a**) Punch biopsy of a microcystic adnexal carcinoma. (**b**) Solid aggregates and small keratinous cysts. (**c**) The same case immunohistochemically studied for BerEp4. (**d**) Weak immunoexpression of neoplastic cells for BerEp4

luminal surfaces and secretions. Myoepithelial differentiation (S-100 protein, actin, positivity) is a constant feature. The basement membrane material is composed of a mixture of collagens IV and V and laminin [165].

Disclosures We do not have any conflict of interest to declare.

We do not have any financial support.

References

1. Prieto VG, O'shea CR, Celebes JT, Busam KJ. Adnexal Tumors. In: Busam KJ, editor. Dermatopathology. 1st ed. Philadelphia: Saunders Elsevier; 2010. p. 381–436.
2. Obaidat NA, Alsaad KO, Ghazarian D. Skin adnexal neoplasms-part 2: An approach to tumours of cutaneous sweat glands. J Clin Pathol. 2007;60:145–59.
3. Saga K. Structure and function of human sweat glands studied with histochemistry and cytochemistry. Prog Histochem Cytochem. 2002;37:323–86.
4. Kazakov DV, Michal M, Kacerovska D, Mckee PH. Lesions with predominant apocrine and eccrine differentiation. In: Kazakov DV, Michal M, Kacerovska D, Mckee PH, editors. Cutaneous adnexal tumors. 1st ed. Philadelphia: Wolters Kluwer Health; 2012. p. 1–171.
5. van der Putte SC. Apoeccrine glands in nevus sebaceus. Am J Dermatopathol. 1994;16:23–30.
6. van der Putte SC. Mammary-like glands of the vulva and their disorders. Int J Gynecol Pathol. 1994;13:150–60.
7. Weedon D. Tumors of cutaneous appendages. In: Weedon D, editor. Skin pathology. 3rd ed. Edinburgh: Churchill Livingstone; 2010. p. 398–440.
8. Busam KJ, Tan LK, Granter SR, Kohler S, Junkins-Hopkins J, Berwick M, Rosen PP. Epidermal growth factor, estrogen, and progesterone receptor expression in primary sweat gland carcinomas and primary and metastatic mammary carcinomas. Mod Pathol. 1999;12:786–93.
9. Mirza I, Kloss R, Sieber SC. Malignant eccrine spiradenoma. Arch Pathol Lab Med. 2002;126:591–4.
10. Sato K, Leidal R, Sato F. Morphology and development of an apoeccrine sweat gland in human axillae. Am J Physiol. 1987;252:166–80.
11. Kamada A, Saga K, Jimbow K. Apoeccrine sweat duct obstruction as a cause for Fox-Fordyce disease. J Am Acad Dermatol. 2003;48:453–5.
12. Abbott JJ, Ahmed I. Adenocarcinoma of mammary-like glands of the vulva: report of a case and review of the literature. Am J Dermatopathol. 2006;28:127–33.
13. Nishie W, Sawamura D, Mayuzumi M, Takahashi S, Shimizu H. Hidradenoma papilliferum with mixed histopathologic features of syringocystadenoma papilliferum and anogenital mammary-like glands. J Cutan Pathol. 2004;31:561–4.
14. Sarabi K, Khachemoune A. Hidrocystomas-a brief review. Med Gen Med. 2006;8:57.
15. Monk BE, Pieris S, Soni V. Schöpf-Schulz-Passarge syndrome. Br J Dermatol. 1992;127:33–5.
16. Mallaiah U, Dickinson J. Photo essay: bilateral multiple eyelid apocrine hidrocystomas and ectodermal dysplasia. Arch Ophthalmol. 2011;119:1866–7.
17. Buchner SA, Itin P. Focal dermal hypoplasia syndrome in a male patient. Report of a case and histologic and immunohistochemical studies. Arch Dermatol. 1992;128:1078–82.
18. Alessi E, Gianotti R, Coggi A. Multiple apocrine hidrocystomas of the eyelids. Br J Dermatol. 1997;137:642–5.
19. Fariña MC, Piqué E, Olivares M, Escalonilla P, Martín L, Requena L, Sarasa JL. Multiple hidrocystoma of the face: three cases. Clin Exp Dermatol. 1995;20:323–7.
20. Sugiyama A, Sugiura M, Piris A, Tomita Y, Mihm MC. Apocrine cystadenoma and apocrine hidrocystoma: examination of 21 cases with emphasis on nomenclature according to proliferative features. J Cutan Pathol. 2007;34:912–7.
21. Ohnishi T, Watanabe S. Immunohistochemical analysis of cytokeratin expression in apocrine cystadenoma or hidrocystoma. J Cutan Pathol. 1999;26:295–300.
22. de Viragh PA, Szeimies RM, Eckert F. Apocrine cystadenoma, apocrine hidrocystoma, and eccrine hidrocystoma: three distinct tumors defined by expression of keratins and human milk fat globulin 1. J Cutan Pathol. 1997;24:249–55.
23. Requena L, Kiryu H, Ackerman AB. Neoplasms with apocrine differentiation. Philadelphia, PA: Lippincott-Raven; 1998.
24. Kanitakis J, Kyamidis K, Toussinas A, Tsoïtis G. Pure apocrine nevus: immunohistochemical study of a new case and literature review. Dermatology. 2011;222:97–101.
25. Neill JS, Park HK. Apocrine nevus: light microscopic, immunohistochemical and ultrastructural studies of a case. J Cutan Pathol. 1993;20:79–83.
26. Cordero SC, Royer M, Rush WL, Hallman JR, Lupton GP. Pure apocrine nevus: a report of 4 cases. Am J Dermatopathol. 2012;34:305–9.
27. Koga T, Kubota Y, Nakayama J. Syringocystadenoma papilliferum without an antecedent naevus sebaceus. Acta Derm Venereol. 1999;79:237.
28. Karg E, Korom I, Varga E, Ban G, Turi S. Congenital syringocystadenoma papilliferum. Pediatr Dermatol. 2008;25:132–3.
29. Ishida-Yamamoto A, Sato K, Wada T, Takahashi H, Iizuka H. Syringocystadenocarcinoma papilliferum: case report and immunohistochemical comparison with its benign counterpart. J Am Acad Dermatol. 2001;45:755–9.
30. Yamamoto O, Doi Y, Hamada T, Hisaoka M, Sasaguri Y. An immunohistochemical and ultrastructural study of syringocystadenoma papilliferum. Br J Dermatol. 2002;147:936–45.

31. Boni R, Xin H, Hohl D, Panizzon R, Burg G. Syringocystadenoma papilliferum: a study of potential tumor suppressor genes. Am J Dermatopathol. 2001;23:87–9.

32. Calonje E, Brenn T, Lazar A, McKee PH. Tumors of the sweat glands. In: Calonje E, Brenn T, Lazar A, McKee PH, editors. McKee's pathology of the skin. 4th ed. Philadelphia: Saunders Elsevier; 2012. p. 1508–70.

33. Konohana I, Niizeki H, Ikutomi M. A case of tubular apocrine adenoma located on the genital area. Rinshouhifuka. 1991;45:809–12.

34. Ishiko A, Shimizu H, Inamoto N, Nakmura K. Is tubular apocrine adenoma a distinct clinical entity? Am J Dermatopathol. 1993;15:482–7.

35. Kazakov DV, Bisceglia M, Calonje E, Hantschke M, Kutzner H, Mentzel T, Michal M, Mukensnabl P, Spagnolo DV, Rütten A, Rose C, Urso C, Vazmitel M, Zelger B. Tubular adenoma and syringocystadenoma papilliferum: a reappraisal of their relationship. An interobserver study of a series, by a panel of dermatopathologists. Am J Dermatopathol. 2007;29:256–63.

36. Mizuoka H, Senzaki H, Shikata N, Uemura Y, Tsubura A. Papillary eccrine adenoma: immunohistochemical study and literature review. J Cutan Pathol. 1998;25:59–64.

37. Requena L, Peña M, Sánchez M, Sánchez Yus E. Papillary eccrine adenoma. Light microscopic and immunohistochemical study. Clin Exp Dermatol. 1990;15:425–8.

38. Megahed M, Hölzle E. Papillary eccrine adenoma. A case report with immunohistochemical examination. Am J Dermatopathol. 1993;15:150–5.

39. Loane J, Kealy WF, Mulcahy G. Perianal hidradenoma papilliferum occurring in a male: a case report. Ir J Med Sci. 1998;167:26–7.

40. Handa Y, Yamanaka N, Inagaki H, Tomita Y. Large ulcerated perianal hidradenoma papilliferum in a young female. Dermatol Surg. 2003;29:790–2.

41. Pelosi G, Martignoni G, Bonetti F. Intraductal carcinoma of mammary-type apocrine epithelium arising within a papillary hidradenoma of the vulva. Report of a case and review of the literature. Arch Pathol Lab Med. 1991;115:1249–54.

42. Tamaki K, Furue M, Matsukawa A, Ohara K, Mizoguchi M, Hino H. Presence and distribution of carcinoembryonic antigen and lectin-binding sites in benign apocrine sweat gland tumours. Br J Dermatol. 1985;113:565–71.

43. Ansai S, Koseki S, Hozumi Y, Kondo S. An immunohistochemical study of lysozyme, Cd-15 (Leu M1), and gross cystic disease fluid protein-15 in various skin tumors. Assessment of the specificity and sensitivity of markers of apocrine differentiation. Am J Dermatopathol. 1995;17:249–55.

44. Thompson LD, Nelson BL, Barnes EL. Ceruminous adenomas: a clinicopathologic study of 41 cases with a review of the literature. Am J Surg Pathol. 2004;28:308–18.

45. Lott Limbach AA, Hoschar AP, Thompson LD, Stelow EB, Chute DJ. Middle ear adenomas stain for two cell populations and lack myoepithelial cell differentiation. Head Neck Pathol. 2012;6:345–53.

46. Fernandez-Flores A, Suarez-Peñaranda JM. Immunophenotype of nipple adenoma in a male patient. Appl Immunohistochem Mol Morphol. 2011;19:190–4.

47. Ohnishi T, Watanabe S. Histogenesis of clear cell hidradenoma: immunohistochemical study of keratin expression. J Cutan Pathol. 1997;24:30–6.

48. Biernat W, Kordek R, Woźniak L. Phenotypic heterogeneity of nodular hidradenoma. Immunohistochemical analysis with emphasis on cytokeratin expression. Am J Dermatopathol. 1996;18:592–6.

49. Vodovnik A. Coexpression of S-100 and smooth muscle actin in nodular hidradenoma. Am J Dermatopathol. 2003;25:361–2.

50. Behboudi A, Winnes M, Gorunova L, van den Oord JJ, Mertens F, Enlund F, Stenman G. Clear cell hidradenoma of the skin-a third tumor type with a t(11;19)-associated TORC1-MAML2 gene fusion. Genes Chromosomes Cancer. 2005;43:202–5.

51. Winnes M, Mölne L, Suurküla M, Andrén Y, Persson F, Enlund F, Stenman G. Frequent fusion of the CRTC1 and MAML2 genes in clear cell variants of cutaneous hidradenomas. Genes Chromosomes Cancer. 2007;46:559–63.

52. Behboudi A, Enlund F, Winnes M, Andrén Y, Nordkvist A, Leivo I, Flaberg E, Szekely L, Mäkitie A, Grenman R, Mark J, Stenman G. Molecular classification of mucoepidermoid carcinomas-prognostic significance of the MECT1-MAML2 fusion oncogene. Genes Chromosomes Cancer. 2006;45:470–81.

53. Kallam AR, Krishna R, Thumma RR, Setty VK. Mixed tumour of ala-nasi: a rare case report and review. J Clin Diagn Res. 2013;7:2019–20.

54. Alsaad KO, Obaidat NA, Ghazarian D. Skin adnexal neoplasms—part 1: an approach to tumours of the pilosebaceous unit. J Clin Pathol. 2006;60:129–44.

55. Satter EK, Graham BS. Chondroid syringoma. Cutis. 2003;71:49–52.

56. Metze D, Grunert F, Neumaier M, Bhardwaj R, Amann U, Wagener C, Luger TA. Neoplasms with sweat gland differentiation express various glycoproteins of the carcinoembryonic antigen (CEA) family. J Cutan Pathol. 1996;23:1–11.

57. Kazakov DV, Kacerovska D, Hantschke M, et al. Cutaneous mixed tumor, eccrine variant: a clinicopathologic and immunohistochemical study of 50 cases, with emphasis on unusual histophatological features. Am J Dermatopathol. 2011;33:557–68.

58. González-Guerra E, Kutzner H, Rutten A, Requena L. Immunohistochemical study of calretinin in normal skin and cutaneous adnexal proliferations. Am J Dermatopathol. 2012;34:491–505.

59. Bahrami A, Dalton JD, Krane JF, Fletcher CD. A subset of cutaneous and soft tissue mixed tumors are genetically linked to their salivary gland counterpart. Genes Chromosomes Cancer. 2012;51:140–8.

60. Flucke U, Palmedo G, Blankenhorn N, Slootweg PJ, Kutzner H, Mentzel T. EWSR1 gene rearrangement occurs in a subset of cutaneous myoepithelial tumors: a study of 18 cases. Mod Pathol. 2011;24:1444–50.

61. Seo SH, Oh CK, Ks K, Kim MB. A case of milium-like syringoma with focal calcification in Down syndrome. Br J Dermatol. 2007;157:612–4.

62. Schepis C, Siragusa M, Palazzo R, Batolo D, Romano C. Perforating milia-like idiopathic calcinosis cutis and periorbital syringomas in a girl with Down syndrome. Pediatr Dermatol. 1994;11:258–60.

63. Eckert F, Nilles M, Schmid U, Altmannsberger M. Distribution of cytokeratin polypeptides in syringomas. An immunohistochemical study on paraffin-embedded material. Am J Dermatopathol. 1992;14:115–21.

64. Ohnishi T, Watanabe S. Immunohistochemical analysis of keratin expression in clear cell syringoma. A comparative study with conventional syringoma. J Cutan Pathol. 1997;24:370–6.

65. Mazoujian G, Margolis R. Immunohistochemistry of gross cystic disease fluid protein (GCDFP-15) in 65 benign sweat gland tumors of the skin. Am J Dermatopathol. 1988;10:28–35.

66. Zhu L, Okano S, Takahara M, Chiba T, Tu Y, Oda Y, Furue M. Expression of S100 protein family members in normal skin and sweat gland tumors. J Dermatol Sci. 2013;70:211–9.

67. Saggar S, Chernoff KA, Lodha S, Horev L, Kohl S, Honjo RS, Brandt HR, Hartmann K, Celebi JT. CYLD mutations in familial skin appendage tumours. J Med Genet. 2008;45:298–302.

68. Szepietowski JC, Wasik F, Szybejko-Machaj G, Bieniek A, Schwartz RA. Brooke-Spiegler syndrome. J Eur Acad Dermatol Venereol. 2001;15:346–69.

69. Weyers W, Nilles M, Eckert F, Schill WB. Spiradenomas in Brooke–Spiegler syndrome. Am J Dermatopathol. 1993;15:156–61.

70. Tellechea O, Reis JP, Ilheu O, Baptista AP. Dermal cylindroma. An immunohistochemical study of thirteen cases. Am J Dermatopathol. 1995;17:260–5.

71. Penneys NS, Kaiser M. Cylindroma expresses immunohistochemical markers linking it to eccrine coil. J Cutan Pathol. 1993;20:40–3.

72. Pfaltz M, Bruckner-Tuderman L, Schnyder UW. Type VII collagen is a component of cylindroma basement membrane zone. J Cutan Pathol. 1989;16:388–95.

73. Bruckner-Tuderman L, Pfaltz M, Schnyder UW. Cylindroma overexpresses collagen VII, the major anchoring fibril protein. J Invest Dermatol. 1991;96:729–34.

74. Kurokawa I, Nishimura K, Tarumi C, Hakamada A, Isoda K, Mizutani H, Tsubura A. Eccrine spiradenoma: co-expression of cytokeratin and smooth muscle actin suggesting differentiation toward myoepithelial cells. J Eur Acad Dermatol Venereol. 2007;21:121–3.

75. Sima R, Vanecek T, Kacerovska D, Trubac P, Cribier B, Rutten A, Vazmitel M, Spagnolo DV, Litvik R, Vantuchova Y, Weyers W, Pearce RL, Pearn J, Michal M, Kazakov DV. Brooke-Spiegler syndrome: report of 10 patients from 8 families with novel germline mutations: evidence of diverse somatic mutations in the same patient regardless of tumor type. Diagn Mol Pathol. 2010;19:83–91.

76. Kazakov DV, Carlson JA, Vanecek T, Vanecek T, Vazmitel M, Kacerovska D, Zelger B, Calonje E, Michal M. Expression of p53 and TP53 mutational analysis in malignant neoplasms arising in preexisting spiradenoma, cylindroma, and spiradenocylindroma, sporadic or associated with Brooke-Spiegler syndrome. Am J Dermatopathol. 2010;32:215–21.

77. Kamiya H, Oyama Z, Kitajima Y. "Apocrine" poroma: review of the literature and case report. J Cutan Pathol. 2001;28:101–4.

78. Kakinuma H, Miyamoto R, Iwasawa U, Baba S, Suzuki H. Three subtypes of poroid neoplasia in a single lesion: eccrine poroma, hidroacanthoma simplex, and dermal duct tumor. Histologic, histochemical, and ultrastructural findings. Am J Dermatopathol. 1994;16:66–72.

79. Yamamoto O, Hisaoka M, Yasuda H, Kasai T, Hashimoto H. Cytokeratin expression of apocrine and eccrine poromas with special reference to its expression in cuticular cells. J Cutan Pathol. 2000;27:367–73.

80. Tateyama H, Eimoto T, Tada T, Inagaki H, Nakamura T, Yamauchi R. p53 protein and proliferating cell nuclear antigen in eccrine poroma and porocarcinoma. An immunohistochemical study. Am J Dermatopathol. 1995;17:457–64.

81. Ichihashi N, Kitajima Y. Loss of heterozygosity of adenomatous polyposis coli gene in cutaneous tumors as determined by using polymerase chain reaction and paraffin section preparations. J Dermatol Sci. 2000;22:102–6.

82. Hornick JL, Fletcher CD. Cutaneous myoepithelioma: a clinicopathologic and immunohistochemical study of 14 cases. Hum Pathol. 2004;35:14–24.

83. Hornick JL, Fletcher CD. Myoepithelial tumors of soft tissue: a clinicopathologic and immunohistochemical study of 101 cases with evaluation of prognostic parameters. Am J Surg Pathol. 2003;27: 1183–96.

84. Fernández-Figueras MT, Puig L, Trias I, Lorenzo JC, Navas-Palacios JJ. Benign myoepithelioma of the skin. Am J Dermatopathol. 1998;20:208–12.

85. Requena L. Cutaneous myoepithelioma? Am J Dermatopathol. 2000;22:360–1.

86. Mentzel T, Requena L, Kaddu S, Soares de Almeida LM, Sangueza OP, Kutzner H. Cutaneous myoepithelial neoplasms: clinicopathologic and immunohistochemical study of 20 cases suggesting a continuous spectrum ranging from benign mixed tumor of the skin to cutaneous myoepithelioma and myoepithelial carcinoma. J Cutan Pathol. 2003;30:294–302.

87. Numata M, Hosoe S, Itoh N, Munakata Y, Hayashi S, Maruyama Y. Syringadenocarcinoma papilliferum. J Cutan Pathol. 1985;12:3–7.

88. Arslan H, Diyarbakrl M, Batur S, Demirkesen C. Syringocystadenocarcinoma papilliferum with squamous cell carcinoma differentiation and with locoregional metastasis. J Craniofac Surg. 2013;24:38–40.

89. Satter E, Grady D, Schlocker CT. Syringocystadenocarcinoma papilliferum with locoregional metastases. Dermatol Online J. 2014;20:22335.

90. Leeborg N, Thompson M, Rossmiller S, Gross N, White C, Gatter K. Diagnostic pitfalls in syringocystadenocarcinoma papilliferum: case report and review of the literature. Arch Pathol Lab Med. 2010;134:1205–9.

91. Peterson J, Tefft K, Blackmon J, Rajpara A, Fraga G. Syringocystadenocarcinoma papilliferum: a rare tumor with a favorable prognosis. Dermatol Online J. 2013;19:19620.

92. Park SH, Shin YM, Shin DH, Choi JS. Kim KH. Syringocystadenocarcinoma papilliferum: A case report. J Korean Med Sci. 2007;22:762–5.

93. Woestenborghs H, Van Eyken P, Dans A. Syringocystadenocarcinoma papilliferum in situ with pagetoid spread: a case report. Histopathology. 2006;48:869–70.

94. Rütten A, Kutzner H, Mentzel T, Hantschke M, Eckert F, Angulo J, Rodríguez Peralto JL, Requena L. Primary cutaneous cribriform apocrine carcinoma: A clinicopathologic and immunohistochemical study of 26 cases of an under-recognized cutaneous adnexal neoplasm. J Am Acad Dermatol. 2009;61:644–51.

95. Standley E, Dujardin F, Arbion F, Touzé A, Machet L, Velut S, Guyétant S. Recurrent primary cutaneous mucinous carcinoma with neuroendocrine differentiation: case report and review of the literature. J Cutan Pathol. 2014;41:686–91.

96. Karimipour DJ, Johnson TM, Kang S, Wang TS, Lowe L. Mucinous carcinoma of the skin. J Am Acad Dermatol. 1997;36:323–6.

97. Kazakov DV, Suster S, LeBoit PE, Calonje E, Bisceglia M, Kutzner H, Rütter A, Mentzel T, Schaller J, Zelger B, Baltaci M, Leivo I, Rose C, Fukunaga M, Simpson RH, Yang Y, Carlson JA, Cavazza A, Hes O, Mukensnabl P, Vanecek T, Fidalgo A, Pizinger K, Michal M. Mucinous carcinoma of the skin, primary, and secondary: a clinicopathologic study of 63 cases with emphasis on the morphologic spectrum of primary cutaneous forms: homologies with mucinous lesions in the breast. Am J Surg Pathol. 2005;29:764–82.

98. Kwatra KS, Prabhakar BR, Jain S. Oestrogen and progesterone receptors in primary mucinous carcinoma of skin. Australas J Dermatol. 2005;46:246–9.

99. Han S-E, Lim SY, Lim HS. Neuroendocrine differentiation of primary mucinous carcinoma of the cheek skin. Arch Plast Surg. 2013;40:159–62.

100. Kim J-B, Choi J-H, Kim J-H, Park HJ, Lee JS, Joh OJ, Song KY. A case of primary cutaneous mucinous carcinoma with neuroendocrine differentiation. Ann Dermatol. 2010;22:472–7.

101. Bellezza G, Sidoni A, Bucciarelli E. Primary mucinous carcinoma of the skin. Am J Dermatopathol. 2000;22:166–70.

102. Levy G, Finkelstein A, McNiff JM. Immunohistochemical techniques to compare primary vs. metastatic mucinous carcinoma of the skin. J Cutan Pathol. 2010;37:411–5.

103. Ivan D, Nash JW, Prieto VG, Calonje E, Lyle S, Diwan AH, Lazar AJ. Use of p63 expression in distinguishing primary and metastatic cutaneous adnexal neoplasms from metastatic adenocarcinoma to skin. J Cutan Pathol. 2007;34:474–80.

104. Flieder A, Koerner FC, Pilch BZ, Maluf HM. Endocrine mucin-producing sweat gland carcinoma. A cutaneous neoplasm analogous to solid papillary carcinoma of the breast. Am J Surg Pathol. 1997;21:1501–6.

105. Zembowicz A, Garcia CF, Tannous ZS, Mihm MC, Koerner F, Pilch BZ. Endocrine mucin-producing sweat gland carcinoma. Twelve new cases suggest that it is a precursor of some invasive mucinous carcinomas. Am J Surg Pathol. 2005; 9:1330–9.

106. Bulliard C, Murali R, Maloof A, Adams S. Endocrine mucin-producing sweat gland carcinoma: report of a case and review of the literature. J Cutan Pathol. 2006;33:812–6.

107. Emanuel PO, De Vinck D, Waldorf HA, et al. Recurrent endocrine mucin-producing sweat gland carcinoma. Ann Diagn Pathol. 2007;11:448–52.

108. Mehta S, Thiagalingam S, Zembovicz A, et al. Endocrine mucin-producing sweat gland carcinoma of the eyelid. Ophthal Plast Reconstr Surg. 2008;24:164–5.

109. Inozume T, Kawasaki T, Harada K, et al. A case of endocrine mucin-producing sweat gland carcinoma. Pathol Int. 2012;62:344–6.

110. Salim AA, Karim RZ, McCarthy SW, et al. Endocrine mucin-producing sweat gland carcinoma: a clinicopathological analysis of three cases. Pathology. 2012;44:568–71.

111. Dhaliwal CA, Torgersen A, Ross JJ, Ironside JW, Biswas A. Endocrine mucin-producing sweat gland carcinoma: report of two cases of an under-recognized malignant neoplasm and review of literature. Am J Dermatopathol. 2013;35:117–24.

112. Hoguet A, Warrow D, Milite J, et al. Mucin-producing sweat gland carcinoma of the eyelid: diagnostic and prognostic considerations. Am J Ophthalmol. 2013;155:585–92.

113. Koike T, Mikami T, Maegawa J, et al. Recurrent endocrine mucin-producing sweat gland carcinoma in the eyelid. Australas J Dermatol. 2013;54:e46–9.

114. Castro CY, Deavers M. Ductal carcinoma in-situ arising inmammary-like glands of the vulva. Int J Gynecol Pathol. 2001;20:277–83.

115. Shah SS, Adelson M, Mazur MT. Adenocarcinoma in situ arising in vulvar papillary hidradenoma: report of 2 cases. Int J Gynecol Pathol. 2008;27:453–6.

116. Vazmitel M, Spagnolo DV, Nemcova J, et al. Hidradenoma papilliferum with a ductal carcinoma in situ component: case report and review of the literature. Am J Dermatopathol. 2008;30:392–4.

117. Kazakov DV, Spagnolo DV, Kacerovska D, Michal M. Lesions of anogenitalmammary-like glands: an update. Adv Anat Pathol. 2011;18:1–28.

118. Duke WH, Sherrod TT, Lupton GP. Aggressive digital papillary adenocarcinoma. (Aggressive digital papillary adenoma and adenocarcinoma revisited.). Am J Surg Pathol. 2000;24:775–84.

119. Kao GF, Helwig EB, Graham JH. Aggressive digital papillary adenoma and adenocarcinoma. A clinicopathological study of 57 patients, with histochemical immunopathological and ultrastructural observations. J Cutan Pathol. 1987;14:129–46.

120. Hsu HC, Ho CY, Chen CH, Yang CH, Hong HS, Chuang YH. Aggressive digital papillary adenocarcinoma: a review. Clin Exp Dermatol. 2010;35:113–9.

121. Chen S, Asgari M. Is aggressive digital papillary adenocarcinoma really aggressive digital papillary adenocarcinoma? Dermatol Pract Concept. 2014;4:33–5.

122. Suchak R, Wang WL, Prieto VG, Ivan D, Lazar AJ, Brenn T, Calonje E. Cutaneous digital papillary adenocarcinoma: a clinicopathologic study of 31 cases of a rare neoplasm with new observations. Am J Surg Pathol. 2012;36:1883–91.

123. Crain N, Nelson BL, Barnes EL, Thompson LD. Ceruminous gland carcinomas: a clinicopathologic and immunophenotypic study of 17 cases. Head Neck Pathol. 2009;3:1–17.

124. Kazakov DV, Belousova IE, Bisceglia M, Calonje E, Emberger M, Grayson W, Hantschke M, Kempf W, Kutzner H, Michal M, Spagnolo DV, Virolainen S, Zelger B. Apocrine mixed tumor of the skin ('mixed tumor of the folliculosebaceous-apocrine complex'). Spectrum of differentiations and metaplastic changes in the epithelial, myoepithelial, and stromal components based on a histopathologic study of 244 cases. J Am Acad Dermatol. 2007;57:467–83.

125. Schulhof Z, Anastassov GE, Lumerman H, Mashadian D. Giant benign chondroid syringoma of the cheek: case report and review of the literature. J Oral Maxillofac Surg. 2007;65:1836–9.

126. Nather A, Sutherland IH. Malignant transformation of a benign cutaneous mixed tumor. Br J Hand Surg. 1986;11:139–43.

127. Scott A, Metcalf JS. Cutaneous malignant mixed tumor. Am J Dermatopathol. 1988;10:335–42.

128. Trown K, Heenan PJ. Malignant mixed tumor of the skin (malignant chondroid syringoma). Pathology. 1994;26:237–43.

129. Metzler G, Schaumburg-Lever G, Hornstein O, Rassner G. Malignant chondroid syringoma: immunohistopathology. Am J Dermatopathol. 1996;18:83–9.

130. Kiely JL, Dunne B, McCabe M, McNicholas WT. Malignant chondroid syringoma presenting as multiple pulmonary nodules. Thorax. 1997;52:395–6.

131. Robson A, Lazar AJ, Ben Nagi J, Hanby A, Grayson W, Feinmesser M, Granter SR, Seed P, Warneke CL, McKee PH, Calonje E. Primary cutaneous apocrine carcinoma: a clinico-pathologic analysis of 24 cases. Am J Surg Pathol. 2008;32:682–90.

132. Robson A, Greene J, Ansari N, et al. Eccrine porocarcinoma (malignant eccrine poroma): a clinicopathologic study of 69 cases. Am J Surg Pathol. 2001;25:710–20.

133. Claudy AL, Garcier F, Kanitakis J. Eccrine porocarcinoma. Ultrastructural and immunological study. J Dermatol. 1984;11:282–6.

134. Wollina U, Castelli E, Rülke D. Immunohistochemistry of eccrine poroma and porocarcinoma more than acrosyringeal tumors? Recent Results Cancer Res. 1995;139:303–16.

135. Kurisu Y, Tsuji M, Yasuda E, Shibayama Y. A case of eccrine porocarcinoma: usefulness of immunostain for S-100 protein in the diagnoses of recurrent and metastatic dedifferentiated lesions. Ann Dermatol. 2013;25:348–51.

136. Mahalingam M, Richards JE, Selim MA, Muzikansky A, Hoang MP. An immunohistochemical comparison of cytokeratin 7, cytokeratin 15, cytokeratin 19, CAM 5.2, carcinoembryonic antigen, and nestin in differentiating porocarcinoma from squamous cell carcinoma. Hum Pathol. 2012;43:1265–72.

137. Gu LH, Ichiki Y, Kitajam Y. Aberrant expression of p16 and RB protein in eccrine porocarcinoma. J Cutan Pathol. 2002;29:473–9.

138. Holden CA, Shaw M, McKee PH, et al. Loss of membrane B2 microglogulin in eccrine porocarcinoma. Its association with the histopathologic and clinical criteria for malignancy. Arch Dermatol. 1984;120:732–5.

139. Diaz de Leon E, Carcangiu ML, Prieto VG, McCue PA, Burchette JL, To G, Norris BA, Kovatich AJ, Sanchez RL, Krigman HR, Gatalica Z. Extramammary Paget disease is characterized by the consistent lack of estrogen and progesterone receptors but frequently expresses androgen receptor. Am J Clin Pathol. 2000;113:572–5.

140. Liegl B, Horn LC, Moinfar F. Androgen receptors are frequently expressed in mammary and extramammary Paget's disease. Mod Pathol. 2005;18:1283–8.

141. Goldblum JR, Hart WR. Vulvar Paget's disease: a clinicopathologic and immunohistochemical study of 19 cases. Am J Surg Pathol. 1997;21:1178–87.

142. Ohnishi T, Watanabe S. Immunohistochemical analysis of human milk fat globulin expression in extramammary Paget's disease. Clin Exp Dermatol. 2001;26:192–5.

143. Inoguchi N, Matsumara Y, Kanazawa N, Morita K, Tachibana T, Sakurai T. UtaniA, Miyachi Y. Expression of prostate-specific antigen and androgen receptor in extramammary Paget's disease and carcinoma. Clin Exp Dermatol. 2007;32:91–4.

144. Kuivanen T, Tanskanen M, Jahkola T, Impola U, Asko-Seljavaara S, Saarialho-Kere U. Matrilysin-1

(MMP-7) and MMP-19 are expressed by Paget's cells in extramammary Paget's disease. J Cutan Pathol. 2004;31:483–91.

145. Liu H, Moroi Y, Yasumoto S, Kokuba H, Imafuku S, Koga T, Masuda T, Tu Y. FurueM, Urabe K. Expression of insulin-like growth factor-1 receptor, p-AKT and p-ERK1/2 protein in extramammary Paget's disease. Br J Dermatol. 2006;155:586–91.

146. Liu H, Urabe K, Uchi H, Takeuchi S, Nakahara T, Dainichi T, Tu Y, Furue M, Moroi Y. Expression and prognostic significance of Stat5a and E-cadherin in extramammary Paget's disease. J Cutan Pathol. 2007;34:33–8.

147. Liu HJ, Moroi Y, Masuda T, Yasumoto S, Kokuba H, Imafuku S, Koga T, Tetsuya T, Tu YT, Aburatani H, Furue M, Urabe K. Expression of phosphorylated Stat3, cyclin D1 and bcl-xl in extramammary Paget disease. Br J Dermatol. 2006;154:926–32.

148. Sellheyer K, Krahl D. Ber-EP4 enhances the differential diagnostic accuracy of cytokeratin 7 in pagetoid cutaneous neoplasms. J Cutan Pathol. 2008; 35:366–72.

149. Kuan SF, Montag AG, Hart J, Krausz T, Recant W. Differential expression of mucin genes in mammary and extramammary Paget's disease. Am J Surg Pathol. 2001;25:1469–77.

150. Pizinger K, Michal M. Malignant cylindroma in Brooke-Spiegler syndrome. Dermatology. 2000;201: 255–7.

151. Durani BK, Kurzen H, Jaeckel A, Kuner N, Naeher H, Hartschuh W. Malignant transformation of multiple dermal cylindromas. Br J Dermatol. 2001;145: 653–6.

152. Argenyi ZB, Nguyen AV, Balogh K, Sears JK, Whitaker DC. Malignant eccrine spiradenoma: a clinicopathologic study. Am J Dermatopathol. 1992;14:181–390.

153. Crowson AN, Magro CM, Mihm MC. Malignant adnexal neoplasms. Mod Pathol. 2006;19:93–126.

154. Ohtsuka H, Nagamatsu S. Microcystic adnexal carcinoma: review of 51 Japanese patients. Dermatology. 2002;204:190–3.

155. Callahan EF, Vidimos AT, Bergfeld WF. Microcystic adnexal carcinoma (MAC) of the scalp with extensive pilar differentiation. Dermatol Surg. 2002;28:536–9.

156. Ongenae KC, Verhaegh ME, Vermeulen AH, Naeyaert JM. Microcystic adnexal carcinoma: an uncommon tumor with debatable origin. Dermatol Surg. 2001;27:979–84.

157. Hoang MP, Dresser KA, Kapur P, High WA, Mahalingam M. Microcystic adnexal carcinoma: an immunohistochemical reappraisal. Mod Pathol. 2008;21:178–85.

158. Krahl D, Sellheyer K. Monoclonal antibody BerEP4 reliable discriminates between microcystic adnexal carcinoma and basal cell carcinoma. J Cutan Pathol. 2007;34:782–7.

159. Requena L, Marquina A, Alegre V, Aliaga A, Sanchez YE. Sclerosing-sweat-duct (microcystic adnexal) carcinoma—a tumor from a single eccrine origin. Clin Exp Dermatol. 1990;15:222–4.

160. Smith KJ, Williams J, Corbett D, Skelton H. Microcystic adnexal carcinoma. An immunohistochemical study including markers of proliferation and apoptosis. Am J Surg Pathol. 2001; 25:464–71.

161. van der Kwast TH, Vuzevski VD, Ramaekers F, Bousema MT, Van Joost T. Primary cutaneous adenoid cystic carcinoma: case report, immunohistochemistry, and review of the literature. Br J Dermatol. 1988;118:567–77.

162. Chu SS, Chang YL, Lou PJ. Primary cutaneous adenoid cystic carcinoma with regional lymph node metastasis. J Laryngol Otol. 2001;115:673–5.

163. Eckert F, Pfau A, Landthaler M. Adenoid cystic sweat gland carcinoma: a clinicopathologic and immunohistochemical study. Hautarzt. 1994;45:318–23.

164. Matsumura T, Kumakiri M, Ohkaware A, Yoshida T. Adenoid cystic carcinoma of the skin: an immunohistochemical and ultrastructural study. J Dermatol. 1993;20:164–70.

165. Fukai K, Ishii M, Kobayashi H, et al. Primary cutaneous adenoid cystic carcinoma: ultrastructural study and immunolocalization of types I, II, IV, V collagens and laminin. J Cutan Pathol. 1990;17: 374–80.

Immunohistology and Molecular Studies of Follicular Tumors

3

Olayemi Sokumbi and Jose A. Plaza

Introduction

Follicular neoplasms are epithelial tumors with differentiation toward the hair follicle. These tumors include hamartomas, benign and malignant neoplasms and hyperplasias. Making the specific diagnosis is of importance clinically as some of the lesions are cutaneous signs of underlying hereditary tumor syndromes (Birt–Hogg–Dube syndrome, Cowden's disease). In this chapter, we focus on the utility of immunohistochemistry sorting out the challenging differential diagnosis often encountered in dermatopathology.

Tumor of the Follicular Infundibulum (Infundibuloma)

Clinical

Clinical findings are usually subtle and presenting lesions are solitary thin papules or plaques with little palpable substance. The lesion occurs most frequently on the head and neck. Clinically the differential diagnosis is often that of a seborrheic keratosis and superficial basal cell carcinoma.

Histology

Recent literature has suggested that TFI might represent a histologic reactive process analogous to focal acantholytic dyskeratosis, epidermolytic hyperkeratosis, and cornoid lamellation [1]. This is based on findings of an increased association with other cutaneous lesions. The salient diagnostic features for TFI were originally described by Ackerman [2]. These features include a distinctive silhouette with a plate-like proliferation of characteristic neoplastic epithelial cells with small monomorphic nuclei and abundant pink cytoplasm in which the keratinocytes are all interconnected. Peripheral palisading may be noted in well-developed lesions. The glycogen in the cells can be highlighted with PAS stain and an orecin stain typically highlights the presence of elastic fiber network at the periphery of the tumor. Other histologic features which may be observed include horn cyst, squamous eddies, ductal differentiation, sebaceous differentiation, thickened eosinophilic cuticle, cornoid lamellation and rudimentary follicular germinative structure formation [3–8].

O. Sokumbi, M.D. (✉)
Department of Dermatology, Section of Dermatopathology, Medical College of Wisconsin, Milwaukee, WI, USA
e-mail: osokumbi@mcw.edu

J.A. Plaza, M.D.
Miraca Life Sciences, Dermatopathology Division, 6655 MacArthur Boulevard, Dallas, Texas 75039, USA
e-mail: jplaza@miracals.com

© Springer International Publishing Switzerland 2016
J.A. Plaza, V.G. Prieto (eds.), *Applied Immunohistochemistry in the Evaluation of Skin Neoplasms*, DOI 10.1007/978-3-319-30590-5_3

Differential Diagnosis

The histologic differential diagnosis of TFI includes superficial basal cell carcinoma, clear cell seborrheic keratosis, eccrine syringofibroadenoma of Mascaro, superficial lesions of fibroepithelioma of Pinkus and acanthomatous superficial sebaceous hamartoma. While a superficial basal cell carcinoma and fibroepithelioma of pinkus both exhibit plate-like growth with multiple epidermal connections and peripheral palisading similar to TFI the absence of pale cells and the presence of cytologic atypia, frequent mitosis, apoptotic cells and fibromyxoid stroma go against TFI. The presence of pseudo-horn cyst and a broader interconnecting rete pattern without the peritumoral elastic fibers. Syringocystadenoma has slender anastamosing epithelial cords with foci of ductal differentiation in a fibrovascular stroma. Finally, although acanthomatous superficial sebaceous hamartoma is characterized by plate-like proliferation similar to TFI, the cells are basaloid rather than pale, and exhibit with varying degrees of sebaceous differentiation differentiating the two entities.

Immunohistochemistry

The origin of tumor of infundibulum (TFI) is largely unclear. However, there are at least two school of thoughts attributed to the histopathology of the neoplasm. The first hypothesis proposes that the origin of TFI is the follicular infundibulum. This theory is supported by Mehregan and Buttler, who originally described this entity, and is based on the glycogen content of the lesional cells and the plate like nature of the proliferation [3]. The second theory believes that TFI is a misnomer and favor the tumor cells being isthmic in origination with derivation from the upper part of the outer root sheath exhibiting trichilemmal differentiation [2]. Although in clinical practice the diagnosis of TFI does not require immunohistochemistry, the absence of staining might be helpful. In reviewing the differential diagnosis of superficial basal cell carcinoma and TFI the absence of strong Ber-Ep4 staining typical of a basal cell carcinoma can be helpful in ruling out a BCC. In addition, CK20 expression of Merkel cells is seen in TFI while notably absent in BCC [4].

Pilar Sheath Acanthoma

Clinical

Solitary asymptomatic, small skin-colored nodule with a central pore containing keratinous debris. Most commonly located on the upper lip. No gender predilection.

Histology

There is a multilobulated cystic invagination arising from the epidermis with numerous tumor lobules extending into the surrounding dermis. The cystic wall is composed of keratinizing stratified squamous epithelium with granular cell layer. The tumor stroma is usually inconspicuous.

Differential Diagnosis

The histologic differential diagnosis includes dilated pore of Winer and trichofolliculoma. In a trichofolliculoma there are radiating small hair follicles in variable stable states of maturity extending from the central cystic structure. A dilated pore of Winer contains a patulous opening surrounded by radiating small digitate projections from the follicular epithelium into the surrounding connective tissue as opposed to lobular arrangement of pilar sheath acanthoma.

Immunohistochemistry

The diagnosis of a pilar sheath acanthoma does not require immunohistochemistry. This neoplasm arises from the infundibular portion of the pilar apparatus as supported by the superficial nature of the growth, the connection with the epidermis, a pore-like opening, proliferation of the outer sheath epithelium, infundibular keratinization, and connection with pilosebaceous structure [9, 10].

Trichofolliculoma

Clinical

Trichofolliculomas are benign hamartomatous lesions that develop at any age, and typically involve the face. It represents abortive differentiation of cutaneous pluripotent stem cells towards hair follicles. They present as skin-colored, single or multiple small nodules with central epidermal ostium, in which hair emerge.

Histology

They consist of centrally located, keratin-filled, unilocular or multilocular cystic cavities, usually connected to the epidermis, and lined by infundibular squamous epithelium with prominent granular layer [11, 12]. There are numerous surrounding secondary and tertiary hair follicles surrounded by variable numbers of sebaceous glands bud out and branch out radially from the central cavity into a fibrotic stroma (Fig. 3.1). Sebaceous trichofolliculoma is a variant of trichofolliculoma characterized by prominent lobules of well-differentiated sebaceous glands within the tumors and lacking the vellus hair component [13].

Differential Diagnosis

The differential diagnosis of a sebaceous trichofolliculoma is folliculosebaceous cystic hamartoma (FSCH). Unlike the sebaceous trichofolliculoma this lesion characterized by a folliuolosebaceous proliferation with a cyst-like infundibular dilatation without connection to the overlying epidermis. In addition there is a surrounding stroma composed of dense collagenous tissue containing variable amounts of adipose tissue with vascular and neural proliferation. The lack of epidermal connection and the prominent stromal component are important features distinguishing FSCH from a trichofolliculoma [13, 14].

Both pilar sheath acanthoma and dilated pore of Winer are benign follicular tumors in the differential diagnosis of a trichofolliculoma. See section on "Pilar Sheath Acanthoma" for histologic features differentiating these entities from one another.

Immunohistochemistry

Immunohistochemistry plays a limited role in making a diagnosis of a trichofolliculoma. The presence of Merkel cells as highlighted by CK20 underlies the classification of a trichofolliculoma as a hamartoma with follicular differentiation [15]. The reported immunohistochemical profile of this neoplasm includes CK15 expression in the

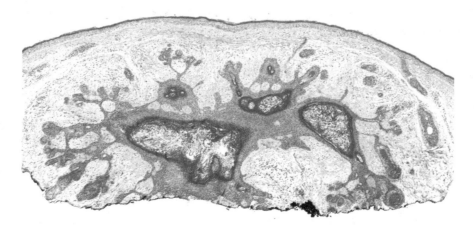

Fig. 3.1 Secondary and tertiary hair follicles radially branching out from a central cavity intro a fibrotic stroma

basal cells of the primary structure and secondary follicles. In the suprabasal layers the cells of the primary cystic structure and the immature secondary follicles express CK16 and CK17 [11]. Ber-Ep4 expression has been reported to be generally weak in the secondary and tertiary hair germ-like structures [11]. As with most benign tumor of the hair follicle, stromal CD10 immunopositivity is not an uncommon finding [16].

Benign Follicular Hamartoma

Clinical

Benign follicular hamartoma (BFH) is a benign adnexal tumor derived from hair follicles that may occur alone or in association with other genodermatosis or diseases including Bazex–Dupre–Christol syndrome (BDCS) and Brown–Crounse syndrome. It has also been reported in association with other systemic diseases such as systemic lupus erythematosus and myasthenia gravis. The pathogenesis of BFH is found to be associated with the patched mutation on chromosomes 9q23 [17–22]. It may manifest as multiple lesions with a generalized or localized distribution, or as a solitary lesion [21]. Solitary BFH may present as a smooth papule or plaque appearing most commonly on the face or scalp. The localized forms may present as plaques with alopecia or as linear unilateral lesions associated with lines of Blaschko [18, 21]. While several forms of generalized BFH have been described, generalized basaloid follicular hamartoma syndrome represents an autosomal dominant familial variant that presents with disseminated milia, palmoplantar pitting, hypotrichosis, and basaloid follicular hamartoma [21–23].

Histology

BFH is characterized by strands and cords of basaloid cells emanating from the infundibular portion of hair follicles embedded in a loose, occasionally mucinous or densely fibrous stroma. The tumor may sometimes be associated with small kerati-

nous cysts. It may take on an adenoid or reticulated pattern, resembling infundibulocystic basal cell carcinoma. Calcification of the tumors may occur. There are no mitotic figures or apoptotic cells.

Differential Diagnosis

The histopathological differential diagnosis includes trichoepithelioma, fibrofolliculoma, fibroepithelioma of Pinkus, and infundibulocystic basal cell carcinoma. In a trichoepithelioma, the tumor islands of basaloid cells may have a lace-like pattern with no branching pattern unlike a BFH. In addition, trichoepitheliomas are usually lager and have a more cellular stroma than BFH. A fibrofolliculoma has an increased amount of stroma with few epithelial strands compared to a BFH. In fibroepithelioma of Pinkus the presence of eccrine ducts, not seen in BFH, may be a helpful clue to differentiate the two entities. Also, unlike BFH, fibroepithelioma of Pinkus is surrounded by a prominent fibrovascular stroma. Histologically BFH can be very difficult to distinguish from IFBCC. IFBCC is formed by cords and strands of basaloid cells in a loose stroma similar to a BFH. In addition, it may also have horn cysts like a BFH. However, unlike a BFH is it not a folliculocentric tumor and may be located in the interfollicular dermis. In addition, pilosebaceous structures are usually destroyed and they are not seen in IFBCC. Deep infiltration and epidermal ulceration usually imply a diagnosis of IFBCC and should not be present in a BFH.

Immunohistochemistry

The most important histopathological differential diagnosis of BFH is infundibulocystic basal cell carcinoma. The similarity between these two entities often poses a diagnostic dilemma in clinical practice. Fortunately, immunostaining profiles have provided some useful clues in differentiating between the two entities. Bcl-2 diffusely stains the tumor nests in IFBCC, but stains only the outermost tumor cells in BFH. In addition, while the stromal cells of BFH stains positive for CD34, the stromal cells IFBCC are negative [23]. Interestingly, a recent study in 2014 by Honarpisheh et al. favored that both BFH and IFBCC were similar lesions. In their series, this conclusion was based on the overall histologic similarity and the diffuse distribution of CK20-positive cells in both neoplasms. Unfortunately, the utility of pleckstrin homology-like domain, family A, member 1 protein (PHLDA1), a protein usually absent in BCC, was inconclusive in supporting this assumption of similarity between BFH and IFBCC [24]. Finally, while CD10 stains both the stroma and BCC tumor cells, it stains only weakly in the stromal cells of BFH [23].

Trichoepithelioma

Trichoepithelioma (TE) is a benign tumor derived from basal cells in the hair follicle. It may be sporadic or as the principal feature of a genetic disorder called Brook-Spiegler syndrome which is inherited in an autosomal dominant pattern. Limited variants of this syndrome include multiple familial trichoepithelioma and familial cylindromatosis. When inherited, the syndrome is due to a germline mutation in the cylindromatosis (CYLD) gene on chromosome 16q12.

Clinical

The tumors are typically small (usually less than 1 cm), firm, round and shiny. They can be solitary or multiple when associated with a syndrome. They usually occur on the face in locations around the nose, eyes and on the cheeks. Clinical differential diagnosis is often that of a basal cell carcinoma.

Histology

Histologically, TE is characterized by a well circumscribed dermal tumor composed of islands, nests and cords of uniform basaloid cells in a cellular fibrous stroma. The tumor may be associated with epithelial structures that resemble hair papillae or abortive hair follicle, small keratocysts (infundibular differentiation) lined by stratified squamous epithelium and foci of calcification Figs. 3.2 and 3.3. Retraction of stroma from adjacent dermis and few mitotic figures are two characteristic features of this tumor.

Differential Diagnosis

The distinction between basal cell carcinoma (BCC) and trichoepithelioma (TE) may be very difficult in some cases because of the close similarities of these two lesions clinically and histopathologically. Both tumors are composed of nests of basaloid cells with follicular differentiation. Sometimes it may be impossible to make a histopathologic differentiation on the basis of routine hematoxylin and eosin staining.

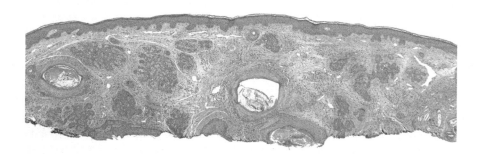

Fig. 3.2 Dermal tumor with islands of uniform basaloid cells in a cellular fibrotic stroma

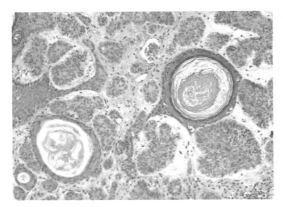

Fig. 3.3 Small keratocysts lined by squamous epithelium

Diagnostic distinction is clinically important because of the differences in prognosis and treatment of these tumors.

Immunohistochemistry

The distinction of TE and basal cell carcinomas (BCCs) from each other is not common nor generally a difficult morphologic problem. However, when these two neoplasms share histologic features, especially in scenarios where the biopsy is partial or incomplete, it can make their differentiation exceedingly difficult to the practicing pathologist. BCCs are the most common human malignancy and tend to be indolent neoplasms that can be controlled with conservative local excision, but have the potential for numerous recurrences and locally aggressive behavior. Trichoepitheliomas, contrastingly, are benign adnexal tumors with the treatment of conservative excision being curative. Due to the major differences in management and prognosis of these two lesions, a correct diagnosis is desirable and expected.

TE in some instances may take on a pattern, resembling BCC, so the differential diagnosis of BCC versus TE can be problematic based on clinical presentation and routine hematoxylin and eosin stained sections. Over the years there have been several attempts to distinguish BCC and trichoepithelioma by immunohistochemistry.

Although most of the antibodies that have been discussed in the literature are not specific for each of these tumors, they represent adjunctive tools that may be useful in resolving the existing problem in clinical histological differentiation of these two entities. Stains reported in dermatopathology literature to be of relevance include androgen receptor, CD34, Bcl-2, CD10, cytokeratin 15, and cytokeratin 20 (CK20).

The recent discovery of androgen receptor (AR) positivity in basal cell carcinomas has been helpful in the evaluation of hair follicle tumors, especially in trichoepitheliomas. Several studies have shown that while AR is expressed in a significant number of basal cell carcinomas, it is seldom expressed in trichoepitheliomas [25–28]. The use of CK20 is one of the most common IHCs used in dermatopathology practice to sort out this differential. CK20 identifies colonizing Merkel cells which are present in trichoepithelioma much more commonly than BCC [29–31] (Fig. 3.4 a, b). In addition, numerous studies have shown that different staining patterns of CD10 staining in these tumors that is basaloid staining in BCC and stromal staining in TE may also be useful in resolving this difficult histologic challenge [16, 32–34]. In regard to the usefulness of CD34 staining in differentiating these two entities there have been conflicting reports. While Tebcherani et al. reported that there was no significant difference in staining with CD34 between BCC and TE, other studies have shown the usefulness of CD34 by showing the lack of CD34 expression by tumor stroma in BCC, but positive in TE [34–37] (Fig. 3.5). Similarly, the role of BCl-2 oncogene has been conflicting. While there are many studies showing that diffuse staining of tumor nests in BCC versus staining of only the outermost layers in TE can be helpful, there are a few studies which question the reliability of this staining pattern [29, 30, 34, 38] (Fig. 3.6). Regarding the use of cytokeratin 15, Choi et al. showed an increase in peripheral localization of cytokeratin 15 expression in TE than BCC while BCCs were found to contain more elastic fibers than TE [39]. More recently, the utilization of pleckstrin homology-like domain family A member 1 protein (PHLDA1)

a

b

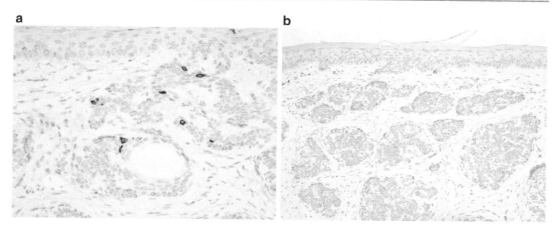

Fig. 3.4 (**a**) CK20 immunohistochemistry highlights the Merkel cells in trichoepithelioma. (**b**) CK20 immunohisto-chemistry is more likely negative for Merkel cells in BCC

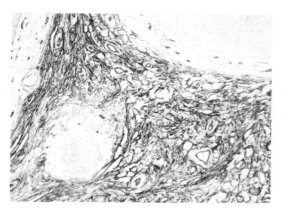

Fig. 3.5 CD34 expression by tumor stroma in trichoepithelioma

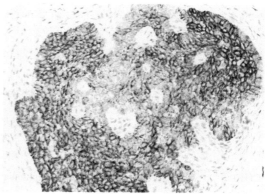

Fig. 3.6 Diffuse BCl-2 staining of tumor nests in BCC unlike the expected staining of only outermost layers in trichoepithelioma

has been reported, however, this likely has more relevance when faced with the differential diagnosis of a desmoplastic variant of trichoepithelioma versus a morpheaform basal cell carcinoma [40–43].

We published the utility of D2-40 (podoplanin) to separate TE from BCC (Immunolabeling pattern of podoplanin (d2-40) may distinguish basal cell carcinomas from trichoepitheliomas: a clinicopathologic and immunohistochemical study of 49 cases) Recently some published studies have found podoplanin to be expressed in the basal cells of the outer root sheath of hair follicles. Ishida et al. studied podoplanin immunoexpression in BCCs and showed that these tumors

focally expressed podoplanin in up to 65 % of their cases and concluded that this expression in BCCs seems to reflect the differentiation towards the outer root sheath of hair follicles. In our study, we found expression of podoplanin in 22.20 % of BCCs (14.8 % of cases showed focal positivity) and 95 % of TE expressed podoplanin (45 % of the cases showed focal positivity). Also, podoplanin expression in TE was noted to be present not only in the basal layer of the tumor cells but also in the suprabasal layer of the tumor cells, as opposed to BCCs in which the positivity was primarily located in the basal layer of the tumor nests (Fig. 3.7 a, b). The overall sensitivity and specificity of podoplanin immuno-

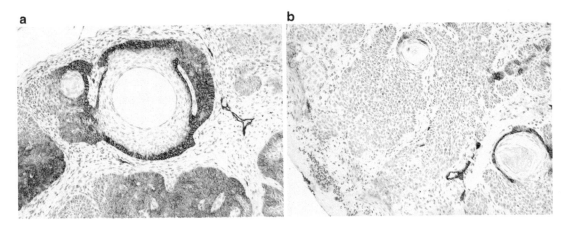

Fig. 3.7 (a) Podoplanin expression in trichoepithelioma present in both basal and suprabasal layers of tumor cells. (b) Podoplanin expression in BCC present only in the basal layer of tumor cells

Table 3.1 Summary of immunohistochemistry of BCC versus TE

Immunohistochemistry	BCC	TE
Cytokeratin 20 (CK20)	Absent	Diffuse staining of the cytoplasm of Merkel cells within the epithelial strands
Androgen receptor	Staining of nuclei of the epithelial proliferation	Absent
Bcl-2	Diffuse staining of tumor nests[a]	Staining of only the outermost layers of the tumor
CD34	Absent[a]	Staining of connective tissue around epithelial proliferations
CD10	Staining of epithelial proliferations	Staining of connective tissue around epithelial proliferations
Cytokeratin 15	Staining in the center of the tumor proliferation	Staining in the periphery of the tumor nests
BerEp4	No difference in pattern	No difference in pattern

[a]Conflicting reports in the literature

reactivity to separate primary BCCs from TE was 95.5 % and 77.8 %, respectively, in this study. An important aspect of this study is that a subset BCCs can express podoplanin and this could embrace the premise that these neoplasms may have the potential for multilinear differentiation. The results of this study may be useful when enough tumor cells are available for interpretation; however, this marker can be of limited diagnostic utility in those cases in which small samples are provided. In our opinion, the application of strict histologic criteria remains the best way to achieve an accurate diagnosis (Table 3.1).

Desmoplastic Trichoepithelioma

Desmoplastic trichoepithelioma (DTE) is an uncommon variant of trichoepithelioma with a predilection for the face.

Clinical

Patients typically present with a stable, firm skin-colored to red, annular (ring-shaped) plaque with a central dimple. The lesion is most commonly located on the upper cheek. Multiple lesions are quite rare.

Histology

DTE is characterized by a well-circumscribed tumor in the superficial and mid dermis that contain cords and nests of basaloid cells within a desmoplastic stroma (Fig. 3.8). The proliferation is frequently associated with foci of dystrophic calcification, keratinous cysts, and keratin granulomas. At scanning magnification a depression in the surface at the lesion may be seen.

Differential Diagnosis

The histologic differential diagnosis of DTE includes syringoma, microcystic adnexal carcinoma and morpheaform basal cell carcinoma. Differentiation between these neoplasms is especially challenging to sort out when dealing with a lesion that is sampled only in part where the silhouette and circumscription of the lesion cannot be assessed.

Unlike DTE, microcystic adnexal carcinoma is typically characterized by a deeper component of smaller nests and strands of basaloid cells embedded in a markedly hyalinized stroma with frequent skeletal muscle, subcutaneous tissue and perineural invasion. In addition, the presence of mitotic figures, ductal differentiation are more likely found in MAC while the presence of keratinous cyst, keratin granulomas, and calcification are specific features of DTE [44]. Horn cysts, epidermal hyperplasia, squamous aggregations, and calcifications are four histologic features that are consistently found in

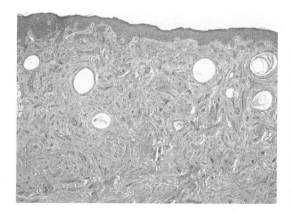

Fig. 3.8 Dermal tumor in superficial and mid dermis containing cords, nests of basaloid cells, and keratocysts within a desmoplastic stroma

DTE but not in MBCC. Tumor aggregates in MBCC typically have cleft between the basaloid cells and stroma versus DTE that has aggregations rimmed by thin bundles of collagen that are separated from the surrounding dermis by a cleft. Despite these clues the differentiation between these two entities remains challenging and often requires immunohistochemistry [45, 46]. Syringoma is a small, symmetrical, well-circumscribed sweat gland neoplasm in a sclerotic stroma that is typically confined to the upper dermis. The nests vary in shape and often adopt a tadpole like morphology. Unlike DTE, syringoma lacks keratinization which is helpful features in distinguishing the two.

Immunohistochemistry

In the published literature misdiagnosis of DTE as MAC and MBCC has been well reported. Therefore, the role of immunohistochemistry in distinguishing between DTE from MAC and MBCC has been extensively studied. To distinguish DTE from MAC stains which have been reported to be of value include BerEP4, carcinoembryonic antigen (CEA), cytokeratin (CK)17, CK19, CK14, CK15, CK20, CD5, CD23, and p63 [4–47]. CEA has been tradicionally the marker of choice in demonstrating ductal differentiation in MAC. This focus of glandular differentiation should be noticeably absent in DTE. Recently the role of CK17, CK19 and epidermal growth factor receptor (EGFR) in differentiating between MAC and DTE has been studied. While CK17 and EGFR were not valuable adjuncts in this distinction, CK19 was strongly expressed in the neoplastic cells of MAC and absent in DTE [44]. Interestingly, CK15 a specific marker of hair follicle-related tumors did not distinguish between MAC and DTE as it is expressed in both neoplasm [44]. In contrast, lymphoid markers CD23 and CD5 may be expressed in MAC while both markers are absent in sclerosing epithelial neoplasms like DTE. Merkel cells are frequently found in neoplasms that are benign tumors and of follicular germinative origin [44]. Hence, CK20 staining is commonly used in dermatopathologic practice to differentiate DTE from MAC [31, 44].

In differentiating MBCC from DTE immunostains such as Bcl-2, cytokeratin 20 (CK20), androgen receptor (AR), CD34, CD10, and PHLDA1 have been extensively studied. Of these, evaluation of androgen receptor (AR) and cytokeratin 20 (CK20) expressions remain one of the most reliable immunohistochemistry panel used in sorting out this distinction in routine dermatopathology practice. The AR−, CK20+ immunophenotype is sensitive (87 %) and specific for DTE (100 %). The AR+, CK20− immunophenotype is specific (100 %) and moderately sensitive (61 %) for mBCC [48, 49]. The presence of both CD34 and CD10 staining in the tumor stroma of DTE and the absence of staining in MBCC tumor stroma may be helpful. However, this finding has been inconsistently reported in the literature making interpretation difficult [23, 32, 33, 36]. Similarly, while some studies have described staining of the periphery of basaloid proliferations of DTE with Bcl-2 and diffuse staining in MBCC basaloid tumor, several studies have also questioned the reliability of this finding as it is inconsistent [30, 37, 38, 48]. Recently, PHLDA1 a follicular stem cell marker has been reported to be useful in differentiating the two neoplasms based on immunoreactivity of the basaloid cells in DTE with PHLDA1 and the absence of staining in MBCC [40–43, 47]. In light of varying reports and the overlap of immunophenotypes, the final diagnosis of DTE should include a careful consideration of clinical and histologic review in additional to the immunoprofile before reaching a final diagnosis (Table 3.2).

Table 3.2 Summary of immunohistochemistry of DTE versus MBCC and DTE Versus MAC

IHC marker	DTE	MBCC
CK20	+	−
Androgen receptor	−	+
Bcl-2	+/−	+/−
CD34	+/−	+/−
CD10	+/−	+/−
PHLDA1	+	−
IHC marker	DTE	MAC
CK20	+	−
CK15	+	+
CD23	−	+/−
CD5	−	+/−
CD19	+/−	+/−
CEA	−	+

Trchoblastoma

Clinical

Rare benign neoplasm with differentiation towards the follicular germinative cells. It appears as a small, well-circumscribed, nonulcerated, skin-colored papules that most commonly affect the face and scalp. There are no specific distinguishing clinical features. It is usually an isolated lesion, but can also appear as multiple lesions.

Histology

The tumor consists of nodules of cords and nests formed of solid basaloid germinative epithelial cells that exhibit peripheral palisading and brisk mitotic activity. Follicular papillae are characteristically present and small keratin cyst may be found. The minimal intervening stromal component separates thee epithelial nodules with absent or inconspicuous cleft artifact (Fig. 3.9 a, b).

Differential Diagnosis

The differential diagnosis between the large nodular variant of trichoblastoma and nodular basal cell carcinoma can be exceedingly difficult. Features favoring a trichoblastoma include sharp circumscription, vertical growth pattern, symmetry, and a dense stroma with focal clefts within the stroma itself. Follicular differentiation in the large nodular variant of trichoblastoma is not a common occurrence as in a basal cell carcinoma and tumor necrosis in the larger nodules of trichoblastoma may be comparable to a basal cell carcinoma. The lack of epidermal connection, a more conspicuous stroma with papillary mesenchymal bodies and minimal retraction artifact are useful features not seen in a basal cell carcinoma.

Compared to a conventional trichoepithelioma, a trichoblastoma is found in the deep dermis and subcutaneous tissue compared to the superficial

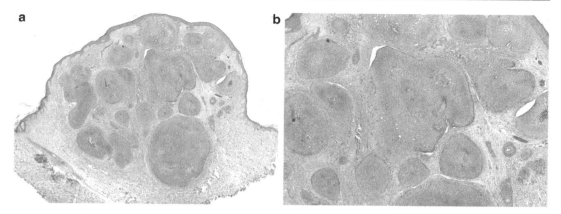

Fig. 3.9 (**a**) Nodules of solid basaloid germinative epithelial cells with peripheral palisading. (**b**) Dense stroma with focal clefts within stroma itself

location of a trichoepithelioma. In addition, at trichoblastoma shows less keratinization and devoid of epidermal or follicular origin compared to a trichoepithelioma.

Immunohistochemistry

Sometimes the histological appearance of a trichoblastoma is difficult to distinguish from those of a basal cell carcinoma. In these instances, immunohistochemistry may play a useful role in the differential diagnosis, although the cytokeratin (CK) expression pattern is similar in both entities. This is likely due to shared pattern histiogenesis with both being derived from germinative cells of the hair follicle. The only exception is CK15, which is expressed in most trichoblastomas but not in basal cell carcinoma, which may be of some value [50, 51]. Bcl-2 expression is predominantly in the periphery of the tumor cells in a trichoblastoma while it is expressed in a diffuse pattern in a basal cell carcinoma [30, 38, 52]. P53 nuclear staining and MIB-1 proliferative index are increased in basal carcinoma compared to a trichoblastoma, and androgen receptor is absent in a trichoblastoma while diffusely present in basal cell carcinoma [26]. In regard to the tumor stroma, CD34 and CD10 positive cells are present in a trichoblastoma and largely absent in the tumor stroma of a

basal cell carcinoma. In contrast, CD10 expression is found in the epithelial component of a basal cell component while absent in the trichoblastoma tumor cells [16, 36, 37, 52, 53]. Merkel cells, identified by CK20, are frequently seen in trichoblastoma and absent in basal cell carcinoma [50, 53]. Finally, pleckstrin homology-like domain, family A, member 1 (PHLDA1), a follicular stem cell marker, has been reported to differentiate between trichoblastomas from basal cell carcinoma with strong expression in a trichoblastoma [54]. Although IHC markers may facilitate this challenging differential diagnosis, there are no specific antibodies that can be used reliably (Table 3.3).

Table 3.3 Immunohistochemical profile of trichoblastoma versus basal cell carcinoma

Immunohistochemistry	TB	BCC
Bcl-2	+ peripheral	+ diffuse
CD10 (epithelium)	+/−	+
CD10 (stroma)	+	−
CD34 (stroma)	+/−	+/−
Androgen receptor (epithelium)	−	+
CK20	+	−
34BE12	+/−	++
CK6	+/−	++
PHLDA1	+	−

Trichoadenoma

Clinical

Solitary skin-colored papulonodule often found on the face or buttock. It may appear at any age without any sex predilection.

Histology

The neoplasm is a proliferation of follicular germinative germ cells with inconspicuous basaloid cells, predominance of keratin cysts and without hair shaft formation embedded in a sclerotic stroma (Fig. 3.10a, b). The tumor overlies a normal epidermal and the prominent cyst walls are composed of squamous epithelium, which manifest as epidermoid keratinization.

Differential Diagnosis

The morphologic differentiation of trichoadenoma is situated between a trichofolliculoma and a trichoepithelioma with hair follicle-like direction of differentiation. The tumor may show overlapping histologic features with desmoplastic trichoepithelioma. However, the predominance of the cystic component in the tumor versus the predominant mostly solid neoplasm of desmoplastic trichoepithelioma and trichoepithelioma.

Immunohistochemistry

The tumor differentiates toward the infundibula portion of the pilosebaceous canal. Previous immunohistochemistry studies have shown CK10 and CK15 expression with no expression of CK16 which differs from the phenotype of trichoepitheliomas and trichofolliculomas [55]. In comparing trichoadenoma to desmoplastic trichoepithelioma, immunohistochemical analysis has shown that CK20 expression of Merkel cells and BEr-Ep4 negative, androgen receptor-negative immunophenotype is supportive of a trichoadenoma, while CK20 positive, BEr-Ep4-positive, androgen receptor-negative phenotype is seen in a desmoplastic trichoepithelioma [56]. The absence of EMA and CEA rule out the possibility of a ductal neoplasm [44].

Trichilemmoma

Clinical

Trichilemmoma is a hamartoma of the hair follicle infundibulum, and most are sporadic solitary lesions that occur most commonly on the face.

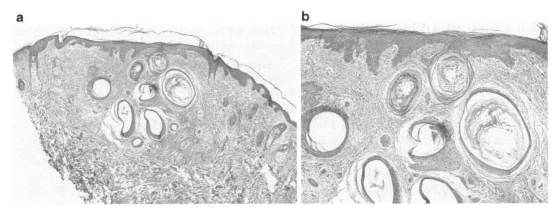

Fig. 3.10 (**a** and **b**) follicular germinative germ cells with inconspicuous basaloid cells and predominant of keratin cysts in a sclerotic stroma

The presence of multiple trichilemmoma is almost invariably associated with Cowden syndrome. Cowden syndrome is a multisystem disorder autosomal dominant disorder caused by a germline inactivating mutation in phosphatase and tensin homolog (PTEN) on chromosome 10, a tumor suppressor gene [57–60]. Patients with Cowden syndrome may present with hamartomatous overgrowth of tissues from all three embryonic developmental lineages—ectodermal, mesodermal, and endodermal. They also have an increased risk of malignancy of the thyroid, breast, and other organs.

Histology

Trichilemmoma is benign follicular tumor that arises from the outer root sheath of the hair follicle. It is usually a well-circumscribed, symmetrical epithelial lobular proliferation with plate-like growth pattern composed of glycogenated clear cells with basal cell peripheral palisading resting on a PAS-positive thickened eosinophilic hyaline basement membrane (Fig. 3.11a, b). The cells are uniform and small with round or oval vesicular nuclei (Fig. 3.12). Pleomorphism and mitosis are not features of this benign tumor. The tumor typically has minimal keratinization which is usually superficial and trichilemmal [59]. There may be overlying mild papillomatosis and hyperkeratosis giving a wart-like configuration in some instances.

Differential Diagnosis

Trichilemmomas can be easily confused with clear cell basal cell carcinoma, hidroacanthoma simplex/poroma, trichilemmal carcinoma, and tumor of the follicular infundibulum. While a clear cell basal carcinoma may be histologically similar to a trichilemmoma, the absence of an eosinophilic hyaline basement membrane and the presence of a tumor with numerous mitotically active cells set in a mucinous stroma are features of a clear cell basal

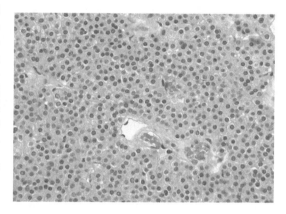

Fig. 3.12 Small uniform cells with round or oval vesicular nuclei

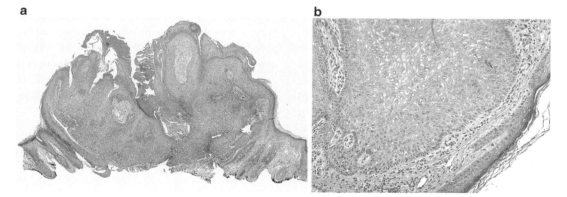

Fig. 3.11 (**a**) Lobular proliferation with plate-like growth composed of glycogenated clear cells. (**b**) Basal cell peripheral palisading resting on thickened eosinophilic hyaline basement membrane

carcinoma that distinguish the two entities. The presence of distinct peripheral palisade and an eosinophilic hyaline basement membrane, the absence of ductal differentiation and/or intracytoplasmic lumina are helpful clues that distinguish a trichilemmoma from hidroacanthoma simplex/poroma. The lack of nuclei pleomorphism, absence of conspicuous mitotic activity, and the presence of an invading pushing border are all features that separate a trichilemmoma from a trichilemmal carcinoma. While a tumor of the follicular infundibulum may appear similar to a trichilemmoma with its pale staining tumor cells with peripheral palisade and as eosinophilic basement membrane, however, it lacks the lobular configuration of a trichilemmoma and instaead has a fenestrated epithelial which is not seen in a trichilemmoma.

Immunohistochemistry

The follicular derivation of a trichilemmoma is supported by studies which have shown that the tumor cells are highlighted with nestin and cytokeratin 15 both of which are hair follicle stem cells. In fact, nestin-expressing hair follicle cells often give rise to the outer root sheath also confirming the precise derivation of the neoplasm [61]. In routine dermatopathology practice, the use of immunohistochemistry is rarely indicated in making a diagnosis of a trichilemmoma. However, IHCs may be helpful when differentiating this tumor from histologically similar tumors. The ductal differentiation and intracytotoplasmic lumina of hidroacanthoma simplex/poroma are highlighted with EMA and CEA. This is helpful when distinguishing this tumor from a trichilemmoma [62]. Recently, the use of PTEN IHC has been reported to help differentiate between a trichilemmoma arising sporadically versus a tumor presenting as a manifestation of Cowden's syndrome. The complete loss of PTEN IHC is suggestive of Cowden's syndrome in a patient presenting with multiple trichilemmomas and may serve as a helpful

screen prior to performing germline testing of PTEN mutation [63, 64].

Desmoplastic Trichilemmoma

Clinical

Solitary, slowly growing, skin-colored, dome-shaped papule. Lesions are predominantly found on the face. This is a rare variant of trichilemmoma with no association with Cowden's disease. The tumor generally occurs in men after the fifth decade of life.

Histology

The neoplasm has a characteristic biphasic tumor cell population. In the center of the lesion there are irregular epithelial strands of tumor cells entrapped in a dense, pale eosinophilic hypocellular and fibrotic dermis containing diastase-resistant, PAS-positive/diastase resistant and Alcian blue-positive material. At the periphery of the lesion there are typical lobules of conventional trichilemmoma Fig 3.13a–c.

Differential Diagnosis

The prominent desmoplastic component in the central zone with irregular epithelial strands simulates invasive squamous cell carcinoma and morpheaform basal cell carcinoma. However, the presence of conventional trichilemmoma at the periphery of a desmoplastic lesion is an important feature favoring this benign diagnosis over a carcinoma. In addition, the perilobular hyaline mantle enables DT to be differentiated from trichilemmal carcinoma [65].

Immunohistochemistry

Immunohistochemical analysis is of value when considering the histologic differential diagnosis of DT. In all cases of DT, the

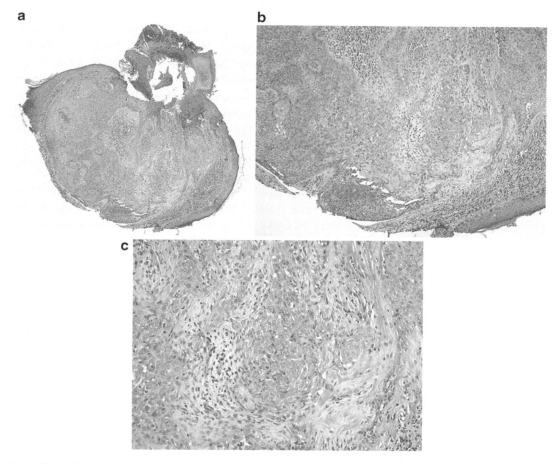

Fig. 3.13 (**a**) Biphasic tumor population with typical lobules of conventional trichilemmoma in periphery. (**b** and **c**) irregular epithelial strands of tumor cells in a dense, pale eosinophilic hypocellular and fibrotic dermis

epithelial tumor cells show CD34 immunostaining unlike CD34 negativity in basal cell carcinoma and squamous cell carcinoma [66]. The negative staining with EMA and CEA distinguish this neoplasm from tumors of ductal origination.

Trichilemmal Carcinoma

Clinical

Trichielemmal carcinoma (TLC) Rare cutaneous adnexal tumor of the outer root sheath, considered as the malignant counterpart of a trichilemmoma. Most commonly occurs on the sun-exposed, hair-

bearing anatomic sites of older Caucasians. It presents as unremarkable solitary papules, nodules and plaques, which are frequently ulcerated and sometimes crusted. Lesion often resemble a basal cell carcinoma.

Histology

Lobular proliferation of atypical, glycogen-heavy clear cells lacking mucin and palisading around a pilosebaceous unit. There is tendency towards trichilemmal keratinization. There is variable nuclear pleomorphism from mild to high-grade tumors. There is brisk mitotic activity and some tumors may have hemorrhage or necrosis.

A hyaline mantle may be found on the nuclear periphery with nuclear palisading and subnuclear vacuolation (Fig. 3.14 a–c). The tumor typically has a pushing border rather than the infiltrative growth pattern typical of a squamous cell carcinoma.

Differential Diagnosis

Although trichilemmal carcinoma resembles a trichilemmoma in the presence of a plate-like endophytic nodules extending into the dermis, it differs with respect to the occurrence of frequent mitosis and cellular atypia. Malignant proliferating trichilemmal tumors (PTT) are often confused with TLC. However, PTT usually arise in a preexisting trichilemmal cyst and demonstrate sharply circumscribed convoluted lobules with pushing margins, deep dermal extensions, extensive areas of tumor necrosis, abrupt keratinization, and low mitotic activity. Malignant clear cell tumors including clear cell squamous carcinoma, clear cell porocarcinoma, clear cell hidradenocarcinoma and malignant melanoma with clear cell change should be considered in the differential diagnosis. Unlike the pushing border of trichilemmal carcinoma, squamous cell carcinoma has an infiltrative growth pattern and typically lacks the peripheral palisading, hyaline mantle, lobular proliferation and trichilemmal keratinization typical of trichilemmal carcinoma. The absence of ductal differentiation and intracytoplasmic lumen formation in trichilemmal carcinoma are helpful clues in ruling out the diagnosis of porocarcinoma and hidradenocarcinoma.

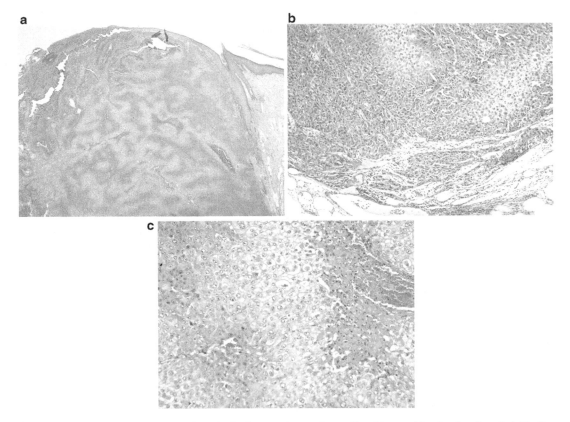

Fig. 3.14 (**a**) Lobular proliferation of atypical, glycogen-heavy clear cells with a pushing border. (**b** and **c**) Hyaline mantle in the nuclear periphery with nuclear palisading and subnuclear vacuolation

Immunohistochemistry

The utility of ummunohostochemical studies is limited in this neoplasm Cytokeratin expression of CK1, 10, 14, and 17 suggest that trichilemmal carcinoma differentiates towards the follicular infundibulum. The absence of CK15 and CK16 staining in TLC versus the presence of these cytokeratin in trichilemmoma may be a result of malignant transformation [67]. Although the expression of CD34 as a marker of differentiation from the outer hair root sheath can be a helpful adjunct in making the diagnosis, it is often negative in TLC [65, 66, 68–70]. Unlike squamous cell carcinoma, EMA is negative in trichilemmal carcinoma. Furthermore, the absence of CEA and EMA highlighting ductal differentiation rule out ductal neoplasms such as porocarcinoma and hidradenocarcinoma [62].

Benign Proliferating Pilar Tumor

Clinical

This tumor, also referred to proliferating trichilemmal cyst (PTC), is a usually benign tumor of outer root sheath differentiation that often develops within the wall of a preexisting pilar cyst. It usually presents as a solitary nodulocystic lesion ranging in size from 1 to 10 cm in diameter. It is most commonly found on the scalp s of elderly women. Occasionally patients may present with multiple tumors.

Histology

The neoplasm exhibits differentiation towards the isthmic portion of the outer root sheath and consists of well-defined lobulated solid and cystic mass of proliferating squamous epithelium, surrounded by thick hyalinized basement membrane and involves the deep dermis and subcutaneous tissue (Fig. 3.15a). Epithelial growth extension into the lumen and peripheral palisading of small basaloid cells may be seen. Widespread trichilemmal keratinization associated with necrosis is characteristic. Keratinous debris is associated with a foreign body giant cell reaction and calcification may be present. Some areas may have epidermoid keratinization with individual cell keratinization and squamous eddy formation may be features (Fig. 3.15b). The squamous cells exhibit blank or mildly atypical cytonuclear features, and inconspicuous, basally located mitotic activity. Focus of residual pilar cysts may be identified.

Differential Diagnosis

The two most important histologic differential diagnosis include squamous cell carcinoma and

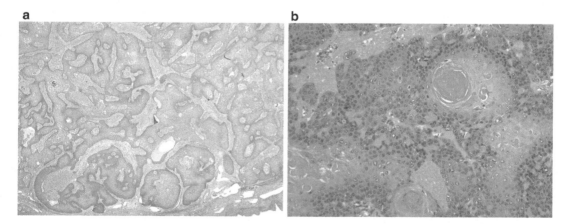

Fig. 3.15 (**a**) Solid lobulated and cystic mass of proliferating squamous epithelium involving the deep dermis and subcutaneous tissue. (**b**) Epithelial growth extension into the lumen and peripheral palisading of small basaloid cells

malignant proliferating pilar cyst, its malignant counterpart (see section on "Malignant Proliferating Pilar Tumor" below) [71]. PTC can be distinguished from a squamous cell carcinoma by the presence of well circumscribed nodules showing a noninfiltrative palisaded border and the presence of a hyaline basement membrane showing abundant trichilemmal keratinization. The absence or inconspicuous cytonuclear atypia and minimal mitotic activity are additional helpful clues to sort out this differential diagnosis.

Immunohistochemistry

There is limited role for immunohistochemistry is differentiating PTC from squamous cell carcinoma. In fact, a study over a decade ago demonstrated similar p53 staining pattern in both neoplasms favoring the consideration of PTC as a low-grade carcinoma [72]. However, a more recent study showed negative p53 staining in PTC in contrast to malignant proliferating trichilemmal tumor and squamous cell carcinoma [71]. Finally, the localized presence of ki67 staining to a few basal cells of the tumor supports the benignity of this neoplasm [71–73].

Malignant Proliferating Pilar Tumor

Clinical

Clinically this tumor is more likely to present in non-scalp location, with a rapid growth and size greater than 5 cm.

Histology

This neoplasm often presents with a varied histologic spectrum which may range from focal in situ lesion to frankly invasive neoplasm accompanied by a destructive growth pattern. Focal necrosis and ulceration with infiltrative growth, abundant mitotic figures and marked cytological atypia are some notable features. Perineural and lymphovascular invasion may be present in neoplasms with metastatic potential [74, 75].

Differential Diagnosis

This histologic differential diagnosis includes PTT and squamous cell carcinoma. The rapid increase in size, tumor greater size greater than 5 cm, the infiltrative growth pattern and significant cytonuclear atypia and brisk mitotic activity are features that favor malignancy over the benign PTC. The presence of lobulated expansile masses of squamous cells with non-lamellated trichilemmal keratinization are clues of the pilar origin of the neoplasm over a squamous cell carcinoma.

Immunohistochemistry

In difficult cases immunohistochemistry may provide a useful tool to differentiate between benign proliferating trichilemmal tumors from MPTT or to differentiate PTT and MPTT from squamous cell carcinoma. MPTTs exhibit CD34 immunohistochemical staining, indicating trichilemmal differentiation while CD34 is negative in squamous cell carcinoma [71, 74, 75]. Calcretinin, a marker of companion layer of the outer rot sheath, positivity has been described in MPTT supporting the outer root sheath origin of the tumor [76]. In addition, p53 and ki67 are helpful adjuncts in differentiating PPT from MPTT. Both an increase in p53 and ki67 expression can assist in stratifying these pilar neoplasms into benign versus malignant [71–73].

Pilomatrix Carcinoma

Clinical

Rare neoplasm considered to be the malignant counterpart of a pilomatricoma. The tumor shows a male predilection and more than 60% of cases occur on the head and neck region. The tumor is considered locally aggressive and occasionally shows rapid progression to infiltration to the muscle, bone and blood vessels. Recurrences are common and there have been reports of metastases to the lymph nodes, lungs and bone.

Histology

Similar to pilomatricomas, pilomatrix carcinoma harbors mutations in exon 3 of CTNNB1, a gene that encodes beta catenin, a downstream effector in the WNT-signaling pathway [77]. The presence of similar mutations in both benign and malignant pilomatricomas suggest a common pathogenesis, consistent with the notion that a pilomatrix carcinoma may arise through transformation of a pilomatricoma [77–79].

On histology there is a large, asymmetric, poorly circumscribed, nodular proliferation of basaloid cells with nuclear pleomorphism, prominent nucleoli, atypical mitosis figures, tumor necrosis, and desmoplastic stroma with an infiltrating border often with involvement of the fascia or skeletal muscle (Fig. 3.16a, b). There may be lymphatic, vascular, and perineural invasion.

Differential Diagnosis

The differential diagnosis includes a basal cell carcinoma with matrical differentiation and a proliferating matricoma. Basal cell carcinoma with matrical differentiation is a rare variant of a BCC. The tumor will have typical features of a BCC, but also has basaloid nests containing shadow cells. In addition, the higher degree of nuclear pleomorphism and the frequent atypical mitosis in the basaloid cells favor pilomatrix carcinoma over BCC with matrical differentiation [79–81]. Proliferating pilomatricoma is usually symmetrical with expansive growth pattern which is different from the asymmetric infiltrative growth pattern of pilomatrix carcinoma [78, 79, 81].

Immunohistochemistry

Pilomatrix carcinoma is a tumor with differentiation towards the hair matrix. Haasanein and Glanz reviewed 21 cases of pilomatricoma and 5 cases of pilomatrix carcinoma. All cases displayed nuclear and cytoplasmic staining of beta-catenin of the basaloid cells with focal membranous staining. Shadow cells were negative for beta catenin in all tumors [77]. The presence of both nuclear and cytoplasmic staining for beta-catenin in the basaloid tumor cells is consistently found in this neoplasm. In contrast, a basal carcinoma with matrical differentiation demonstrates membranous and cytoplasmic staining of beta-catenin [77]. The absence of nuclear staining is an important discriminating factor.

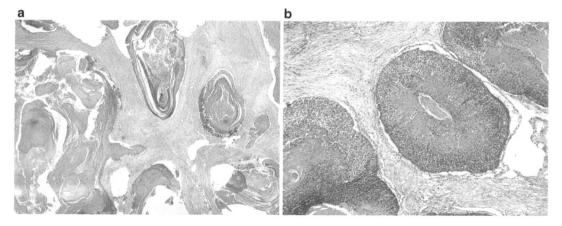

Fig. 3.16 (**a**) Large asymmetric cystic proliferation of basaloid cells with infiltrating border. (**b**) Basaloid cells with nuclear pleomorphism, mitosis. and tumor necrosis

References

1. Abbas O, Mahalingam M. Tumor of the follicular infundibulum: an epidermal reaction pattern? Am J Dermatopathol. 2009;31:626–33.
2. Ackerman AB, Viragh PA, Chongchitnant N. Neoplasms with follicular differentiation. Philadelphia. Lea Febiger. 1993;553.
3. Mehregan AH, Butler JD. A tumor of follicular infundibulum. report of a case. Arch Dermatol. 1961; 83:924–7.
4. Alomari A, Subtil A, Owen CE, McNiff JM. Solitary and multiple tumors of follicular infundibulum: a review of 168 cases with emphasis on staining patterns and clinical variants. J Cutan Pathol. 2013;40:532–7.
5. Kubba A, Batrani M, Taneja A, Jain V. Tumor of follicular infundibulum: an unsuspected cause of macular hypopigmentation. Indian J Dermatol Venereol Leprol. 2014;80(2):141–4.
6. Cribier B, Grosshans E. Tumor of the follicular infundibulum: a clinicopathologic study. J Am Acad Dermatol. 1995;33:979–84.
7. Schnitzler L, Civatte J, Robin F, Demay C. Multiple tumors of the follicular infundibulum with basocellular degeneration. Apropos of a case. Ann Dermatol Venereol. 1987;114:551–6.
8. Kolivras A, Moulonguet I, Ruben BS, Sass U, Cappelletti L, André J. Eruptive tumors of the follicular infundibulum presenting as hypopigmented macules on the buttocks of two Black African males. J Cutan Pathol. 2012;39:444–8.
9. Kushner JA, Thomas RS, Young RJ. An unusual location of a pilar sheath acanthoma. Int J Trichol. 2014;6(4):185–6.
10. Mehregan AH, Brownstein MH. Pilar sheath acanthoma. Arch Dermatol. 1978;114(10):1495–7.
11. Misago N, Kimura T, Toda S, Mori T, Narisawa Y. A revaluation of trichofolliculoma: the histopathological and immunohistochemical features. Am J Dermatopathol. 2010;32(1):35–43.
12. Gokalp H, Gurer MA, Alan S. Trichofolliculoma: a rare variant of hair follicle hamartoma. Dermatol Online J. 2013;19(8):19264.
13. Abdou AG, Asaad NY. Sebaceous trichofolliculoma of the cheek in a 65-year-old man. Pol J Pathol. 2014;65(3):253–4.
14. Merklen-Djafri C, Batard ML, Guillaume JC, Kleinclauss I, Cribier B. Folliculosebaceous cystic hamartoma: anatomo-clinical study. Ann Dermatol Venereol. 2012;139(1):23–30.
15. Hartschuh W, Schulz T. Immunohistochemical investigation of the different developmental stages of trichofolliculoma with special reference to the Merkel cell. Am J Dermatopathol. 1999;21(1):8–15.
16. Sengul D, Sengul I, Astarci MH, Ustun H, Mocan G. CD10 for the distinct differential diagnosis of basal cell carcinoma and benign tumours of cutaneous appendages originating from hair follicle. Pol J Pathol. 2010;61(3):140–6.
17. Gumaste P, Ortiz AE, Patel A, Baron J, Harris R, Barr R. Generalized basaloid follicular hamartoma syndrome: a case report and review of the literature. Am J Dermatopathol. 2015;37(3):e37–40.
18. Huang SH, Hsiao TF, Lee CC. Basaloid follicular hamartoma: a case report and review of the literature. Kaohsiung J Med Sci. 2012;28(1):57–60.
19. Mills O, Thomas LB. Basaloid follicular hamartoma. Arch Pathol Lab Med. 2010;134(8):1215–9.
20. Patel AB, Harting MS, Smith-Zagone MJ, Hsu S. Familial basaloid follicular hamartoma: a report of one family. Dermatol Online J. 2008;14(4):14.
21. Brownstein MH. Basaloid follicular hamartoma: solitary and multiple types. J Am Acad Dermatol. 1992;27(2 Pt 1):237–40.
22. Morton S, Stevens A, Powell RJ. Basaloid follicular hamartoma, total body hair loss and SLE. Lupus. 1998;7(3):207–9.
23. Ramos-Ceballos FI, Pashaei S, Kincannon JM, Morgan MB, Smoller BR. Bcl-2, CD34 and CD10 expression in basaloid follicular hamartoma, vellus hair hamartoma and neurofollicular hamartoma demonstrate full follicular differentiation. J Cutan Pathol. 2008;35(5):477–83.
24. Honarpisheh H, Glusac EJ, Ko CJ. Cytokeratin 20 expression in basaloid follicular hamartoma and infundibulocystic basal cell carcinoma. J Cutan Pathol. 2014;41(12):916–21.
25. Bayer-Garner IB, Givens V, Smoller B. Immunohistochemical staining for androgen receptors:a sensitive marker of sebaceous differentiation. Am J Dermatopathol. 1999;21:426–31.
26. Izikson L, Bhan A, Zembowicz A. Androgen receptor expression helps to differentiate basal cell carcinoma from benign trichoblastic tumors. Am J Dermatopathol. 2005;27:91–5.
27. Katona TM, Ravis SM, Perkins SM, et al. Expression of androgen receptor by fibroepithelioma of Pinkus: evidence supporting classification as a basal cell carcinoma variant? Am J Dermatopathol. 2007;29:7–12.
28. Arits AH, Van Marion AM, Lohman BG, Thissen MR, Steijlen PM, Nelemans PJ, Kelleners-Smeets NW. Differentiation between basal cell carcinoma and trichoepithelioma by immunohistochemical staining of the androgen receptor: an overview. Eur J Dermatol. 2011;21(6):870–3.
29. Poniecka AW, Alexis JB. An immunohistochemical study of basal cell carcinoma and trichoepithelioma. Am J Dermatopathol. 1999;21:332–6.
30. Abdelsayed RA, Guijarro-Rojas M, Ibrahim NA, et al. Immunohistochemical evaluation of basal cell carcinoma and trichoepithelioma using Bcl-2, Ki67, PCNA and P53. J Cutan Pathol. 2000;27:169–75.
31. Abesamis-Cubillan E, El-Shabrawi-Caelen L, LeBoit PE. Merkel cells and sclerosing epithelial neoplasms. Am J Dermatopathol. 2000;22:311–5.
32. Heidarpour M, Rajabi P, Sajadi F. CD10 expression helps to differentiate basal cell carcinoma from trichoepithelioma. J Res Med Sci. 2011;16(7):938–44.

33. Pham TT, Selim MA, Burchette Jr JL, Madden J, Turner J, Herman C. CD10 expression in trichoepithelioma and basal cell carcinoma. J Cutan Pathol. 2006;33:123–8.

34. Tebcherani AJ, de Andrade Jr HF, Sotto MN. Diagnostic utility of immunohistochemistry in distinguishing trichoepithelioma and basal cell carcinoma: evaluation using tissue microarray samples. Mod Pathol. 2012;25(10):1345–53.

35. Illueca C, Monteagudo C, Revert A, et al. Diagnostic value of CD34 immunostaining in desmoplastic trichilemmoma. J Cutan Pathol. 1998;25:435–9.

36. Kirchmann TT, Prieto VG, Smoller BR. CD34 staining pattern distinguishes basal cell carcinoma from trichoepithelioma. Arch Dermatol. 1994;130:589–92.

37. Basarab T, Orchard G, Russell-Jones R. The use of immunostaining for Bcl-2 and CD34 and the lectin peanut agglutinin in differentiating between basal cell carcinomas and trichoepitheliomas. Am J Dermatopathol. 1998;20:448–52.

38. Smoller BR, Van de Rijn M, Lebrun D, et al. Bcl-2 expression reliably distinguishes trichoepitheliomas from basal cell carcinomas. Br J Dermatol. 1994;131:28–31.

39. Choi CW, Park HS, Kim YK, Lee SH, Cho KH. Elastic fiber staining and cytokeratin 15 expression pattern in trichoepithelioma and basal cell carcinoma. J Dermatol. 2008;35(8):499–502.

40. Sellheyer K, Krahl D. PHLDA1 (TDAG51) is a follicular stem cell marker and differentiates between morphoeic basal cell carcinoma and desmoplastic trichoepithelioma. Br J Dermatol. 2011;164(1):141–7.

41. Battistella M, Carlson JA, Osio A, Langbein L, Cribier B. Skin tumors with matrical differentiation: lessons from hair keratins, beta-catenin and PHLDA-1 expression. J Cutan Pathol. 2014;41(5):427–36.

42. Sellheyer K, Nelson P. Follicular stem cell marker PHLDA1 (TDAG51) is superior to cytokeratin-20 in differentiating between trichoepithelioma and basal cell carcinoma in small biopsy specimens. J Cutan Pathol. 2011;38(7):542–50.

43. Sellheyer K, Nelson P, Kutzner H, Patel RM. The immunohistochemical differential diagnosis of microcystic adnexal carcinoma, desmoplastic trichoepithelioma and morpheaform basal cell carcinoma using BerEP4 and stem cell markers. J Cutan Pathol. 2013;40(4):363–70.

44. Tse JY, Nguyen AT, Le LP, Hoang MP. Microcystic adnexal carcinoma versus desmoplastic trichoepithelioma: a comparative study. Am J Dermatopathol. 2013;35(1):50–5.

45. Krahl D, Sellheyer K. Monoclonal antibody Ber-EP4 reliably discriminates between microcystic adnexal carcinoma and basal cell carcinoma. J Cutan Pathol. 2007;34:782–7.

46. Hoang MP, Dresser KA, Kapur P, et al. Microcystic adnexal carcinoma: an immunohistochemical reappraisal. Mod Pathol. 2008;21:178–85.

47. Yeh I, McCalmont TH, LeBoit PE. Differential expression of PHLDA1 (TDAG51) in basal cell carcinoma and trichoepithelioma. Br J Dermatol. 2012;167(5):1106–10.

48. Costache M, Bresch M, Böer A. Desmoplastic trichoepithelioma versus morphoeic basal cell carcinoma: a critical reappraisal of histomorphological and immunohistochemical criteria for differentiation. Histopathology. 2008;52(7):865–76.

49. Katona TM, Perkins SM, Billings SD. Does the panel of cytokeratin 20 and androgen receptor antibodies differentiate desmoplastic trichoepithelioma from morpheaform/infiltrative basal cell carcinoma? J Cutan Pathol. 2008;35(2):174–9.

50. Misago N, Satoh T, Miura Y, Nagase K, Narisawa Y. Merkel cell-poor trichoblastoma with basal cell carcinoma-like foci. Am J Dermatopathol. 2007;29(3):249–55.

51. Kurzen H, Esposito L, Langbein L, Hartschuh W. Cytokeratins as markers of follicular differentiation: an immunohistochemical study of trichoblastoma and basal cell carcinoma. Am J Dermatopathol. 2001;23(6):501–9.

52. Córdoba A, Guerrero D, Larrinaga B, Iglesias ME, Arrechea MA, Yanguas JI. Bcl-2 and CD10 expression in the differential diagnosis of trichoblastoma, basal cell carcinoma, and basal cell carcinoma with follicular differentiation. Int J Dermatol. 2009;48(7):713–7.

53. Vega Memije ME, Luna EM, de Almeida OP, Taylor AM, Cuevas González JC. Immunohistochemistry panel for differential diagnosis of Basal cell carcinoma and trichoblastoma. Int J Trichol. 2014;6(2):40–53.

54. Battistella M, Peltre B, Cribier B. PHLDA1, a follicular stem cell marker, differentiates clear-cell/granular-cell trichoblastoma and clear-cell/granular cell basal cell carcinoma: a case-control study, with first description of granular-cell trichoblastoma. Am J Dermatopathol. 2014;36(8):643–50.

55. Kurokawa I, Mizutani H, Nishijima S, Kato N, Yasui K, Tsubura A. Trichoadenoma: cytokeratin expression suggesting differentiation towards the follicular infundibulum and follicular bulge regions. Br J Dermatol. 2005;153(5):1084–6.

56. Shimanovich I, Krahl D, Rose C. Trichoadenoma of Nikolowski is a distinct neoplasm within the spectrum of follicular tumors. J Am Acad Dermatol. 2010;62(2):277–83.

57. Blumenthal GM, Dennis PA. PTEN hamartoma tumor syndromes. Eur J Hum Genet. 2008;16:1289–300.

58. Brownstein MH, Mehregan AH, Bikowski JP. Trichilemmomas in Cowden's disease. JAMA. 1977;238:267.

59. Brownstein MH, Mehregan AH, Bikowski JBB, Lupulescu A, Patterson JC. The dermatopathology of Cowden's syndrome. Br J Dermatol. 1979;100:667–73.

60. Tsai JH, Huang WC, Jhuang JY, Jeng YM, Cheng ML, Chiu HY, Kuo KT, Liau JY. Frequent activating HRAS mutations in trichilemmoma. Am J Dermatopathol. 2013;35(6):637–40.

61. Kanoh M, Amoh Y, Sato Y, Katsuoka K. Expression of the hair stem cell-specific marker nestin in epidermal and follicular tumors. Eur J Dermatol. 2008; 18(5):518–23.

62. Alsaad KO, Obaidat NA, Ghazarian D. Skin adnexal neoplasms—part 1: An approach to tumours of the pilosebaceous unit. J Clin Pathol. 2007;60:129–44.

63. Jin M, Hampel H, Pilarski R, Zhou X, Peters S, Frankel WL. Phosphatase and tensin homolog immunohistochemical staining and clinical criteria for Cowden syndrome in patients with trichilemmoma or associated lesions. Am J Dermatopathol. 2013;35(6):637–40.

64. Al-Zaid T, Ditelberg JS, Prieto VG, Lev D, Luthra R, Davies MA, Diwan AH, Wang WL, Lazar AJ. Trichilemmomas show loss of PTEN in Cowden syndrome but only rarely in sporadic tumors. J Cutan Pathol. 2012;39(5):493–9.

65. Hunt SJ, Kilzer B, Santa Cruz DJ. Desmoplastic trichilemmoma: histologic variant resembling invasive carcinoma. J Cutan Pathol. 1990;17(1):45–52.

66. Illueca C, Monteagudo C, Revert A, Llombart-Bosch A. Diagnostic value of CD34 immunostaining in desmoplastic trichilemmoma. J Cutan Pathol. 1998;25(8):435–9.

67. Kurokawa I, Senba Y, Nishimura K, Habe K, Hakamada A, Isoda K, Yamanaka K, Mizutani H, Tsubura A. Cytokeratin expression in trichilemmal carcinoma suggests differentiation towards follicular infundibulum. In Vivo. 2006;20(5):583–5.

68. Wong TY, Suster S. Tricholemmal carcinoma: a clinicopathologic study of 13 cases. Am J Dermatopathol. 1994;16:463–73.

69. Poblet E, Jiménez F. CD34 in human hair follicle. J Invest Dermatol. 2003;121:1220–1.

70. Sajin M, Luchian MC, Hodorogea Prisăcaru A, Dumitru A, Pătraşcu OM, Costache D, Dumitrescu D, Oproiu AM, Simionescu O, Costache M. Trichilemmal carcinoma - a rare cutaneous malignancy: report of two cases. Rom J Morphol Embryol. 2014;55(2 Suppl):687–91.

71. Chaichamnan K, Satayasoontorn K, Puttanupaab S, Attainsee A. Malignant proliferating trichilemmal tumors with CD34 expression. J Med Assoc Thai. 2010;93 Suppl 6:S28–34.

72. Fernández-Figueras MT, Casalots A, Puig L, Llatjós R, Ferrándiz C, Ariza A. Proliferating trichilemmal tumor: p53 immunoreactivity in association with p27 Kip1 over-expression indicates a low-grade carcinoma profile. Histopathology. 2001;38:454–7.

73. Rangel-Gamboa L, Reyes-Castro M, Dominguez-Cherit J, Vega-Memije E. Proliferating trichilemmal cyst: the value of ki67 immunostaining. Int J Trichol. 2013;5(3):115–7.

74. Alici O, Keles MK, Kurt A. A rare cutaneous adnexal tumor: malignant proliferating trichilemmal tumor. Case Rep Med. 2015;2015:742920.

75. Malhotra KP, Shukla S, Singhal A, Husain N. Proliferating trichilemmal cyst with nodal enlargement mimicking metastatic squamous cell carcinoma. Indian J Dermatol Venereol Leprol. 2015;81:418–20.

76. González-Guerra E, Requena L, Kutzner H. Immunohistochemical study of calretinin in normal hair follicles and tumors with follicular differentiation. Actas Dermosifiliogr. 2008;99(6):456–63.

77. Hassanein AM, Glanz SM. Beta-catenin expression in benign and malignant pilomatrix neoplasms. Br J Dermatol. 2004;150(3):511–6.

78. Czerniawska E, Pogrzebielski A, Romanowska-Dixon B. Malherbe's calcifying epithelioma (pilomatrixoma). Klin Oczna. 2011;113(7-9):274–6.

79. Nishioka M, Tanemura A, Yamanaka T, Tani M, Miura H, Asakura M, Tamai N, Katayama I. Pilomatrix carcinoma arising from pilomatricoma after 10-year senescent period: Immunohistochemical analysis. J Dermatol. 2010;37(8):735–9.

80. Haskell HD, Haynes HA, McKee PH, Redston M, Granter SR, Lazar AJ. Basal cell carcinoma with matrical differentiation: a case study with analysis of beta-catenin. J Cutan Pathol. 2005;32(3):245–50.

81. Sorin T, Eluecque H, Gauchotte G, De Runz A, Chassagne JF, Mansuy L, Gisquet H, Simon E. Pilomatrix Carcinoma of the scalp. A case report and review of the literature. Ann Chir Plast Esthet. 2015;60(3):242–6.

Use of Immunohistochemical and Molecular Studies in the Evaluation of the Sebaceous Neoplasms

Doina Ivan, Victor G. Prieto, and Phyu Aung

Introduction

Sebaceous glands are widely distributed on the body, with the exception of hands and feet. They vary in size and density depending on the anatomic areas and there are more numerous on the head and neck, especially on nose, forehead, and scalp, but also on the midline of the back, external auditory canal, and anogenital area. With few exceptions, sebaceous glands are associated with follicular structures and are connected to the follicular infundibulum. There are also "free sebaceous glands" or "ectopic" which lack the association with the follicular structures and involve the vermillion border of lips, areola, glans penis or labia minora, and even less common, the esophagus and tongue [1–5].

A mature sebaceous gland is composed of sebaceous lobules connected to the follicular infundibulum with a sebaceous duct. At the periphery of the sebaceous lobules there is an outer layer of germinative, immature sebocytes with a basaloid appearance and scant cytoplasm and centrally located are maturing or mature sebocytes cells with abundant multivacuolated cytoplasm and centrally placed, scalloped nuclei. The sebaceous duct is lined by keratinizing stratified squamous epithelium and a compact cornified layer [1, 6].

Sebaceous neoplasms are composed of variable proportion of germinative cells and sebocytes, more or less mature. Usually, the sebaceous nature of a cutaneous adnexal neoplasm is established on the basis of the presence of cells resembling mature sebocytes (i.e., cells with multivacuolated cytoplasm and centrally placed, scalloped nuclei) (Fig. 4.1). However, in some sebaceous tumors (such as poorly differentiated sebaceous carcinomas or some sebaceomas) the predominant cells are those recapitulating the germinative sebaceous cells and their origin is very difficult or impossible to recognize. The less mature sebocytes have rather few intracytoplasmic vacuoles and the cytoplasm is either eosinophilic or finely granular while the nucleus is either displaced to periphery or it is round and centrally placed [1, 6]. The identification of sebaceous duct differentiation and its distinction from other types of ductal differentiation may be difficult, but the presence of unequivocal mature

D. Ivan, M.D. (✉) • V.G. Prieto, M.D., Ph.D.
Department of Pathology, University of Texas – MD Anderson Cancer Center, 1515 Holcombe Blvd, Houston, TX 77030, USA

Department of Dermatology, University of Texas – MD Anderson Cancer Center, Houston, TX 77030, USA
e-mail: dsivan@mdanderson.org

Phyu Aung, M.D., Ph.D.
Department of Pathology, University of Texas – MD Anderson Cancer Center, 1515 Holcombe Blvd, Houston, TX 77030, USA

© Springer International Publishing Switzerland 2016
J.A. Plaza, V.G. Prieto (eds.), *Applied Immunohistochemistry in the Evaluation of Skin Neoplasms*, DOI 10.1007/978-3-319-30590-5_4

sebocytes in vicinity is very helpful in the diagnosis.

Considering all these challenges, histochemical and immunohistochemical studies may be used to aid the diagnosis and confirm the sebaceous differentiation of an adnexal neoplasm. Immunohistochemical markers for sebaceous differentiation are further discussed in this chapter along with other immunohistochemical markers that have been reported to have prognostic significance or therapeutic implications.

The ectopic and some benign sebaceous lesions, such as sebaceous hyperplasia, are almost exclusively sporadic and there is no currently described their association with systemic syndromes. However, other types of sebaceous neoplasms (especially adenomas, sebaceomas, and less often sebaceous carcinomas) may represent the cutaneous manifestations of systemic syndromes and are best known for their association with Muir–Torre syndrome (MTS), which is an autosomal dominantly inherited phenotypic variant of hereditary nonpolyposis colorectal cancer syndrome (HNPCC) or Lynch Syndrome [7–9]. The potential association of sebaceous tumors with internal malignancies and Muir–Torre syndrome was increasingly recognized in the recent years and their distinction is of utmost clinical significance. Well-characterized genetic alterations have been described and implicated in Muir–Torre syndrome pathogenesis and a detailed description of these along with current recommendations for patient's genetic testing and potential strategies for targeted therapies are provided in this chapter (see Fig. 4.2).

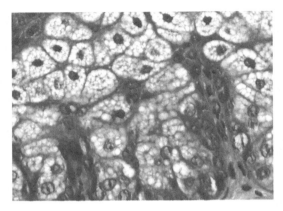

Fig. 4.1 The presence of mature sebocytes in cutaneous adnexal neoplasm is the hallmark for sebaceous differentiation. The cells have multivacuolated cytoplasm and centrally placed, scalloped nuclei

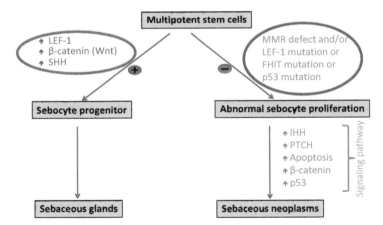

Fig. 4.2 Schematic presentation of the molecular mechanisms involved in the formation of sebaceous neoplasms. The left side of the figure represents the development of the normal sebaceous glands from the multipotent stem cells by normal regulation of β-catenin (Wnt), through Lef-1 transcription factor and sonic hedgehog signaling pathway. In contrast, the right side of the figure demonstrates abnormal proliferation of sebaceous glands (tumorigenesis) by loss of MMR proteins/MSI and/or mutations in *LEF1*, *FHIT* and/or *p53*, leading to activation of the Indian hedgehog and patched pathways, as well as inhibition of p53 and β-catenin (Wnt) signaling pathways.

Clinical Presentation and Histologic Features of Sebaceous Neoplasms

There is a wide spectrum of sebaceous neoplasms ranging from hamartomatous to benign to malignant entities that derive from the sebaceous glands. The classification and the nomenclature of sebaceous neoplasms are relatively confusing and often considered controversial. Sebaceous differentiation in other tumors, other than sebaceous tumors per se, can be encountered in cutaneous adnexal neoplasms with multilineage differentiation as well as in other epithelial lesions, such as squamous cell or basal cell carcinoma, verruca vulgaris or seborrheic keratoses, especially occurring on the face and head and neck area.

Some of the most commonly encountered sebaceous lesions are:

Ectopic Sebaceous Lesions

Sebaceous glands are usually part of the "pilosebaceous unit" and are found in association with hair follicle [1, 2]. However, especially at the mucosal sites, they lack this association and present as small yellow papules, commonly known as Fordyce spots [2, 10]. Their incidence increases with age and since their prevalence is high in general population are considered a normal physiologic variant. They are frequently noted at the vermillion border of the lip, buccal mucosa, medial aspect of labia majora, labia minora, penis (also called Tyson's glands), and rarely in the uterine cervix, vagina, esophagus, or gastroesophageal junction [2–5, 10–13]. They may be also found on the breast areolae, where they are known as Montgomery's tubercules [2, 14, 15]. Histologically the ectopic glands are characterized by sebaceous lobules or small clusters of sebocytes that open directly onto the epithelial surface and lack association with a follicular structure (Fig. 4.3).

Hamartomatous Sebaceous Lesions

Hamartomatous lesions, such nevus sebaceus of Jadassohn, described originally in 1895, repre-

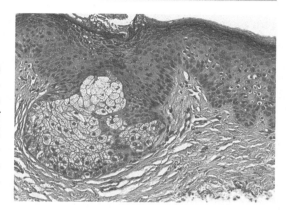

Fig. 4.3 Fordyce spots are ectopic sebaceous glands characterized by lobules or small clusters of sebocytes that open directly onto the epithelial surface and lack association with a follicular structure

sent complex hamartomas involving not only sebaceous glands but also epidermis and dermis. Nevus sebaceus of Jadassohn is also referred to as "organoid nevus" is commonly seen on head and neck area, especially on the scalp, but also forehead, face, postauricular and less commonly the trunk, extremities, oral or perianal region [16–18]. It usually presents since birth as an area of alopecia with a cerebriform appearance and yellow discoloration and it usually enlarges during adolescence under the influence of pubescent hormonal stimulation. In the adults it may also change due to the development of mostly benign and rarely malignant tumors of variable differentiation [17]. It is estimated that about 10–20 % of nevus sebaceus of Jadassohn are complicated by additional proliferations, often multiple and syringocystadenoma papilliferum is the most common association [19–21]. Sebaceous carcinoma arising in nevus sebaceus of Jadassohn is a rare and late occurrence, mostly encountered in the 6th or 7th decade of life [22–24].

Histologically, nevus sebaceus of Jadassohn is characterized by epidermal acanthosis, papillomatosis with an abnormal hair papillae-like proliferations and connections of the sebaceous lobules directly onto the surface epidermis or to the infundibulum of vellus hair follicles. Nevus sebaceus of Jadassohn has a variable number of sebaceous glands, ranging from hyperplastic, increased in number to diminished in number or even absent and characteristically there is a variation in the morphology and distribution of sebaceous glands. A common finding is the absence or significant reduction in the number of mature hair follicles. Induction of hair follicles also occurs, especially on the scalp lesions, as numerous follicular germinative cells (basaloid cells) proliferate and form basaloid hyperplasia or incipient forms of trichoblastoma. Glandular changes, especially increased number and size of apocrine glands were described in approximately 80 % of cases of nevus sebaceus of Jadassohn [16, 17].

In majority of the cases nevus sebaceus of Jadassohn occurs in a sporadic fashion. However, familial cases have been described and sometimes nevus sebaceus of Jadassohn, especially when has a linear appearance, may be part of epidermal nevus syndromes family. and associated with other abnormalities, particularly neurological syndromes, such as mental retardation and seizures, but also with ocular and musculoskeletal deficiencies. The epidermal nevus syndromes that comprises nevus sebaceus of Jadassohn are Schimmelpenning–Feuerstein–Mims syndrome phakomatosis pigmentokeratotica and SCALP (sebaceous nevus, central nervous system malformations, aplasia cutis congenital, limbal dermoid, and pigmented nevus) [25–29].

The pathogenesis of nevus sebaceus of Jadassohn is thought to be caused by genetic mosaicism, but a specific gene responsible for its clinical manifestations is unknown. Loss of heterozygosity of the *PTCH1*(*Drosophila* patched) gene has been described in nevus sebaceus of Jadassohn by Xin et al. but this finding was not supported by subsequent studies [30, 31]. Based on the whole exome sequencing, sebaceous nevi are associated with activating HRAS p.Gly13Arg and KRAS p.Gly12Asp mutations [32].

Steatocystoma Multiplex

Steatocystoma multiplex is characterized by multiple small, yellowish, dome-shaped papules or cysts, usually found in the axillae, chest but also on face, scalp, trunk, extremities, etc. [33, 34]

On histology, there are cysts with undulating, stratified, thin squamous epithelium without a granular layer and with characteristic presence of flattened sebaceous lobules either within or adjacent to the cystic wall [33, 34].

When single (steatocystoma simplex), the lesion occurs in a sporadic fashion. Familial cases of steatocystoma multiplex with autosomal dominant inheritance are well described. Mutations in *KRT17* on chromosome 17 have been documented in families with steatocystoma multiplex and are similar with those seen in pachyonychia congenita type 2 (Jackson–Lawer syndrome) [35, 36]. Rarely multiple steatocystomas have been reported in association with familial syringoma, trichoblastomas, keratoacanthomas, hypertrophic lichen planus, and also hypohidrosis and hypotrichosis [37].

Benign Sebaceous Lesions

Sebaceous Hyperplasia

The most common sebaceous neoplasm is represented by sebaceous hyperplasia which occurs as asymptomatic, solitary or multiple, umbilicated yellow papules on the forehead and face of older individuals and occasionally in younger individuals [1, 38]. Familial cases with early onset have been described. There is a significant increased incidence of sebaceous hyperplasia following renal transplantation, and it was described as being related to therapy with cyclosporine A [39, 40]. The histologic examination reveals an enlarged sebaceous gland with numerous lobules grouped around a centrally located duct.

It is known that the sebaceous gland development is affected by androgens. Sebaceous hyperplasia may also occur after trauma and it is thought that this is due to upregulation of the EGF-EGFR (epidermal growth factor receptor) and the Hedgehog-PTCH signaling pathway [41–43]. There are also studies that show that sebaceous hyperplasia in transgenic mice may be induced by the overexpression of a member of tumor necrosis factor (TNF) ligand family [43].

Sebaceous Adenoma

Sebaceous adenomas are benign tumors derived from sebaceous glands that occur commonly on the head and neck region of older individuals as slowly growing, tan-yellow or pink, small (less than 5 mm) papules [1, 38, 44]. Histologically, they have a lobular, organoid growth pattern, are well-circumscribed and often connected to epithelial surface. Sebaceous adenomas have an increased number of undifferentiated basaloid cells at the periphery of the lobules and more mature sebocytes centrally located. The proportion between these two cell types is variable but sebaceous adenoma is comprised by at least 50 % mature sebocytes [1, 38, 44] (Fig. 4.4).

The association between the presence of usually multiple sebaceous adenomas, often outside of a head and neck location and possible cystic appearance, and Muir–Torre syndrome has been extensively described and is further presented.

It has been recently described that a subset of sebaceous adenomas may harbor inactivating mutations in LEF1, the gene encoding a transcription factor in the Wnt/β-catenin pathway [45]. It was also reported that the Hedgehog and c-Myc pathways may also be involved in the tumorigenesis of sebaceous adenomas [43, 46].

Sebaceoma

The nomenclature of this entity is often confusing and controversial. The term of "sebaceous epithelioma" has been used interchangeably but this mostly refers to cases of basal cell carcinoma with sebaceous differentiation [47, 48]. Sebaceoma appears to be the established nomenclature of choice for this distinctive sebaceous neoplasm which has an increased number of basaloid cells that outnumbers the mature sebaceous component.

Clinically, sebaceomas are usually larger (ranging from 5 to 30 mm), fleshy-yellow, slow-growing, circumscribed nodules or plaques. They often occur in the head and neck region, mostly on the face or scalp, but they were also described on the ear canal or eyelid. There is a female predominance and mostly affect older individuals [47, 48].

On histologic examination, sebaceomas have a lobular growth pattern, similar to sebaceous adenomas, but differ from them by the increased number of basaloid, germinative cells (representing more than 50 % of the lesion) (Fig. 4.5). Often sebaceomas involve dermis but sometimes, connection with epidermal surface is noted. Sebaceomas exhibit numerous histologic patterns, including reticulated, cribriform, cystic, rippled patterns, etc. [47–49] Importantly, sebaceomas are relatively well-circumscribed and

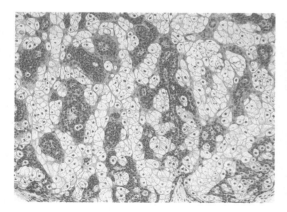

Fig. 4.4 Sebaceous adenomas have a lobular growth pattern and are composed of mature sebocytes (at least 50 % of cells) and an increased number of undifferentiated basaloid cells at the periphery of the lobules

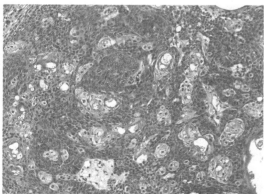

Fig. 4.5 Sebaceomas have a lobular growth pattern, similar to sebaceous adenomas, but differ from them by the increased number of basaloid, germinative cells (representing more than 50 % of the lesion)

lack significant cytologic atypia or an increased number of mitotic figures [50]. However, due to its higher proportion of basaloid, germinative cells and sometimes less obvious presence of mature sebocytes, sebaceomas may be difficult to distinguish from other lesions, such as basal cell carcinomas. The lack of peripheral retraction artifact or associated myxoid stoma is helpful in the differential diagnosis.

Association of multiple sebaceomas with Muir–Torre syndrome has been extensively described and is further discussed.

Malignant Sebaceous Lesions— Sebaceous Carcinoma

Sebaceous carcinomas are relatively uncommon tumors and they may potentially develop from any sebaceous gland and occur at ocular or extraocular sites. Approximately 75 % of cases occur on the eyelids (most common on the upper eyelid), arising mainly from meibomian glands of the tarsal plate and less commonly from the glands of Zeis [51–56]. Extraocular sebaceous carcinomas are predominantly seen in the head and neck area, but can also arise on the trunk, extremities, vulva, penis, etc. [53, 55–57] It was originally believed that the tumors with extraocular location were less aggressive, but it has been shown that these cases have similar metastatic and fatality rates with their ocular counterparts [57, 58]. A recent retrospective review of a large series of cases from the Surveillance, Epidemiology and End-Results (SEER) database of the National Cancer Institute showed no difference in the overall survival between patients with ocular and non-ocular sebaceous carcinoma [58]. Interestingly, the ocular sebaceous carcinomas have a lower likelihood of association with Muir–Torre syndrome than their extraocular counterpart. [57]

Although rare, sebaceous carcinoma is a malignancy with potentially aggressive behavior. Local recurrence complicates 6–29 % of periocular sebaceous cell carcinoma cases [52–56].

Regional or distal metastases affect 14–25 % of patients with a 5-year mortality ranging from 30 % (7–8) to 50–67 % according to different reports [52–58]. The metastatic and mortality rates can be significantly lowered with early detection and treatment but the clinical presentation is notoriously varied and clinical diagnosis is often delayed [59].

Histologically, sebaceous carcinomas are characterized by lobules or sheets of cells with an infiltrative growth pattern in dermis and subcutaneous tissue, or even the underlying skeletal muscle (mostly in the cases involving the eyelid). Sebaceous cell carcinoma in situ often demonstrates pagetoid upward migration of tumor cells, extension into the adnexal structures and may be difficult to distinguish from squamous cell carcinoma. (Fig. 4.6a) The tumor cells of sebaceous carcinoma have often marked cytologic atypia and conspicuous mitotic figures, occasionally atypical (Fig. 4.6b). The degree of sebaceous differentiation varies greatly; in well-differentiated tumors the sebaceous differentiation is usually easily recognized, but in the poorly differentiated forms, mature sebocytes are not conspicuous and the diagnosis is often challenging (Fig. 4.6c, d) Pagetoid intraepithelial spread of neoplastic cells is a common feature and tumor necrosis (sometimes with comedo-like appearance) is often noted [52–58]. Reports of histologically discordant sebaceous neoplasms with architectural features of a benign lesion but significant cytologic atypia have been described in the literature. The authors suggest that these lesions are best fully excised and followed over time, as their behavior is uncertain [56].

Poor prognostic indicators include multicentricity, size greater than 1 cm in diameter, extensive infiltrative growth pattern, and lymphovascular invasion [58].

Sebaceous tumor may occur de novo, but their potential association with internal malignancies and Muir–Torre syndrome has been increasingly recognized in the recent years and this distinction is of utmost clinical significance and is further discussed.

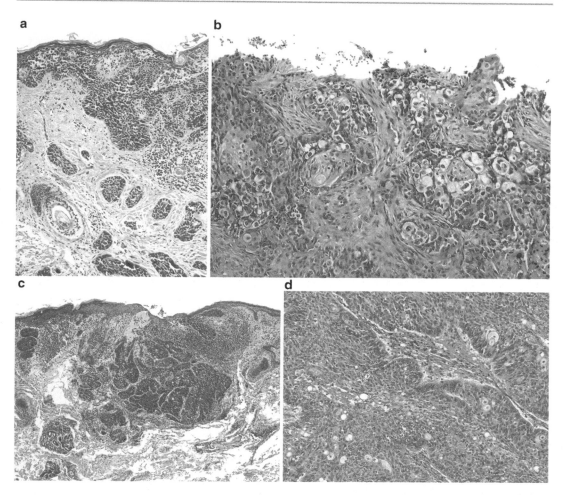

Fig. 4.6 (**a**) Sebaceous carcinomas have an infiltrative growth pattern, extension into adnexal structures, (**b**) demonstrates pagetoid upward migration of tumor cells, and have marked cytologic atypia, conspicuous mitotic figures, and sometimes necrosis. In the poorly differentiated sebaceous carcinoma the mature sebocytes are not conspicuous and the diagnosis is often challenging: (**c**) low power view (magnification 4×) and (**d**) high power view (magnification 4×)

Use of Immunohistochemical Studies in Evaluation of Sebaceous Neoplasms

Immunohistochemical Studies that Support the Sebaceous Differentiation

The presence of mature sebocytes is the hallmark of sebaceous neoplasms. Histologically, the mature sebocytes are recognized by their characteristically centrally placed, indented nuclei and numerous intracytoplasmic lipid droplets (scalloped morphology). However, this distinction may not be so obvious and they may confused with other cells with clear cell histology, such as the clear cells derived from the follicular outer root sheath cells that contain a large amount of glycogen that usually pushes the nucleus to the periphery [2]. These clear cells may be encountered in squamous cell or basal cell carcinomas and their distinction from poorly differentiated sebaceous carcinomas can be difficult. However, this differential diagnosis has a paramount importance in view of the distinct prognostic features of these lesions.

Traditionally, Oil-Red O and Sudan Black IV have been used to identify intracytoplasmic lipid droplets in the sebocytes of the sebaceous lesions. However, these stains require fresh, frozen tissue for analysis and have a relatively low sensitivity, of approximately 40 % [60].

There is a large number of reports in the literature that describe the use of immunohistochemical studies performed on formalin-fixed paraffin-embedded sections to distinguish sebaceous differentiation, with widely variable results. Single markers or panels of antibodies including CK7, AR, CAM 5.2, EMA and Ber-EP4 were used, but numerous limitations were noted and sometimes contradictory results were obtained.

The androgen receptors (AR) are nuclear proteins that frequently are expressed in normal skin and the sebaceous glands, and their greater prominence in the pilosebaceous units of men than in that of women has led to investigations of their influence on the development of male pattern baldness [61]. Among skin tumors, AR have been found in both benign and malignant sebaceous tumors and it was suggested that the presence of AR by immunohistochemical studies is a reliable and highly sensitive marker of sebaceous differentiation [62]. However, further studies reveal that AR may also be present in up to 60 % of basal cell carcinomas [63, 64].

The recommendation to use CK7 to differentiate ocular sebaceous carcinoma from both squamous and basal cell carcinoma has been reported [60, 65, 66]. However, later studies showed that all these tumors can be positive for CK7, in variable proportions, and there is no definite diagnostic utility of this marker in the differential diagnostic of these tumors, especially when trying to distinguish sebaceous carcinoma from basal cell carcinoma [65, 66].

EMA (epithelial membrane antigen) is a cell membrane-associated glycoprotein that is positive in a number of glandular or secretory tumors, including sebaceous lesions. Several studies have been published describing the usefulness of EMA antibodies in diagnosing sebaceous carcinoma, as most of the sebaceous tumors are positive for EMA. Currently, it appears that the immunohistochemical detection of EMA is useful in differentiating sebaceous carcinoma from basal cell carcinoma (which labels less often for EMA), but not from squamous cell carcinoma. One study showed that all cases of squamous cell carcinoma and 80 % of sebaceous carcinomas were positive for EMA, while the marker was negative in all basal cell carcinoma cases. However, in poorly) differentiated cases of sebaceous carcinoma, EMA can be negative or only focally positive [60, 66].

Ber-EP4 expression has been reported in up to 80 % of sebaceous carcinomas. Fan et al. reported that the use of an immunohistochemical panel using EMA and Ber-EP4 may be especially useful [65]. While sebaceous carcinomas are EMA-positive and Ber-EP4-positive, an immunophenotype with EMA-negative and Ber-EP4-positive supports the diagnosis of basal cell carcinoma. The authors also noted that EMA-positive and Ber-EP4-negative labeling favors squamous cell carcinoma [66, 67].

Undifferentiated basaloid cells situated at the periphery of the sebaceous lobules or part of the sebaceous neoplasms express CK15, a stem cell marker, and also D2-40 and p63 [68–70]. Germinative sebaceous cells are positive for androgen receptors and variably positive for CK8/18, CK19 and also stain for SOX9, while the mature sebocytes are usually negative for the marker [71, 72].

Recently, the use of antibodies against the lipid droplet-associated proteins, including adipophilin and perilipin, has gained interest and has been proven to have a significant role in the identification of sebaceous differentiation and the differential diagnosis of these tumors.

Adipophilin is present in milk fat globule membranes and on the surface of lipid droplets in various normal cell types, including the cells of lactating mammary epithelium, adrenal cortex, steatotic hepatocytes in alcoholic cirrhosis, renal cell carcinoma, hepatocellular carcinomas, pancreatic carcinomas, prostatic carcinomas, and liposarcomas, thus suggesting that lipid droplet accumulation is not an uncommon feature of neoplastic cells. The perilipins are a family of phosphoproteins found on the surface of intracellular lipid droplets and in the adrenal gland, Leydig cells, and both brown and white fat [73, 74].

A monoclonal antibody against adipophilin can be used on paraffin-embedded tissue assisting the identification of intracytoplasmic lipids, and it has been proven to be very helpful in identifying sebaceous differentiation, including in poorly differentiated neoplasms. Muthusamy et al. showed that adipophilin and perilipin were positive in 88 % (23/26) and respectively 38 % (10/26) of sebaceous carcinomas [73]. Osler et al. studied the expression of adipophilin in 117 sebaceous lesions and other cutaneous tumors with clear cell histology which may mimic sebaceous tumors and noted that adipophilin was positive in 92 % of sebaceous carcinomas and all cases of sebaceous adenoma, xanthelasmas, and 65 % of metastatic renal cell carcinomas [75]. Subsequent studies similarly have shown remarkable sensitivity of adipophilin in detection of sebaceous carcinoma (97–100 %), but a lower specificity (ranging from 35 to 77 %) than the one originally noted. This discrepancy stems in part from differences in the interpretation of what constitutes true positive staining [76–78]. Ostler et al. noted the membranous and vesicular ("mulberry") staining of intracytoplasmic lipid vacuoles in sebocytes (Fig. 4.7) and also a "granular, non-specific" labeling in the background stroma or other cells. This was originally attributed to possible cross-reactivity with keratohyalin granules and Odland bodies (lamellar bodies, composed of phospholipids associated with lysosomal membranes) [75]. However, Boussahmain and colleagues proposed that "granular" staining is not nonspecific, but rather reflects reactivity with small intracytoplasmic lipid droplets, which show clustering and localization to the outer nuclear membrane in a reproducible pattern. It was also noted the presence of lipid droplets in a wide variety of normal metabolically active cells and in cells altered by neoplastic processes [76]. Straub and colleagues found that adipophilin is nearly ubiquitously expressed in normal human tissues, including in the basal keratinocytes of epidermis with a "dot-like" or "granular" pattern

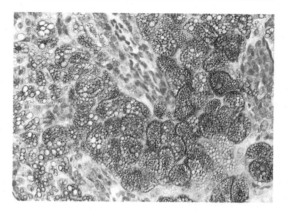

Fig. 4.7 Adipophilin—membranous and vesicular staining of intracytoplasmic lipid vacuoles in sebocytes

and further demonstrated in normal sebocytes and sebaceous neoplasms the "vacuolar" adipophilin labeling of the lipid droplets, by far exceeding the extent expected by light microscopy [73] (Fig. 4.8a, b). Recently, Milman et al. supports the observation on frequent expression of lipid droplet-associated proteins in neoplastic cells due to steatogenesis, but concurs with Ostler et al. that the pattern of adipophilin expression can be useful in distinguishing sebaceous carcinoma from other masquerading periocular neoplasms. [78] They found that the presence of greater than 5 % vacuoles and less than 95 % granules to be 100 % sensitive and 100 % specific in distinguishing sebaceous carcinoma from other periocular and ocular carcinomas [78]. In a recent study of Plaza et al. it has been noted adipophilin expression in all cases of sebaceous carcinoma with a membranous labeling of intracytoplasmic lipid globules and granular uptake in the cytoplasm of 76 % of basal cell carcinoma and 50 % of squamous cell carcinoma (none of those cases showed membranous labeling of intracytoplasmic lipid globules) [66].

In conclusion, when attempting to differentiate tumors with clear cell histology in periocular area, especially sebaceous cell carcinoma from squamous cell or basal cell carcinoma with clear cell features, adipophilin is a very useful immunohistochemical marker, with particular attention being given to the pattern of staining: intracytoplasmic membranous and vesicular type.

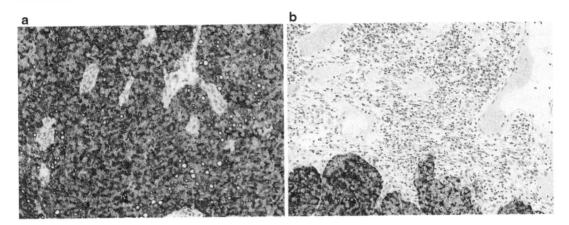

Fig. 4.8 (a) Adipohilin expression in poorly differentiated sebaceous carcinoma with membranous and vesicular labeling of intracytoplasmic lipid vacuoles and (b) adipophilin background, granular, "nonspecific" labeling

Recent work suggests the differential diagnostic value in sebaceous neoplasms of immunohistochemical studies for proteins involved in lipid synthesis and/or processing, namely alpha/beta hydrolase domain-containing protein 5 (ABHD5), progesterone receptor membrane component-1 (PGRMC1) and squalene synthase (SQS) [73, 79]. Perilipin regulates lipolysis by physically binding to the co-lipase ABHD5, thus reducing the interaction of ABHD5 with adipose triglyceride lipase. Mutations in *ABHD5* results in decreased lipid degradation. PGRMC1 is part of a multiprotein complex that binds to progesterone and other steroids to link extracellular signals to P450 activation. It plays an important role in regulating cholesterol and hormone synthesis and turnover. SQS, also known as farnesyldiphosphate farnesyltransferase 1, catalyzes the biosynthesis of squalene and cholesterol, the major lipid components of sebum [73].

Plaza et al. found that these markers are very specific, but not very sensitive for sebaceous carcinoma, since PGRMC1 was expressed in 81.4 %, SQS in 51.8 %, and ABHD5 in 70.3 % of cases. None of basal cell or squamous cell carcinoma included in the study expressed any of these markers [66].

In conclusion, it is recommended that an immunohistochemical panel consisting of adipophilin, EMA and possibly AR to be used for the highest sensitivity and specificity for the differential diagnosis of periocular sebaceous carcinoma from basal or squamous cell carcinoma with clear cell differentiation.

Immunohistochemical Studies with Prognostic Significance or Potential Therapeutic Implications in Sebaceous Neoplasms

P53 is a transcription factor protein encoded by the p53 tumor suppressor gene that induces apoptosis or cell cycle arrest in cells with damaged DNA. Mutation of p53 in non-melanoma skin cancers and previous reports noting p53 staining in sebaceous carcinomas are well documented [80]. Aberrant or absent p53 signaling was identified as potential mediator of an alternative mechanism of malignant sebaceous tumorigenesis (distinct from the microsatellite instability pathway) [57, 80]. Cabral et al. examined 27 benign and malignant sebaceous lesions and found statistically significant increased percentages of p53-positive cells in carcinomas compared with adenomas and a trend for the intensity of p53 staining to be greater in carcinomas compared with benign lesions [81]. Shalin et al. showed that nearly one-quarter of examined carcinomas showed p53 staining, whereas all adenomas were negative and only 1 sebaceoma was positive [57]. Moreover, the same study demonstrated a strong association between p53 dysregulation and periocular tumor location. Interestingly, when p53 staining was compared with expression of DNA mismatch repair proteins in sebaceous lesions, in cases with p53 overexpression, mismatch repair proteins were intact, confirming microsatellite stability, suggesting a divergent signaling mechanisms can contribute to sebaceous neoplasia [57].

A recent study by Kiyosaki et al. found a high percentage of p53 mutations in a small group of eyelid sebaceous carcinomas, but the mutations were not the typical tandem mutations induced by UV damage, raising the possibility that p53 dysregulation as a mechanism of sebaceous tumorigenesis may occur independent of UV damage [82]. In the same study, there was no significant correlation between p53 expression and clinical-pathologic findings, but p21, an inhibitor of cyclin-dependent kinases, induced by p53-dependent and independent pathways, has been shown that inversely correlates with disease stage and lymph node metastases of sebaceous carcinoma. Therefore, it was suggested that p21 immunoreactivity may be used as a tool for prediction of nodal metastasis in sebaceous carcinoma of the eyelid [82].

Dysregulation of cell cycle progression is strongly associated with the development of cancer and tumor progression. Kim et al. showed that high expression of p21, p27, cyclin E, and p16 was found in the majority of cells of sebaceous carcinoma, whereas these proteins were rarely expressed in the normal sebaceous glands [83]. Notably, it was reported that decreased p27 expression correlate with poor prognosis and increased metastatic potential [83]. Loss of $p21^{WAF1}$ compartmentalization in sebaceous carcinoma has been described being helpful for the differential diagnosis from sebaceous adenomas when used as a part of the panel including p53, Ki67, bcl-2, and p21 [84].

Proliferative markers, including PCNA and Ki-67 (MIB-1), are typically elevated in sebaceous carcinomas, and Hasebe et al. showed that carcinomas with a PCNA index greater than 20 % had a worse prognosis [85]. Cabral et al. found that carcinomas had statistically significantly increased levels of p53 in comparison with sebaceous adenomas (50 % versus 11 %, respectively) and Ki-67 (30 % versus 10 %). The carcinomas also had significantly reduced levels of bcl-2 (7 % versus 56 %) and p21 (16 % versus 34 %) compared to the adenomas [81].

Survivin is a member of the inhibitor of apoptosis family of proteins implicated in the inhibition of apoptosis and cell cycle control, both crucial in the progression to malignancy. A study of Calder et al. shows that survivin is expressed more often in sebaceous carcinoma in comparison with sebaceous adenoma and hyperplasia but the study has limitations due the relatively small number of cases studied [86].

Epithelial–mesenchymal transition (EMT) plays an important role in tumor invasion and metastasis in various malignancies and ZEB2/SIP1 is an important EMT regulator and downregulates E-cadherin expression [87]. A recent study reported cytoplasmic overexpression of ZEB2 and membranous loss of E-cadherin were seen in 68 % and respectively 66 % of 65 cases of eyelid sebaceous carcinomas ($P=0.002$) and correlated with high-risk features such as advanced tumor stages and large tumor size. Overexpression of ZEB2 also showed significant association with lymph node metastasis ($P=0.046$), orbital invasion ($P=0.049$) and poor survival [88].

Epidermal growth factor receptor (EGFR), a tyrosine kinase growth factor receptor is normally expressed in periocular surface epithelium, in the conjunctival goblet cells and sebocytes. Ivan et al. showed that EGFR expression is greater in extraocular than periocular sebaceous carcinomas in terms of both distribution and intensity, suggesting a different pathogenic mechanism. Interestingly, the sebaceous carcinomas associated with Muir–Torre syndrome showed a trend towards lower expression of EGFR since they also tend to behave in less aggressive fashion than their microsatellite-stable counterpart. *EGFR* gene mutations were not identified in the study [89].

Human epidermal growth factor receptor 2 protein (HER2) is a transmembrane receptor protein with tyrosine kinase activity that once is activated could potentially inhibit apoptosis, promote cellular proliferation, stimulate tumor-induced neovascularization, and activate invasion and metastasis . A recent study showed that increased copies of the HER2 gene were identified in 5 of 42 ocular sebaceous carcinoma samples (11.9 %), including two with amplification. The study also demonstrated EGFR amplification. HER2 protein overexpression and *HER2* amplification in 2 of 33 (6.1 %) cases of sebaceous carcinoma [90]. This study is of particular importance, since potential targeted therapies against HER2 and EGFR might be beneficial for a subset of patients with sebaceous carcinomas.

Molecular Aspects of Sebaceous Neoplasms

Muir–Torre Syndrome

Muir Torre Syndrome (MTS) is a rare autosomal dominant genodermatosis with a high degree of penetrance and variable expressivity, which was originally reported by Muir and Torre in 1967 and 1968, respectively [7, 91, 92]. MTS is recognized as a phenotypic variant of hereditary non-polyposis colorectal cancer (HNPCC) or Lynch syndrome [8]. It is characterized by the occurrence of sebaceous neoplasms such as adenoma, sebaceoma, sebaceous carcinoma, and/or kerato-acanthomas with visceral malignancies, including gastrointestinal and genitourinary cancers [8]. In almost 40 % of MTS patients a sebaceous neoplasm was the first clinical manifestation of the syndrome and it was reported that as many as 63 % of the MTS patients presenting with a sebaceous neoplasm have a concurrent internal malignancy or develop an additional one [57]. Therefore, early diagnosis of MTS is crucial not only for the patient, but also may prompt familial genetic testing. Colorectal carcinoma and uterine carcinomas are the most commonly associated internal malignancies when associated with MTS and occur in younger patients (typically <50 years old) in comparison with sporadic cases. Tumors of the renal pelvis and breast have also been recognized as being part of the syndrome. One of the cutaneous manifestation of MTS is keratoacanthoma, that occurs in up to 20 % of MTS patients with or without a concurrent sebaceous neoplasm [9]. Hybrid lesions (keratoacanthoma and sebaceous adenoma), called "seboacanthoma" are rare, but considered to be highly suggestive of MTS [7, 8, 93].

Genetic Aspects of Muir–Torre Syndrome

The deoxyribonucleic acid (DNA) mismatch repair (MMR) genes are essential for the maintenance of genomic integrity. These genes eliminate mismatches in base pairing occurring during DNA replication [7, 94]. Microsatellites are repeated sequences of DNA of 1–6 base pairs in length that are normally constant for a given individual. Certain tumors, as is the case in MTS, will show variation in the size of the microsatellite repeats when compared to normal cells from the same individual. The abnormal length of microsatellites occurs as a result of microsatellite instability (MSI) due to defects in the DNA repair process [7, 95, 96]. A germline mutation in one or more of MMR genes, combined with a second somatic mutational "hit" of the remaining functional allele usually causes genetically unstable tumors by the accumulation of replication errors in microsatellite sequences in patients with MTS [97]. The mismatch repair system is composed of human mutL homolog 1 (hMLH1), human mutS homolog 2 (hMSH2), human mutS homolog 6 (hMSH6), human mutS homolog 3 (hMSH3), human post meiotic segregation increased 2 (hPMS2) proteins, among others. Initially a complex of hMSH2 and hMSH6 binds to erroneous DNA segment and then recruits hMLH1 and hPMS2 leading to excision of DNA segment. Many of the patients with HNPCC demonstrate germ-line mutations in genes encoding DNA MMR proteins MLH1 and/or MSH2 and, less commonly, MSH6, MSH3, MLH3, PMS1, and PMS2 [98, 99]. In MTS mutation of *MHS2* locus are more commonly seen (90 %) that *MLH1* gene mutations [57]. The lack of expression of MSH6 in sebaceous lesions of MTS patients suggests that a *MSH6* gene mutation is also common and considering that MSH6 forms a heterodimer with MSH2, it is conceivable that mutations of

MSH2 lead to MSH6 loss and is not necessary representing a germline mutation in *MSH6* [57]. Isolated mutations in *MSH6* are exceptionally noted. MTS is not definitely yet linked to isolated loss of MSH3 or PMS. [57]

Sebaceous lesions that may be potentially associated with MTS include both benign lesions, such as adenomas and sebaceomas as well as malignant (sebaceous carcinoma). Given the frequent occurrence of sebaceous hyperplasia in the general population and its rare association with MTS (0–10%) reported by some studies, the association of sebaceous hyperplasia with MTS is still clinically insignificant [7, 8, 100–102]. In contrast, the remaining other sebaceous neoplasms are reported to play an important role as markers of MTS. Among them, sebaceous adenoma seems to be the most common tumor found in association with MTS, with a reported frequency of 25–60% [7, 100, 101]. On the other hand, association of MTS with sebaceoma and carcinoma ranges from 31 to 86% and from 66 to 100%, respectively [101].

Several reports have documented that loss of MMR proteins in sebaceous tumors occurring outside of the head and neck region, in patients less than 50 years old, multiple sebaceous neoplasms, with keratoacanthoma-like and cystic changes, and/or increased intratumoral lymphocytes may be a strong indicator for MTS [93, 102–104]. However, there are different opinions in this matter; for instance one of the reports did not find cystic change to be statistically associated with sebaceous tumors demonstrating loss of mismatch repair protein expression [93].

Molecular and Immunohistochemical Testing for Muir–Torre Syndrome

The test of choice for identifying genetic instability of tumors in MTS, caused by defects in MMR genes, is the detection of microsatellite instability (MSI) by polymerase chain reaction (PCR). Most studies assess MSI in MTS using the five Bethesda markers, which were recommended by the National Cancer Institute as the standard screen for assessing MSI in tumors from patients with HNPCC [105]. The markers include three dinucleotide repeats (D2S123, D5S346, and D17S250) and two mononucleotide tracts (BAT25, BAT26). If MSI is detected in any two of the five markers, it is considered a positive result and indicative of a high probability of MSI [7, 96, 106].

However, in the daily pathology practice this PCR testing is costly and not always available. Immunohistochemical studies have become the preferred initial screen test, as studies have shown them to be excellent surrogates of underlying MMR gene function although it is not well established as in the case of colonic adenocarcinomas [107]. This technique, which is the initial screening test, uses antibodies directed against the MMR proteins, such as MLH1, MSH2, MSH6, and PMS1, and it is relatively easy to perform and interpret because of their nuclear staining pattern. Loss of MMR protein expression is indicated by complete absence of nuclear staining in the lesional tissue [7, 95, 106] (Fig. 4.9a–d).

In studies on unselected sebaceous neoplasms, the positive predictive value of lack of expression of each of the MMR proteins for MTS varies from 33 to 88% for MLH1, 55 to 66% for MSH2, and is approximately 67% for MSH6 [57, 100]. The positive predictive value for MTS increases when the markers are used in combination: is 55% for MTS tumors with combined loss of MSH2 and MSH6, and 100% for neoplasms with either dual loss of MLH1 and MSH6, or loss of all three (MLH1, MSH2, and MSH6) markers [105]. In their functional state, the MMR proteins form heterodimers. MSH2 dimerizes with MSH6, forming the functional complex, MutSα; and MLH1 dimerizes with PMS2, forming MutLα. It has been shown that the MSH2 and MLH1 proteins are the obligatory partners of their respective heterodimer. Due to this heterodimeric nature of the MMR proteins, loss of expression of a particular protein may in fact be due to the loss of expression of its paired obligatory partner protein. For example, loss of PMS2 alone indicates a defect in PMS2, whereas, when expression of both MLH1 and PMS2 are lost, this is likely due to loss of MLH1 and results in unstable PMS2. The same is true for MSH6 and MSH2, respectively [50]. Therefore, some authors say that MSH6 and PMS2 may be enough and there

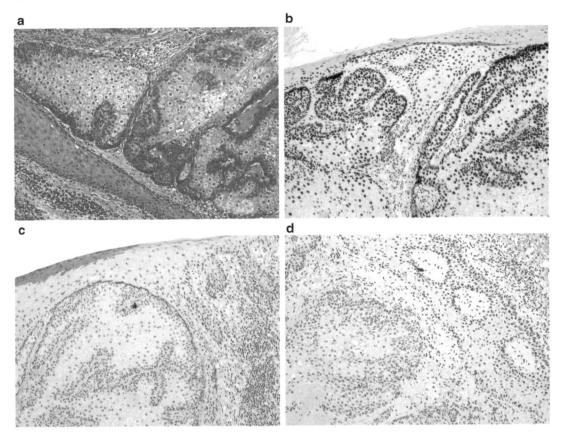

Fig. 4.9 Immunohistochemical studies are used as an initial screening test to determine the loss of MMR protein expression in patients with Muir–Torre syndrome and show: (**a**) Histologic image of sebaceous adenoma (hema- toxylin and eosin) with preservation of nuclear labeling of (**b**) MLH1 and loss of nuclear expression for (**c**) MSH2 and (**d**) MSH6

is no need for testing for MSH2 and MLH1 respectively.

Loss of nuclear staining of MLH1 and MSH2 in tumor cells are more commonly found in Lynch syndrome and MTS, although sporadic, non-germline mutated tumors may also show loss of staining. To distinguish sporadic vs. germline MMR loss, hypermethylation of the upstream MLH1 promoter (and subsequent silencing of the MLH1 gene) or BRAF (V600E) mutation testing can be performed on a tumor sample. Presence of either BRAF mutation or hypermethylation is strongly suggestive of sporadic loss of MMR. [108]

In addition to MSI, there must be other mechanisms involved in the pathogenesis of MTS because not all patients with sebaceous neoplasia and/or a characteristic internal malignancy demonstrate MSI. One study reported that 80 % of the internal malignancy-associated sebaceous neoplasms showed loss of expression of MSH-2 or MLH-1 by immunohistochemical method [109]. For instance, it has been reported that the presence of sebaceous neoplasms in patients with MYH (mutY Homolog) mutation-associated gastrointestinal polyposis syndrome did not exhibit MSI [108]. MYH is a protein involved in DNA base excision repair following DNA oxidative damage. The mechanisms by which the genomic instability due to loss of MMR proteins promotes sebaceous tumorigenesis are not well understood.

Studies in mouse models have shown that Wnt/β-catenin, Indian hedgehog, and p53 signaling pathways along with mutations in numerous tumor suppressor genes such as FHIT (Fragile Histidine Triad), DNA mismatch repair genes, and P53 may contribute to sebaceous tumor formation. After translocation of β-catenin to the nucleus by activation of Wnt signaling, it binds to proteins such as lymphocyte enhancing factor 1 (Lef-1) for gene transcription. A defective β-catenin binding site in the Lef-1 protein in a transgenic mouse causes sebaceous skin tumors due to defective transcriptional activity [110]. Upregulation of Indian hedgehog protein expression occurs in Lef-1 transgenic mice, which increases proliferation of sebaceous precursor cells [43]. This study also suggests that aberrations in β-catenin and hedgehog signaling pathways may promote various cutaneous tumors [108]. Takeda and colleagues found double-nucleotide substitutions in the same *LEF1* allele, irrespective of DNA mismatch repair status, in one-third of human sebaceous adenomas and sebaceomas, resulting in impaired β-catenin binding and decreased transcriptional activity [45].

In addition, the FHIT gene, a tumor suppressor, is a member of the histidine triad proteins and it has been shown that gastrointestinal malignancies and sebaceous lesions develop in transgenic heterozygous Fhit mice, when exposed to carcinogens [111]. Interestingly, no MSI was detected in these tumors [112]. FHIT mutations caused defective programmed cell death, and inhibit β-catenin transcriptional activity [45, 113]. FHIT mutations have), been found in human periocular sebaceous carcinomas regardless of MSI status [114, 115].

Mutations in the DNA-binding regions of p53 are common in skin cancers associated with ultraviolet irradiation [116]. Some sebaceous neoplasms showed increased nuclear immunoreactivity for p53 due to mutations and/or dysregulation of p53 signaling [117]. In contrast, sebaceous tumors developed in transgenic Lef-1 mutated mice showed no expression of p53 protein because of downregulation of its binding partner ARF, a tumor suppressor protein [36]. It has been hypothesized that p53 signaling alterations may represent an early, primary event in a subset of sebaceous malignancies with p53 expression. On the other hand, *LEF1* (a downstream gene) mutations may indicate the secondary effect within the other sebaceous neoplasms with LEF1 mutations [57].

Genetic Testing for Muir–Torre Syndrome

It has been recommended by some authors that the diagnosis of a sebaceous neoplasm located outside the head and neck area in a young patient (<50 years of age) should undergo additional testing for MSI [93]. Immunohistochemical analysis is used as a first line to detect the expression of MMR proteins (especially the more common ones such as MSH2, MLH1 and MSH6). Lack of expression of any one of these proteins should be followed by MSI analyses. If MSI is detected, it should be followed by germline mutation analysis. In a patient with positive results in all the tests mentioned above, cancer surveillance will be required in both the patient and family members. However, not all tumors with loss of these proteins are associated with MTS, and the positive predictive value of a loss of one of these markers is poor unless the clinical setting is taken into consideration. When patients with a positive family history of colon cancer in at least one relative are chosen for testing, the positive predictive value of loss of MMR proteins increased from 22 % to 92 % [105]. If there is a high clinical suspicion of MTS, germline mutation analysis should be done even after a normal finding in the first line immunohistochemical test for MMR proteins and/or the second line MSI PCR analysis [103, 118, 119]. However, if MSI is not detected in a patient with a negative family history, additional genetic tests are not required.

References

1. Rulon DB, Helwig EB. Cutaneous sebaceous neoplasms. Cancer. 1974;33:82–102.
2. Steffen CH, Ackerman AB. Ectopic sebaceous glands. In: Neoplasms with sebaceous differentiation. Philadelphia: Lea & Febiger; 1994. p. 71–88.
3. Daley TD. Intraoral sebaceous hyperplasia. Diagnostic criteria. Oral Surg Oral Med Oral Pathol. 1993 Mar;75(3):343–7.

4. Nakada T, Inoue F, Iwasaki M, Nagayama K, Tanaka T. Ectopic sebaceous glands in the esophagus. Am J Gastroenterol. 1995;90(3):501–3.

5. Robledo MC, Vazquez JJ, Contreras-Mejuto F, Lopez-Garcia G. Sebaceous glands and hair follicles in the cervix uteri. Histopathology. 1992;21(3):278–80.

6. Steffen CH, Ackerman AB. Embrologic, anatomic and histologic aspects. In: Neoplasms with sebaceous differentiation. Philadelphia: Lea & Febiger; 1994. p. 25–52.

7. Ponti G, Ponz de Leon M. Muir-Torre syndrome. Lancet Oncol. 2005;6(12):980.

8. Schwartz RA, Torre DP. The Muir-Torre syndrome: a 25 years retrospect. J Am Acad Dermatol. 1995;33:90.

9. Cohen PR, Kohn SR, Kurzrock R. Association of sebaceous gland and internal malignancy: the Muir-Torre syndrome. Am J Med. 1991;90:606.

10. Arnold HL. Fordyce spots. Arch Dermatol. 1974;110:811.

11. Bakaris S, Kiran H, Kiran G. Sebaceous gland hyperplasia of the vulva. Aust N Z J Obstet Gynaecol. 2004;44:75–6.

12. Belousova IE, Kazakov DV, Michal M. Ectopic sebaceous glands in the vagina. Int J Gynecol Pathol. 2005;24:193–5.

13. Hyman AB, Brownstein MH. Tyson's "glands." Ectopic sebaceous glands and papillomatosis penis. Arch Dermatol. 1969 Jan;99(1):31–6.

14. Krisp A, Krause W. Areolar sebaceous hyperplasia. Acta Derm Venereol. 2003;83:61–2.

15. Catalano PM, Ioannides A. Areolar sebaceous hyperplasia. J Am Acad Dermatol. 1985;13:867–8.

16. Mehregan AH, Pinkus H. Life history of organoid nevi. Special reference to nevus sebaceus of Jadassohn. Arch Dermatol. 1965;91:574–88.

17. Morioka S. The natural history of nevus sebaceus. J Cutan Pathol. 1985;12:200–13.

18. Weng CJ, Tsai YC, Chen TJ. Jadassohn's nevus sebaceous of the head and face. Ann Plast Surg. 1990;25:100–2.

19. Idriss MH, Elston DM. Secondary neoplasms associated with nevus sebaceus of Jadassohn: a study of 707 cases. J Am Acad Dermatol. 2014;70(2):332–7.

20. Cribier B, Scrivener Y, Grosshans E. Tumors arising in nevus sebaceus: a study of 596 cases. J Am Acad Dermatol. 2000;42(2 Pt 1):263–8.

21. Rosenblum GA. Nevus sebaceus, syringocystadenoma papilliferum, and basal cell epithelioma. J Dermatol Surg Oncol. 1985;11:1018–20.

22. Izumi M, Tang X, Chiu C, et al. Ten cases of sebaceous carcinoma arising in nevus sebaceus. J Dermatol. 2008;35:704–11.

23. Matsuda K, Doi T, Kosaka H, et al. Sebaceous carcinoma arising in nevus sebaceus. J Dermatol. 2005;32:641–4.

24. Kazakov DV, Calonje E, Zelger B, et al. Sebaceous carcinoma arising in nevus sebaceus of Jadassohn: a clinicopathological study of five cases. Am J Dermatopathol. 2007;29:242–8.

25. van de Warrenburg BP, van Gulik S, Renier WO, et al. The linear naevus sebaceus syndrome. Clin Neurol Neurosurg. 1998;100:126–32.

26. Happle R. Gustav Schimmelpenning and the syndrome bearing his name. Dermatology. 2004;209:84–7.

27. Warnke PH, Hauschild A, Schimmelpenning G, et al. The sebaceous nevus as part of the Schimmelpenning-Feuerstein-Mims syndrome – an obvious phacomatosis first documented in 1927. J Cutan Pathol. 2003;30:470–2.

28. Feuerstein RC, Mims LC. Linear nevus sebaceus with convulsions and mental retardation. Am J Dis Child. 1962;104:675–9.

29. Happle R. The group of epidermal nevus syndromes Part I. Well defined phenotypes. J Am Acad Dermatol. 2010;63:1–22.

30. Xin H, Matt D, Qin JZ, et al. The sebaceous nevus: a nevus with deletions of the PTCH gene. Cancer Res. 1999;59:1834–6.

31. Takata M, Tojo M, Hatta N, et al. No evidence of deregulated patched-hedgehog signaling pathway into trichoblastomas and other tumors arising within nevus sebaceous. J Invest Dermatol. 2001;117:1666–70.

32. Jonathan LL, Li CT, Lynn MB, et al. Whole exome sequencing reveals somatic mutations in *HRAS* and *KRAS* which cause nevus sebaceous. J Invest Dermatol. 2013 Mar;133(3):827–30.

33. Hurley HJ, LoPresti PJ. Steatocystoma multiplex. Arch Dermatol. 1965;92:110–11.

34. Cho S, Chang SE, Choi JH, et al. Clinical and histologic features of 64 cases of steatocystoma multiplex. J Dermatol. 2002;29:152–6.

35. Covello SP, Smith FJ, SillevisSmitt JH, Paller AS, Munro CS, Jonkman MF, et al. Keratin 17 mutations cause either steatocystoma multiplex or pachyonychia congenita type 2. Br J Dermatol. 1998;139(3):475–80.

36. Smith FJ, Corden LD, Rugg EL, et al. Missense mutations in keratin 17 cause either pachyonychia congenita type 2 or a phenotype resembling steatocystoma multiplex. J Invest Dermatol. 1997;108:220–3.

37. Gianotti R, Cavicchini S, Alessi E. Simultaneous occurrence of multiple trichoblastomas and steatocystoma multiplex. Am J Dermatopathol. 1997;19:294–8.

38. Steffen C, Ackerman AB. Neoplasms with sebaceous differentiation. Philadelphia: Lea & Febiger; 1994. 751p.

39. Salim A, Reece SM, Smith AG, et al. Sebaceous hyperplasia and skin cancer in patients undergoing renal transplant. J Am Acad Dermatol. 2006; 55:878–81.

40. Pang SM, Chau YP. Cyclosporine-induced sebaceous hyperplasia in renal transplant patients. Ann Acad Med Singapore. 2005;34:391–3.

41. Requena L, Roo E, Sanchez YE. Plate-like sebaceous hyperplasia overlying dermatofibroma. J Cutan Pathol. 1992;19:253–5.

42. Dahlhoff M, de Angelis MH, Wolf E, Schneider MR. Ligand-independent epidermal growth factor receptor hyperactivation increases sebaceous gland size

and sebum secretion in mice. Exp Dermatol. 2013;22:667–9.

43. Niemann C, Unden AB, Lyle S, Zouboulis Ch C, Toftgard R, Watt FM. Indian hedgehog and beta-catenin signaling: role in the sebaceous lineage of normal and neoplastic mammalian epidermis. Proc Natl Acad Sci USA. 2003;100 Suppl 1:11873–80.

44. Mehregan AH, Rahbari H. Benign epithelial tumors of the skin II: benign sebaceous tumors. Cutis. 1977;19:317–20.

45. Takeda H, Lyle S, Lazar AJF, et al. Human sebaceous tumors harbor inactivating mutations in LEF1. Nature Medicine. 2006;12:395–7.

46. Lo CC, Berta MA, Braun KM, et al. Characterization of bipotential epidermal progenitors derived from human sebaceous gland: contrasting roles of c-Myc and beta-catenin. Stem Cells. 2008;26:1241–52.

47. Troy JL, Ackerman AB. Sebaceoma. A distinctive benign neoplasm of adnexal epithelium differentiating toward sebaceous cells. Am J Dermatopathol. 1984;6:7–13.

48. Misago N, Mihara I, Ansai S, Narisawa Y. Sebaceoma and related neoplasms with sebaceous differentiation: a clinicopathologic study of 30 cases. Am J Dermatopathol. 2002;24:294–304.

49. Misago N, Narisawa Y. Rippled-pattern sebaceoma. Am J Dermatopathol. 2001;23:437–43.

50. Richman S. Deficient mismatch repair: read all about it (Review). Int J Oncol. 2015 Aug;12.

51. Rao NA, Hidayat AA, McLean IW, Zimmerman LE. Sebaceous carcinomas of the ocular adnexa: a clinicopathologic study of 104 cases, with five-year follow-up data. Hum Pathol. 1982;13:113–22.

52. Shields JA, Demirci H, Marr BP, Eagle Jr RC, Shields CL. Sebaceous carcinoma of the eyelids: personal experience with 60 cases. Ophthalmology. 2004;111:2151–7.

53. Wick MR, Goellner JR, Wolfe JT, et al. Adnexal carcinomas of the skin. II Extraocular sebaceous carcinomas Cancer. 1985;56:1163–72.

54. Bailet JW, Zimmerman MC, Arnstein DP, et al. Sebaceous carcinoma of the head and neck: case report and literature review. Arch Otolaryngol Head Neck Surg. 1992;118:1245–9.

55. Nelson BR, Hamlet KR, Gillard M, et al. Sebaceous carcinoma. J Am Acad Dermatol. 1995;33:1–15.

56. Kazakov DV, Kutzner H, Spagnolo DV, et al. Discordant architectural and cytologic features in cutaneous sebaceous neoplasms – a classification dilemma: report of 5 cases. Am J Dermatopathol. 2009;31(1):31–6.

57. Shalin SC, Lyle S, Calonje E, Lazar AJL. Sebaceous neoplasia and the Muir–Torre syndrome: important connections with clinical implications. Histopathology. 2010 Jan;56(1):133–47.

58. Dasgupta T, Wilson LD, Yu JB. A retrospective review of 1349 cases of sebaceous carcinoma. Cancer. 2009;115:158–65.

59. Yeatts RP, Waller RR. Sebaceous carcinoma of the eyelid: pitfalls in diagnosis. Ophthal Plast Reconstr Surg. 1985;1:35–42.

60. Ansai S, Takeichi H, Arase S, et al. Sebaceous carcinoma: an immunohistochemical reappraisal. Am J Dermatopathol. 2011;33:579–87.

61. Ruizeveld de Winter JA, Trapman J, Vermey M, et al. Androgen receptor expression in human tissues: an immunohistochemical study. J Histochem Cytochem. 1991;39:927–36.

62. Bayer-Garner IB, Givens V, Smoller B. Immunohistochemical staining for androgen receptors: a sensitive marker of sebaceous differentiation. Am J Dermatopathol. 1999;21:426–31.

63. Mulay K, White VA, Shah SJ, Honavar SG. Sebaceous carcinoma: clinicopathologic features and diagnostic role of immunohistochemistry (including androgen receptor). Can J Ophthalmol. 2014;49(4):326–32.

64. Asadi-Amoli F, Khoshnevis F, Haeri H, et al. Comparative examination of androgen receptor reactivity for differential diagnosis of sebaceous carcinoma from squamous cell and basal cell carcinoma. Am J Clin Pathol. 2010;134:22–6.

65. Fan YS, Carr RA, Sanders DSA, et al. Characteristic Ber-EP4 and EMA expression in sebaceoma is immunohistochemically distinct from basal cell carcinoma. Histopathology. 2007;51:80–6.

66. Plaza JA, Mackinnon A, Carrillo L, Prieto VG, Sangueza M, Suster S. Role of Immunohistochemistry in the diagnosis of sebaceous carcinoma: A Clinicopathologic and Immunohistochemical Study. Am J Dermatopathol. 2015;37(11):809–21.

67. Beer TW, Shepherd P, Theaker JM. Ber EP4 and epithelial membrane antigen aid distinction of basal cell, squamous cell and basosquamous carcinomas of the skin. Histopathology. 2000; 37:218–23.

68. Liu Y, Lyle S, Yang Z, Cotsarelis G. Keratin 15 promoter targets putative epithelial stem cells in the hair follicle bulge. J Invest Dermatol. 2003;121:963–8. doi:10.1046/j.1523-1747.2003.12600.

69. Yang HM, Cabral E, Dadras SS, Cassarino DS. Immunohistochemical expression of D2-40 in benign and malignant sebaceous tumors and comparison to basal and squamous cell carcinomas. Am J Dermatopathol. 2008;30(6):549–54.

70. Misago N, Narisawa Y. Cytokeratin 15 expression in neoplasms with sebaceous differentiation. J Cutan Pathol. 2006;33:634–41.

71. Krahl D, Sellheyer K. Basal cell carcinoma and pilomatrixoma mirror human follicular embryogenesis as reflected by their differential expression patterns of SOX9 and β-catenin. Br J Dermatol. 2010;162(6):1294–301.

72. Heyl J, Mehregan D. Immunolabeling pattern of cytokeratin 19 expression may distinguish sebaceous tumors from basal cell carcinomas. J Cutan Pathol. 2008;35:40–5.

73. Straub BK, Herpel E, Singer S, et al. Lipid droplet-associated PAT-proteins show frequent and differential expression in neoplastic steatogenesis. Mod Pathol. 2010;23:480–92.

74. Muthusamy K, Halbert G, Roberts F. Immunohistochemical staining for adipophilin, perilipin and TIP47. J Clin Pathol. 2006;59:1166–70.

75. Ostler DA, Prieto VG, Reed JA, et al. Adipophilin expression in sebaceous tumors and other cutaneous lesions with clear cell histology: an immunohistochemical study of 117 cases. Mod pathol. 2010;23:567–73.

76. Boussahmain C, Mochel MC, Hoang MP. Perilipin and adipophilin expression in sebaceous carcinoma and mimics. Hum Pathol. 2013;44:1811–6.

77. Jakobiec FA, Mendoza PR. Eyelid sebaceous carcinoma: clinicopathologic and multiparametric immunohistochemical analysis that includes adipophilin. Am J Ophthalmol. 2014;157:186.e2–208.e2.

78. Milman T, Schear MJ, Eagle Jr RC. Diagnostic utility of adipophilin immunostain in periocular carcinomas. Ophthalmology. 2014;121:964–71.

79. Chen WS, Chen PL, Li J, et al. Lipid synthesis and processing proteins ABHD5, PGRMC1 and squalene synthase can serve as novel immunohistochemical markers for sebaceous neoplasms and differentiate sebaceous carcinoma from sebaceoma and basal cell carcinoma with clear cell features. J Cutan Pathol. 2013;40:631–8.

80. Gonzalez-Fernandez F, Kaltreider SA, Patnaik BD, Retief JD, Bao Y, Newman S, Stoler MH, Levine PA. Sebaceous carcinoma: tumor progression through mutational inactivation of p53. Ophthalmology. 1998;105:497–506.

81. Cabral ES, Auerbach A, Killian JK, Barrett TL, Cassarino DS. Distinction of benign sebaceous proliferations from sebaceous carcinomas by immunohistochemistry. Am J Dermatopathol. 2006;28:465–71.

82. Kiyosaki K, Nakada C, Hijiya N, et al. Analysis of p53 mutations and the expression of p53 and p21WAF1/CIP1 protein in 15 cases of sebaceous carcinoma of the eyelid. Invest Ophthalmol Vis Sci. 2010;51:7–11.

83. Kim N, Kim JE, Choung HK, Lee MJ, Khwarg SI. Expression of cell cycle regulatory proteins in eyelid sebaceous gland carcinoma: low p27 expression predicts poor prognosis. Exp Eye Res. 2014;118:46–52.

84. McBride SR, Leonard N, Reynolds NJ. Loss of p21(WAF1) compartmentalisation in sebaceous carcinoma compared with sebaceous hyperplasia and sebaceous adenoma. J Clin Pathol. 2002;55:763–6.

85. Hasebe T, Mukai K, Yamaguchi N, et al. Prognostic value of immunohistochemical staining for PCNA, p53, and c-erbB-2 in sebaceous gland carcinoma and sweat gland carcinoma: comparison with histopathological parameter. Mod Pathol. 1994;7:37–43.

86. Calder KB, Khalil FK, Schlauder S, Cualing HD, Morgan MB. Immunohistochemical expression of survivin in cutaneous sebaceous lesions. Am J Dermatopathol. 2008;30:545–8.

87. Vandewalle C, Van Roy F, Berx G. The role of the ZEB family of transcription factors in development and disease. Cell Mol Life Sci. 2009;66:773–87.

88. Bhardwaj M, Sen S, Sharma A, Kashyap S, Chosdol K, Pushker N, Bajaj MS, Bakhshi S. ZEB2/SIP1 as novel prognostic indicator in eyelid sebaceous gland carcinoma. Hum Pathol. 2015;46(10):1437–42.

89. Ivan D, Prieto VG, Esmaeli B, Wistuba II, Tang X, Lazar AJ. Epidermal growth factor receptor (EGFR) expression in periocular and extraocular sebaceous carcinoma. J Cutan Pathol. 2010 Feb;37(2):231–6.

90. Lee MJ, Kim N, Choung HK, Choe JY, Khwarg SI, Kim JE. Increased gene copy number of HER2 and concordant protein overexpression found in a subset of eyelid sebaceous gland carcinoma indicate HER2 as a potential therapeutic target. J Cancer Res Clin Oncol. 2015;4.

91. Muir EG, Bell AJY, Barlow KA. Multiple primary carcinoma of the colon, duodenum and larynx associated with keratoacanthoma of the face. Br J Surg. 1967;54:191.

92. Torre D. Multiple sebaceous gland tumors. Arch Dermatol. 1968;98:549.

93. Singh RS, Grayson W, Redston M, et al. Site and tumor type predicts DNA mismatch repair status in cutaneous sebaceous neoplasia. Am J Surg Pathol. 2008;32(6):936.

94. Peltomaki P. Role of DNA mismatch repair defects in the pathogenesis of human cancer. J Clin Oncol. 2003;21:1174.

95. Kruse R, Ruzicka T. DNA mismatch repair and the significance of a sebaceous skin tumor for visceral cancer prevention. Trends Mol Med. 2004;10:136.

96. Dietmaier W, Wallinger S, Bocker T, et al. Diagnostic microsatellite instability: definition and correlation with mis-match repair protein expression. Cancer Res. 1997;57:4749.

97. Kruse R, Rütten A, Hosseiny-Malayeri HR, et al. "Second hit" in sebaceous tumors from Muir–Torre patients with germline mutations in MSH2: allele loss is not the preferred mode of inactivation. J Invest Dermatol. 2001;116:463.

98. Abdel-Rahman WM, Peltomaki P. Lynch syndrome and related familial colorectal cancers. Crit Rev Oncog. 2008;14:1–22.

99. Lucci-Cordisco E, Zito I, Gensini F, Genuardi M. Hereditary nonpolyposis colorectal cancer and related conditions. Am J Med Genet A. 2003;122A:325–34.

100. Popnikolov NK, Gatalica Z, Colome-Grimmer MI, et al. Loss of mismatch repair proteins in sebaceous gland tumors. J Cutan Pathol. 2003;30:178.

101. Kruse R, Rutten A, Schweiger N, et al. Frequency of microsatellite instability in unselected sebaceous gland neoplasias and hyperplasias. J Invest Dermatol. 2003;120:858.

102. Cesinaro AM, Ubiali A, Sighinolfi P, et al. Mismatch repair proteins expression and microsatellite instability in skin lesions with sebaceous differentiation: a study in different clinical subgroups with and without extracutaneous cancer. Am J Dermatopathol. 2007;29:351.

103. Chhibber V, Dresser K, Mahalingam M. MSH-6: extending the reliability of immunohistochemistry

as a screening tool in Muir-Torre syndrome. Mod Pathol. 2008;21:159.

104. Orta L, Klimstra DS, Qin J, et al. Towards identification of hereditary DNA mismatch repair deficiency: sebaceous neoplasm warrants routine immunohistochemical screening regardless of patient's age or other clinical characteristics. Am J Surg Pathol. 2009;33:934–44.

105. Abbas O, Mahalingam M. Cutaneous sebaceous neoplasms as markers of Muir-Torre syndrome: a diagnostic algorithm. J Cutan Pathol. 2009;36:613–9.

106. Marazza G, Masouye I, Taylor S, et al. An illustrative case of Muir-Torre syndrome: contribution of immunohistochemical analysis in identifying indicator sebaceous lesions. Arch Dermatol. 2006;142:1039.

107. Roberts ME, Rigert-Johnson DL, Thomas BC, et al. Screening for Muir-Torre syndrome using mismatch repair protein immunohistochemistry of sebaceous neoplasms. J Genet Counsel. 2013;22:393–405.

108. Ponti G, Venesio T, Losi L, et al. BRAF mutations in multiple sebaceous hyperplasias of patients belonging to MYH-associated polyposis pedigrees. J Invest Dermatol. 2007;127:1387–91.

109. Morales-Burgos A, Sánchez JL, Figueroa LD, De Jesús-Monge WE, Cruz-Correa MR, González-Keelan C, Nazario CM. MSH-2 and MLH-1 protein expression in Muir Torre syndrome-related and sporadic sebaceous neoplasms. P R Health Sci J. 2008;27(4):322–7.

110. Niemann C, Owens DM, Hulsken J, Birchmeier W, Watt FM. Expression of DeltaNLef1 in mouse epidermis results in differentiation of hair follicles into squamous epidermal cysts and formation of skin tumours. Development. 2002;129:95–109.

111. Zanesi N, Croce CM. Fragile histidine triad gene and skin cancer. Eur J Dermatol. 2001;11:401–4.

112. Fong LY, Fidanza V, Zanesi N, et al. Muir–Torre-like syndrome in Fhit-deficient mice. Proc Natl Acad Sci USA. 2000;97:4742–7.

113. Weiske J, Albring KF, Huber O. The tumor suppressor Fhit acts as a repressor of beta-catenin transcriptional activity. Proc Natl Acad Sci USA. 2007;104:20344–9.

114. Goldberg M, Rummelt C, Foja S, Holbach LM, Ballhausen WG. Different genetic pathways in the development of periocular sebaceous gland carcinomas in presumptive Muir–Torre syndrome patients. Hum Mutat. 2006;27:155–62.

115. Holbach LM, von Moller A, Decker C, Junemann AG, Rummelt-Hofmann C, Ballhausen WG. Loss of fragile histidine triad (FHIT) expression and microsatellite instability in periocular sebaceous gland carcinoma in patients with Muir–Torre syndrome. Am J Ophthalmol. 2002;134:147–8.

116. Benjamin CL, Ananthaswamy HN. p53 and the pathogenesis of skin cancer. Toxicol Appl Pharmacol. 2007;224:241–8.

117. Niemann C, Owens DM, Schettina P, Watt FM. Dual role of inactivating Lef1 mutations in epidermis: tumor promotion and specification of tumor type. Cancer Res. 2007;67:2916–21.

118. Umar A, Boland CR, Terdiman JP, et al. Revised Bethesda guidelines for hereditary nonpolyposis colorectal cancer (Lynch syndrome) and microsatellite instability. J Natl Cancer Inst. 2004;96:261–8.

119. Aung PP, Batrani M, Mirzabeigi M, Goldberg LJ. Extraocular sebaceous carcinoma in situ: report of three cases and review of the literature. J Cutan Pathol. 2014;41:592–6.

Part III

Immunohistology of Cutaneous Metastases and Its Simulators

Cutaneous Metastasis

5

Danielle M. Wehle, Martin Sangueza, and Sadia Salim

Introduction

Cutaneous metastasis, the spread of a primary malignancy to the skin, occurs in 0.6–10.4% of patients with a malignancy [1]. Metastases represent approximately 2% of all cutaneous tumors [1]. They are notoriously difficult to identify for a number of reasons. They may occur from several months up to 5 years after the diagnosis of a primary malignancy with an average of 33 months from primary diagnosis [2]. It is helpful to recognize that the majority of skin metastases tend to occur in close proximity to the primary tumor. For example, breast and lung carcinomas tend to metastasize to the chest wall [3]. Colorectal, ovarian and bladder carcinomas tend to metastasize to the abdomen. Additionally, metastases are known to occur at incisional sites from surgeries related to the primary malignancy [3]. However, a retrospective review of 4020 patients with metastatic dis-

ease (10% of which had cutaneous metastasis) showed 39% of those with cutaneous metastasis had distant metastasis. Although all tumor types were represented among those with distant metastasis, the tumors most likely to result in remote disease were melanoma, lung carcinoma, and breast carcinoma. Additionally, scalp metastases were more common in those with metastatic renal cell carcinoma [3].

In addition to the delay in the emergence of skin metastasis after diagnosis of a primary malignancy and the frequent occurrence of distant cutaneous metastasis, an additional challenge in recognizing a skin metastasis is that it may be the first sign of malignancy (37% men, 6% women) [1]. Lastly, even when a primary diagnosis is available this information is often not added to the clinical history a pathologist receives.

Due to the difficulties inherent to identifying cutaneous metastases the pathologist must not only gather as much clinical information as possible but also employ a panel of immunostains. We examine the various immunohistochemical markers that aid a pathologist in narrowing the differential diagnosis and or pinpointing the primary site of a cutaneous metastasis.

Metastatic Carcinoma

Given the difficulties in recognizing a cutaneous metastasis, knowledge of the most frequent primary tumors metastasizing to skin can be very useful.

Authors' note The introduction and section on metastatic carcinoma is written by Danielle M. Wehle, M.D.M.S. The abstract and section on metastatic melanoma is written by Sadia Salim, M.D. Photomicrographs in this chapter are reproduced with the permission of Dr. Jose Plaza.

D.M. Wehle, M.D., M.S. (✉) • S. Salim, M.D.
Department of Dermatopathology, Miraca Life Sciences, 6655 N. MacArthur Blvd, 76262 Irving, TX, USA
e-mail: daniellemwehle@gmail.com

M. Sangueza, M.D.
Department of Pathology, Hospital Obrero Nro 1, Avda Brazil S/n, 6541 La Paz, Bolivia

© Springer International Publishing Switzerland 2016
J.A. Plaza, V.G. Prieto (eds.), *Applied Immunohistochemistry in the Evaluation of Skin Neoplasms*, DOI 10.1007/978-3-319-30590-5_5

The primary tumor types which give rise to skin metastases vary by gender and age. One study showed that in men the most common skin metastases are lung carcinoma (24 %), colorectal carcinoma (19 %), melanoma (13 %), and oral squamous cell carcinoma (12 %) and in women breast carcinoma (69 %), colorectal carcinoma (9 %), melanoma (5 %), and ovarian carcinoma (5 %) [4]. Another study demonstrated that in men melanoma was the most frequent source of skin metastasis (32 %) followed by lung (11.8 %), colon and rectum (11 %), oral cavity (8.7 %), larynx (5.5 %), and kidney (4.7 %) [3]. In this study as in the previous study breast was the most frequent source of cutaneous metastasis in women (70.7 %), followed by melanoma (12.0 %), ovary (3.3 %), oral cavity (2.3 %), and lung (2.0 %). The high incidence of skin metastasis from breast carcinoma relative to other tumor types may be explained in part by the superficial location of the breast as compared to internal visceral malignancies. In both male and female children the most common skin metastases are neuroblastoma, rhabdomyosarcoma, and leukemia [4].

The diverse expression patterns of cytokeratins (CK) have been correlated with different pathways of epithelial differentiation and allow the pathologist to subtype epithelial cells and identify the origin of metastatic carcinomas [5]. Keratins are differentially expressed in human tissues and when tissue undergoes malignant transformation this keratin expression pattern is retained [6]. As a result, many studies have been performed to examine these expression patterns for the purpose of identifying metastatic malignancies of unknown primary. Cytokeratin 7 (CK7) and CK20 expression patterns have been shown to be the most discriminating in this regard [5–7]. Some important lessons and useful expression patterns have been gleaned from studying CK7 and CK20 (Table 5.1).

As described above, breast adenocarcinoma is the most frequent type of malignancy to metastasize to skin. Twenty five percent of women with breast carcinoma develop cutaneous metastasis [8]. This poses a problem not only due to the morphologic similarities between breast adenocarcinomas and primary cutaneous adnexal neoplasms but also due to the immunohistochemical staining similarities. Common breast markers such as ER, PR, and GCDFP also stain primary cutaneous adnexal neoplasms. As a result, epithelial markers such as p63 and p40 have been employed to aid in this distinction.

p63 is a protein encoded by the p63 gene, a member of the p53 gene family. p63 is expressed in the basal cells and adnexal structures of normal skin. The p63 antibody recognizes all six of the p63 protein isoforms and has been used as a marker of epithelial and squamous differentiation in tumors from several sites of origin such as lung, esophagus, and head and neck.

p63 has been shown to be valuable in distinguishing adnexal neoplasms, both primary and metastatic, from metastatic adenocarcinomas which are typically negative for p63 [9] (Figs. 5.1 and 5.2). Exceptions to this pattern are mucinous carcinomas (both primary and metastatic) and apocrine carcinomas which are typically negative for p63 [9].

The use of p63 antibody coupled with podoplanin (D240) has also been shown to be useful in distinguishing primary cutaneous neoplasms from metastatic adenocarcinomas [10] (Figs. 5.1, 5.2, 5.3 and 5.4). One study stained 37 primary cutaneous neoplasms including adnexal tumors and basal and squamous cell carcinomas as well as 42 metastatic adenocarcinomas. Primary lesions showed variable positivity with podoplanin but all metastatic lesions were negative. In addition all primary cutaneous tumors were positive for p63 and all metastatic lesions were negative [10] (Figs. 5.3, 5.4, 5.5, 5.6, 5.7, and 5.8). However other studies report p63 expression in 11–22 % and podoplanin expression in 4 % of cutaneous metastases [11, 12].

p40 antibody recognizes 3 of the 6 p63 protein isoforms and recently has been touted as having a sensitivity similar to that of p63 while being more specific for identifying primary cutaneous lesions. One study compared the utility of p63, CK5/6, p40, and Gata 3 in a total of 143 cases including 67 primary adnexal tumors and 76 cutaneous metastases. P40, p63, CK5/6, and GATA3 expression was observed in 80 %, 84 %, 86 %, and 47 % of primary adnexal tumors,

Table 5.1 CK7/CK20 expression patterns

Tumor type	CK7+/CK20+ (%)		CK7+/CK20− (%)		CK7−/CK20+ (%)		CK7−/CK20− (%)	
	Weiss et al.	Wang et al.	Weiss et al.	Wang et al.	Weiss et al.	Wang et al.	Weiss et al.	Wang et al.
Breast, ductal carcinoma	0 (0/20)	16 (6/38)	95 (19/20)	82 (31/38)	0 (0/20)	3 (1/38)	5 (1/20)	0 (0/38)
Breast, lobular carcinoma	0 (0/6)	9 (1/11)	100 (6/6)	91 (10/11)	0 (0/6)	0 (0/11)	0 (0/6)	0 (0/11)
Colorectum, adenocarcinoma	5 (1/20)	10 (4/40)	0 (0/20)	0 (0/40)	95 (19/20)	75 (30/40)	0 (0/20)	15 (6/40)
Esophagus, squamous cell carcinoma	0 (0/14)	NA	21 (3/14)	NA	0 (0/14)	NA	79 (11/14)	NA
Head and neck, squamous cell carcinoma	0 (0/30)	NA	27 (8/30)	NA	6 (2/30)	NA	67 (20/30)	NA
Kidney, renal cell carcinoma	0 (0/19)	0 (0/17)	11 (2/19)	24 (4/17)	0 (0/19)	6 (1/17)	89 (17/19)	71 (12/17)
Liver, hepatocellular	0 (0/11)	7 (2/30)	9 (1/11)	17 (5/30)	9 (1/11)	0 (0/30)	82 (9/11)	77 (23/30)
Lung, adenocarcinoma	10 (1/10)	N/A	90 (9/10)	N/A	0 (0/10)	N/A	0 (0/10)	N/A
Lung, small cell carcinoma	0 (0/7)	0 (0/11)	43 (3/7)	18 (2/11)	0 (0/7)	0 (0/11)	57 (4/7)	82 (9/11)
Lung, squamous cell carcinoma	0 (0/15)	0 (0/12)	47 (7/15)	0 (0/12)	0 (0/15)	8 (1/12)	53 (8/15)	89 (11/12)
Ovary, adenocarcinoma	4 (1/24)	0 (0/19)	96 (23/24)	100 (19/19)	0 (0/24)	0 (0/19)	0 (0/24)	0 (0/19)
Skin, Merkel cell carcinoma	0 (0/9)	N/A	0 (0/9)	N/A	78 (7/9)	N/A	12 (2/9)	N/A

Data adapted from Chu P, et al. Mod Pathol 2000; 13(9):962–72

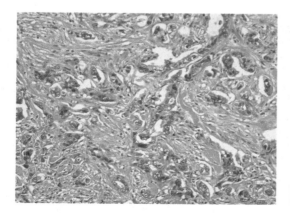

Fig. 5.1 Metastatic carcinoma. *H&E* hematoxylin and eosin stain

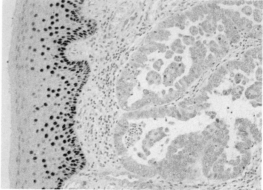

Fig. 5.2 Metastatic carcinoma negative p63 immunohistochemistry (IHC)

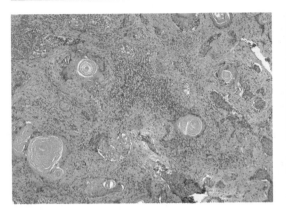

Fig. 5.3 Microcystic adnexal carcinoma H&E

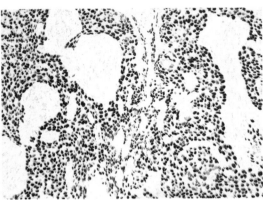

Fig. 5.6 Poorly differentiated squamous cell carcinoma positive p63 IHC

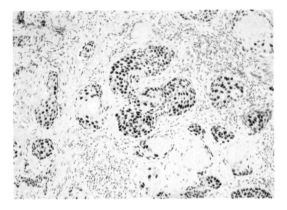

Fig. 5.4 Microcystic adnexal carcinoma positive p63 IHC

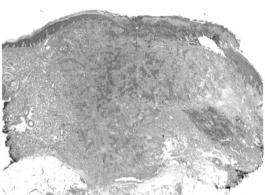

Fig. 5.7 Poorly differentiated adnexal carcinoma H&E

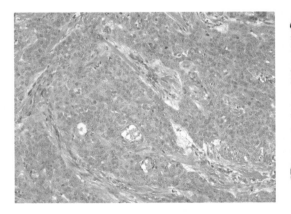

Fig. 5.5 Poorly differentiated squamous cell carcinoma H&E

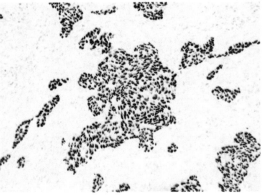

Fig. 5.8 Poorly differentiated adnexal carcinoma positive p63

respectively, and in 8 %, 17 %, 26 %, and 40 % of cutaneous metastasis, respectively. P63, p40, and CK5/6 have similar sensitivity (84 %, 80 %, and 86 %, respectively) in detecting primary adnexal tumors. However, p40 antibody had a 92 % specificity as compared to p63 (84 %) and CK5/6 (86 %) and p40 had the best positive predictive value (90 %) [13].

Another of the most frequent cutaneous metastases is colorectal adenocarcinoma which may metastasize to the skin producing nodules, plaques or ulcerated lesions on the abdomen, umbilicus (Sister Mary Joseph nodule) or perineum as well as in sites of previous surgical incision. Glandular dermal tumor nodules are commonly seen as well as single cell necrosis with many neutrophils (dirty necrosis). The typical immunohistochemical pattern seen is CK7 negative, CK20 positive (82 %) [5]. However, 10 % may be CK7 and CK20 negative [5]. Interestingly if CK7 and CK20 are both positive it has been reported that the primary site is more commonly rectum rather than colon [7]. This is important information as one review reports that most colorectal tumors with skin metastases originate in the rectum [1]. In short, one should remember to consider a rectal primary when identifying a CK7 and CK20 positive cutaneous metastasis.

Not only may CK7 and CK20 prove helpful in identifying colorectal cutaneous metastasis but CDX2 has been reported to be a highly sensitive and specific marker of colorectal adenocarcinomas [14]. The CDX2 antibody targets an intestine specific transcription factor expressed in the nuclei of epithelial cells from the duodenum to the rectum. A review of 476 tumors from colon, duodenum and rectum using the monoclonal antibody CDX2-88 showed that CDX2 was expressed in 76–100 % of tumor cells in all but one tumor evaluated. However CDX2 staining was seen in rare examples of mucinous carcinoma of the ovary and adenocarcinoma of the bladder [14]. Another more recent study reviewed 118 cases of colorectal carcinoma and showed that CDX2 stained 114 of 118 (97 %) of them [15].

Lung carcinomas are the most common cutaneous metastasis in men and the leading cause of death from carcinoma in men. Approximately 50 % of non-small cell carcinomas (adenocarcinoma and squamous cell carcinoma) and 80 % of small cell carcinomas are metastatic at the time of diagnosis [4]. Lung adenocarcinomas in particular may be difficult to distinguish from primary cutaneous adnexal neoplasms. It is useful to recognize that 90 % of lung adenocarcinomas are CK7 positive and CK20 negative. Additionally, 78 % of metastatic lung carcinomas stain with TTF-1 according to one study [16]. In this study 11/11 (100 %) of metastatic lung adenocarcinomas stained with TTF-1 while 6/7 (86 %) of small cell carcinomas were positive for TTF-1. The so-called large cell carcinomas were also studied and 15/19 (79 %) stained with TTF-1. All metastatic squamous cell carcinomas (3) were negative. Lung squamous cell carcinomas are also usually CK7 and CK20 negative (70 %) and may be difficult if not impossible to distinguish from primary cutaneous squamous cell carcinoma [6].

It is also important to note that 76 % of small cell carcinomas of the lung are negative for both CK7 and CK20 [5]. These lesions are also Cam 5.2 positive and negative for Merkel cell polyoma virus (MCPyV) distinguishing them from Merkel cell carcinoma.

Although ovarian carcinomas rarely metastasize to the skin, they are one of the most common types of skin metastasis in women. Late in the course of the disease 3–4 % of patients with ovarian cancer will develop metastasis [1]. Metastases from ovarian carcinomas, like colorectal metastases, occur on the abdomen, in prior surgical incisions and on the umbilicus (Sister Mary Joseph nodule). The histology of these metastases typically demonstrates a glandular or papillary architecture. 98 % of ovarian carcinomas are CK7+/CK20−. Only 2 % of ovarian adenocarcinomas are CK7+ and CK20+ [6]. CA125 is positive in 90 % of ovarian carcinomas while WT1 is positive in 76 % [17].

Squamous cell carcinomas of the oral cavity are one of the most common sources of metastasis to skin in men [1]. These tumors usually metastasize to the neck or face. Typically these patients have a known primary tumor and the metastasis occurs at the site of surgery for the primary tumor. Otherwise these tumors may be indistinguishable from primary cutaneous squamous cell carcinomas. Both P63 and MNF116 have shown high sensitivity for squamous cell carcinomas and are useful in identifying poorly differentiated squamous cell carcinomas [18]. However, an important pitfall to keep in mind is that MNF116 has shown false positivity in leiomyosarcoma and p63 may show nonspecific cytoplasmic staining in leiomyosarcomas [19]. It has been reported that p40 has comparable specificity for cutaneous sarcomatoid squamous cell carcinoma but that p40 is less sensitive than p63 in this regard (56 % and 81 % respectively) [20].

Metastatic Melanoma

Malignant melanoma is a highly aggressive tumor accounting for approximately 3 % of all tumors [21]. The ability of melanoma to metastasize is well known which most commonly occurs through lymphatic and hematogenous spread followed by direct extension. The most common presentation of metastatic melanoma is locoregional and occurs in the vicinity of the primary melanoma. In-transit metastasis is defined as the occurrence of metastatic deposit greater than 5 cm away from the primary lesion within the areas served by the same lymphatic drainage. This type of metastasis occurs most frequently on the extremities and scalp. Melanoma can also metastasize to distant sites anywhere on the body [21, 22]. Plaza et al. studied 115 cases of metastatic melanoma and reported the most frequent sites of cutaneous metastasis included the legs, scalp, arm, and face [23]. Another study conducted by Marcoval et al. investigated the metastatic behavior in malignant melanoma including metastasis to visceral sites. Their study showed that visceral metastases occurred in 92 of the 1083 patients and the most common sites of visceral metastases were lung, brain, liver, and bone. Metastatic melanoma predicts a poor clinical outcome with a 5-year relative overall survival rate of only about 16 % [24]. Patients with locoregional, distant nodal, and soft tissue metastasis

have a better survival rate (1-year survival rate of 62 %) than the patients with visceral metastasis (1-year survival rate for pulmonary metastasis 53 %, 1-year survival for non-pulmonary visceral metastases 33 %) [24, 25].

Skin metastases from melanoma represent a relatively frequent event in the natural history of the disease and can develop in both early and late stages of disease. Various studies show that cutaneous or subcutaneous lesions arise in 10–17 % of patients affected by melanoma and approximately 50 % of patients with metastatic disease develop skin involvement [21, 26–29]. In up to 5 % of patients, a metastatic deposit is the first manifestation of the disease. Wolf et al. reported that cutaneous metastasis may be the first clue that lymphatic or hematogenous spread has occurred [30].

In most cases, the diagnosis of metastatic melanoma is made easier by the recurrence being detected during routine follow-up after treatment of primary disease. This is particularly true when the metastasis presents at or close to the site of excision. Occasionally, difficulties in diagnosis can arise when the metastasis occurs many years after diagnosis of primary melanoma. The metastatic deposits can be distant from the original melanoma site and adopt unusual clinical appearances mimicking other benign or malignant cutaneous lesions. Such cases may be mistaken both clinically and histologically with non-melanoma skin cancer, primary melanoma or with benign melanocytic nevi. Distinction of skin metastasis from primary melanoma is of paramount importance because the therapeutic management and the implications for disease stage can be drastically different.

Melanoma metastatic to the skin usually involves the dermis and subcutaneous fat; however, in some cases, the lesions may be located superficially. The typical histologic appearance of metastatic melanoma is a tumor deposit in the dermis or subcutis, without epidermotropism (Fig. 5.9). The cytology is usually epithelioid and scattered mitoses may be noted. Cytoplasmic pigment may be seen. The depth of the dermal nodule is typically more than the width of the lesion. Less commonly, epidermotropic metastatic melanoma can be seen (Fig. 5.10). Studies have documented

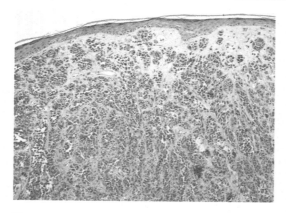

Fig. 5.9 Metastatic melanoma. *H&E* hematoxylin and eosin

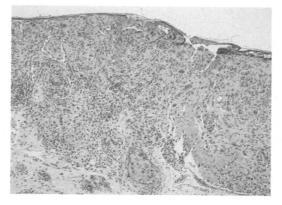

Fig. 5.10 Epidermotropic metastatic melanoma. *H&E* hematoxylin and eosin

the histopathologic features of melanomas metastatic to the skin [31, 33]. These studies have shown that in some cases, secondary melanomas in the skin cannot be distinguished reliably from lesions arising there, because of the overlapping histologic features. A study by White and Hitchcock summarized characteristics of metastatic melanoma, which make it challenging to distinguish metastatic melanoma from primary melanoma at that site and even a benign melanocytic nevus [31]. These characteristics include the ability for epidermotropic growth beyond the lateral confines of a dermal component, formation of epidermal collarettes around nodules in the dermis, the ability for solely intraepidermal growth with the appearance of in situ melanoma, tumor symmetry, nevoid cytological features, and apparent dermal "maturation." Metastatic melanoma with spindled cytology and cytoplasmic pigment may be mistaken for a blue nevus (Fig. 5.11). Similarly, nevoid cytology and "maturation" in metastatic melanoma be misleading and the findings interpreted as an intradermal nevus (Fig. 5.12). The cells in metastatic melanoma show uniform atypia compared to the heterogeneous cytology and pleomorphism seen in primary melanoma.

Metastatic melanoma my mimic various epithelial and soft tissue lesions. Plaza et al. in their study observed unusual features in cutaneous metastatic melanoma that closely simulated metastatic carcinoma (Fig. 5.13), dermatofibroma,

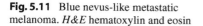

Fig. 5.11 Blue nevus-like metastatic melanoma. *H&E* hematoxylin and eosin

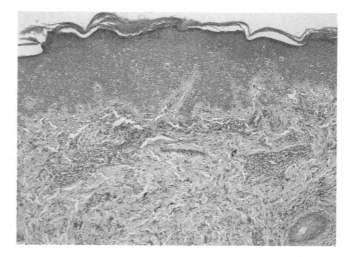

Fig. 5.12 Metastatic melanoma with nevoid configuration and "maturation." *H&E* hematoxylin and eosin

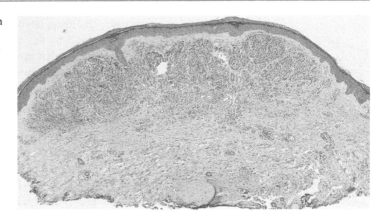

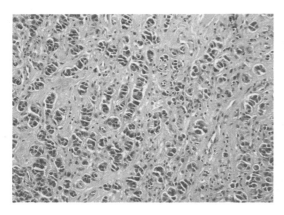

Fig. 5.13 Carcinoma-like metastatic melanoma with cord and single cells infiltrating the dermis mimicking metastatic breast carcinoma. *H&E* hematoxylin and eosin

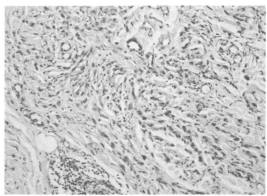

Fig. 5.15 Metastatic melanoma with pseudovascular structures and angiosarcoma like features. *H&E* hematoxylin and eosin

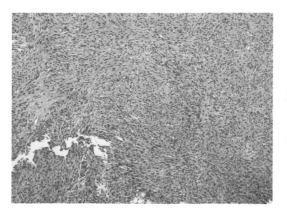

Fig. 5.14 Metastatic melanoma with spindle cells arranged in long fascicles mimicking leiomyosarcoma. *H&E* hematoxylin and eosin

leiomyosarcoma (Fig. 5.14), angiosarcoma (Fig. 5.15), nevoid melanoma, halo nevus, blue nevi, atypical fibroxanthoma (Fig. 5.16), and lym-

phoma. Metastatic melanomas with small cell, rhabdoid, signet ring, and balloon cell cytology have also been described (Fig. 5.17). Stromal changes may exhibit myxoid change or osseous metaplasia [23]. Metastatic melanoma should always be considered in the differential diagnosis of a new cutaneous lesion in patients who present with a malignancy of unknown origin.

Immunohistochemical staining is extensively used to differentiate melanomas from tumors that they mimic in conventionally stained sections. No stains can reliably differentiate metastatic melanoma from a primary lesion. Another commonly recognized confounding feature of some melanoma metastases is the loss of classic melanocyte differentiation markers such as S-100, HMB-45, Melan-A, and tyrosinase, sometimes described as an "antigenic shift" in tumor pro-

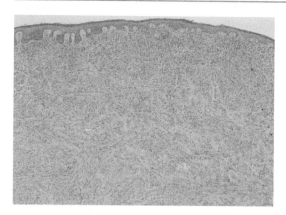

Fig. 5.16 Metastatic melanoma with features of atypical fibroxanthoma. *H&E* hematoxylin and eosin

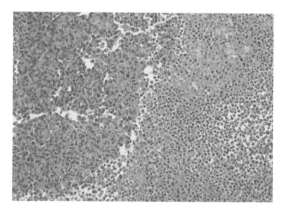

Fig. 5.17 Metastatic melanoma with rhabdoid cytology. *H&E* hematoxylin and eosin

gression [30, 32, 35] (Table 5.2). In the evaluation of a tumor as possible metastatic melanoma, a carefully selected, broad-spectrum panel of immunohistochemical stains should be performed.

S100 is a 21 kDa acidic calcium-binding protein and is widely used as a marker of melanocytic differentiation. S100 has 97–100% sensitivity as a melanocytic marker [34]. It is nuclear and cytoplasmic stain and greater than 95% of melanomas stain with this antibody. When compared to staining with other melanocytic markers, it is the most sensitive marker for spindle cell/desmoplastic melanomas. The specificity of S100 is reported to be 75–87% for melanocytic tumors and it stains numerous other non-melanocytic tumors including those derived

Table 5.2 Melanocytic marker expression in metastatic melanoma

Markers	Expression in metastatic melanoma	Comment
S100	97–100%	Sensitive marker for spindle/desmoplastic melanoma
Mart-1/Melan A	75–92%	
HMB-45	63–93%	Can be used to distinguish spindle/desmoplastic melanoma from blue nevus
MiTF	81–100%	Stains tumor of many lineage. Most useful in highlighting intraepidermal melanocytes in primary melanoma
SOX-10	99–100%	Does not stain dendritic melanocytes which helps distinguish pigmented melanophages from melanocytes in the evaluation nodal metastasis. Similar sensitivity to S100 for spindle/demoplastic melanoma. Stains neural and myoepithelial cells

Data Source: Ohsie et al. Immunohistochemical characteristics of melanoma. J Cutan Pathol. 2008

from nerve sheath cells, myoepithelial cells, adipocytes, chondrocytes and Langerhans cells [34]. It can also stain spindle cells in dermal scars and should be used with caution in the evaluation of melanoma re-excision, especially desmoplastic melanoma. S100 should be used in parallel with other more specific melanocytic markers to reliably distinguish melanoma form other S100 positive malignancies.

Human melanoma black (HMB-45) a marker of the cytoplasmic premelanosomal glycoprotein gp100, was one of the first melanoma "specific" markers discovered. It is a cytoplasmic stain with reported sensitivity of HMB-45 for melanoma ranging from 69% to 90%. The expression of HMB-45 is reported to be maximal in primary melanoma specimens (77–100%) and less in metastases (58–83%) [34, 40]. HMB-45 shows a zonal staining pattern in benign melanocytic nevi. The most intense staining is seen in the epidermal melanocytes of compound nevi with a gradual and subsequent loss of stain from top to bottom of the dermal component. Ordinary dermal nevi are HMB-45 negative. Uniform staining is seen in melanoma without any gradient. However, there are exceptions to this staining pattern, particularly in the setting of certain nevic variants of melanoma. Therefore interpretation of HMB-45 staining should be done with caution, the pattern of expression should not be the only criterion in classifying a melanocytic lesion as benign versus a malignant lesion. There is strong and uniform staining in blue nevi. This can be helpful feature as spindle cell and desmoplastic melanomas tend to be HMB-45 negative.

Melanoma antigen recognized by T-cells-1 (MART-1) and Melan-A are synonyms for a cytoplasmic protein of melanosomal differentiation recognized by T-cells. Two monoclonal antibodies, A103, generally referred to as Melan-A and M2-7C10 referred to as Mart-1, have been raised against this protein. Both are cytoplasmic stains and have a 100 % correlation with regard to staining in melanoma. The staining is more specific than S100 and is reported to be 95–100 %. There is also diffuse and intense staining of the dermal component of melanoma. The sensitivity is reported 75–92 % for melanocytic neoplasms [34, 35]. In addition to melanocytes, there is staining of PEComas (angiomyolipomas, lymphangiomyomatosis, pulmonary "sugar" tumors), some clear cell sarcoma. Clone A103 (Melan-A) also shows positive staining in adrenocortical tumors as well as testicular Leydig cell tumors and ovarian Sertoli–Leydig tumors.

MiTF (Microopthalmia transcription factor) is a gene essential in the development and survival of melanocytes. It is a nuclear stain with a reported sensitivity of 81–100 % for melanocytes. Although initially thought to be highly specific, it is now reported to stain many tumors including renal cell carcinoma, neurothekeoma, breast carcinoma, and spindle cell neoplasms. Busam et al. reported in a study that MiTF shows positive staining in dermal histiocytes, fibroblasts, Schwann cells and smooth muscle cells in addition to melanocytes and should be interpreted with caution [36].

In recent years, SOX-10 (SRY (Sex Determining Region Y)-Box 10), a nuclear transcription factor that plays an important role in the differentiation of neural crest progenitor cells to melanocytes, has emerged as a reliable marker of neural crest differentiation. It is consistently expressed in tumors of schwannian and melanocytic lineage and reportedly been shown to be a sensitive and specific marker of primary and metastatic malignant melanoma. In comparing the expression of SOX-10 in melanoma of various histologic subtypes versus carcinoma, benign nevi, and non-neoplastic tissue, Mohamed et al. reported the sensitivity and specificity for SOX-10 in the diagnosis of melanoma as 1.0 and 0.93, respectively and the positive and negative predictive values as 0.87 and 1.0, respectively [37]. In a separate study, Willis et al. evaluated the expression of SOX-10 in melanoma metastatic to lymph node and compared it with S100, HMB-45 and Mart-1 [41]. In their study SOX-10 staining showed a staining intensity which was statistically significant when compared with S100 protein, HMB-45, and Melan-A. Their study also showed that a higher percentage of tumor cells stained with SOX-10, compared to S100 protein, HMB-45, and Melan-A. SOX-10 is a nuclear stain with a crisp nuclear staining superior to both S100 and Mart-1 stain. In addition to schwannian and melanocytic tumors, SOX-10 also stains tumors of myoepithelial origin.

Ki-67 a proliferation marker and is expressed in proliferating cells. Benign nevi show reactivity less than 1 % of cells, typically in the epidermal component or the very superficial portion of the lesion. Melanoma, on the other hand shows greater than 10 % reactivity with a more random pattern of staining, particularly in the deep dermal portion of the lesion. The combined pattern of reactivity of HMB-45 and Ki-67, which show maturation with descent in the dermal component, is helpful in differentiating a benign nevus from nevoid melanoma.

A 2004 study by Kovach et al. assessed whether selected immunohistochemistry might permit more confident separation of malignant primary and secondary metastatic melanoma of the skin [28]. They studied several immunohistochemical markers including p53, bcl-2, CD117/c-kit, and Ki67. They observed differences in reference to CD117/c-kit expression and showed

Table 5.3 Immunohistochemical panel for evaluation of metastatic melanoma

Markers	Metastatic melanoma	Carcinoma	Leiomyosarcoma	Merkel cell carcinoma	Lymphoma	Atypical fibroxanthoma
S100	+	−	−	−	−	−
SOX-10	+	−	−	−	−	−
Mart-1	+	−	−	−	−	−
Cytokeratin	−	+	−	+	−	−
Desmin	−	−	+	−	−	−
Myogenin/Myo-D1	Not well studied in melanoma	−	+	−	−	−
CD31	−	−	−	−	−	−
CD45 (LCA)	−	−	−	−	+	−
CK20	−	−	−	+	−	−
CD68	−/+	−/+	−	−	−/+	+

The table depicts typical positive and negative staining in metastatic melanoma

that secondary deposits of melanoma generally lose CD117. However, there is controversy about whether or not c-kit expression is preserved in cutaneous metastases or is useful in this setting. The specificity of CD117 is low with regard to melanocytic lesions. Many other tumor stain positive with CD117, including clear cell sarcoma, gastrointestinal stromal tumors, mastocytoma, and myeloid leukemia, and is seldom used in the diagnosis of melanocytic lesions.

A broad panel with at least two or more melanocytic markers should be employed when evaluating for unusual presentations of metastatic melanoma. The immunohistochemical stains should be interpreted with caution, since certain histologic variants, such as metastatic melanoma with rhabdoid cytology has been reported to have variable immunoprofile. Also, metastatic melanoma may lose some of the classic melanocytic markers or may have aberrant expression of non-melanocytic markers [32, 38, 39, 42]. Depending on the histologic findings, the panel of immunohistochemical stains may need to include markers for non-melanoma skin metastasis or primary tumors. These include but are not limited to cytokeratin stains (p63, CK5/6, AE1/3, pancytokeratin) for spindled sarcomatoid squamous cell carcinoma, fibrohistiocytic markers (CD34, Factor XIII) for dermatofibrosarcoma protruberans and dermatofibroma, desmin, smooth muscle actin (SMA) myogenin, Myo-D1 for leiomyosarcoma and rhabdomyosarcoma. In cases of melanoma with small cell morphology, LCA (CD45) and CK20 will help differentiate melanoma from a lymphoid malignancy and Merkel cell carcinoma (Table 5.3).

References

1. Alcaraz I, Cerroni L, Rutten A, Kutzner H, Requena L. Cutaneous metastases from internal malignancies: a clinicopathologic and immunohistochemical review. Am J Dermatopathol. 2012;34:347–93.
2. Saeed S, Keehn CA, Morgan MB. Cutaneous metastasis: a clinical, pathologic and immunohistochemical appraisal. J Cutan Pathol. 2004;31:419–30.
3. Lookingbill DP, Spangler N, Helm KF. Cutaneous metastasis: a clinical, pathologic and immunohistochemical appraisal. J Am Acad Dermatol. 1993;29:228–36.
4. Hussein MRA. Skin metastasis: a pathologist's perspective. J Cutan Pathol. 2010;37:e1–20.
5. Chu P, Wu E, Weiss LM. Cytokeratin 7 and cytokeratin 20 expression in epithelial neoplasms: a survey of 435 cases. Mod Pathol. 2000;13(9):962–72.
6. Weiss LM. Keratin expression in human tissues and neoplasms. Histopathology. 2002;40:403–39.
7. Zhang PJ, Shah M, Spiegel GW, Brooks JJ. Cytokeratin 7 immunoreactivity in rectal adenocarcinomas. Appl Immunohistochem Mol Morphol. 2003;11(4):306–10.
8. Rollins-Raval M, Chivukula M, Tseng GC, Jukic D, Dabbs DJ. An immunohistochemical panel to differentiate metastatic breast carcinoma to skin from primary sweat gland carcinomas with a review of the literature. Arch Pathol Lab Med. 2011;135:975–83.

9. Ican D, Nash JW, Prieto VG, Calonje E, Lyle S, Diwan AH, et al. Use of p63 expression in distinguishing primary and metastatic cutaneous adnexal neoplasms from metastatic adenocarcinoma to skin. J Cutan Pathol. 2007;34:474–80.

10. Plaza JA, Ortega PF, Stockman DL, Suster S. Value of p63 and podoplanin (D2-40) immunoreactivity in the distinction between primary cutaneous tumors and adenocarcinomas metastatic to the skin: a clinicopathologic and immunohistochemical study of 79 cases. J Cutan Pathol. 2010;37:403–10.

11. Mahalingam M, Nguyen LP, Richards JE, Muzikansky A, Hoang MP. The diagnostic utility of immunohistochemistry in distinguishing primary skin adnexal carcinomas from metastatic adenocarcinoma to skin: an immunohistochemical reappraisal using cytokeratin 15, nestin, p63, D2-40 and calretinin. Mod Pathol. 2010;23:713–9.

12. Qureshi HS, Ormsby AH, Lee MW, Zarbo RJ, Ma CK. The diagnostic utility of p63, CK 5/6, CK7 and CK20 in distinguishing primary cutaneous adnexal neoplasms from metastatic carcinomas. J Cutan Pathol. 2004;31:145–52.

13. Lee JJ, Mochel MC, Piris A, Boussahmain C, Mahalingam M, Hoang MP. p40 exhibits better specificity than p63 in distinguishing primary skin adnexal carcinomas from cutaneous metastases. Hum Pathol. 2014;45:1078–83.

14. Werling RW, Yaziji H, Bacchi CE, Gown AM. CDX2, a highly sensitive marker of adenocarcinomas of intestinal origin: an immunohistochemical survey of 476 primary and metastatic carcinomas. Am J Surpathol. 2003;27(3):303–10.

15. Bayrak R, Haltas H, Yenidunya S. The value of CDX2 and cytokeratins 7 and 20 expression in differentiating colorectal adenocarcinomas from extraintestinal gastrointestinal adenocarcinomas: cytokeratin 7–/20+ phenotype is more specific than CDX2 antibody. Diagn Pathol. 2012;7:9.

16. Srodon M, Westra WH. Immunohistochemical staining for thyroid transcription factor-1: a helpful aid in discerning primary site of tumor origin in patients with brain metastases. Hum Pathol. 2002; 33(6):642–5.

17. Tornos C, Soslow R, Chen S, Akram M, Hummer AJ, Abu-Rustum N, et al. Expression of WT1, CA125 and GCDFP-15 as useful markers in the differential diagnosis of primary ovarian carcinomas versus metastatic breast cancer to the ovary. Am J Surg Pathol. 2005;29(11):1482–9.

18. Alomari AK, Glusac EJ, Mcniff JM. P40 is a more specific marker than p63 for cutaneous poorly differentiated squamous cell carcinoma. J Cutan Pathol. 2014;41:838–45.

19. Dotto JE, Glusac EJ. p63 is a useful marker for cutaneous spindle cell squamous cell carcinoma. J Cutan Pathol. 2006;33:413–7.

20. Ha Lan TT, Chen SJT, Arps DP, Fullen DR, Patel RM, Siddiqui J, et al. Expression of the p40 isoform of p63 has high specificity for cutaneous sarcomatoid squamous cell carcinoma. J Cutan Pathol. 2014; 41:831–8.

21. Tas F. Metastatic behavior in melanoma: timing, pattern, survival, and influencing factors. J Oncol. 2012;2012:647–84. Published online 2012 June 27.

22. Soong SJ, Harrison RA, McCarthy WH, Urist MM, Balch CM. Factors affecting survival following local, regional, or distant recurrence from localized melanoma. J Surg Oncol. 1998;67(4):228–33.

23. Plaza JA, Torres-Cabala C, Evans H, Diwan HA, Suster S, Prieto VG. Cutaneous metastases of malignant melanoma: a clinicopathologic study of 192 cases with emphasis on the morphologic spectrum. Am J Dermatopathol. 2010;32(2):129–36.

24. Marcoval J, Ferreres JR, Martín C, Gómez S, Penín RM, Ochoa de Olza M, et al. Patterns of visceral metastasis in cutaneous melanoma: a descriptive study. Actas Dermosifiliogr. 2013;104(7):593–7.

25. Gershenwald JE, Balch CM, Soong SJ, Thompson JF. Prognostic factors and natural history of melanoma. In: Balch CM, Houghton AN, Sober AJ, Soong SJ, Atkins MB, Thompson JF, editors. Cutaneous melanoma. 5th ed. St. Louis, MO: Quality Medical Publishing; 2009. p. 35–64.

26. Atkins MB, Hauschild A, Wahl RL, Balch CM. Diagnosis of Stage IV melanoma. In: Balch CM, Houghton AN, Sober AJ, Soong SJ, Atkins MB, Thompson JF, editors. Cutaneous melanoma. 5th ed. St. Louis, MO: Quality Medical Publishing; 2009. p. 573–602.

27. Savoia P, Fava P, Nardò T, Osella-Abate S, Quaglino P, Bernengo MG. Skin metastases of malignant melanoma: a clinical and prognostic survey. Melanoma Res. 2009;19(5):321–6.

28. Guerriere-Kovach PM, Hunt EL, Patterson JW, Glembocki DJ, English 3rd JC, Wick MR. Primary melanoma of the skin and cutaneous melanomatous metastases: comparative histologic features and immunophenotypes. Am J Clin Pathol. 2004;122(1):70–7.

29. Balch CM, Gershenwald JE, Soong SJ, Thompson JF, Atkins MB, Byrd DR, et al. Final version of 2009 AJCC melanoma staging and classification. J Clin Oncol. 2009;27(36):6199–206.

30. Wolf IH, Richtig E, Kopera D, Kerl H. Locoregional cutaneous metastases of malignant melanoma and their management. Dermatol Surg. 2004;30:244–7.

31. White WL, Hitchcock MG. Dying dogma: the pathological diagnosis of epidermotropic metastatic malignant melanoma. Semin Diagn Pathol. 1998;15(3):176–88.

32. Pulitzer M, Brady MS, Blochin E, Amin B, Teruya-Feldstein J. Anaplastic large cell lymphoma: a potential pitfall in the differential diagnosis of melanoma. Arch Pathol Lab Med. 2013;137(2):280–3.

33. Damsky WE, Rosenbaum LE, Bosenberg M. Decoding melanoma metastasis. Cancers (Basel). 2010;3(1):126–63.

34. Prieto VG, Shea CR. Immunohistochemistry of melanocytic proliferations. Arch Pathol Lab Med. 2011;135(7):853–9.

35. Plaza JA, Suster D, Perez-Montiel D. Expression of immunohistochemical markers in primary and metastatic malignant melanoma: a comparative study in 70 patients using a tissue microarray technique. Appl Immunohistochem Mol Morphol. 2007;15(4):421–5.

36. Busam KJ, Iversen K, Coplan KC, Jungbluth AA. Analysis of microphthalmia transcription factor expression in normal tissues and tumors, and comparison of its expression with S-100 protein, gp100, and tyrosinase in desmoplastic malignant melanoma. Am J Surg Pathol. 2001;25(2):197–204.

37. Mohamed A, Gonzalez RS, Lawson D, Wang J, Cohen C. SOX10 expression in malignant melanoma, carcinoma, and normal tissues. Appl Immunohistochem Mol Morphol. 2013;21(6):506–10.

38. Aisner DL, Maker A, Rosenberg SA, Berman DM. Loss of S100 antigenicity in metastatic melanoma. Hum Pathol. 2005;36(9):1016–9.

39. Ko CJ, Mcniff JM, Glusac EJ. Squamous cell carcinomas with single cell infiltration: a potential diagnostic pitfall and the utility of MNF116 and p63. J Cutan Pathol. 2008;35:353–7.

40. Rothberg BE, Moeder CB, Kluger H, Halaban R, Elder DE, Murphy GF, et al. Nuclear to non-nuclear Pmel17/gp100 expression (HMB45 staining) as a discriminator between benign and malignant melanocytic lesions. Mod Pathol. 2008;21(9):1121–9.

41. Willis BC, Johnson G, Wang J, Cohen C. SOX10: a useful marker for identifying metastatic melanoma in sentinel lymph nodes. Appl Immunohistochem Mol Morphol. 2015;23(2):109–12.

42. Drier JK, Swanson PE, Cherwitz DL, et al. S100 protein immunoreactivity in poorly differentiated carcinomas. Immunohistochemical comparison with malignant melanoma. Arch Pathol Lab Med. 1987;111:447–52.

Part IV
Immunohistology of Mesenchymal Neoplasms

Immunohistology and Molecular Studies of Fibrohistiocytic and Myofibroblastic Cutaneous Tumors

6

Danny Ghazarian, Sebastien Labonte,
Brendan Craig Dickson, and Ayman Al Habeeb

Introduction

Fibrohistiocytic tumors of the skin and superficial soft tissues form a loosely defined group of mesenchymal lesions with variable fibroblastic and myofibroblastic differentiation. This group includes extremely common tumors (e.g., dermatofibroma) and extremely rare ones (e.g., myxoinflammatory fibroblastic sarcoma). We chose to restrict the scope of this chapter to a limited number of entities with clinical or academic interest. Several excellent reviews on this subject have been published in recent years [1–3].

D. Ghazarian, MB, ChB, PhD, FRCPC (✉)
Laboratory Medicine Program, University Health
Network, 200 Elizabeth St., Toronto, ON,
Canada, M5G 2C4
e-mail: dr.danny.ghazarian@uhn.ca

S. Labonte, MD, FRCP(C)
Department of Pathology,
CHU-L'Hotel-Dieu de Quebec,
11 Cote du Palais, Quebec, QC, Canada, G1R 2J6

B.C. Dickson, BA, BSc, MD, MSc, FCAP, FRCP(C)
Department of Pathology and Laboratory Medicine,
Mount Sinai Hospital, 600 University Ave, Suite
6.500.12.5, Toronto, ON, Canada, M5G 1X5

A. Al Habeeb, MBBS, FRCPC
Department of Laboratory Medicine and
Pathobiology, University Health Network,
UHN, Eaton Wing, 11th Floor, 200 Elizabeth Street,
Toronto, ON, Canada, M5G 2C4

The vast majority of fibrohistiocytic tumors of the skin and superficial soft tissues are easily diagnosed by conventional histopathology, with minimal need for ancillary immunohistochemical or molecular testing like FISH or RT-PCR. The aim of this chapter is to briefly review morphology and expose salient immunohistochemical and molecular features that can be used to resolve diagnostic dilemmas.

Dermatofibroma

Clinical

Dermatofibromas (synonym: benign fibrous histiocytoma) are very common skin tumors. They can occur virtually anywhere on the skin, but tend to favor the extremities. There is a small female predominance. Their size varies from a few millimeters to approximately 2 cm. Palpation reveals a firm nodule, and pinching the lesion can cause "dimpling," a downward movement of the tumor. The biological behavior is benign, with occasional local recurrence/persistence, mainly after incomplete excision, and exceptionally rare metastasis. Cellular dermatofibroma have a recurrence rate of approximately 20–30 %, and probably deserve a more thorough excision, based on clinical considerations that cannot be determined by histopathology.

© Springer International Publishing Switzerland 2016
J.A. Plaza, V.G. Prieto (eds.), *Applied Immunohistochemistry in the Evaluation of Skin Neoplasms*, DOI 10.1007/978-3-319-30590-5_6

Histopathology

Morphologically, dermatofibromas are centered on the dermis and are poorly demarcated. There is occasionally superficial involvement of the hypodermis (Figs. 6.1 and 6.2), either along fibrous septae or as a bulbous rounded protrusion. The fibrous background can be prominent or inconspicuous and the mid-power architecture is typically storiform. The overlying epidermis can be hyperplastic and hyperpigmented, with occasional small basaloid proliferations resembling superficial basal cell carcinoma. At the tumor–dermis interface, there is generally a characteristic "entrapment" of coarse collagen bundles by tumor cells (Fig. 6.3). Many different cell types are found in varying proportions (Fig. 6.4),

creating multiple histological variants (see Table 6.1). Spindle cells resembling fibroblasts, ovoid cells with features of histiocytes, and some multinucleated cells are the basic populations that one can observe. Plump spindle cells with myofibroblastic features, "foam cells," endothelial cells, lymphocytes, and sometimes neutrophils, eosinophils, and plasma cells complete the picture. Occasionally, hemosiderin is abundant, with or without extravasated red blood cells and gaping vascular spaces, or blood-filled cavities without endothelial lining.

Epithelioid dermatofibroma has traditionally been considered as a morphological variant of dermatofibroma. Morphologically it is composed of angulated epithelioid cells that resemble intradermal Spitz nevus.

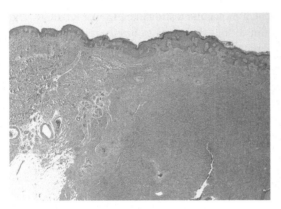

Fig. 6.1 Dermatofibroma, low power H&E. Tumor involves dermis and superficial hypodermis

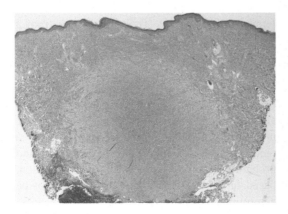

Fig. 6.2 Dermatofibroma, low power H&E. Tumor involves dermis and superficial hypodermis

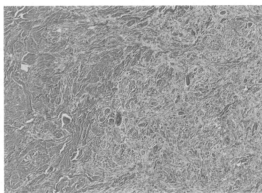

Fig. 6.3 Dermatofibroma, mid power H&E. Entrapment of coarse collagen fibers and storiform architecture

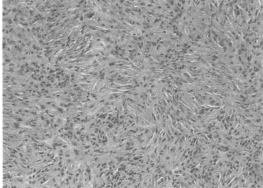

Fig. 6.4 Dermatofibroma, high power H&E. Storiform architecture and mixture of different cell types

Table 6.1 Histologic variants of dermatofibroma (not exhaustive)

– Dermatofibroma with atypical/monster cells
– Atrophic dermatofibroma
– Deep dermatofibroma
– Cellular dermatofibroma
– Aneurysmal dermatofibroma
– Hemosiderotic dermatofibroma
– Dermatofibroma rich in giant cells
– Dermatofibroma with clear cells
– Dermatofibroma with xanthomatous (lipidized) changes
– Dermatofibroma with granular cells
– Dermatofibroma with myxoid changes
– Epithelioid dermatofibroma

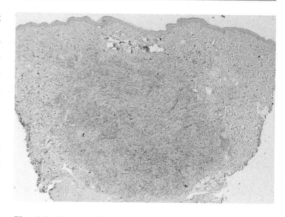

Fig. 6.5 Dermatofibromas, low power factor XIIIa. The tumor is stained stronger than the adjacent dermis

Immunohistochemistry

Dermatofibromas rarely cause any diagnostic difficulty. Immunohistochemistry is generally only required with very limited biopsies, or in unusual cases bearing morphologic overlap with other entities (e.g., dermatofibrosarcoma protuberans, melanocytic lesions, etc.).

Numerous cells express factor XIIIa in dermatofibroma. This is well appreciated at low power where the density of factor XIIIa positive cells is higher in the lesion than in the adjacent dermis (Figs. 6.5 and 6.6). Conversely, CD34 positive cells are rare in dermatofibroma. This can also be well appreciated at low power (Figs. 6.7 and 6.8). In fact, CD34-positive dermal fibroblasts appear to be pushed away by the dermatofibroma, sometimes realizing a peripheral zone rich in CD34-positive cells. Occasionally, fascicles of CD34 positive cells are seen in an otherwise typical dermatofibroma. That should not be interpreted as positivity for CD34 in the lesional cells. Stromelysin 3 and D2-40 (Fig. 6.9) have been reported to stain like factor XIIIa in dermatofibroma [6, 7], while ApoD is negative [8]. It is important to keep in mind that factor XIIIa and other "positive markers" in dermatofibroma actually stain an increased number of cells *when compared to the adjacent dermis*. The assessment is somewhat qualitative and requires some judgment and experience in borderline cases. Finally, CD30 is reported to be positive in epithelioid der-

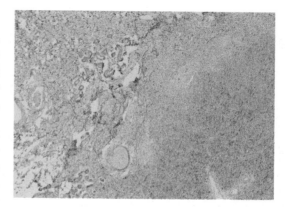

Fig. 6.6 Dermatofibromas, intermediate power factor XIIIa. The tumor is stained stronger than the adjacent dermis

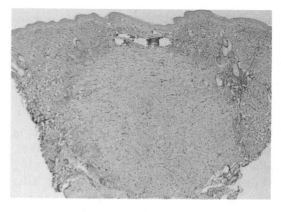

Fig. 6.7 Dermatofibromas, low power CD34. The tumor is stained less strongly than the adjacent dermis

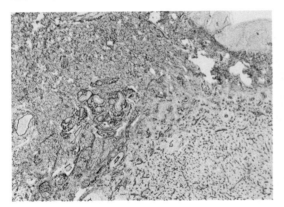

Fig. 6.8 Dermatofibromas, intermediate power CD34. The tumor is stained less strongly than the adjacent dermis

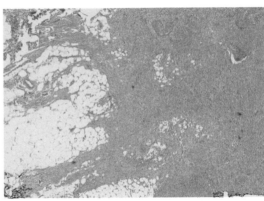

Fig. 6.10 Dermatofibroma, intermediate power H&E. Interstitial infiltration of hypodermis resembling a dermatofibrosarcoma protuberans

Fig. 6.9 Dermatofibroma and adjacent dermis, intermediate power D2-40. The tumor is stained stronger than the adjacent dermis, but weaker than the lymphatic endothelium (small dark brown lines at the upper right)

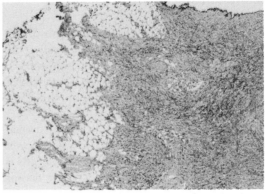

Fig. 6.11 Dermatofibroma, intermediate power factor XIIIa. Same lesion as Figure 6.10 with interstitial infiltration of hypodermis. The tumor stains strongly for factor XIIIa and is negative for CD34 (not shown)

matofibroma [4], and Doyle et al. [5] demonstrated that the majority are also ALK-1 positive (29/33; 88%).

Pitfalls

Sometimes, cellular dermatofibromas extend in the hypodermis, creating a focally "interstitial" infiltration of fat, resembling a DFSP (Fig. 6.10). In these cases, immunostaining for factor XIIIa (Fig. 6.11) and CD34 can be helpful, keeping in mind the peripheral zone of compressed CD34-positive fibroblasts in dermatofibroma. Other second line markers that can be useful are D2-40

and ApoD. In case of doubt, FISH or RT-PCR can be performed to exclude a DFSP.

There are occasional dermal fibrohistiocytic tumors with high cellularity and convincing positivity for CD34 and factor XIIIa (Figs. 6.12–6.17). To designate them, the name "indeterminate fibrohistiocytic lesion" has been proposed [9]. These lesions behave like cellular dermatofibromas, with a recurrence rate of approximately 15–20% when incompletely excised. Although the concept of an indeterminate fibrohistiocytic lesion with features of both dermatofibroma and dermatofibrosarcoma is probably not warranted, the descriptive term can be useful in clinical practice.

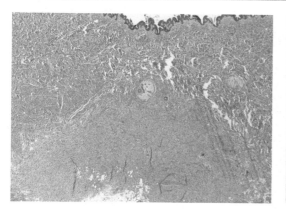

Fig. 6.12 Indeterminate fibrohistiocytic lesion, low power H&E

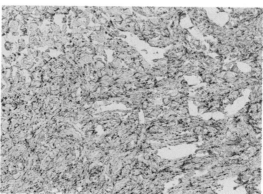

Fig. 6.15 Indeterminate fibrohistiocytic lesion, mid power factor XIIIa

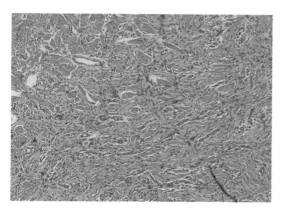

Fig. 6.13 Indeterminate fibrohistiocytic lesion, mid power H&E

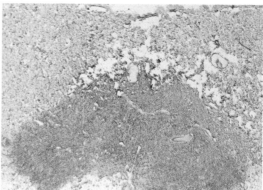

Fig. 6.16 Indeterminate fibrohistiocytic lesion, low power CD34

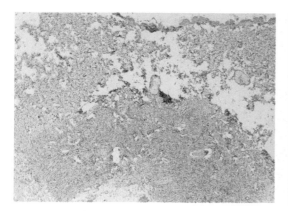

Fig. 6.14 Indeterminate fibrohistiocytic lesion, low power factor XIIIa

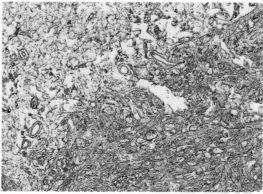

Fig. 6.17 Indeterminate fibrohistiocytic lesion, mid power CD34

Dermatofibrosarcoma Protuberans

Clinical

Dermatofibrosarcoma protuberans (DFSP) is a locally aggressive superficial fibroblastic neoplasm carrying a COL1A1-PDGFB fusion gene. It is relatively rare and favors young to middle-aged adults. It can be found in young children where it sometimes takes the morphology of a giant cell fibroblastoma. It occurs mainly on the trunk and proximal extremities, with a predilection for the shoulder and pelvic girdles. It is a slowly growing indurated plaque that eventually forms nodules and takes a red-brown to violaceous color. The tumor is firm on palpation and attached to the subcutaneous tissue. In a minority of cases, areas of tumor progression ("fibrosarcomatous transformation") to a higher grade spindle cell sarcoma are encountered. Fibrosarcomatous transformation of DFSP is associated with a 10–15 % risk of metastasis, whereas usual DFSP virtually never metastasizes.

Histopathology

Morphologically, DFSP shows a diffuse dermal infiltration by bland spindle cells arranged in a tight storiform pattern (Figs. 6.18 and 6.19). There is typically a diffuse "interstitial" infiltration of the hypodermis (Fig. 6.20), sometimes leaving large fat lobules uninvolved between layers of tumor. The epidermis is spared. The most superficial portion of the lesion can be relatively hypocellular and thus difficult to recognize on a small superficial biopsy. Morphological variants exist: myxoid DFSP, DFSP with myoid differentiation, pigmented DFSP (Bednar tumor, Fig. 6.21). Fibrosarcomatous transformation is loosely defined, but hypercellular areas forming long fascicles instead of a tight storiform pattern are worrisome, especially in the presence of increased nuclear atypia and mitotic activity (Figs. 6.22 and 6.23) [10].

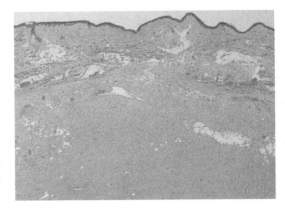

Fig. 6.18 Dermatofibrosarcoma protuberans, low power H&E

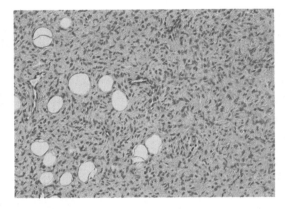

Fig. 6.19 Dermatofibrosarcoma protuberans, high power H&E

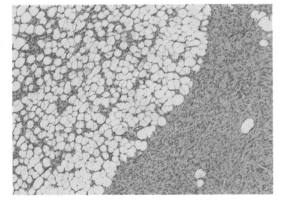

Fig. 6.20 Dermatofibrosarcoma protuberans, mid power H&E. Interstitial pattern of fat infiltration

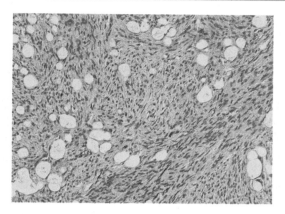

Fig. 6.21 Dermatofibrosarcoma protuberans, high power H&E. Pigmented cells containing melanin and positive for melanocytic markers are embedded in the tumor (pigmented dermatofibrosarcoma protuberans/Bednar tumor)

Fig. 6.22 Dermatofibrosarcoma protuberans with fibrosarcomatous transformation, low power H&E. Darker areas are hypercellular. This case was confirmed with RT-PCR for COL1A1-PDGFB fusion transcript

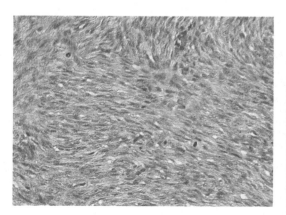

Fig. 6.23 Dermatofibrosarcoma protuberans with fibrosarcomatous transformation, high power H&E. Hypercellularity, fascicular architecture, and two mitotic figures in this 400X field (same tumor as Figure 6.22)

Immunohistochemistry

DFSP are virtually always CD34-positive, ApoD-positive, Factor XIIIa-negative, stromelysin 3-negative, and D2-40-negative in a nonequivocal manner (see discussion regarding dermatofibroma) (Figs. 6.24–6.27). These immunostains in combination can be very helpful in occasional cases where one hesitates between a dermatofibroma and a DFSP. Areas of fibrosarcomatous transformation can express CD34 and ApoD less strongly [11]. Pigmented DFSP contains melanocytes stained for conventional melanocytic markers (S100, Melan-A, HMB45).

Molecular

DFSP are characterized by supernumerary ring chromosomes containing sequences derived from chromosomes 17 and 22 and reciprocal translocation of t(17;22)(q22;q13) [12]. Both yield fusion of COL1A1 with PDGFB [13], placing exon 2 of PDGFB under the control of the COL1A1 promoter [14, 15]. The fusion product can be detected by RT-PCR [16], but FISH offers greater sensitivity, in part because it better encompasses the multitude of potential breakpoints that can occur within COL1A1 [16–18]. The chimeric fusion protein is believed to induce tumor proliferation via autocrine/paracrine stimulation of the PDGF receptor [15]. A majority of cases are characterized by this gene fusion [19], with other primary forms of rearrangement rarely reported [20].

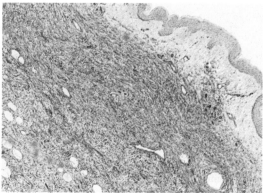

Fig. 6.24 Dermatofibrosarcoma protuberans, mid power CD34. Strong diffuse expression of CD34 is typical

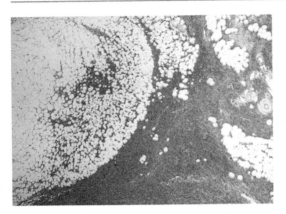

Fig. 6.25 Dermatofibrosarcoma protuberans, mid power CD34. Strong diffuse expression of CD34 enhances the interstitial infiltration of hypodermis

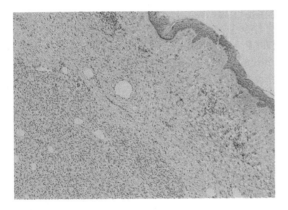

Fig. 6.26 Dermatofibrosarcoma protuberans, mid power factor XIIIa. Same area as Figure 6.24. Notice scattered positive cells outside the tumor, in the superficial dermis

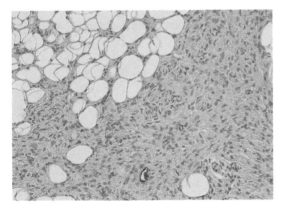

Fig. 6.27 Dermatofibrosarcoma protuberans, high power D2-40. Tumor cells are negative. Notice the small lymphatic channel stained strongly (lower center)

Pitfalls

DFSP can be very similar to other mesenchymal lesions: diffuse neurofibroma, spindle cell lipoma, plaque-like CD34-positive dermal fibroma.

Clues to Differentiate DFSP Versus Diffuse Neurofibroma

Both tumors can look disturbingly similar (Figs. 6.28–6.30), and the differential diagnosis can be challenging. Clinically, DFSP is firm and neurofibroma is soft. Careful scrutiny can sometimes detect an increased density of distorted nerve bundles in diffuse neurofibroma (Figs. 6.31 and 6.32). S100 and SOX10 are negative in DFSP and *sometimes focally positive* in neurofibroma, but this depends on the percentage of Schwann cells present. That percentage can be very low, so it is not always useful and negative staining is inconclusive (Figs. 6.33 and 6.34). Intralesional axons positive for synaptophysin (Fig. 6.35), neurofilament protein and PGP9.5 can be seen occasionally in neurofibroma; their presence is useful but their absence is inconclusive. In difficult cases, RT-PCR or preferably FISH should be used

Clues to Differentiate DFSP Versus Spindle Cell Lipoma

This is rarely a problem, but it may be difficult on a core biopsy, particularly in the absence of appropriate clinical information. DFSP are dermal-based and firm whereas spindle-cell lipoma are deeper and generally softer. Immunohistochemistry for androgen receptor is almost always positive in spindle cell lipoma [21] but no large series of DFSP has been assessed for expression of this marker. In select cases, molecular tests can help rule out a DFSP (Table 6.2).

Clues to Differentiate DFSP Versus Plaque-Like CD34-Positive Dermal Fibroma

This is an interesting problem (see section on CD34-positive dermal fibroma below), and the so-called atrophic variant of DFSP is very similar morphologically. Ultimately, molecular tests are required [22].

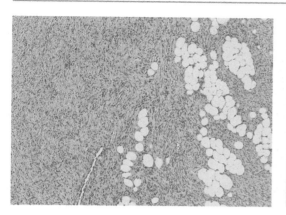

Fig. 6.28 Diffuse neurofibroma, mid power H&E. Diffuse neurofibroma can resemble dermatofibrosarcoma protuberans to a great extent, with storiform architecture and interstitial infiltration of fat

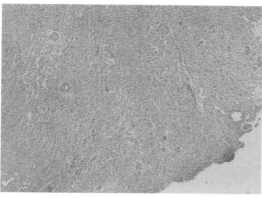

Fig. 6.31 Diffuse neurofibroma, low power H&E. Observation of distorted nerve bundles in the tumor is a strong clue to a diffuse neurofibroma. They are generally not as obvious as in this case however

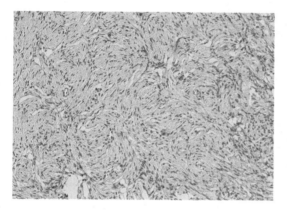

Fig. 6.29 Diffuse neurofibroma, high power factor XIIIa. Absence of staining for factor XIIIa and strong diffuse positivity for CD34 can mimic dermatofibrosarcoma protuberans almost to perfection

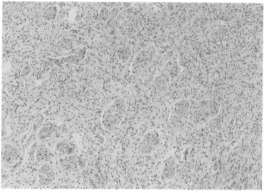

Fig. 6.32 Diffuse neurofibroma, mid power H&E. Observation of distorted nerve bundles in the tumor is a strong clue to a diffuse neurofibroma. They are generally not as obvious as in this case however

Atypical Fibroxanthoma

Clinical

Atypical fibroxanthoma (AFX) is in the overwhelming majority of cases a tumor of elderly people, predominantly males, occurring on sun damaged skin of the head and neck. Other locations can also be involved rarely (ocular conjunctiva, cornea, limbs, trunk) [23]. It occurs as a rapidly growing polypoid lesion with frequent ulceration, and a diameter generally less than 2 cm [24]. Despite cellular pleomorphism and worrisome histopathological features, the biological behavior is essentially benign, with cure

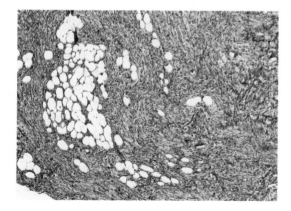

Fig. 6.30 Diffuse neurofibroma, mid power CD34. Absence of staining for factor XIIIa and strong diffuse positivity for CD34 can mimic dermatofibrosarcoma protuberans almost to perfection

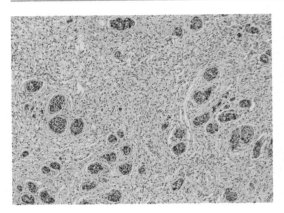

Fig. 6.33 Diffuse neurofibroma, mid power S100. The distorted nerve bundles contain numerous Schwann cells and are highlighted by S100. The rest of the neurofibroma however, is nearly devoid of S100-positive Schwann cells. Thus, the absence of Schwann cells does not exclude a diffuse neurofibroma

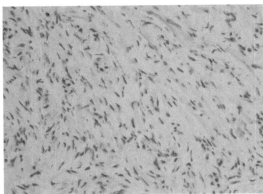

Fig. 6.35 Diffuse neurofibroma, high power synaptophysin. There are scattered synaptophysin-positive axons in the tumor (also positive for neurofilament and PGP9.5) ; a strong clue in favor of a neurofibroma. The absence of such axons, however, does not exclude a diffuse neurofibroma, since they are generally not as numerous as in the actual case

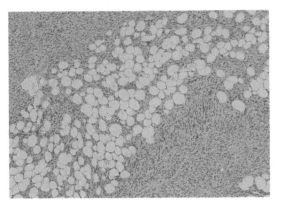

Fig. 6.34 Diffuse neurofibroma, mid power SOX10. Large fields of the tumor show a complete absence of SOX10-positive Schwann cells. This is not an unusual finding and the absence of Schwann cells does not exclude a diffuse neurofibroma

Table 6.2 Dermatofibroma versus dermatofibrosarcoma (immunohistochemistry)

	Dermatofibroma	Dermatofibrosarcoma
CD34	Negative	Positive
Factor XIIIa	Positive	Negative
Stromelysin 3	Positive	Negative
D2-40	Positive	Negative
ApoD	Negative	Positive
CD10	Positive	Focally positive

Histopathology

The low power silhouette is often polypoid with an epidermal collarette, but can also be plaque-like. The borders are usually circumscribed and the lesion commonly abuts on the lower epidermis. Ulceration is commonly observed (Fig. 6.36). There are varying combinations of spindle cells, plump ovoid cells, epithelioid cells, bizarre pleomorphic cells and multinucleated giant cells (Fig. 6.37). Mitotic figures are numerous and can be atypical. Other changes can be found (clear cells, granular cells, myxoid changes, keloidal changes, hemosiderin deposition, xanthomatization, lymphocytic infiltrate, pseudoangiomatous changes). The proliferation is centered in the dermis and can extend to a limited degree in the superficial hypodermis. The architecture can be

being achieved by a simple but complete excision. Recurrence after incomplete excision is well documented but rare [23]. Metastatic spread in incompatible with a diagnosis of AFX, and these cases are best designated as pleomorphic dermal sarcoma (see histopathology below). [24, 25] There is still some controversy as to the histogenesis of AFX, some evidence supporting a connection between AFX and sarcomatoid squamous cell carcinoma [26]. The debate is beyond the scope of this chapter.

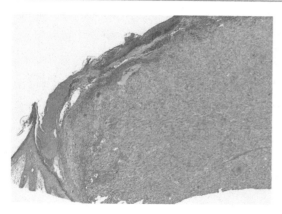

Fig. 6.36 Atypical fibroxanthoma, low power H&E. An ulcerated spindle cell tumor of the dermis with an epidermal collarette. Immunohistochemistry is necessary to resolve the differential diagnosis (see text)

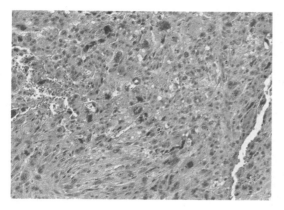

Fig. 6.37 Atypical fibroxanthoma, high power H&E. Pleomorphic spindle and epithelioid cells with a few monstrous nuclei consistent with an atypical fibroxanthoma. This is a diagnosis of exclusion and immunohistochemistry is required, as well as an excisional biopsy to assess the amount of necrosis, depth of invasion, perineural involvement, and vascular invasion

fascicular or storiform. The following are not acceptable in AFX: significant necrosis, vascular invasion, perineural invasion, significant involvement of hypodermis or deeper tissue. If present, those features warrant a diagnosis of pleomorphic dermal sarcoma [24]. Pleomorphic dermal sarcomas have a higher rate of recurrence (28 %) and can metastasize, albeit rarely (10 %) [25]. From a strictly histopathological point of view, the differential diagnosis includes: AFX, sarcomatoid squamous cell carcinoma (S-SCC), spin-

dle cell melanoma, angiosarcoma of the scalp, leiomyosarcoma, myxofibrosarcoma, and dermatofibroma with monster cells/atypical dermatofibroma. Immunohistochemistry is essential to resolve the issue since the diagnosis of AFX is one of exclusion.

Immunohistochemistry

By definition, cytokeratins must be negative, the commonly used antibodies or antibody cocktails being: AE1/3, MNF116, CAM5.2, 34BE12, CK5/6, CK14 (Figs. 6.38 and 6.39). EMA can be focally positive (16–24 %) [25, 27]. Likewise, focal p63 positivity is described in AFX (up to 15 %) [28]. In this regard, p40 seems to be better than p63 because of virtually absent staining in AFX and excellent sensitivity for S-SCC detection [28–30]. Melanocytic markers must be negative (S100, SOX10), but focal nonspecific staining for Melan-A/MART1 and HMB45 has been described in tumor giant cells (Figs. 6.40 and 6.41). Smooth muscle actin is frequently expressed (45–70 %) and can be strong and diffuse, but desmin and caldesmon are negative. Among vascular markers, CD34 and ERG are consistently negative [24]. CD31, FLI1 and D2-40 can be expressed in AFX [27, 31], and this should not be considered a sign of angiosarcoma or other vascular tumor. Much has been written about CD10 and CD99 expression in AFX [23, 28, 32–34]. Indeed, one can very often find strong and diffuse staining for these markers in AFX (Figs. 6.42 and 6.43), whereas the probability of staining in S-SCC or melanoma is much lower, but not insignificant. In other words, positivity for CD10 and CD99 does not exclude S-SCC or melanoma, and appropriate "negative staining" must be demonstrated with conventional epithelial and melanocytic markers to render a diagnosis of AFX. In clinical practice, the author uses four antibodies for initial screening: AE1/3, CK5/6, S100, and desmin. If the result is equivocal or the morphology suspicious, p63 or p40, 34BE12, SOX10, and ERG are added as necessary (Table 6.3).

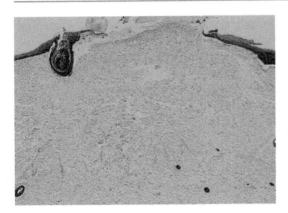

Fig. 6.38 Atypical fibroxanthoma, low power AE1/3. Tumor is negative, with crisp positive internal control

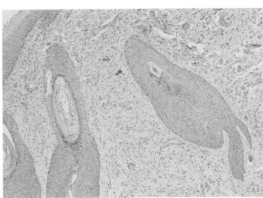

Fig. 6.41 Atypical fibroxanthoma, mid power SOX10. Tumor is negative with positive internal controls (SOX10 stains a few melanocytic nuclei at the upper left)

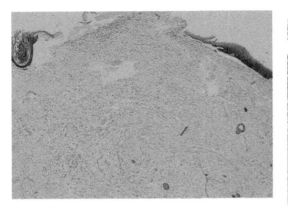

Fig. 6.39 Atypical fibroxanthoma, low power CK5/6. Tumor is negative, with crisp positive internal control

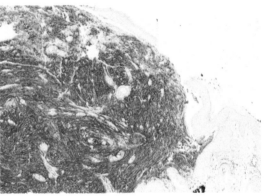

Fig. 6.42 Atypical fibroxanthoma, low power CD10. Strong diffuse staining for these markers is almost always observed in atypical fibroxanthoma and this can be valuable information. Unfortunately, it is not specific for atypical fibroxanthoma (positivity for CD10 and CD99 can be seen in sarcomatoid squamous cell carcinoma and spindle cell melanoma), so one still has to stain for keratins and S100

Molecular

No specific molecular findings exist. There are often genetic changes consistent with ultraviolet irradiation.

Pitfalls

The biological behavior of AFX is essentially benign, and thus, treatment must be conservative.

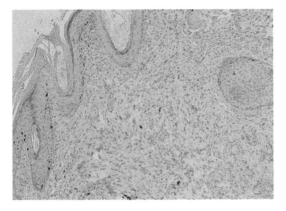

Fig. 6.40 Atypical fibroxanthoma, mid power S100. Tumor is negative with positive internal controls

AFX is a diagnosis of exclusion, and it requires an excisional biopsy and appropriate immunohistochemistry. One must also exclude deep tissue invasion, vascular invasion, perineural invasion, and significant necrosis. These features warrant a diagnosis of pleomorphic dermal sarcoma, which behaves like a "low-grade malignancy" (28% recurrence, 10% metastasis, mostly locoregional). Interestingly, S-SCC has a biological behavior similar to pleomorphic dermal sarcoma [26]. A diagnosis of angiosarcoma or spindle cell melanoma portends a much worse prognosis. A myxofibrosarcoma can resemble a myxoid AFX, but it is less well circumscribed, generally involves deeper soft tissue, is larger and has a different anatomic distribution. A dermatofibroma with monster cells/atypical dermatofibroma can be distinguished from an AFX by its occurrence in younger individuals, in a different anatomic distribution and by the presence of more typical areas of dermatofibroma.

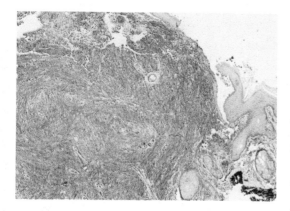

Fig. 6.43 Atypical fibroxanthoma, low power CD99. Strong diffuse staining for these markers is almost always observed in atypical fibroxanthoma and this can be valuable information. Unfortunately, it is not specific for atypical fibroxanthoma (positivity for CD10 and CD99 can be seen in sarcomatoid squamous cell carcinoma and spindle cell melanoma), so one still has to stain for keratins and S100

Plaque-Like CD34-Positive Dermal Fibroma

Clinical

Plaque-like CD34-positive dermal fibroma (PDF), also known as medallion-like dermal dendrocyte hamartoma, is a rare and recently described lesion [22, 35–37]. Initial reports focused on presentation in very young children as an erythematous slightly atrophic rounded or triangular plaque measuring between 0.5 and 8 cm,

Table 6.3 Immunohistochemical characteristics of AFX

Antibody	Finding	Comment
CD10	Diffuse positive	Not specific, interpret with caution
CD99	Diffuse positive	Not specific, interpret with caution
S100	Negative	Interstitial S100+ cells can be seen
Melan-A/MART1	Negative	Nonspecific staining in giant cells
HMB45	Negative	
SOX10	Negative	
MiTF	Focally positive	Interpret with caution if other melanocytic markers are negative
SMA	Can be positive	Interpret with caution if other muscular markers are negative
Desmin	Negative	
h-Caldesmon	Negative	
CD31	Often positive	Nonspecific staining
CD34	Negative	
ERG	Negative	
EMA	Focally positive	Interpret in light of keratins
Keratins	Negative	Use multiple antibodies (AE1/3, MNF116, 34BE12, CK5/6, etc.)
p63	Rare positive cells	Diffusely positive in S-SCC
p40	Negative	Positive in S-SCC, better specificity than p63

on the chest. Other reports and small series expanded the spectrum and sites of involvement. Currently, it is accepted that PDF can present in adults and be non-atrophic. The clinical behavior is benign and treatment is thus conservative when a firm diagnosis can be established. Resemblance to DFSP can be striking.

Histopathology

There is a diffuse infiltration of the dermis by bland spindle cells, with a rich vascular network including dilated venules (Figs. 6.44–6.47). Densely packed collagen fibers are present, with a decrease in the density of elastic fibers (Fig. 6.48). The spindle cells tend to be oriented perpendicular to the skin surface at the upper portion of the infiltrate, whereas their orientation becomes rather parallel to the skin surface in the deeper part. An increased number of mast cells is observed. There is some concentric arrangement of cells around vessels and small nerves. In some cases, the lesion is limited to the upper two-thirds of the dermis, while in others, mainly congenital, there is involvement of the deep dermis and hypodermis.

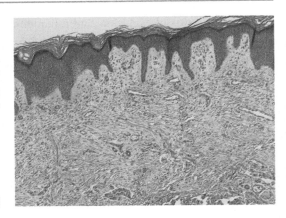

Fig. 6.45 Plaque-like CD34-positive dermal fibroma, mid power H&E. A "busy dermis" with epidermal hyperplasia and dilated venules in the superficial dermis. Bland spindle cells in a vaguely storiform architecture can mimic an "atrophic" form of dermatofibrosarcoma protuberans

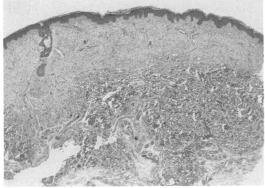

Fig. 6.46 Plaque-like CD34-positive dermal fibroma, low power H&E. Another case showing a "busy dermis" with dilated venules in the superficial dermis. Once again, there is resemblance to an "atrophic" form of dermatofibrosarcoma protuberans

Immunohistochemistry

Spindle cells are strongly and diffusely positive for CD34 (Figs. 6.49–6.51). Positivity for Factor XIIIa was initially reported, but this was not confirmed in later reports. S100, Melan-A, and smooth-muscle actin are negative.

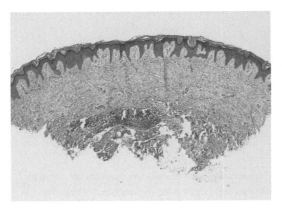

Fig. 6.44 Plaque-like CD34-positive dermal fibroma, low power H&E. A "busy dermis" with epidermal hyperplasia and dilated venules in the superficial dermis. Bland spindle cells in a vaguely storiform architecture can mimic an "atrophic" form of dermatofibrosarcoma protuberans

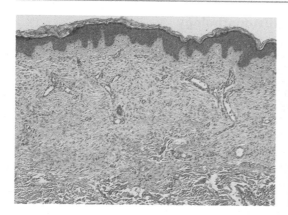

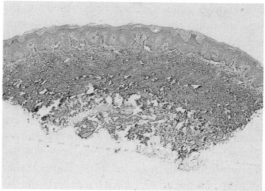

Fig. 6.47 Plaque-like CD34-positive dermal fibroma, mid power H&E. Another case showing a "busy dermis" with dilated venules in the superficial dermis. Once again, there is resemblance to an "atrophic" form of dermatofibrosarcoma protuberans

Fig. 6.49 Plaque-like CD34-positive dermal fibroma, low power CD34. There is striking positivity for CD34 in tumor cells. The mid power photograph shows a pattern vaguely resembling fingerprints

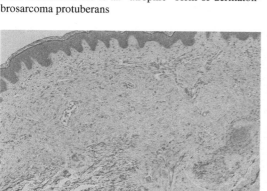

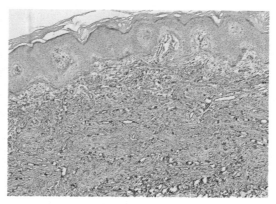

Fig. 6.48 Plaque-like CD34-positive dermal fibroma, mid power Giemsa–Weigert. Elastic fibers (stained purple, look lower left for internal positive control) are completely absent in the lesion

Fig. 6.50 Plaque-like CD34-positive dermal fibroma, mid power CD34. There is striking positivity for CD34 in tumor cells. The mid power photograph shows a pattern vaguely resembling fingerprints

Molecular

No specific molecular alteration is described for PDF. The most significant differential diagnosis is with an atrophic DFSP. Thus, RT-PCR or preferably FISH for COL1A1/PDGFB fusion is essential to rule out a DFSP in suspected cases.

Pitfalls

As stated above, PDF can be indistinguishable from an atrophic DFSP, and the reader is invited to review the pitfalls section under DFSP. Other

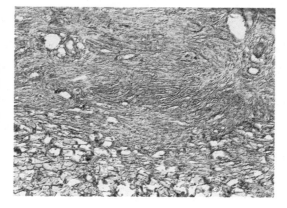

Fig. 6.51 Plaque-like CD34-positive dermal fibroma, high power CD34. There is striking positivity for CD34 in tumor cells. The mid power photograph shows a pattern vaguely resembling fingerprints

differential diagnoses include certain melanocytic nevi, neurofibroma, dermal scar, and circumscribed storiform collagenoma. Melanocytic markers (S100, Melan-A) are positive in melanocytic tumors and negative in PDF. Ruling out a neurofibroma can be challenging, but finding significant numbers of S100 and SOX10 positive cells and/or convincing intralesional axons favors a neurofibroma (their absence is however inconclusive). Circumscribed storiform collagenoma is less cellular and more sclerotic, and contains collagen bundles arranged in a laminated fashion, sometimes resembling fingerprints.

Plexiform Fibrohistiocytic Tumor

Clinical

Plexiform fibrohistiocytic tumor (PFHT) is a neoplasm composed of fibroblasts and histiocyte-like cells, which is associated with a high rate of local recurrence and rarely metastasis [3]. Despite its name, a myofibroblastic etiology is generally favored [38]. Tumors show a predilection for children and young adults; however, they may affect a broad range from congenital to the elderly [38–41]. Some reports suggest a higher incidence amongst females [39, 40], but conflicting results were observed in other large series [38, 42]. The extremities, particularly the upper extremity, are the most common sites of involvement, followed by the trunk and head and neck region [39]. The tumor typically presents as a small, ill-defined mass (average less than 3 cm, range 0.3–8.0 cm) [39, 40], which is occasionally centrally umbilicated [39]. It tends to be painless and slow-growing, and it is not unusual for patients to endorse a long-standing history, in the realm of years [39]. Most lesions are marginally excised. The rate of local recurrence is approximately 12–40 % [38–40, 42]. Admittedly uncommon, lymph node [39] and lung metastasis, and disease-related death [42] have been reported.

Histopathology

Histologically, two frequently overlapping patterns of growth may be observed: fibrohistiocytic and fibroblastic (Figs. 6.52 and 6.53) [39]. The fibrohistiocytic pattern is characterized by nests and nodules of epithelioid cells with pale eosinophilic cytoplasm (Fig. 6.54). The nuclei are round and monomorphic, with one or more small nucleoli; mitotic activity is generally low. Interspersed there are often numerous multinucleate osteoclast-type giant cells (Fig. 6.55). The fibro-

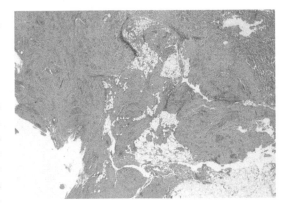

Fig. 6.52 Plexiform fibrohistiocytic tumor, low power H&E. Irregular nodules invading adipose tissue

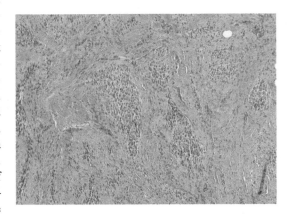

Fig. 6.53 Plexiform fibrohistiocytic tumor, mid power H&E. Ovoid nodules of histiocyte-like cells separates by bland fibroblastic stroma

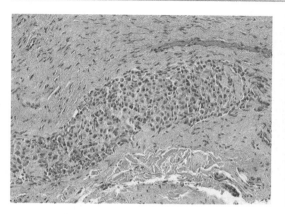

Fig. 6.54 Plexiform fibrohistiocytic tumor, high power H&E. Nodule of histiocyte-like cells

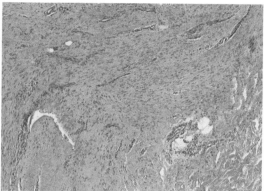

Fig. 6.56 Plexiform fibrohistiocytic tumor, mid power H&E. Fibrous area that can resemble a fibromatosis if taken out of context

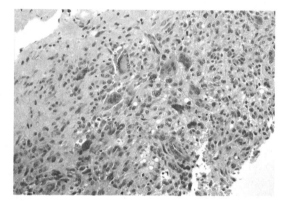

Fig. 6.55 Plexiform fibrohistiocytic tumor, high power H&E. Giant cells can be numerous in some of these tumors

blastic pattern (Fig. 6.56) is characterized by intersecting fascicles of spindle shaped cells yielding a distinct plexiform pattern. The cytoplasm is generally eosinophilic with indistinct cell borders. The nuclei are ovoid with minimal atypia and rare mitotic activity (usually less than 3 per 10 HPFs). Rarely, tumors show moderate-marked pleomorphism, and atypical mitosis have very rarely been reported [42]. Areas of dense fibrosis and stromal hyalinization are common. Likewise, interstitial hemorrhage, hemosiderin deposition and chronic inflammation are often observed. Rarely metaplastic bone formation may occur. Vascular invasion may be encountered. Necrosis is not a typical finding. There

does not appear to be a relationship between mitotic activity and clinical behavior [39]. Wide excision is typically advised [39].

Immunohistochemistry

There is ubiquitous staining for vimentin. The myofibroblastic cells are generally positive for smooth muscle actin, with variable staining for muscle specific actin. CD68 is positive amongst multinucleated giant cells (Fig. 6.57), and in some cases this also highlights fibrohistiocytic cells [42]. Tumors are negative for S100, desmin, keratin and epithelial membrane antigen.

Molecular

Plexiform fibrohistiocytic tumor remains poorly characterized at the genetic level. There are reported cases with abnormal karyotypes [43–45]. No known molecular test is useful at this time.

Pitfalls

The differential diagnosis of plexiform fibrohistiocytic tumor varies depending on the predominant growth pattern present. Potential pitfalls for

Fig. 6.57 Plexiform fibrohistiocytic tumor, mid power CD68. Fibrohistiocytic areas are lightly stained whereas fibrous areas are not

Dermatofibroma, in the absence of previous incomplete sampling, is typically circumscribed and lacks the presence of multinodular growth. PFHT, on the other hand, tends to be more ill-defined and varied in its arrangement. Both tumors may show an architecture that ranges from storiform to fascicular; however, the former tends to be more conspicuous in dermatofibroma, whereas the fibrohistiocytic PFHT is more whorled and the fibroblastic pattern characterized by fascicles extending along native fibrous septae. PFHT may additionally exhibit immunoreactivity for neuron specific enolase, PGP9.5, and CD56 [46]; however, these markers are known for their promiscuity and the reader is advised not to place undue reliance on them.

a fibrohistiocytic pattern of PFHT largely include dermatofibroma, giant cell tumor of soft tissue and cellular neurothekeoma. Potential pitfall for a fibroblastic pattern of PFHT include superficial fibromatosis. Many of the challenges in achieving a definitive diagnosis arise as a result of limited sampling. Given that many of the lesions in the differential diagnosis are small and superficial—and the implications to the patient tremendous, both in terms of risk of local recurrence and possible underlying genetic traits—an excisional biopsy can frequently be recommended without causing significant morbidity to the patient. In the context of adequate sampling, the following serve as a means of avoiding potential pitfalls.

Clues to Differentiate PFHT Versus Dermatofibroma

PFHT and dermatofibroma exhibit cytologic and immunophenotypic overlap. This, in part, is owing to the protean morphologies of the various dermatofibroma subtypes. Both lesions, for example, consist of spindle-epithelioid cells that are often admixed with multinucleated giant cells. Moreover, both have the potential to show immunoreactivity for CD68, actin and Factor XIIIa. The key to resolving the differential often rests with a low-magnification examination.

Clues to Differentiate PFHT Versus Giant Cell Tumor of Soft Tissue

Giant cell tumor of soft tissue (GCT-ST) is morphologically analogous to its bone counterpart, and likewise shares its risk of local recurrence and rarely metastasis. Morphologically it has the potential for prominent multinodular growth that, with limited sampling may be next to impossible to differentiate from PFHT. GCT-ST, however, is frequently larger and deeper situated than PFHT, and lacks a plexiform pattern. In the case of small and superficial lesions, the presence of more prominent sheets of evenly distributed osteoclast-type giant cells—as opposed to the more central aggregation of smaller numbers of osteoclast-like cells—often aids in the recognition of GCT-ST. Similar to PFHT, GCT-ST may be associated with metaplastic bone formation; this is more common in the latter, and often found peripherally. On higher magnification, the mononucleated stromal component of GCT-ST typically contains a rate of mitotic activity that far exceeds that typical of PFHT. Immunohistochemistry is rarely of benefit in resolving the differential diagnosis as both show significant overlap. It remains to be fully established whether giant cell tumor of soft tissue contains the same H3F3A driver mutation arising in its bone counterpart [47].

Clues to Differentiate PFHT Versus Cellular Neurothekeoma

There is appreciable clinical, morphologic and immunohistochemical overlap between cellular neurothekeoma (CN) and PFHT, leading to speculation of a shared histogenesis [42, 46]. There is reasonable evidence to support this assertion rendering in depth discussion of the differential moot. That being said, it should be mentioned this link is not universally accepted, with some believing CN and PFHT represent distinct entities that can, in part, be differentiated immunohistochemically. The former has been described as consistently positive for MiTF and the latter negative [48]. However, given that MiTF is typically expressed in monocyte-derived giant cells [49], these findings are somewhat unexpected, and suggest a need for broader understanding from characterization at the level of molecular pathogenesis.

Clues to Differentiate PFHT Versus Fibromatosis

Fibromatosis can generally be readily differentiated from PFHT based on its typically deep soft tissue involvement. Superficial disease, as in the palmar/plantar variants, are likewise typically characterized by an anatomic distribution that shows minimal overlap with PFHT. In the absence of an adequate clinical history, some confusion may arise as superficial fibromatosis may exhibit multinodular growth and even contain osteoclast-like giant cells. Fibromatosis often has more prominent stromal collagen, particularly in more mature lesions. Early lesions may have more plump cells that lack abundant collagen and wavy nuclei. In these instances immunohistochemistry may be of use, since a majority of cases of fibromatosis exhibit nuclear staining for B-catenin.

Myxoinflammatory Fibroblastic Sarcoma

Clinical

Myxoinflammatory fibroblastic sarcoma (MIFS), also known as inflammatory myxohyaline tumor of the distal extremities with virocyte/Reed-

Sternberg-like cells, is a low-grade locally aggressive fibroblastic neoplasm [3, 50]. It is rare and predominates in adults, but can affect any age, without an obvious sex predilection [49–51]. The vast majority of tumors arise in the distal extremities, particularly the hands and feet [50, 52]. Rarely, however, they may arise at other sites. The lesion is generally painless and slow growing, with some patients giving a history of 20 years duration [50, 51]. There is a very high rate of local recurrence—owing in part to incomplete excision—and very rarely lymph node and lung metastasis [50, 53, 54]. Tumors are generally around 3 cm in size (range 0.5–15 cm) [53], multinodular and poorly circumscribed [50].

Histopathology

Tumors are often centered in subcutis (Fig. 6.58), lobulated or ill-defined, and tend to extend along native connective tissue planes [53]. The stroma is frequently fibrosclerotic with variably sized areas of myxoid matrix (Fig. 6.59). Important for the diagnosis is the presence of, sometimes rare, ganglion-like cells with macronucleoli (Fig. 6.60). Areas of myxoid-rich stroma are often accompanied by pseudolipoblasts (Fig. 6.61) and emperipolesis. Cellular regions often contain spindle-epithelioid cells with abundant pale cytoplasm. The nuclei range from small and ovoid, to large and pleomorphic, and often contain prominent clefts;

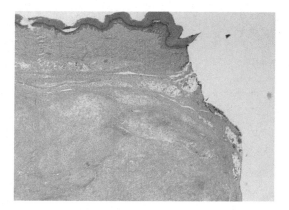

Fig. 6.58 Myxoinflammatory fibroblastic sarcoma, low power H&E. A lobulated tumor centered in subcutaneous tissue/hypodermis

Fig. 6.59 Myxoinflammatory fibroblastic sarcoma, mid power H&E. Myxoid and fibrous areas with a focal inflammatory infiltrate

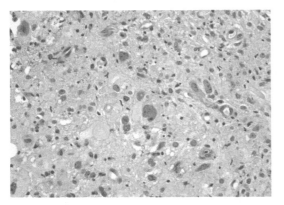

Fig. 6.60 Myxoinflammatory fibroblastic sarcoma, high power H&E. Characteristic tumor cells with large nucleus and macro-nucleolus, vaguely resembling ganglion cells

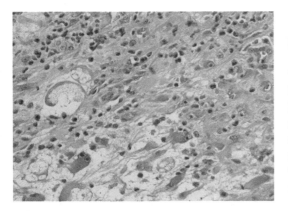

Fig. 6.61 Myxoinflammatory fibroblastic sarcoma, high power H&E. Areas of myxoid-rich stroma with by pseudolipoblasts and inflammatory infiltrate rich in eosinophils

mitotic activity tends to be sparse, and atypical forms may be observed [50]. Tumors are also characterized by the presence of a prominent inflammatory infiltrate largely consisting of lymphocytes, plasma cells, neutrophils, and eosinophils [50]. Lymphocytes may be associated with lymphoid follicles, and microabscesses formed by neutrophils [53]. Thick hyalinized vessels may be observed, and tumors may have prominent hemosiderin deposition. Hyalinized and fibrous septae are also commonly observed [52]. Necrosis can occasionally be present. Hybrid tumors bearing morphologic overlap with so-called hemosiderotic fibrolipomatous tumor (HFT) have been reported; indeed, analogous to atypical lipomatous tumor and dedifferentiated liposarcoma, these tumors are thought to fall on a histologic continuum [53, 55, 56]. More recently it has been recognized that these tumors may be associated with high grade sarcomas, including those reminiscent of myxofibrosarcoma and undifferentiated pleomorphic sarcoma [55]. Atypical features, including increased mitotic activity, thick-walled arcuate vasculature, and cellular fascicles, have also been reported and may portend a more aggressive clinical course [53].

Immunohistochemistry

Tumors are positive for vimentin, with variable immunoreactivity for D2-40, CD34 (Fig. 6.62), smooth muscle actin, and keratin [50, 51, 53].

Molecular

Two genetic pathways have been reported in MIFS. The most commonly described is a translocation t(1;10) (p22; q24) involving unbalanced rearrangements of TFGBR3 and MGEA5; these are transcribed in opposite directions, thereby failing to result in a fusion product [55, 57, 58]. This, nevertheless, appears to be associated with increased expression of a closely related gene on 10q, FGF8 [58]. In addition, amplification of 3p11-12, corresponding to *VGLL3*, has been described [55, 58, 59].

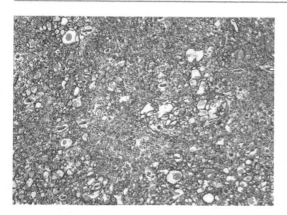

Fig. 6.62 Myxoinflammatory fibroblastic sarcoma, high power CD34. There is often strong positivity for this marker, which lacks specificity

Pitfalls

The differential diagnosis for MIFS is broad, and nowhere is this better illustrated than amongst the original descriptions of this entity, where originating consultants queried the possibility of reactive, infectious, benign neoplasms (e.g., tenosynovial giant cell tumor, nodular and proliferative fasciitis, myxoma) and malignant neoplasms (e.g., Hodgkin's disease, myxofibrosarcoma, liposarcoma, dermatofibrosarcoma protuberans, undifferentiated pleomorphic sarcoma) [50–52]. Many such considerations are obviated with foreknowledge of the HFT-MIFS continuum.

Clues to Differentiate HFT-MIFS Versus Tenosynovial Giant Cell Tumor
In both the diffuse and localized forms of tenosynovial giant cell tumor (TS-GCT), the low power examination bears some resemblance to MIFS. Exceedingly more common, TS-GCT also typically involves the soft tissues of the tendon sheath and joints. On low-power examination tumors range from lobulated to ill-defined and often contain nests of cells divided by prominent hyalinized septa that are not dissimilar from those observed in MIFS. Additionally, these lesions are often associated with an obscuring infiltrate of lymphocytes and histiocytes, along with prominent aggregates of hemosiderin.

However, closer examination almost inevitably reveals the presence of numerous osteoclast-type giant cells, aggregates of foamy macrophages and a bland cytomorphology amongst the mononucleated cell component. Immunohistochemistry offers limited assistance in resolving the differential diagnosis; however, it is worth noting that TS-GCT is genetically characterized by translocation involving rearrangement of CSF1 [60, 61].

Clues to Differentiate HFT-MIFS Versus Pleomorphic Hyalinizing Angiectatic Tumor
Pleomorphic hyalinizing angiectatic tumor (PHAT) is a curious neoplasm with a marked propensity for superficial regions of the lower extremities. Tumors are characterized, at low magnification, by the presence of ectatic vascular spaces containing hyalinized wall and endothelium lined by fibrin (Figs. 6.63 and 6.64). At higher magnification tumors contain spindle to pleomorphic cells arranged in sheets and fascicles, with a conspicuous dearth of mitotic activity (Fig. 6.65) [62]. There is usually diffuse positivity for CD34 (Fig. 6.66) In and of themselves, these findings are nonspecific. Similar such changes may be observed in MIFS, as well as myxofibrosarcoma. An association between PHAT and HFT [63], and, by extension MIFS [64], has been proposed based on overlapping clinical and histopathologic attributes. There appears to be some genetic support to substantiate this assertion, with some cases exhibiting evidence of *TGFBR3* and/or *MGEA5* rearrangement, which would render the need to differentiate these entities moot [64, 65]. However, the fact that not all cases contain this finding, and contradictory results from other groups [58, 66], indicate that further research into this topic is warranted.

Clues to Differentiate HFT-MIFS Versus Myxofibrosarcoma
Myxofibrosarcoma represents an important consideration in the differential diagnosis of MIFS, and accurate recognition is essential based on its potential for more aggressive behavior. It is relatively common, particularly amongst the

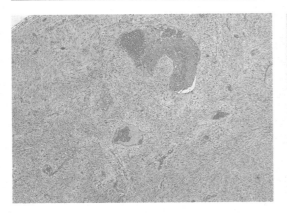

Fig. 6.63 Pleomorphic hyalinizing angiectatic tumor, low power H&E. Ectatic vascular spaces containing hyalinized wall and endothelium lined by fibrin

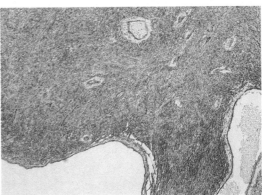

Fig. 6.66 Pleomorphic hyalinizing angiectatic tumor, low power CD34. Diffuse positivity for CD34 is the rule, but it lacks specificity

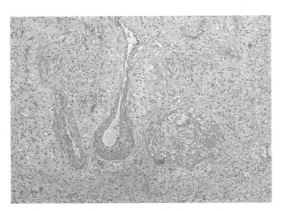

Fig. 6.64 Pleomorphic hyalinizing angiectatic tumor, mid power H&E. Ectatic vascular spaces containing hyalinized wall and endothelium lined by fibrin

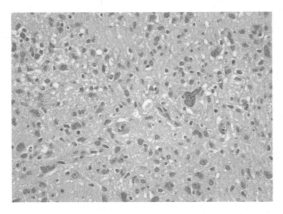

Fig. 6.65 Pleomorphic hyalinizing angiectatic tumor, high power H&E. Spindle to pleomorphic cells, without significant mitotic activity

elderly, and often superficially situated; in contrast to MIFS, while also showing a predilection for the extremities, myxofibrosarcoma only rarely involve the hands and feet. Not only is this tumor frequently superficial, it may exhibit a spectrum of morphologies that overlap with MIFS. Myxofibrosarcoma is frequently lobulated and ranges from hypocellular to hypercellular, with varying degrees of pleomorphism that on the far spectrum can be indistinguishable from an undifferentiated pleomorphic sarcoma. Cases of MIFS with atypical histologic features—including hypercellularity, sarcoma-like vasculature, and abnormal mitotic figures [53]—may be virtually indistinguishable from myxofibrosarcoma without extensive sampling. In the case of low to intermediate grade lesions differentiation is less challenging. Myxofibrosarcoma often contains pseudolipoblasts, but these tend to be smaller and lack the presence of complex eosinophilic interdigitations that are often conspicuous in MIFS. Additionally, myxofibrosarcoma can typically be correctly identified based on the presence of only thin fibrous septa rather than areas of prominent hyalinization, a "quiet" background that typically lacks obscuring inflammation, a delicate curvilinear vasculature, and the absence of bizarre virocyte-like cells.

References

1. Gru AA, Santa Cruz DJ. Atypical fibroxanthoma: a selective review. Semin Diagn Pathol. 2013;30(1): 4–12.

2. Luzar B, Calonje E. Cutaneous fibrohistiocytic tumours – an update. Histopathology. 2010;56(1): 148–65.

3. Fletcher CDM, World HH. WHO classification of tumours of soft tissue and bone. Lyon: IARC Press; 2013.

4. Szablewski V, Laurent-Roussel S, Rethers L, Rommel A, Van Eeckhout P, Vaneechout P, et al. Atypical fibrous histiocytoma of the skin with CD30 and p80/ALK1 positivity and ALK gene rearrangement. J Cutan Pathol. 2014;41(9):715–9.

5. Doyle LA, Mariño-Enriquez A, Fletcher CD, Hornick JL. ALK rearrangement and overexpression in epithelioid fibrous histiocytoma. Mod Pathol. 2015;28(7): 904–12.

6. Kim HJ, Lee JY, Kim SH, Seo YJ, Lee JH, Park JK, et al. Stromelysin-3 expression in the differential diagnosis of dermatofibroma and dermatofibrosarcoma protuberans: comparison with factor XIIIa and CD34. Br J Dermatol. 2007;157(2):319–24.

7. Bandarchi B, Ma L, Marginean C, Hafezi S, Zubovits J, Rasty G. D2-40, a novel immunohistochemical marker in differentiating dermatofibroma from dermatofibrosarcoma protuberans. Mod Pathol. 2010; 23(3):434–8.

8. West RB, Harvell J, Linn SC, Liu CL, Prapong W, Hernandez-Boussard T, et al. Apo D in soft tissue tumors: a novel marker for dermatofibrosarcoma protuberans. Am J Surg Pathol. 2004;28(8):1063–9.

9. Horenstein MG, Prieto VG, Nuckols JD, Burchette JL, Shea CR. Indeterminate fibrohistiocytic lesions of the skin: is there a spectrum between dermatofibroma and dermatofibrosarcoma protuberans? Am J Surg Pathol. 2000;24(7):996–1003.

10. Goldblum JR, Folpe AL, Weiss SW, Enzinger FMSTT, Weiss SWEASTT. Enzinger and Weiss's soft tissue tumors. Philadelphia, PA: Saunders/Elsevier; 2014.

11. Palmerini E, Gambarotti M, Staals EL, Zanella L, Sieberova G, Longhi A, et al. Fibrosarcomatous changes and expression of CD34+ and apolipoprotein-D in dermatofibrosarcoma protuberans. Clin Sarcoma Res. 2012;2(1):4.

12. Pedeutour F, Simon MP, Minoletti F, Barcelo G, Terrier-Lacombe MJ, Combemale P, et al. Translocation, t(17;22)(q22;q13), in dermatofibrosarcoma protuberans: a new tumor-associated chromosome rearrangement. Cytogenet Cell Genet. 1996; 72(2–3):171–4.

13. Simon MP, Pedeutour F, Sirvent N, Grosgeorge J, Minoletti F, Coindre JM, et al. Deregulation of the platelet-derived growth factor B-chain gene via fusion with collagen gene COL1A1 in dermatofibrosarcoma

protuberans and giant-cell fibroblastoma. Nat Genet. 1997;15(1):95–8.

14. O'Brien KP, Seroussi E, Dal Cin P, Sciot R, Mandahl N, Fletcher JA, et al. Various regions within the alpha-helical domain of the COL1A1 gene are fused to the second exon of the PDGFB gene in dermatofibrosarcomas and giant-cell fibroblastomas. Genes Chromosomes Cancer. 1998;23(2):187–93.

15. Sirvent N, Maire G, Pedeutour F. Genetics of dermatofibrosarcoma protuberans family of tumors: from ring chromosomes to tyrosine kinase inhibitor treatment. Genes Chromosomes Cancer. 2003;37(1):1–19.

16. Wang J, Hisaoka M, Shimajiri S, Morimitsu Y, Hashimoto H. Detection of COL1A1-PDGFB fusion transcripts in dermatofibrosarcoma protuberans by reverse transcription-polymerase chain reaction using archival formalin-fixed, paraffin-embedded tissues. Diagn Mol Pathol. 1999;8(3):113–9.

17. Salgado R, Llombart B, Pujol RM, Fernández-Serra A, Sanmartín O, Toll A, et al. Molecular diagnosis of dermatofibrosarcoma protuberans: a comparison between reverse transcriptase-polymerase chain reaction and fluorescence in situ hybridization methodologies. Genes Chromosomes Cancer. 2011;50(7):510–7.

18. Karanian M, Pérot G, Coindre JM, Chibon F, Pedeutour F, Neuville A. Fluorescence in situ hybridization analysis is a helpful test for the diagnosis of dermatofibrosarcoma protuberans. Mod Pathol. 2015; 28(2):230–7.

19. Patel KU, Szabo SS, Hernandez VS, Prieto VG, Abruzzo LV, Lazar AJ, López-Terrada D. Dermatofibrosarcoma protuberans COL1A1-PDGFB fusion is identified in virtually all dermatofibrosarcoma protuberans cases when investigated by newly developed multiplex reverse transcription polymerase chain reaction and fluorescence in situ hybridization assays. Hum Pathol. 2008;39(2):184–93.

20. Bianchini L, Maire G, Guillot B, Joujoux JM, Follana P, Simon MP, et al. Complex t(5;8) involving the CSPG2 and PTK2B genes in a case of dermatofibrosarcoma protuberans without the COL1A1-PDGFB fusion. Virchows Arch. 2008;452(6):689–96.

21. Syed S, Martin AM, Haupt H, Podolski V, Brooks JJ. Frequent detection of androgen receptors in spindle cell lipomas. Arch Pathol Lab Med. 2008;132:81–3.

22. Kutzner H, Mentzel T, Palmedo G, Hantschke M, Rütten A, Paredes BE, et al. Plaque-like cd34-positive dermal fibroma ("medallion-like dermal dendrocyte hamartoma"): clinicopathologic, immunohistochemical, and molecular analysis of 5 cases emphasizing its distinction from superficial, plaque-like dermatofibrosarcoma protuberans. Am J Surg Pathol. 2010; 34(2):190–201.

23. Mirza B, Weedon D. Atypical fibroxanthoma: a clinicopathological study of 89 cases. Australas J Dermatol. 2005;46(4):235–8.

24. Brenn T. Pleomorphic dermal neoplasms: a review. Adv Anat Pathol. 2014;21(2):108–30.

25. Miller K, Goodlad JR, Brenn T. Pleomorphic dermal sarcoma: adverse histologic features predict aggressive behavior and allow distinction from atypical fibroxanthoma. Am J Surg Pathol. 2012;36(9): 1317–26.

26. Nonaka D, Bishop PW. Sarcoma-like tumor of head and neck skin. Am J Surg Pathol. 2014;38(7): 956–65.

27. Luzar B, Calonje E. Morphological and immunohistochemical characteristics of atypical fibroxanthoma with a special emphasis on potential diagnostic pitfalls: a review. J Cutan Pathol. 2010;37(3):301–9.

28. Kanner WA, Brill LB, Patterson JW, Wick MR. CD10, p63 and CD99 expression in the differential diagnosis of atypical fibroxanthoma, spindle cell squamous cell carcinoma and desmoplastic melanoma. J Cutan Pathol. 2010;37(7):744–50.

29. Alomari AK, Glusac EJ, McNiff JM. P40 is a more specific marker than p63 for cutaneous poorly differentiated squamous cell carcinoma. J Cutan Pathol. 2014;41(11):839–45.

30. Henderson SA, Torres-Cabala CA, Curry JL, Bassett RL, Ivan D, Prieto VG, Tetzlaff MT. P40 is more specific than p63 for the distinction of atypical fibroxanthoma from other cutaneous spindle cell malignancies. Am J Surg Pathol. 2014;38(8):1102–10.

31. Cuda J, Mirzamani N, Kantipudi R, Robbins J, Welsch MJ, Sundram UN. Diagnostic utility of fli-1 and D2-40 in distinguishing atypical fibroxanthoma from angiosarcoma. Am J Dermatopathol. 2013;35(3): 316–8.

32. Bull C, Mirzabeigi M, Laskin W, Dubina M, Traczyc T, Guitart J, Gerami P. Diagnostic utility of low-affinity nerve growth factor receptor (P 75) immunostaining in atypical fibroxanthoma. J Cutan Pathol. 2011;38(8):631–5.

33. Wieland CN, Dyck R, Weenig RH, Comfere NI. The role of CD10 in distinguishing atypical fibroxanthoma from sarcomatoid (spindle cell) squamous cell carcinoma. J Cutan Pathol. 2011;38(11):884–8.

34. Monteagudo C, Calduch L, Navarro S, Joan-Figueroa A, Llombart-Bosch A. CD99 immunoreactivity in atypical fibroxanthoma: a common feature of diagnostic value. Am J Clin Pathol. 2002;117(1):126–31.

35. Rodríguez-Jurado R, Palacios C, Durán-McKinster C, Mercadillo P, Orozco-Covarrubias L, Saez-de-Ocariz Mdel M, Ruiz-Maldonado R. Medallion-like dermal dendrocyte hamartoma: a new clinically and histopathologically distinct lesion. J Am Acad Dermatol. 2004;51(3):359–63.

36. Shah KN, Anderson E, Junkins-Hopkins J, James WD. Medallion-like dermal dendrocyte hamartoma. Pediatr Dermatol. 2007;24(6):632–6.

37. Marque M, Bessis D, Pedeutour F, Viseux V, Guillot B, Fraitag-Spinner S. Medallion-like dermal dendrocyte hamartoma: the main diagnostic pitfall is congenital atrophic dermatofibrosarcoma. Br J Dermatol. 2009;160(1):190–3.

38. Hollowood K, Holley MP, Fletcher CD. Plexiform fibrohistiocytic tumour: clinicopathological, immuno-histochemical and ultrastructural analysis in favour of a myofibroblastic lesion. Histopathology. 1991;19(6): 503–13.

39. Enzinger FM, Zhang RY. Plexiform fibrohistiocytic tumor presenting in children and young adults: an analysis of 65 cases. Am J Surg Pathol. 1988; 12(11):818–26.

40. Remstein ED, Arndt CA, Nascimento AG. Plexiform fibrohistiocytic tumor: clinicopathologic analysis of 22 cases. Am J Surg Pathol. 1999;23(6):662–70.

41. Muezzinoglu B, Tohumcu A, Ekingen G. An unusual occurrence of plexiform fibrohistiocytic tumour: congenital tumour diagnosed at 7 years of age. Pathology. 2011;43(4):380–1.

42. Moosavi C, Jha P, Fanburg-Smith JC. An update on plexiform fibrohistiocytic tumor and addition of 66 new cases from the armed forces institute of pathology, in honor of Franz M. Enzinger, MD. Ann Diagn Pathol. 2007;11(5):313–9.

43. Smith S, Fletcher CD, Smith MA, Gusterson BA. Cytogenetic analysis of a plexiform fibrohistiocytic tumor. Cancer Genet Cytogenet. 1990;48(1):31–4.

44. Redlich GC, Montgomery KD, Allgood GA, Joste NE. Plexiform fibrohistiocytic tumor with a clonal cytogenetic anomaly. Cancer Genet Cytogenet. 1999;108(2):141–3.

45. Leclerc-Mercier S, Pedeutour F, Fabas T, Glorion C, Brousse N, Fraitag S. Plexiform fibrohistiocytic tumor with molecular and cytogenetic analysis. Pediatr Dermatol. 2011;28(1):26–9.

46. Jaffer S, Ambrosini-Spaltro A, Mancini AM, Eusebi V, Rosai J. Neurothekeoma and plexiform fibrohistiocytic tumor: mere histologic resemblance or histogenetic relationship? Am J Surg Pathol. 2009;33(6): 905–13.

47. Behjati S, Tarpey PS, Presneau N, Scheipl S, Pillay N, Van Loo P, et al. Distinct H3F3A and H3F3B driver mutations define chondroblastoma and giant cell tumor of bone. Nat Genet. 2013;45(12):1479–82.

48. Fox MD, Billings SD, Gleason BC, Moore J, Thomas AB, Shea CR, et al. Expression of MiTF may be helpful in differentiating cellular neurothekeoma from plexiform fibrohistiocytic tumor (histiocytoid predominant) in a partial biopsy specimen. Am J Dermatopathol. 2012;34(2):157–60.

49. Seethala RR, Goldblum JR, Hicks DG, Lehman M, Khurana JS, Pasha TL, Zhang PJ. Immunohistochemical evaluation of microphthalmia-associated transcription factor expression in giant cell lesions. Mod Pathol. 2004;17(12):1491–6.

50. Meis-Kindblom JM, Kindblom LG. Acral myxoinflammatory fibroblastic sarcoma: a low-grade tumor of the hands and feet. Am J Surg Pathol. 1998;22(8):911–24.

51. Montgomery EA, Devaney KO, Giordano TJ, Weiss SW. Inflammatory myxohyaline tumor of distal extremities with virocyte or Reed-Sternberg-like cells: a distinctive lesion with features simulating inflammatory conditions, Hodgkin's disease, and various sarcomas. Mod Pathol. 1998;11(4):384–91.

52. Michal M. Inflammatory myxoid tumor of the soft parts with bizarre giant cells. Pathol Res Pract. 1998;194(8):529–33.

53. Laskin WB, Fetsch JF, Miettinen M. Myxoinflammatory fibroblastic sarcoma: a clinicopathologic analysis of 104 cases, with emphasis on predictors of outcome. Am J Surg Pathol. 2014;38(1):1–12.

54. Lombardi R, Jovine E, Zanini N, Salone MC, Gambarotti M, Righi A, et al. A case of lung metastasis in myxoinflammatory fibroblastic sarcoma: analytical review of one hundred and thirty eight cases. Int Orthop. 2013;37(12):2429–36.

55. Hallor KH, Sciot R, Staaf J, Heidenblad M, Rydholm A, Bauer HC, et al. Two genetic pathways, t(1;10) and amplification of 3p11-12, in myxoinflammatory fibroblastic sarcoma, haemosiderotic fibrolipomatous tumour, and morphologically similar lesions. J Pathol. 2009;217(5):716–27.

56. Elco CP, Mariño-Enríquez A, Abraham JA, Dal Cin P, Hornick JL. Hybrid myxoinflammatory fibroblastic sarcoma/hemosiderotic fibrolipomatous tumor: report of a case providing further evidence for a pathogenetic link. Am J Surg Pathol. 2010;34(11):1723–7.

57. Lambert I, Debiec-Rychter M, Guelinckx P, Hagemeijer A, Sciot R. Acral myxoinflammatory fibroblastic sarcoma with unique clonal chromosomal changes. Virchows Arch. 2001;438(5):509–12.

58. Antonescu CR, Zhang L, Nielsen GP, Rosenberg AE, Dal Cin P, Fletcher CD. Consistent t(1;10) with rearrangements of TGFBR3 and MGEA5 in both myxoinflammatory fibroblastic sarcoma and hemosiderotic fibrolipomatous tumor. Genes Chromosomes Cancer. 2011;50(10):757–64.

59. Mansoor A, Fidda N, Himoe E, Payne M, Lawce H, Magenis RE. Myxoinflammatory fibroblastic sarcoma with complex supernumerary ring chromosomes composed of chromosome 3 segments. Cancer Genet Cytogenet. 2004;152(1):61–5.

60. West RB, Rubin BP, Miller MA, Subramanian S, Kaygusuz G, Montgomery K, et al. A landscape effect in tenosynovial giant-cell tumor from activation of CSF1 expression by a translocation in a minority of tumor cells. Proc Natl Acad Sci U S A. 2006; 103(3):690–5.

61. Panagopoulos I, Brandal P, Gorunova L, Bjerkehagen B, Heim S. Novel CSF1-S100A10 fusion gene and CSF1 transcript identified by RNA sequencing in tenosynovial giant cell tumors. Int J Oncol. 2014;44(5):1425–32.

62. Smith ME, Fisher C, Weiss SW. Pleomorphic hyalinizing angiectatic tumor of soft parts. A low-grade neoplasm resembling neurilemoma. Am J Surg Pathol. 1996;20(1):21–9.

63. Folpe AL, Weiss SW. Pleomorphic hyalinizing angiectatic tumor: analysis of 41 cases supporting evolution from a distinctive precursor lesion. Am J Surg Pathol. 2004;28(11):1417–25.

64. Carter JM, Sukov WR, Montgomery E, Goldblum JR, Billings SD, Fritchie KJ, Folpe AL. TGFBR3 and MGEA5 rearrangements in pleomorphic hyalinizing angiectatic tumors and the spectrum of related neoplasms. Am J Surg Pathol. 2014;38(9):1182–992.

65. Wei S, Pan Z, Siegal GP, Winokur TS, Carroll AJ, Jhala D. Complex analysis of a recurrent pleomorphic hyalinizing tumor of soft parts. Hum Pathol. 2012;43(1):121–6.

66. Mohajeri A, Kindblom LG, Sumathi VP, Brosjö O, Magnusson L, Nilsson J, et al. SNP array and FISH findings in two pleomorphic hyalinizing angiectatic tumors. Cancer Genet. 2012;205(12):673–6.

Immunohistology and Molecular Studies of Smooth Muscle and Neural Cutaneous Tumors

Tammie Ferringer

Cutaneous Smooth Muscle Tumors

Smooth muscle is noted in the gastrointestinal, respiratory, and genitourinary tracts. In skin, locations include arrector pili muscles, vascular smooth muscle, and smooth muscle of genital skin (vulva, areola, and dartos of the scrotum). Benign tumors arising at these sites are known as piloleiomyoma, angioleiomyoma, and leiomyoma of genital skin, respectively.

Piloleiomyomas

Introduction

Piloleiomyomas can occur as solitary lesions, but typically present as multiple small, clustered or grouped lesions on the trunk or extensors of young adults (Fig. 7.1a). Clinically they present as red-brown firm papulonodules that may be tender with minimal trauma or cold exposure.

Zosteriform and plaque-like variants have been reported [1]. Multiple piloleiomyomas can be inherited in association with uterine leiomyomas in an autosomal dominant syndrome that results from a germline mutation in fumarate hydratase. Twenty percent of patients with this syndrome, now known as hereditary leiomyomatosis and renal cell cancer (HLRCC) (OMIM 150800), develop type II papillary renal cell carcinoma [2].

Microscopic Features

These ill-defined dermal tumors are composed of fascicles of elongate cells with eosinophilic cytoplasm and blunt-ended or cigar-shaped nuclei with a small perinuclear, clear vacuole (Fig. 7.1b, c).

Immunohistochemistry

Several immunohistochemical markers identify smooth muscle cells. Some can assist in differentiation from myofibroblasts and myoepithelial cells (Table 7.1).

Smooth muscle actin (SMA) recognizes the alpha-smooth muscle isoform of actin and thus is expressed in arrector pili, vascular and genital smooth muscle, as well as myofibroblasts, myoepithelial cells, pericytes, and glomus cells [3]. However, myofibroblasts tend to show a parallel subplasmalemmal pattern of SMA expression in a "tram-track" pattern (Fig. 7.2) unlike the more diffuse cytoplasmic pattern in smooth muscle cells (Fig. 7.1d).

T. Ferringer, M.D. (✉)
Department of Dermatology, Geisinger Medical Center, 115 Woodbine Lane, MC 52-06, Danville, PA 17822, USA

Department of Laboratory Medicine, Geisinger Medical Center, 100 N. Academy Ave, MC 19-20, Danville, PA 17822, USA
e-mail: tferringer@geisinger.edu

© Springer International Publishing Switzerland 2016
J.A. Plaza, V.G. Prieto (eds.), *Applied Immunohistochemistry in the Evaluation of Skin Neoplasms*, DOI 10.1007/978-3-319-30590-5_7

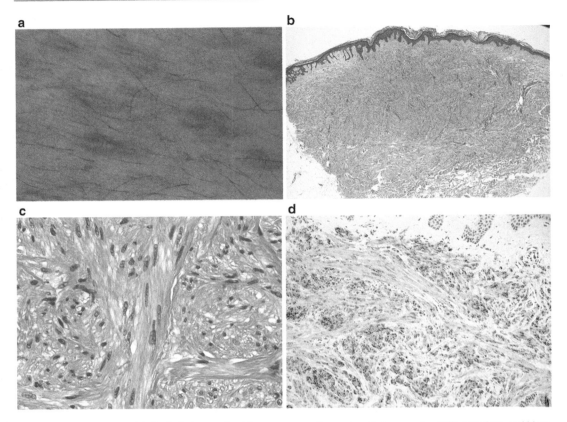

Fig. 7.1 Piloleiomyoma. (**a**) Typical cluster of red-brown piloleiomyomas on the flank of an adult male. (**b**) Ill-defined dermal tumor composed of fascicles of spindle cells. (**c**) The smooth muscle cells have eosinophilic cytoplasm and blunt-ended or cigar-shaped nuclei with a small perinuclear, clear vacuole. (**d**) Diffuse cytoplasmic SMA expression

Table 7.1 Immunohistochemical muscle markers

	Smooth muscle	Skeletal muscle	Myofibroblasts	Myoepithelial cells
MSA	+	+	+	+
Desmin	+ except vascular	+	±	−
SMMS	+	−	±	+
h-Caldesmon	+	−	−	Normal myoepithelial cells
SMA	+	−	+	+
Calponin	+	−	+	+

MSA muscle-specific actin, *SMMS* smooth muscle myosin, *SMA* smooth muscle actin

Caldesmon is a cytoskeletal protein that is thought to regulate cellular contraction in muscle cells. It is present in many cell types in a low molecular weight form but the high molecular weight form (h-caldesmon) is expressed in smooth muscle cells and normal myoepithelial cells. It also strongly stains glomus cells [3]. Anti-h-caldesmon can help distinguish smooth muscle tumors from myofibroblastic lesions such as nodular fasciitis and pleomorphic sarcoma, in which it is absent [4, 5].

Calponin preferentially binds with actin. It is observed in myofibroblasts, smooth muscle, glomus, and myoepithelial cells [4]. Immunoreactivity has also been reported in neurothekeomas [6].

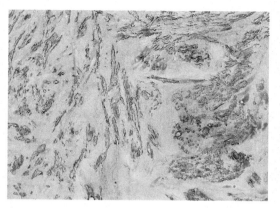

Fig. 7.2 Myofibroma. Parallel subplasmalemmal pattern of SMA expression in a "tram-track" pattern in the myofibroblasts of a myofibroma

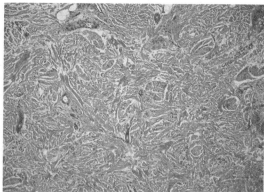

Fig. 7.3 Smooth muscle hamartoma. Discrete bundles of smooth muscle fibers in various directions separated by collagen

Smooth muscle myosin (SMMS) heavy chain is a cytoplasmic structural protein of the contractile apparatus in smooth muscle cells that is also expressed in myoepithelial cells but is typically negative in myofibroblastic lesions [4].

Desmin is an intermediate filament found in skeletal, cardiac, and smooth muscle cells, with the exception of some vascular smooth muscle [7]. It is weak and focal in myofibroblasts [3] and negative in myoepithelial cells [8].

MSA (HHF35) is an antibody common to skeletal and smooth muscle, as well as myoepithelial cells, myofibroblasts, and glomus cells [5, 7]. Piloleiomyomas theoretically are MSA positive but this has not been reported in the literature. They are reportedly positive with SMMS, SMA, calponin, desmin, and h-caldesmon [3, 4].

Myogenin and MyoD1 are transcription factors involved in myogenic differentiation that are expressed earlier than myoglobin and show nuclear expression in skeletal muscle [3]. Any focal expression in smooth muscle tumors is likely due to entrapped or regenerating skeletal muscle fibers [9].

Caveolin is a scaffolding protein in endothelial cells but expression has also been reported in adipocytic and smooth muscle tumors [10].

Molecular Studies

Accumulation of fumarate in HLRCC tumor cells results in aberrant succination and forma-

tion of S-(2-succino)-cysteine (2SC), which can be detected immunohistochemically. Immunoexpression of 2SC has served as a metabolic biomarker for fumarate deficiency in noncutaneous tumors of HLRCC and could potentially serve as a screening tool for this syndrome in piloleiomyomas [2, 11, 12].

Differential Diagnosis

In contrast to piloleiomyomas, smooth muscle hamartomas are typically congenital plaques consisting of discrete bundles of smooth muscle fibers in various directions separated by collagen (Fig. 7.3).

Leiomyomas of the Genital Skin

Introduction

Leiomyomas derived from the smooth muscle found in the areola, scrotum, and vulva are uncommon.

Microscopic Features

While leiomyomas of the nipple share similar histopathologic features as piloleiomyoma, scrotal and vulvar tumors are typically larger and better circumscribed [13]. Vulvar leiomyomas predominantly contain spindled cells but some can be epithelioid with hyalinized or myxoid stroma. Nielsen et al. characterized vulvar smooth muscle tumors based on the presence or absence of the following features: over 5 cm in size, infiltrative margins, five or more mitotic figures in ten high power fields, and moderate to severe cytologic atypia. They recommended diagnosing tumors with one or none of these characteristics as leiomyoma, those with two features as atypical leiomyomas, and those with three or more as leiomyosarcoma [14].

Similarly atypical scrotal leiomyomas have been variably reported as "symplastic" or "bizarre" leiomyomas. These lesions share with usual scrotal leiomyomas small size, low cellularity, minimal to no mitotic activity, and low Ki-67 proliferation rate. Matoso et al. separated these atypical lesions based on the presence of cytologic atypia but with degenerative multinucleated or smudgy chromatin. High cellularity, nuclear to cytoplasmic ratio, or mitotic activity should be considered leiomyosarcoma [15].

Immunohistochemistry
Genital leiomyomas show similar smooth muscle reactivity to piloleiomyomas. However, leiomyomas of the nipple are reportedly estrogen- and progesterone-receptor positive [16], unlike piloleiomyomas [17]. Similarly, scrotal lesions express androgen receptor [18].

Molecular Studies
Pericentric inversion (12)(p12q13–14) and t(7;9) (p13;q11.2) have each been reported in a leiomyoma of the vulva but consistent findings have not been reported thus far [19, 20].

Differential Diagnosis
In contrast to vulvar leiomyoma, aggressive angiomyxoma is less cellular and the spindle cells are separated by mucin. The thick, hyalinized vessel walls and lack of desmin expression also help distinguish them from leiomyoma. Angiomyofibroblastoma could also be considered in the differential and do express desmin but generally are negative with SMA and have multinucleated giant cells in an edematous stroma.

Angioleiomyomas

Introduction
Angioleiomyomas are deep dermal and/or subcutaneous tumors that arise from vascular smooth muscle. They tend to occur as solitary nodules on the lower extremities of middle-aged adults with a female predominance. Lesions usually are less than 2 cm in size and often are tender.

Microscopic Features
These encapsulated tumors are composed of bundles of smooth muscle cells between vascular channels. Angioleiomyomas are generally separated into solid, cavernous, and venous types. The vessels in the solid type are reduced to small slit-like channels in a background of compact muscle bundles, while the vessels of the cavernous type are dilated. The layers of smooth muscle surrounding the vessels merge with the intervascular fascicles (Fig. 7.4a, b). Vascular channels

a

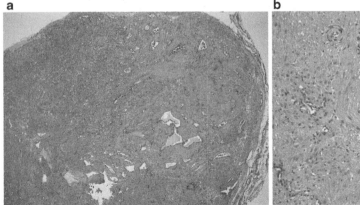

b

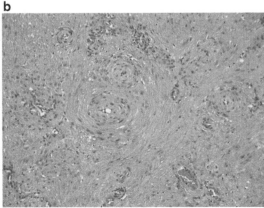

Fig. 7.4 Angioleiomyoma. (**a**) Encapsulated tumor composed of bundles of smooth cells between vascular channels. (**b**) Layers of smooth muscle surrounding the vessels merge with intervascular fascicles

distinct from the intervascular muscle are seen in the venous type [21].

While convincing malignant transformation has not been reported, lesions containing scattered atypical cells with large, pleomorphic, bizarre, and vacuolar nuclei have been reported as pleomorphic angioleiomyomas. These lesions remain circumscribed and lack necrosis and significant mitotic activity [22].

Immunohistochemistry

Immunohistochemical expression includes diffuse reactivity for SMA, calponin, and h-caldesmon. Desmin is less consistent with reactivity reportedly in only 10–20 % of angioleiomyomas [23]. This is not surprising given that desmin expression in vascular smooth muscle varies based on the size and site of the vessel [24].

Molecular Studies

Variable cytogenetic abnormalities have been reported in some studied angioleiomyomas with the most consistent being a regional loss in chromosome 22 [25].

Differential Diagnosis

Lesions that resemble angioleiomyomas but contain collections of mature adipose tissue are designated as angiomyolipomas (Fig. 7.5). Unlike renal angiomyolipomas, these tumors are HMB-45 negative and are not associated with tuberous sclerosis.

Myopericytomas are characterized by round myoid cells in a concentric pattern around vessels. There is reactivity to calponin, h-caldesmon, and SMA, similar to angioleiomyomas and thus are considered by some in the same spectrum. Although desmin expression reportedly differs; subsequent reports have shown reactivity in only 10–20 % of both lesions [23].

Superficial Leiomyosarcomas

Introduction

Primary superficial leiomyosarcomas typically occur in the fifth decade or later on the extremities. The cutaneous lesions that predominately are situated in the dermis differ prognostically from subcutaneous forms. The dermal lesions derive from the arrector pili muscle, while the subcutaneous lesions presumably arise from vascular smooth muscle. Both lesions can recur locally but subcutaneous tumors are much more likely to metastasize [26]. The skin, particularly of the scalp, is the most common site for distant metastasis followed by the lungs [26]. The latency period until metastasis can be as long as 20 years after initial diagnosis [26].

EBV-associated smooth muscle tumors in immunodeficient patients, particularly children, have been reported. Most EBV-associated leiomyosarcomas are deep but dermal involvement has rarely been reported [27].

Microscopic Features

Cutaneous leiomyosarcomas are ill-defined predominantly dermal tumors consisting of interlacing bundles of smooth muscle cells with blunt-ended vesicular nuclei and a high nuclear to cytoplasmic ratio (Fig. 7.6a). Focal extension into the subcutaneous tissue can occur. Variable cytologic atypia and nuclear pleomorphism is noted but tumor necrosis is rare. Perinuclear clear zones, typical of smooth muscle, can be present (Fig. 7.6b). Emphasis has been placed by some authors on the presence of mitoses, particularly atypical forms [28–30]. Subcutaneous lesions are

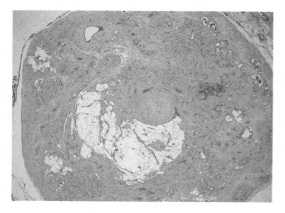

Fig. 7.5 Angiomyolipoma. Resemble angioleiomyoma but contain collections of mature adipose tissue

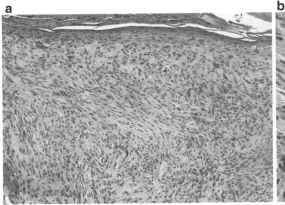
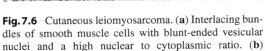
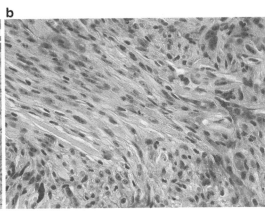

Fig. 7.6 Cutaneous leiomyosarcoma. (**a**) Interlacing bundles of smooth muscle cells with blunt-ended vesicular nuclei and a high nuclear to cytoplasmic ratio. (**b**) Cytologic atypia, nuclear pleomorphism, and perinuclear clear zones, typical of smooth muscle cells

more nodular but are locally infiltrative. They often have a prominent vascular pattern. Rare variants include lesions with epithelioid or granular cells [31, 32].

The relatively indolent behavior of cutaneous leiomyosarcomas has led to the proposed alternative name "atypical intradermal smooth muscle neoplasm" [33, 34]; however, metastases have been reported in up to 12 % in one recent study, with two deaths due to disease [26]. High mitotic count, increased tumor depth or size, and increased grade have been reported to suggest poor outcomes; however, studies have been varied [28, 29, 33, 35–41].

Immunohistochemistry

Most cases of leiomyosarcoma are positive with SMA, MSA, and calponin. Desmin and h-caldesmon are less consistent [4, 34]. Expression of desmin can be focal and tends to occur less frequently in higher grade and subcutaneous lesions [42, 43].

Cytokeratin and S100 expression may be present, but usually focal, creating an important pitfall in differentiation from other atypical spindle cell tumors of the skin [42, 44, 45]. In contrast, atypical fibroxanthomas (AFXs) can have myofibroblastic differentiation and therefore show reactivity with some myogenic markers, particularly calponin and SMA (Fig. 7.7a, b) [45–49].

Desmin (Fig. 7.7c) and h-caldesmon are negative in AFX and may be required for differentiation [45, 46, 48, 49].

Molecular Studies

Comparative genomic hybridization has revealed varying amplifications and losses in leiomyosarcomas with losses in 13q being most notable in one study [50].

Differential Diagnosis

Secondary leiomyosarcoma from a uterine or retroperitoneal primary tends to be multifocal, spheroid in outline and may present within the vessel lumen [35].

Dermal leiomyosarcomas can mimic other atypical spindle cell tumors of the skin and immunohistochemistry may be required to differentiate from spindle cell melanoma, carcinoma, and atypical fibroxanthoma with the above discussed pitfalls in mind.

Cutaneous Neural and Neuroendocrine Tumors

Most neural tumors are benign and arise from or differentiate toward various combinations of the peripheral nerve components: Schwann cell, perineurial cells, neurofilaments, and fibroblasts.

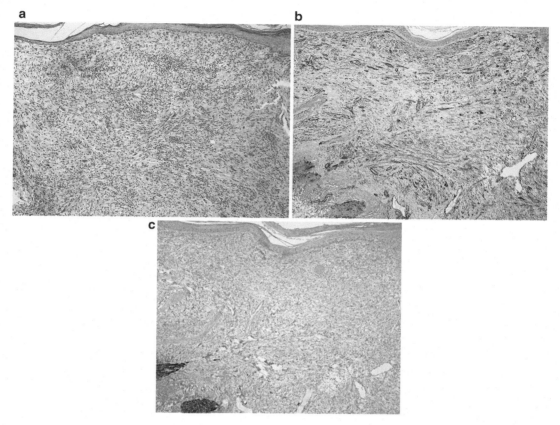

Fig. 7.7 Atypical fibroxanthoma. (**a**) Atypical spindle cell neoplasm. (**b**) Focal SMA reactivity but (**c**) absence of desmin expression with internal control staining of pili arrector muscle

Recently hybrid tumors containing conspicuous components of more than one portion of the peripheral nerve sheath have been reported, most commonly hybrid schwannoma/perineurioma. In contrast, most neuroendocrine tumors are malignant.

Solitary Circumscribed Neuroma

Introduction
Solitary circumscribed neuroma, also known as palisaded encapsulated neuroma, typically arises in adulthood as a solitary skin-colored dome-shaped, nodule involving the central face, particularly bordering the mucocutaneous junction [51, 52]. They also frequent the oral mucosa and have been reported on acral skin and the penis [53–

55]. These nodular lesions tend to pop out on shave biopsy [52].

While rarely multiple [54] they are not associated with neurofibromatosis or multiple endocrine neoplasia, type 2b.

Microscopic Features
Solitary circumscribed neuromas, despite the original name, are only partially encapsulated and rarely show palisading. Historically, neuromas are defined by a 1:1 ratio of axons to Schwann cell fascicles [52].

Typically, there is a well-circumscribed dermal nodule composed of intersecting Schwann cell fascicles with interfascicular clefting (Fig. 7.8a) [51]. The spindled Schwann cells have wavy tapered nuclei. There can be a plexiform pattern [54, 56]. In many cases the nerve of origin

a

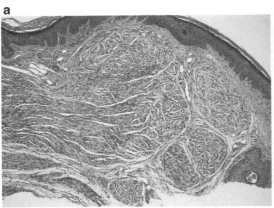

b

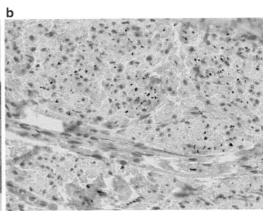

Fig. 7.8 Solitary circumscribed neuroma. (**a**) Well-circumscribed dermal nodule composed of intersecting Schwann cell fascicles with interfascicular clefting. (**b**) With neurofilament protein, the axon to Schwann cell fascicle ratio approaches 1:1

is present at the base of the lesion [53]. Mitoses and pleomorphism are not readily identified [53]. Vascular [57], epithelioid [56, 58] and myxoid variants have been reported [59].

Immunohistochemistry

S100 is positive but glial fibrillary acidic protein (GFAP) is negative [53, 60], in contrast to the positivity in one-third to half of neurofibromas and schwannomas [61–63]. EMA, claudin-1, and GLUT-1 highlight the partial capsule. With neurofilament protein (NFP), the axon to Schwann cell fascicle ratio approaches 1:1 (Fig. 7.8b) [60].

Differential Diagnosis

Angioleiomyomas (Fig. 7.4a, b) do not have clefts between the fascicles of smooth muscle cells and the nuclei are blunt-ended instead of tapered.

In neurofibroma, axons are present in some Schwann cell fascicles but do not approach the 1:1 ratio seen in neuromas [52]. However, in practice distinction is difficult to appreciate. Neurofibromas lack the compact bundles of cells with interfascicular clefting [52].

Schwannomas are usually in the subcutis rather than primarily in the dermis. Unlike, schwannoma, palisading is unusual and verocay bodies and Antoni A and B areas are not identified in solitary circumscribed neuroma.

Multiple mucosal neuromas is one of the first manifestations of the autosomal dominant disorder, multiple endocrine neoplasia syndrome (type 2b) due to a mutation in the RET gene on chromosome 10q11. This syndrome is also characterized by medullary thyroid carcinoma and pheochromocytoma [64]. Histologically, mucosal neuromas can resemble solitary circumscribed neuromas but they can also consist of tortuous hyperplastic nerves with a thick perineurium [52].

Traumatic neuroma is a hyperplastic response to nerve injury. These neuromas occur in a background of fibrous scar tissue that ultimately surrounds haphazardly arranged, newly formed nerve fascicles [52]. EMA positive perineurial cells surround each fascicle, in contrast to the peripheral, partial capsule in solitary circumscribed neuroma [65].

Pacinian neuroma usually occurs on the digit and histologically is composed of numerous pacinian corpuscles admixed with nerve fibers and fibrous tissue [66].

Morton's neuroma is a degenerative response to chronic low grade tissue damage, typically overlying the metatarsal heads of women. Histologically, marked fibrosis distorts the nerve trunk [67].

Neurofibromas

Introduction

Neurofibromas are essentially a hyperplasia of all components of the nerve fascicle. They are composed of Schwann cells and supporting elements of nerve fibers, including endoneurial fibroblasts and perineurial cells. Mast cells are a conspicuous component and may be a major player in neurofibroma formation [68].

Cutaneous neurofibromas are soft, flesh-colored protuberant to pedunculated papules. Most neurofibromas are solitary and are unassociated with other systemic features but multiple lesions form one of the primary features of neurofibromatosis type I (von Recklinghausen's disease) (Fig. 7.9a). This is an autosomal dominant disorder but spontaneous germline mutations occur in half of cases. The mutation is in the NF1 gene on chromosome 17q11.2 that encodes the protein neurofibromin. Other diagnostic findings include Lisch nodules of the iris, multiple café-au-lait macules, optic gliomas, axillary freckling, and skeletal dysplasia [69].

Plexiform neurofibromas, as defined clinically, are virtually pathognomonic for neurofibromatosis, type I [70]. This large, soft exophytic dermal and subcutaneous proliferation has been likened to a "bag of worms" on palpation and is typically present at birth or shortly thereafter. Overlying hyperpigmentation and hypertrichosis may be present (Fig. 7.9b) [71]. Rapid growth or persistent pain may herald malignant transformation [72].

Diffuse neurofibromas produce local thickening and induration of the skin. Up to a third of cases are associated with neurofibromatosis type I [73, 74].

Microscopic Features

Neurofibromas are nonencapsulated dermal or subcutaneous proliferations of spindle cells with scant cytoplasm and small wavy or comma-shaped nuclei in a pale fibrillar, myxoid, or collagenous stroma (Fig. 7.9c, d). CD34+/S100− multinucleated floret-like giant cells may be focally present [75].

Histological variants of neurofibroma include cellular, myxoid, hyalinized, epithelioid, plexiform, diffuse, pigmented, clear cell, lipomatous, sclerosing, granular, and dendritic cell tumor with pseudorosettes [73, 76–80].

Plexiform lesions are dermal and/or subcutaneous and are composed of tortuous, large nerve fascicles in a hypocellular and myxomatous stroma (Fig. 7.9e). The fascicles are surrounded by perineurium. Small cutaneous neurofibromas with this histopathologic pattern are not necessarily associated with neurofibromatosis [81]. Presence of high cellularity, necrosis, pleomorphism, and especially, mitoses should raise concern for malignant transformation which can occur in 2–13 % of plexiform neurofibromas [71].

Diffuse lesions are ill-defined and infiltrate the dermis and subcutis, often extending along septa (Fig. 7.9f). The stroma is often more collagenous and Meissner bodies may be identified [74]. Similar to pigmented neurofibromas, focal cells with melanocytic differentiation have been noted in nonpigmented diffuse neurofibromas [82, 83].

Dendritic cell neurofibroma with pseudorosettes consists of small, dark cells with little cytoplasm concentrically grouped around a second type of larger cell with copious cytoplasm [80].

Hybrid peripheral nerve sheath tumors containing focal areas with distinct perineurial or Schwannian differentiation have been reported in neurofibroma [84–87].

Atypical sporadic neurofibromas show nuclear pleomorphism, variable cellularity, but only very rare mitotic figures [88]. This may represent degenerative or ancient change similar to that in ancient schwannoma.

Immunohistochemistry

Neurofibromas express S100 in a diffuse, sharp, wavy pattern [89] but label only 40–50 % of the cells [90]. Sox10, a neural crest transcription factor, is positive in neurofibromas [91, 92], while GFAP is positive in 11–50 % of these lesions [62, 63]. CD34 highlights the endoneurium of normal nerve and neurofibroma [93]. Because of the long, delicate staining between collagen bundles in a whorled pattern with

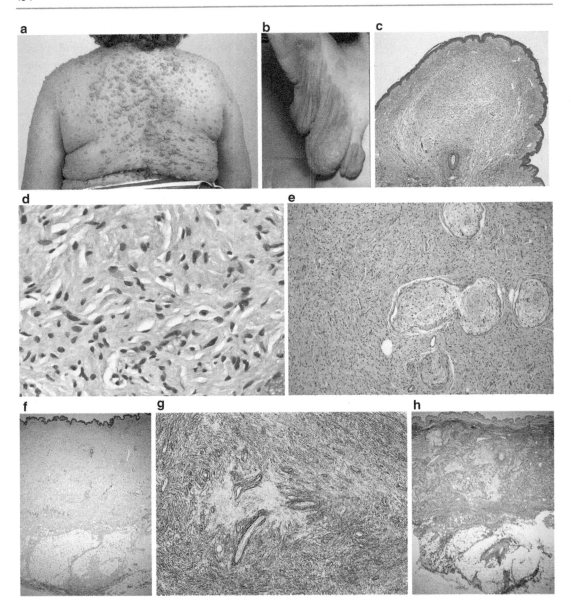

Fig. 7.9 Cutaneous neurofibroma. (**a**) Multiple soft, flesh-colored protuberant to pedunculated neurofibromas in a patient with neurofibromatosis, type I. (**b**) Large, soft exophytic plexiform neurofibroma that has been likened to a "bag of worms" in a patient with neurofibromatosis, type I. (**c**) Nonencapsulated proliferation of spindle cells with scant cytoplasm in a pale fibrillar, myxoid, and collagenous stroma. (**d**) Small cells with wavy or comma-shaped nuclei with admixed mast cells. (**e**) Tortuous, large nerve fascicles in the hypocellular and myxomatous stroma of a plexiform neurofibroma. (**f**) Diffuse neurofibroma with ill-defined infiltration of the dermis and subcutis, along septa. (**g**) Long, delicate CD34 staining of a neurofibroma in a whorled pattern resembling a human fingerprint. (**h**) CD34 expression in a diffuse neurofibroma can mimic dermatofibrosarcoma protuberans

CD34, it has been likened to a human fingerprint (Fig. 7.9g) [94]. Given the cellular composition of neurofibromas, it is not surprising that some lesions show EMA positive perineurial cells, particularly plexiform lesions [71, 93]. Entrapped axons are NFP positive.

Molecular Studies

Chromosomal imbalance, particularly losses, is more common in neurofibromatosis type I associated lesions than in sporadic neurofibromas. The most frequent losses in neurofibromatosis associated lesions are in chromosomes 17 where the NF1 gene resides and 19p but losses are also found in 19q and 22q [95].

Differential Diagnosis

Old neurotized nevi may resemble neurofibroma histopathologically, but residual nevus cells or an epidermal component can declare their true nature.

The fingerprint pattern of CD34 in a neurofibroma (Fig. 7.9g) can help distinguish it from early desmoplastic melanoma where it is absent or rarely focal [94].

At low power, diffuse neurofibroma (Fig. 7.9f) and pigmented neurofibroma can mimic dermatofibrosarcoma protuberans (DFSP) and Bednar tumor, respectively, and both can be CD34 positive (Fig. 7.9h), but DFSP and Bednar are S100 negative [74, 96].

Atypical or cellular neurofibromas may be confused with malignant peripheral nerve sheath tumors (MPNST); however, mitoses, particularly in the setting of neurofibromatosis type I, should favor the later. Increased p53 and Ki-67 staining also indicates MPNST [88].

Perineuriomas

Introduction

Perineurioma can be intraneural or extraneural; the later including soft tissue, sclerosing, plexiform, and reticular variants. Intraneural perineuriomas develop primarily in named nerves of the extremities and rarely involve skin. Soft tissue perineuriomas present as painless nodules of the extremities or trunk without obvious associated identifiable nerve. Sclerosing perineuriomas typically occur on the digits and palm of young adults [97].

Microscopic Features

Soft tissue perineuriomas are well-circumscribed but unencapsulated tumors composed of elongate spindle cells with long, slender bipolar processes and occasional epithelioid cells. The lesion is organized in fascicles, whorls, or a storiform pattern [98]. The stroma can be collagenous or more myxoid. Atypical lesions have been reported with scattered pleomorphic cells and infiltrative margins but appear to be indolent and likely represent degenerative change similar to what is seen in ancient schwannomas [98].

The retiform or reticular variant is composed of anastomosing cords of cells with bipolar cytoplasmic process that wrap around islands of fibromyxoid stroma in a net-like pattern [99].

Sclerosing perineuriomas can involve the dermis and/or subcutis and are characterized by epithelioid and spindle cells in a trabecular or whorled (onion skin) pattern within a dense sclerotic, collagenous stroma (Fig. 7.10a, b) [97].

Malignant perineuriomas are very rare and are considered a perineurial variant of malignant peripheral nerve sheath tumor [100].

Immunohistochemistry

Like normal perineurium, perineuriomas are positive with epithelial membrane antigen (EMA) (Fig. 7.10c), glucose transporter-1 (GLUT-1) (Fig. 7.10d), and the tight junction protein, claudin-1 but are negative with S-100 protein, GFAP, and NFP [101]. Given the extremely thin cytoplasmic processes of perineurial cells and the abundant fibrous component, EMA can appear negative and GLUT-1 and claudin-1 may be of greater use [98, 102]. As many as 60 % of perineuriomas express SMA and CD34 [97, 98, 103, 104].

Molecular Studies

Studies of perineuriomas to date have predominantly focused on abnormalities in the region of the NF2 gene on chromosome 22. Giannini et al. identified deletion of part or all of chromosome 22 in two cases of soft tissue perineurioma and recently another such lesion was reported in a patient with neurofibromatosis type 2 [105, 106]. Two other groups demonstrated mutations in the NF2 gene by molecular analyses in four sclerosing perineurioma and one soft tissue perineurioma [107, 108]. In contrast, loss of chromosome 13 was the sole abnormality in another soft tissue lesion [109]. Two cases of sclerosing perineuri-

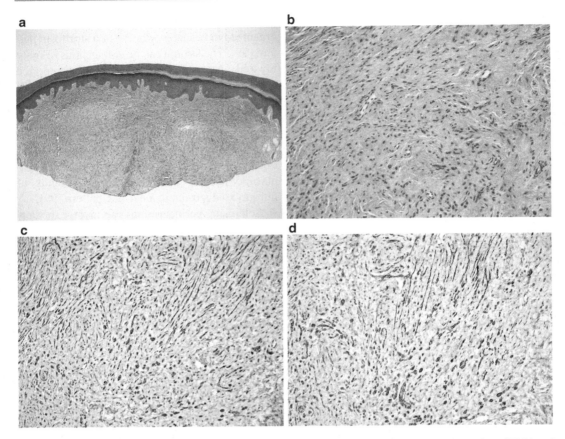

Fig. 7.10 Sclerosing perineurioma. (**a**) Dermal tumor on acral skin characterized by cells in a trabecular or whorled pattern within a dense sclerotic, collagenous stroma. (**b**) Epithelioid and spindled cells. (**c**) Expression of EMA and (**d**) GLUT-1

oma have been reported that demonstrate rearrangement and deletion of chromosome 10q [108, 110]. Molecular studies currently are of greatest value in excluding important lesions in the differential of perineurioma.

Differential Diagnosis

DFSP can be EMA positive and enter the differential diagnosis of a soft tissue perineurioma. This is further complicated by the fact that some perineuriomas are CD34 positive. However, most perineuriomas are circumscribed and lack the honeycomb infiltration of fat and t(17;22), seen in DFSP [104].

Similarly, low grade fibromyxoid sarcomas (LGFMS) often immunohistochemically express EMA and can express claudin-1, but typically show alternating hyalinized and myxoid zones and are characterized by t(7;16) [111, 112]. LGFMS has only been studied with GLUT-1 in two cases in which they were completely negative but additional study is required to confirm its potential utility [113].

Solitary fibrous tumors, sclerotic fibromas, and fibromas of the tendon sheath are EMA negative. Schwannoma, neurofibroma, and myxoid neurothekeoma can be distinguished by expression of S100 protein. However, benign peripheral nerve sheath tumors with hybrid features of perineurioma-neurofibroma and perineurioma-schwannoma are increasingly being reported [114].

Schwannomas

Introduction

Schwannomas, formerly known as neurilemmomas, involve cranial or peripheral nerves but also occur in the soft tissue and dermis as solitary, asymptomatic nodules. Lesions may be painful or tender [115]. Cutaneous lesions occur with a predilection for the limbs of young to middle age adults [116]. Multiple lesions occur in neurofibromatosis type 2 (NF2) which is characterized by acoustic schwannomas, often bilateral, as well as cutaneous schwannomas, meningiomas, and cataracts [117]. This autosomal dominant syndrome is due to a mutation in the gene encoding neurofibromin-2, also called merlin, on chromo-

some 22q12.2. Schwannomatosis has been used to refer to patients with multiple subcutaneous, dermal, and internal schwannomas but without the vestibular and central nervous system tumors that characterize NF2 [118].

Microscopic Features

Classic schwannomas are circumscribed, encapsulated, predominantly subcutaneous tumors composed of varying proportions of a cellular component with parallel nuclei (Antoni A tissue) and loose myxoid component (Antoni B tissue) often with hyalinized vessels. The elongate nuclei of the Antoni A area form rows separated by cell processes forming verocay bodies (Fig. 7.11a). Degenerative pleomorphism, microcysts, and

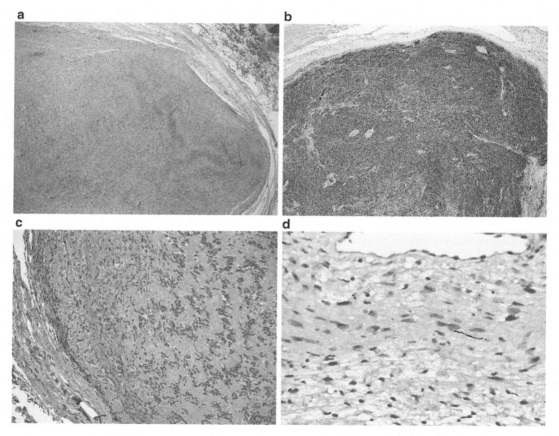

Fig. 7.11 Schwannoma. (**a**) Circumscribed, encapsulated, predominantly subcutaneous tumor composed of a cellular component with parallel nuclei (Antoni A tissue forming verocay bodies) and loose myxoid component (Antoni B tissue). (**b**) S100 protein is strongly expressed. (**c**) EMA highlights the perineurial cells of the capsule. (**d**) Neurofilament protein highlights sparse axons within a schwannoma

hemorrhage can be identified. Prominent degenerative features characterize ancient schwannoma but mitoses are rare [119].

Several histologic variants have been described [120]. Pseudoglandular schwannomas contain prominent microcystic change that resembles glands [121]. However, true glands have been reported in some schwannomas [122]. In the cellular variant, verocay bodies and Antoni B areas are nearly absent [123–125]. The plexiform pattern of multiple interlacing fascicles and nodules is particularly common in cutaneous lesions but lacks correlation with neurofibromatosis and although lesions may be cellular with mild pleomorphism and limited mitotic activity, malignant transformation, as seen in plexiform neurofibroma is not a concern [126–131].

Melanotic schwannomas contain heavily pigmented cells. This variant most commonly involves the spinal nerves from which it can have an aggressive course, while the rarely reported cutaneous lesions have been more indolent [132–134]. Melanotic schwannomas tend to lack a distinct capsule, well-developed Verocay bodies, and distinct Antoni A and B areas [120]. Melanotic schwannomas with prominent psammoma bodies are usually seen in Carney's complex that is comprised of lentigines, myxomas, and endocrinopathy [135–138]. These psammomatous melanotic schwannomas are uncommon in the skin [139].

Epithelioid schwannomas are mainly subcutaneous lesions that contain focal nests and cords of epithelioid cells, in association with areas of classic schwannoma [140–142]. A malignant counterpart of this variant has been described [143, 144]. In contrast, small round cells with little cytoplasm forming rosettes around collagenous cores define the neuroblastoma-like schwannoma [145–147].

Hybrid peripheral nerve sheath tumors containing focal areas with distinct perineurial differentiation have been reported in schwannoma [84, 114, 148, 149]. These areas can be distinct or intimately admixed [150]. Double staining with S100 and EMA may be required to confirm the dual differentiation in the later.

Immunohistochemistry

S100 protein is strongly expressed (Fig. 7.11b), while EMA highlights the perineurial cells of the capsule in schwannomas (Fig. 7.11c). Sox10 is a newer nuclear neural crest marker of Schwann cells and melanocytes that is also positive in schwannomas [91]. GFAP is positive in 33–70% of schwannomas [61, 63].

Originally, schwannomas, unlike neurofibromas, were thought to lack tumoral axons; however, immunohistochemistry for NFP has shown axons both centrally (Fig. 7.11d) and at the periphery in schwannomas of various types, particularly those in patients with NF2 [151–153]. Axons are usually more diffusely distributed in neurofibromas than schwannomas [152].

Most schwannomas lack melanocytic expression with the exception of melanocytic schwannomas that at times, can more strongly express HMB-45 and Melan-a than S100 [133]. Loss of expression of PRKAR1A in a melanotic schwannoma suggests Carney syndrome [133].

Molecular Studies

Mutations involving 22q are the basis of schwannomas, both sporadic and in NF2 [116, 154–158]. Mutations in the NF2 gene have also been detected in one case of hybrid schwannoma-perineurioma [84].

Patients with Schwannomatosis do not have germline mutations in NF2 but somatic mutations have been noted in their cutaneous lesions. Germline mutations in INI-1/SMARCB1 (22q11) have been reported in a small number of these patients [159–163].

Melanotic schwannomas of Carney complex have shown mutations involving 17q22–24, the location of the tumor suppressor gene PRKAR1A that encodes type 1 regulatory subunit of protein kinase A [164–166]. Most of the remaining cases of Carney complex have genetic abnormalities at 2p16 [166].

Differential Diagnosis

Neurofibromas and schwannomas are both S100 positive but it is expressed in a much higher proportion of cells in schwannomas [152]. This is not surprising given that neurofibromas are composed of other cell types in addition to Schwan cells.

Cellular schwannomas, in particular, can be confused with leiomyomas that can also contain Verocay-like structures but lack the blunt-ended nuclei and perinuclear vacuole seen in smooth muscle cells and can be distinguished by the S100 expression in the former and desmin and SMA in the later [116, 120, 167].

MPNSTs are also hypercellular but generally show geographic necrosis and a mitotic count over 4/10 high power fields, unlike cellular schwannomas [120]. Expression of S100 is also less consistent and diffuse in MPNSTs.

Epithelioid schwannomas are mainly subcutaneous lesions that may mimic melanocytic lesions but lack expression of Melan-A and HMB45 [168].

Nerve Sheath Myxomas

Introduction

Although nerve sheath myxoma and neurothekeoma were once considered in the same spectrum, the latter being the more cellular and less myxoid form [169], they are now known to be unrelated [170, 171]. Only the nerve sheath myxoma, formerly known as classic or myxoid neurothekeoma, has proven to be a true peripheral nerve sheath tumor. Nerve sheath myxomas have a propensity for the hands and knee of adults in the fourth decade of life. These tumors are typically solitary and range from 0.5 to 2.5 cm [172]. In contrast, neurothekeomas tend to favor the head, neck, and upper extremities of pediatric and young adult females [170, 173]. Based on immunohistochemical and gene expression, neurothekeomas likely represent a fibrohistiocytic tumor [170, 174].

Microscopic Features

Nerve sheath myxomas are well defined, dermal tumors composed of myxoid lobules separated by fibrous septa (Fig. 7.12a). The lobular cells are typically spindled or stellate and sometimes epithelioid, arranged in a swirling, lamellar, or concentric pattern (Fig. 7.12b). The myxoid stroma reportedly is rich in sulfated acid mucin [175]. Mitotic activity is low but variable hyperchromatism and sometimes nuclear atypia can be present.

Immunohistochemistry

Nerve sheath myxomas express S100, S100A6, NSE, CD57, and GFAP [6, 172, 176]. CD34 and

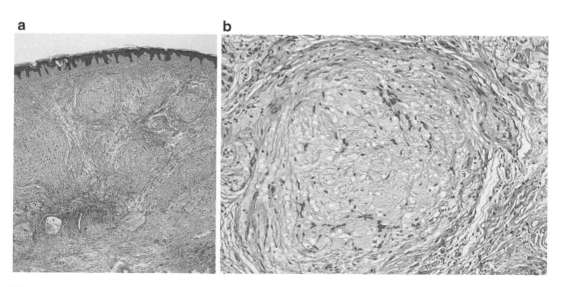

Fig. 7.12 Nerve sheath myxoma. (**a**) Well-defined, dermal tumor composed of myxoid lobules separated by fibrous septa. (**b**) Spindled lobular cells in a swirling pattern within a myxoid stroma

less commonly SMA can highlight scattered spindle cells in the lobules [6]. EMA positive perineurial cells are focally present in the fibrous tissue surrounding the lobules [172]. Usually nerve fibers are not identified within the tumor itself with NFP [6]. Sox10, a Schwannian and melanocytic marker, was expressed in a recently studied nerve sheath myxoma [177].

Molecular Studies

A study of ten spinal nerve sheath myxomas revealed cytogenetic loss of 22q in 80 % of cases but only two involving the NF2 locus [178]. However, there is only one study looking at cutaneous nerve sheath myxomas at the molecular level and they confirmed that nerve sheath myxomas are peripheral nerve sheath tumors, distinct from neurothekeomas [174].

Differential Diagnosis

Superficial angiomyxomas have a vascular component and often epithelial elements, not seen in nerve sheath myxoma. Myxoid neurofibroma may appear similar but typically lack the lobular pattern. Dermal myxoma is less cellular than nerve sheath myxoma. Solitary circumscribed neuroma can show similarities histologically but myxoid change is uncommon [59].

Neurothekeomas are also predominantly dermal, multilobular tumors that can have myxoid foci but are comprised mostly of epithelioid cells (Fig. 7.13a). Cytologic atypia and normal mitotic figures are not uncommon. Despite their prior inclusion in the same spectrum as nerve sheath myxomas, neurothekeomas can be distinguished immunohistochemically. While they are reactive with S100A6 (Fig. 7.13b), they lack

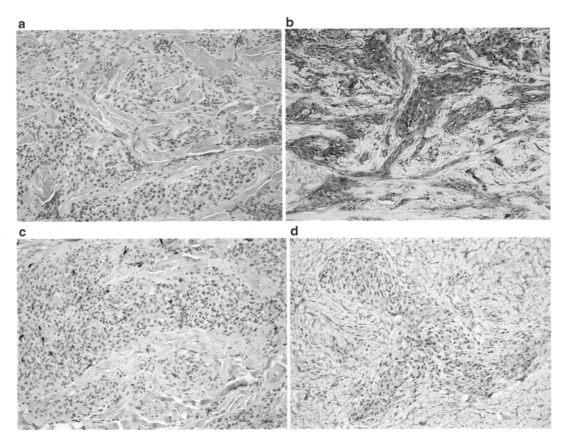

Fig. 7.13 Cellular neurothekeoma. (**a**) Dermal, multilobular tumor composed of epithelioid cells. (**b**) Strongly reactive with S100A6 but (**c**) lacks S100 expression. (**d**) MITF expression can cause confusion with a melanocytic lesion

S100 (Fig. 7.13c) and Sox10 expression. NSE, NKI-C3, CD10, PGP9.5, and podoplanin are positive. A small proportion show focal SMA [170, 173, 177, 179–182]. KBA.62 and MITF (Fig. 7.13d) expression in neurothekeomas can [183, 184] confound distinction from melanocytic lesions but these lesions lack a junctional component and are S100 and Mart-1 negative [177, 180, 181, 185, 186].

Granular Cell Tumors

Introduction

Granular cell tumors (GCTs), previously known as granular cell myoblastoma, can occur at almost any cutaneous or visceral site but occur most on the tongue. They tend to occur in females of the third to sixth decade and have a predilection for the black race [183, 184]. Multiple tumors of the skin and/or viscera occur in up to a quarter of patients [184].

Controversy existed for years over the histogenesis, most likely due to confusion with granular cell change in other types of tumors, but immunohistochemistry is consistent with Schwannian derivation in true GCTs [187–189].

Microscopic Features

These non-encapsulated dermal and/or subcutaneous tumors are composed of sheets or trabeculae of large polyhedral cells with indistinct cell borders, ample granular pink cytoplasm and small, round central nuclei. There are varying numbers of large granules with surrounding clear halo known as pustulo-ovoid bodies of Milian (Fig. 7.14a) [190]. Pseudoepitheliomatous hyperplasia is not uncommonly noted in dermal tumors or those involving the tongue (Fig. 7.14b) [191]. Considering the Schwannian etiology, it is not surprising that perineural spread can be seen (Fig. 7.14c) [192]. Clear cell change and plexiform pattern have been noted [193–195]. Similar to other hybrid peripheral nerve sheath tumors, GCTs with dual perineurial lineage have been reported [196–198].

Immunohistochemistry

Strong S100 (Fig. 7.14d) and Sox10 (Fig. 7.14e) expression in GCTs supports a neuroectodermal origin [199]. These tumors are also positive for NKI-C3, NSE, and CD68 [187, 200, 201]. Studies have also shown expression of calretinin, inhibin-α, PGP9.5, and nerve growth factor receptor [202–206]. Recently, HBME-1, a mesothelial marker, and Galectin-3 reactivity have been noted in GCTs [206]. GCTs are often reactive for MITF but fail to display HMB-45 and only very rarely and focally express Melan-A [207]. Desmin, myoglobin, NFP, and GFAP are negative [200, 208].

Molecular Studies

Molecular studies of GCTs are sparse and have only evaluated oral lesions. Carinci et al. described up- and down-regulation of multiple genes in a GCT from the tongue, many of which were related to neural alterations [209]. However, Gomes et al. noted loss of heterozygosity in five of eight oral granular cell tumors, predominantly involving 9p and 17p [210]. Cytogenetic analysis of three malignant GCTs was inconsistent [211–213] but the findings of one study showed similar alterations as MPNSTs [213].

Differential Diagnosis

The presence of granules in GCT is due to an increased number of lysosomes but it is important to recognize that this can occur focally or more extensively in a variety of other lesions, including dermatofibromas, smooth muscle tumors, basal cell carcinomas, atypical fibroxanthomas, fibrous papules (Fig. 7.15a, b) and dermatofibrosarcoma protuberans [214–228]. Lack of expression of Sox10 and S100 (Fig. 7.15c) may help indicate one of these alternative tumors [199].

Pseudoepitheliomatous hyperplasia of a GCT, particularly in superficial biopsies, can be confused with squamous cell carcinoma [191].

Conventional GCTs differ immunohistochemically from what was initially reported as polypoid granular cell tumor but now is known as

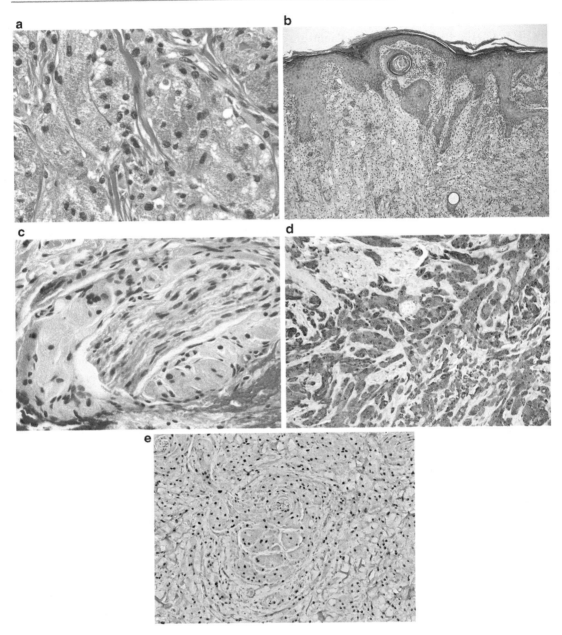

Fig. 7.14 Granular cell tumor. (**a**) Large polygonal cells containing ample granular pink cytoplasm with occasional large granules surrounded by a clear halo, known as pustulo-ovoid bodies of Milian. (**b**) Pseudoepitheliomatous hyperplasia and sheets of large polygonal cells with pink cytoplasm. (**c**) Perineural spread. (**d**) Strong S100 and (**e**) Sox10 expression

primitive or dermal nonneural granular cell tumor (PNGCT) [229–232]. These tumors of the skin mainly involve the trunk. PNGCTs tend to involve the dermis in association with an epidermal collarette (Fig. 7.16a, b) but uncommonly show the pseudoepitheliomatous hyperplasia seen in GCTs. They also tend to be more circumscribed than conventional GCTs [233]. Cytologic

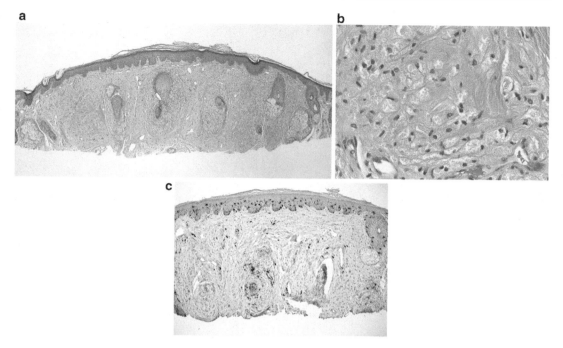

Fig. 7.15 Fibrous papule with granular cell change. (**a**) Dome-shaped papule with perivascular and perifollicular concentric collagenous stroma. (**b**) Cells with granular cytoplasm are noted at higher power. (**c**) The granular cells are S100 negative unlike GCTs

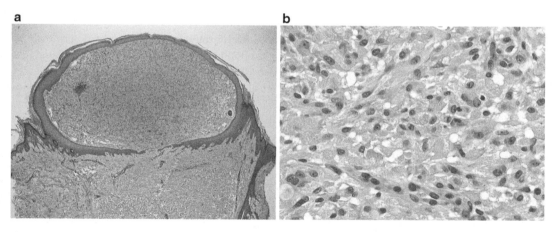

Fig. 7.16 Primitive nonneural granular cell tumor. (**a**) An epidermal collarette surrounds the lesion. (**b**) Ovoid cells with ample granular cytoplasm

features of spindled to ovoid cells with ample granular cytoplasm and expression of lysosomal markers, NKI-C3 and CD68 are similar but PNGCTs are negative with S100 [229–231]. They also lack expression of smooth muscle actin, desmin, cytokeratin, EMA, and Mart-1 [229, 231]. NSE has only been evaluated in one study and was positive in half of cases [231]. Lack of confirmed line of differentiation in these lesions has led some to suggest that they could be granular cell variants of epithelioid histiocytoma [234, 235].

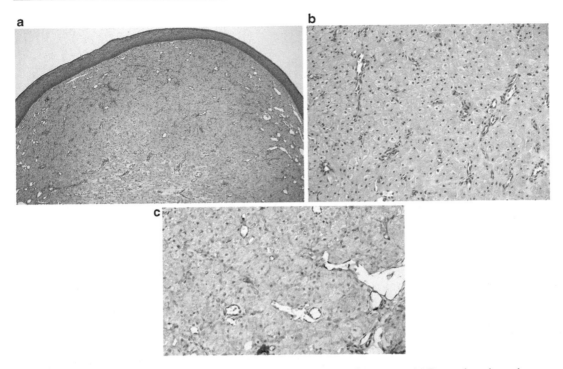

Fig. 7.17 Congenital granular cell epulis of the anterior alveolar ridge of a neonate. (**a**) Dome-shaped papule composed of sheets of pale round cells. (**b**) Ample granular cytoplasm. (**c**) S100 negative unlike GCT

Congenital granular cell epulis has similar cytopathologic features but occurs on the anterior alveolar ridge of neonates and often spontaneously regresses [236]. They tend to show more vascularity than GCTs (Fig. 7.17a, b). Similar to PNGCT, congenital granular cell epulis is S100 negative (Fig. 7.17c), NKI/C3 and variably CD68 positive [237–239]. PGP9.5 and NSE expression has been reported [237, 238].

Malignant behavior has been reported in lesions with only mild atypia and thus criteria diagnostic of malignant GCT is not well defined. Size over 5 cm, rapid growth, and vascular invasion have been considered ominous. Fanburg-Smith et al. offered criteria for categorizing lesions histopathologically. Tumors with two or less of the following are classified as atypical and those with three or more, as malignant: necrosis, spindling of tumor cells, vesicular nuclei with large nucleoli, mitotic rate over two in ten high power fields, high nuclear to cytoplasmic ratio, or pleomorphism [240]. Mitotic

and proliferative rate can also be determined by immunohistochemistry with phosphorylated histone H3 and Ki-67 [241]. More recently Nasser et al. showed that necrosis and mitotic activity alone had similar selectivity for aggressive behavior [242].

Merkel Cell Carcinomas

Introduction

The exact derivation of neuroendocrine carcinoma of the skin is debated. Given the immunohistochemical profile and ultrastructural features, epidermal Merkel cells are the favored histogenesis and thus the more common name, Merkel cell carcinoma (MCC) [243]. Derivation from a dermal neuroendocrine cell or pluripotent epidermal stem cell has also been proposed [244]. Trabecular carcinoma was a former designation for MCC but many lesions do not have a trabecular histologic pattern.

The pathogenesis is not understood but the propensity for involvement of sun-damaged skin of the head, neck, and upper extremities suggests a role for UV irradiation [245]. An altered immune status also is associated with development of disease [245–248]. Integration of viral Merkel cell polyomavirus DNA into the genome of the tumor cells suggests a role for this virus in the etiology of MCC [249].

Presentation is typical in elderly Caucasians as an indistinct, pink to violaceous nodule (Fig. 7.18a). Recurrence and metastases to lymph nodes, liver, bone, and lung are not uncommon [250, 251]. The prognosis is poor, especially with advanced disease. The 10 year survival rate of localized disease is 71% but regional and distant spread drops to 48% and 20%, respectively [252].

Microscopic Features

MCC is primarily a dermal tumor but commonly extends into the subcutaneous fat. It is composed of sheets of round cells with high nuclear to cytoplasmic ratio, stippled nuclei, and prominent nucleoli. Mitotic figures and apoptotic cells are frequent and nuclear molding is notable (Fig. 7.18b). Intraepidermal spread is noted in 10% or more of cases (Fig. 7.18c) and rarely has been reported in the epidermis alone, often in association with squamous cell carcinoma in situ [253–264].

Three variants are reported with the intermediate type being the most common. The intermediate subtype is characterized by nodules and sheets of cells with vesicular nuclei, inconspicuous cytoplasm, and small nucleoli. The trabecular variant is least common, despite the original designation of trabecular carcinoma, and consists of ribbons of tumor cells. In contrast, the small cell variant consists of hyperchromatic small cells that often show crush artifact similar to lymphomas.

It is not uncommon to see intermixed or synchronous MCC with squamous cell carcinoma (Fig. 7.18d) and less commonly basal cell carcinoma [265–267]. Lymphoepithelial-like, melanocytic, glandular, neuroblastic, and sarcomatous

components have been reported [244, 264, 268–275].

Larger tumors with subcutaneous extension, small cell size, high mitotic rate, lymphovascular invasion, and heavy lymphoid infiltrate tend to have a worse prognosis [251, 276, 277]. Although the histopathologic features of prognostic interest are still being studied, the current College of American Pathologists protocol for reporting a primary MCC includes: tumor size, thickness, lymphovascular invasion, invasion of bone/muscle/ fascia/cartilage, mitotic rate, tumor-infiltrating lymphocytes, nodular versus infiltrative growth pattern, and secondary malignancy. However, the current pathologic staging of MCC only takes in to account maximum tumor dimension (2 cm or less is pT1, over 2 cm but less than 5 cm is pT2, and over 5 cm is pT3) and invasion of bone, muscle, fascia, or cartilage (pT4) [278].

Immunohistochemistry

As the name implies, MCC (primary cutaneous neuroendocrine carcinoma of the skin), these lesions express neuroendocrine markers as well as epithelial markers, especially lower molecular weight keratins. Most MCCs are CK20 (Fig. 7.18e) and NFP (Fig. 7.18f) positive in a paranuclear dot-like pattern but staining can be more diffuse [279–284]. Unlike metastatic small cell carcinoma of the lung, MCC is typically negative with MASH-1 (mammalian achaete-scute homolog-1), CK7, and thyroid transcription factor 1 (TTF-1) [285–287]. However, exceptions occur and CK20–/CK7+ MCCs, even rarely with TTF-1 expression, have been noted [288, 289]. NSE, chromogranin, and synaptophysin are variably expressed [279, 290, 291].

Markers often associated with various lymphomas can also be reactive in MCC, including: Alk-1 (depending on the clone used), bcl-2, terminal deoxynucleotidyl transferase (TdT), PAX5, and CD56 [292–300]. Other immunohistochemical markers important when considering entities in the histopathologic differential diagnosis include: PAX-8 [301] and Ber-EP4 [290, 302] that are positive in most reported

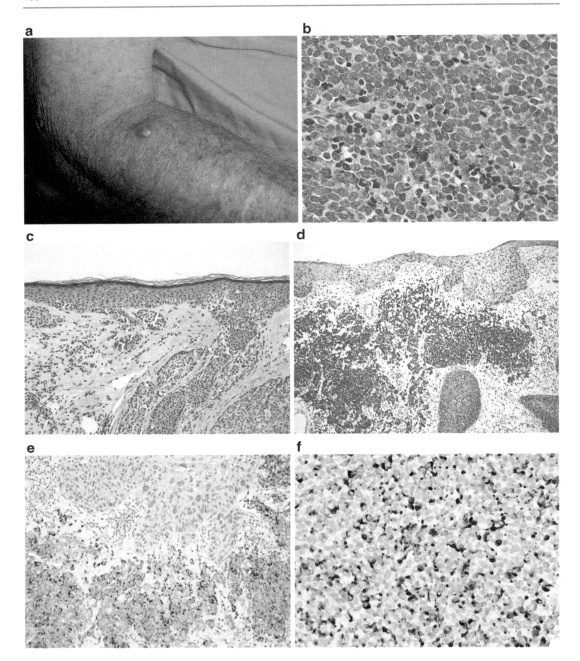

Fig. 7.18 Merkel cell carcinoma. (**a**) Pink to violaceous nodule on an elderly man's arm. (**b**) Round cells with high nuclear to cytoplasmic ratio, stippled nuclei, mitotic figures, apoptotic cells, and nuclear molding. (**c**) Intraepidermal spread. (**d**) Intermixed squamous cell carcinoma. (**e**) Paranuclear dot like pattern with CK20 in the MCC but absent in the squamous cell carcinoma. (**f**) Paranuclear dot like pattern with neurofilament protein. (**g**) Small metastatic focus in a sentinel lymph node. (**h**) Tumor in the lymph node highlighted with CK20

g h

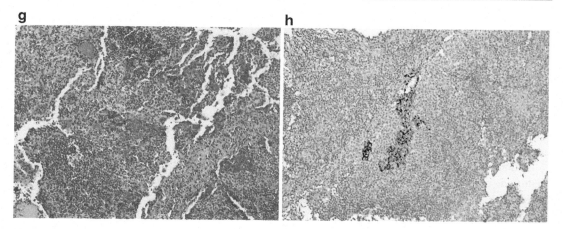

Fig. 7.18 (continued)

cases and Fli-1 [303–305] and CD99 [305–307] that show expression in up to half of reported MCCs. In contrast, CD45 is negative and S100 expression is only very rarely reported in MCCs [290, 308].

In 2008, a polyomavirus, dubbed Merkel cell polyomavirus (MCV), was identified in 80 % of MCCs [249]. Although real-time PCR is more reliable for identification, Merkel cell polyomavirus (MCV) large T (LT) antigen can be detected immunohistochemically with the antibodies CM2B4 and Ab3 with significant correlation relative to copy number of MCV per cell. Approximately 70–80 % of MCCs are positive with the commercially available CM2B4 but this may vary geographically [309–312]. Matsushita et al. recently studied a new polyclonal antibody to the MCV small T antigen (ST-1) with improved specificity but lower sensitivity [313]. Immunohistochemical identification may suggest the diagnosis of MCC; however, given the low incidence of the virus in Australian MCCs and reports of viral presence by PCR and rarely CM2B4 expression in non-Merkel cell skin cancers, further study is warranted [312, 314–317].

Increased Ki-67 proliferative index and although with some controversy, presence of p63 expression, have been associated with a worse prognosis [305, 317–324]. Similar to small cell lung cancer, MCCs often express CD117 (KIT receptor); however, they do not seem to contain the activating mutations in exons 9, 13, or 17 and response to the c-kit inhibitor, imatinib has been limited in MCCs [325–329].

Immunohistochemistry improves detection of small metastatic foci in sentinel lymph nodes (Fig. 7.18g) [330, 331]. CK20 is popular in this setting (Fig. 7.18h) and although expression can change in metastatic foci, it is important to consider the staining pattern of the primary tumor when selecting markers for evaluation, as all MCCs are not CK20 positive [288, 289, 332].

Molecular Studies

Based on the demographics affected, MCC development is associated with ultraviolet exposure and immunosuppression but discovery of integration of MCV DNA into the genome of MCC cells suggests that it has at least a part in the pathogenesis [249, 333, 334].

Studies using PCR have typically identified MCV in 60–90 % of MCCs; however, most of these studies have been in North America or Europe while two studies on prevalence in Australia identified MCV in only 20 % of MCCs [312]. Paik et al. proposed that there is a separate MCV independent pathway of oncogenesis in many MCCs arising in chronically sun-exposed skin [312]. Presence of the virus by PCR has been associated with a better prognosis but subsequent studies have found no such association [309, 317, 320, 335–339].

Presence of the virus alone is not diagnostic of MCC given that it is ubiquitous in the population [340–342]. It is also infrequently found in metastatic neuroendocrine tumors from other organs, including the lung, when comprehensive primers are used and in 25–30 % of non-MCC skin cancers [314, 343–345]. However, viral load is much lower than in MCC and often is not detectable by immunohistochemistry [314, 346].

Although a signature mutation has not been identified, multiple chromosomal abnormalities have been demonstrated in MCC, including increased copies of chromosomes 1, 3q, 5p, and 6 as well as losses in 3p, 4, 5q, 7, 10, and 13 [347, 348]. However, studies differ considerably and others have shown deletions in 1p similar to other neoplasms of the neural crest [349–352]. MCC with and without MCV may similarly have inactivation of retinoblastoma (Rb) through differing mechanisms [353]. In lesions with MCV, viral antigens bind, sequester, and inactivate this tumor suppressor [354]. Whereas, RB1 is often downregulated in virus negative tumors, possibly due to deletions or mutations in chromosome 13 in the region of this locus [355, 356].

Differential Diagnosis

The small blue cells of MCC can be confused with extraskeletal Ewing's sarcoma/ primitive neuroectodermal tumor (EWS/PNET), lymphoma, melanoma, and metastatic small cell carcinoma, typically from the lung.

Both small cell melanoma and MCC can show pagetoid epidermal involvement but S100 is expressed in melanoma and only very rare in MCC. CK20 and NFP characterize MCC but not melanoma [308].

While MCC and metastatic small cell carcinoma of the lung can both be NSE positive, the latter is typically CK20 and NFP negative but CK7, TTF-1, and MASH-1 positive [285–287, 357]. However, TTF-1 and CK7 expression has been reported in some MCCs and CK20 has been reported in small cell carcinoma of the lung [289, 358]. Therefore, a panel of these markers is preferred, in addition to clinical correlation.

The small blue cell appearance of MCC in conjunction with Alk-1 or CD56 reactivity can be confused with anaplastic large cell lymphoma or NK-cell lymphoma, respectively [292, 294]. Similarly, expression of bcl-2, TdT, or PAX5 could misguide the unwary pathologist to diagnosis B-cell lymphoma [293, 295–300, 359]. Expression of CD45 (leukocyte common antigen), however, helps distinguish lymphoma from MCC.

NSE and synaptophysin are expressed in both MCC and EWS/PNET. CD99 and Fli-1 reactivity is typical of EWS/PNET but can be expressed in up to half of MCCs [303–307]. Pankeratin is usually absent and CK20 expression has not yet been reported in EWS/PNET and therefore, may be helpful [360]. Fluorescence in situ hybridization for the t(11;22) translocation or PCR for the EWS-Fli-1 fusion in EWS/PNET can confirm the diagnosis [306, 361].

MCC can be confused with basal cell carcinoma (BCC), particularly in small biopsies. Ber-EP4 and/or bcl-2 should not be used alone for distinction given that most MCCs are positive with both and in contrast, BCC can rarely express chromogranin or synaptophysin [290, 302, 359, 362, 363]. CK20 and a larger biopsy may be helpful in distinction.

Melanoma, Paget's disease, Bowen disease, sebaceous carcinoma, and cutaneous T-cell lymphoma enter the differential of the small proportion of cases of MCC with intraepidermal spread. Immunohistochemistry should serve to distinguish these entities [364].

Malignant Peripheral Nerve Sheath Tumors

Introduction

Malignant peripheral nerve sheath tumor (MPNST) is the preferred term for what was previously called neurofibrosarcoma, malignant schwannoma, or neurogenic sarcoma [365, 366]. Most cutaneous cases are thought to arise from a neurofibroma [367]. The extremity is the most common site of involvement, followed by the trunk [368].

Nearly half of MPNSTs occur in patients with neurofibromatosis type I (NF-1), usually within

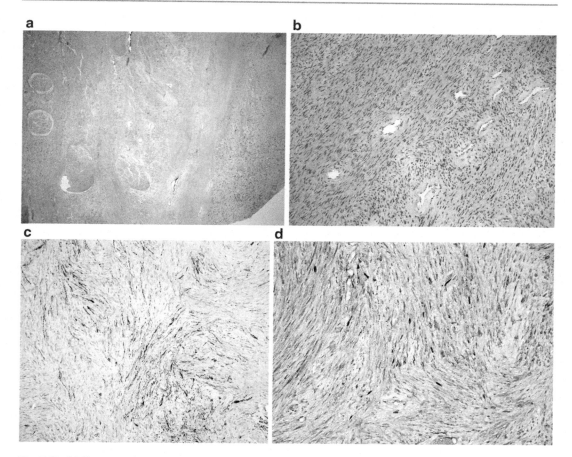

Fig. 7.19 Malignant peripheral nerve sheath tumor. (**a**) MPNST (*right*) occurring in a plexiform neurofibroma (*left*). (**b**) Fascicles of spindle cells with hyper- and hypo-cellular areas with hyperchromatic and pleomorphic nuclei. (**c**) Focal S100 expression. (**d**) Focal Sox-10 expression

plexiform neurofibromas (Fig. 7.19a) that are showing enlargement and pain [72, 369, 370]. In comparison, patients with NF-1 have a less than 10 % lifetime risk of developing a MPNST. When developing in NF-1, it typically occurs at an earlier age than sporadic lesions [369, 371]. Ten percent of MPNSTs, instead arise in the setting of prior therapeutic radiation [368, 372].

Microscopic Features

Classically, MPNSTs arise in the deep soft tissue; however, there have been case reports and small series describing dermal tumors [373–375]. MPNSTs consist of fascicles of spindle cells with hyper- and hypo-cellular areas. The nuclei are variably hyperchromatic and pleomorphic based on the grade of tumor (Fig. 7.19b). Cells with more epithelioid features tend to collect around blood vessels. Myxoid change can be prominent. Normal and atypical mitotic figures are present.

Tumors occasionally show glandular, chondroid, osteoid, vascular, or rhabdomyosarcomatous differentiation [370, 376–378]. The latter is known as a malignant triton tumor. Rare cases of MPNST show perineurial differentiation ("malignant perineuriomas") [100, 379].

Epithelioid MPNST is a rare variant thought to arise from a schwannoma [380–382]. It is characterized by variably sized round to oval cells with eosinophilic cytoplasm in a lobulated pattern [383].

Immunohistochemistry

Up to half of MPNSTs are S100 and Sox-10 positive, but typically only in a focal pattern (Fig. 7.19c, d) [92, 384–386]. Strong diffuse staining should suggest possible alternative diagnoses. However, epithelioid MPNSTs tend to be strongly and diffusely S100 positive [380]. Recently, growth-associated protein 43 (GAP43) expression was noted in 18/21 MPNSTs, but is also positive in neurofibromas, schwannomas, and desmoplastic melanoma [387]. Nestin and p75 (NGFR) are expressed in the majority of tumors [205, 388–390]. While only studied in a limited number of early described tumors, expression of NSE, CD57 (Leu-7), and myelin basic protein (MBP) has been noted in some MPNSTs. PGP9.5, a broad neural marker, is positive in most cases, including some that are S100 negative [391]. GFAP and NFP positivity are reported in a small percentage of studied cases [61, 365, 392–394]. CD99, EMA and other cytokeratins are generally negative [365, 390, 392, 395].

The rhabdomyoid element of the malignant triton tumor can be confirmed with desmin, myoglobin, myogenin, or muscle-specific actin [396, 397]. The perineurial variant is EMA positive and S100 negative [379, 398].

Molecular Studies

MPNSTs show numerous chromosome aberrations and complex karyotype changes with no specific balanced gene rearrangement identified [399, 400]. Common are gains in chromosome arms 8q, 17q, and 7p, and losses in 9p, 11q, and 17p [401–403]. Somatic NF1 mutations in 17q11 are identified in a sizable proportion of MPNSTs regardless of history of neurofibromatosis, type 1 [156, 404–406].

Differential Diagnosis

MPNSTs can be difficult to distinguish from other malignant spindle cell tumors. Fibrosarcoma are also cellular spindle cell tumors but typically have a herringbone pattern and lack S100 reactivity. Leiomyosarcomas contain cells with blunt-ended nuclei and a paranuclear vacuole. Reactivity for desmin and SMA may be necessary to confirm the smooth muscle lineage.

Pleomorphic undifferentiated sarcoma often contains multinucleated pleomorphic cells, in addition to the spindle cell component, and lacks S100 expression. Dermatofibrosarcoma protuberans (DFSP) contains more uniform cells that extend into the fat in a honeycomb pattern.

Desmoplastic or spindle cell melanoma can be difficult to distinguish from MPNSTs given that both are S100 and Sox-10 positive and usually negative with more specific melanocytic markers. Although not always present, melanin or a junctional component suggests melanoma. Strong and diffuse S100 or Sox-10 reactivity also favors melanoma over MPNSTs that tend to be more focal or patchy [407].

Degenerative features of ancient schwannoma, including cytologic atypia and mitoses may be present but these lesions are small and well-delineated. Other degenerative changes such as calcification, cysts, myxoid change, hemorrhage, and siderophages may also be present in ancient schwannomas [383]. Cellular schwannomas are similarly more circumscribed and usually diffusely S100 and Sox-10 positive [388].

Some epithelioid MPNST may need to be distinguished from epithelioid sarcoma or carcinoma, both of which are generally positive with cytokeratins and negative with S100.

MPNSTs, particularly those with a glandular component, should be distinguished from synovial sarcoma, but it is typically S100, nestin, and Sox-10 negative and cytokeratin or EMA positive [384, 390]. The t(X;18) translocation is frequent in synovial sarcoma but has also been reported in MPNSTs [384, 408, 409].

References

1. Sahoo B, Radotra BD, Kaur I, Kumar B. Zosteriform pilar leiomyoma. J Dermatol. 2001;28(12):759–61.
2. Tomlinson IP, Alam NA, Rowan AJ, Barclay E, Jaeger EE, Kelsell D, et al. Germline mutations in FH predispose to dominantly inherited uterine fibroids, skin leiomyomata and papillary renal cell cancer. Nat Genet. 2002;30(4):406–10.
3. Fuertes L, Santonja C, Kutzner H, Requena L. Immunohistochemistry in dermatopathology: a review of the most commonly used antibodies (part I). Actas Dermosifiliogr. 2013;104(2):99–127.

4. Perez-Montiel MD, Plaza JA, Dominguez-Malagon H, Suster S. Differential expression of smooth muscle myosin, smooth muscle actin, h-caldesmon, and calponin in the diagnosis of myofibroblastic and smooth muscle lesions of skin and soft tissue. Am J Dermatopathol. 2006;28(2):105–11.

5. Ceballos KM, Nielsen GP, Selig MK, O'Connell JX. Is anti-h-caldesmon useful for distinguishing smooth muscle and myofibroblastic tumors? An immunohistochemical study. Am J Clin Pathol. 2000;114(5):746–53.

6. Laskin WB, Fetsch JF, Miettinen M. The "neurothekeoma": immunohistochemical analysis distinguishes the true nerve sheath myxoma from its mimics. Hum Pathol. 2000;31(10):1230–41.

7. Rangdaeng S, Truong LD. Comparative immunohistochemical staining for desmin and muscle-specific actin. A study of 576 cases. Am J Clin Pathol. 1991;96(1):32–45.

8. Truong LD, Rangdaeng S, Cagle P, Ro JY, Hawkins H, Font RL. The diagnostic utility of desmin. A study of 584 cases and review of the literature. Am J Clin Pathol. 1990;93(3):305–14.

9. Cessna MH, Zhou H, Perkins SL, Tripp SR, Layfield L, Daines C, et al. Are myogenin and myoD1 expression specific for rhabdomyosarcoma? A study of 150 cases, with emphasis on spindle cell mimics. Am J Surg Pathol. 2001;25(9):1150–7.

10. Bayer-Garner I, Morgan M, Smoller BR. Caveolin expression is common among benign and malignant smooth muscle and adipocyte neoplasms. Mod Pathol. 2002;15(1):1–5.

11. Bardella C, El-Bahrawy M, Frizzell N, Adam J, Ternette N, Hatipoglu E, et al. Aberrant succination of proteins in fumarate hydratase-deficient mice and HLRCC patients is a robust biomarker of mutation status. J Pathol. 2011;225(1):4–11.

12. Chen YB, Brannon AR, Toubaji A, Dudas ME, Won HH, Al-Ahmadie HA, et al. Hereditary leiomyomatosis and renal cell carcinoma syndrome-associated renal cancer: recognition of the syndrome by pathologic features and the utility of detecting aberrant succination by immunohistochemistry. Am J Surg Pathol. 2014;38(5):627–37.

13. Newman PL, Fletcher CD. Smooth muscle tumours of the external genitalia: clinicopathological analysis of a series. Histopathology. 1991;18(6):523–9.

14. Nielsen GP, Rosenberg AE, Koerner FC, Young RH, Scully RE. Smooth-muscle tumors of the vulva. A clinicopathological study of 25 cases and review of the literature. Am J Surg Pathol. 1996;20(7):779–93.

15. Matoso A, Chen S, Plaza JA, Osunkoya AO, Epstein JI. Symplastic leiomyomas of the scrotum: a comparative study to usual leiomyomas and leiomyosarcomas. Am J Surg Pathol. 2014;38(10):1410–7.

16. Chaudhary KS, Shousha S. Leiomyoma of the nipple, and normal subareolar muscle fibres, are oestrogen and progesterone receptor positive. Histopathology. 2004;44(6):626–8.

17. McGinley KM, Bryant S, Kattine AA, Fitzgibbon JF, Googe PB. Cutaneous leiomyomas lack estrogen and progesterone receptor immunoreactivity. J Cutan Pathol. 1997;24(4):241–5.

18. Suarez-Penaranda JM, Vieites B, Evgenyeva E, Vazquez-Veiga H, Forteza J. Male genital leiomyomas showing androgen receptor expression. J Cutan Pathol. 2007;34(12):946–9.

19. Horton E, Dobin SM, Debiec-Rychter M, Donner LR. A clonal translocation (7;8)(p13;q11.2) in a leiomyoma of the vulva. Cancer Genet Cytogenet. 2006;170(1):58–60.

20. Guardiola MT, Dobin SM, Dal Cin P, Donner LR. Pericentric inversion (12)(p12q13-14) as the sole chromosomal abnormality in a leiomyoma of the vulva. Cancer Genet Cytogenet. 2010;199(1):21–3.

21. Holst VA, Junkins-Hopkins JM, Elenitsas R. Cutaneous smooth muscle neoplasms: clinical features, histologic findings, and treatment options. J Am Acad Dermatol. 2002;46(4):477–90. quiz 491–4.

22. Kawagishi N, Kashiwagi T, Ibe M, Manabe A, Ishida-Yamamoto A, Hashimoto Y, et al. Pleomorphic angioleiomyoma. Am J Dermatopathol. 2000;22(3):268–71.

23. Matsuyama A, Hisaoka M, Hashimoto H. Angioleiomyoma: a clinicopathologic and immunohistochemical reappraisal with special reference to the correlation with myopericytoma. Hum Pathol. 2007;38(4):645–51.

24. Johansson B, Eriksson A, Thornell LE. Intermediate filament proteins in developing human arteries. Anat Embryol (Berl). 1999;199(3):225–31.

25. Nishio J, Iwasaki H, Ohjimi Y, Ishiguro M, Kobayashi K, Nabeshima K, et al. Chromosomal imbalances in angioleiomyomas by comparative genomic hybridization. Int J Mol Med. 2004; 13(1):13–6.

26. Winchester DS, Hocker TL, Brewer JD, Baum CL, Hochwalt PC, Arpey CJ, et al. Leiomyosarcoma of the skin: clinical, histopathologic, and prognostic factors that influence outcomes. J Am Acad Dermatol. 2014;71(5):919–25.

27. Ramdial PK, Sing Y, Deonarain J, Hadley GP, Singh B. Dermal Epstein Barr virus-associated leiomyosarcoma: tocsin of acquired immunodeficiency syndrome in two children. Am J Dermatopathol. 2011;33(4):392–6.

28. Stout AP, hill WT. Leiomyosarcoma of the superficial soft tissues. Cancer. 1958;11(4):844–54.

29. Fields JP, Helwig EB. Leiomyosarcoma of the skin and subcutaneous tissue. Cancer. 1981;47(1):156–69.

30. Idriss MH, Kazlouskaya V, Malhotra S, Andres C, Elston DM. Phosphohistone-H3 and Ki-67 immunostaining in cutaneous pilar leiomyoma and leiomyosarcoma (atypical intradermal smooth muscle neoplasm). J Cutan Pathol. 2013;40(6):557–63.

31. Suster S, Rosen LB, Sanchez JL. Granular cell leiomyosarcoma of the skin. Am J Dermatopathol. 1988;10(3):234–9.

32. Suster S. Epithelioid leiomyosarcoma of the skin and subcutaneous tissue. Clinicopathologic, immunohistochemical, and ultrastructural study of five cases. Am J Surg Pathol. 1994;18(3):232–40.

33. Kraft S, Fletcher CD. Atypical intradermal smooth muscle neoplasms: clinicopathologic analysis of 84 cases and a reappraisal of cutaneous "leiomyosarcoma". Am J Surg Pathol. 2011;35(4):599–607.

34. Hall BJ, Grossmann AH, Webber NP, Ward RA, Tripp SR, Rosenthal HG, et al. Atypical intradermal smooth muscle neoplasms (formerly cutaneous leiomyosarcomas): case series, immunohistochemical profile and review of the literature. Appl Immunohistochem Mol Morphol. 2013;21(2):132–8.

35. Dahl I, Angervall L. Cutaneous and subcutaneous leiomyosarcoma. A clinicopathologic study of 47 patients. Pathol Eur. 1974;9(4):307–15.

36. Jensen ML, Jensen OM, Michalski W, Nielsen OS, Keller J. Intradermal and subcutaneous leiomyosarcoma: a clinicopathological and immunohistochemical study of 41 cases. J Cutan Pathol. 1996;23(5):458–63.

37. Fauth CT, Bruecks AK, Temple W, Arlette JP, DiFrancesco LM. Superficial leiomyosarcoma: a clinicopathologic review and update. J Cutan Pathol. 2010;37(2):269–76.

38. Hashimoto H, Daimaru Y, Tsuneyoshi M, Enjoji M. Leiomyosarcoma of the external soft tissues. A clinicopathologic, immunohistochemical, and electron microscopic study. Cancer. 1986;57(10):2077–88.

39. Massi D, Franchi A, Alos L, Cook M, Di Palma S, Enguita AB, et al. Primary cutaneous leiomyosarcoma: clinicopathological analysis of 36 cases. Histopathology. 2010;56(2):251–62.

40. Miyajima K, Oda Y, Oshiro Y, Tamiya S, Kinukawa N, Masuda K, et al. Clinicopathological prognostic factors in soft tissue leiomyosarcoma: a multivariate analysis. Histopathology. 2002;40(4):353–9.

41. Pisters PW, Leung DH, Woodruff J, Shi W, Brennan MF. Analysis of prognostic factors in 1,041 patients with localized soft tissue sarcomas of the extremities. J Clin Oncol. 1996;14(5):1679–89.

42. Kaddu S, Beham A, Cerroni L, Humer-Fuchs U, Salmhofer W, Kerl H, et al. Cutaneous leiomyosarcoma. Am J Surg Pathol. 1997;21(9):979–87.

43. Oliver GF, Reiman HM, Gonchoroff NJ, Muller SA, Umbert IJ. Cutaneous and subcutaneous leiomyosarcoma: a clinicopathological review of 14 cases with reference to antidesmin staining and nuclear DNA patterns studied by flow cytometry. Br J Dermatol. 1991;124(3):252–7.

44. Swanson PE, Stanley MW, Scheithauer BW, Wick MR. Primary cutaneous leiomyosarcoma. A histological and immunohistochemical study of 9 cases, with ultrastructural correlation. J Cutan Pathol. 1988;15(3):129–41.

45. Sakamoto A, Oda Y, Yamamoto H, Oshiro Y, Miyajima K, Itakura E, et al. Calponin and h-caldesmon expression in atypical fibroxanthoma and superficial leiomyosarcoma. Virchows Arch. 2002;440(4):404–9.

46. Ito A, Yamada N, Yoshida Y, Morino S, Yamamoto O. Myofibroblastic differentiation in atypical fibroxanthomas occurring on sun-exposed skin and in a burn scar: an ultrastructural and immunohistochemical study. J Cutan Pathol. 2011;38(8):670–6.

47. Longacre TA, Smoller BR, Rouse RV. Atypical fibroxanthoma. Multiple immunohistologic profiles. Am J Surg Pathol. 1993;17(12):1199–209.

48. Luzar B, Calonje E. Morphological and immunohistochemical characteristics of atypical fibroxanthoma with a special emphasis on potential diagnostic pitfalls: a review. J Cutan Pathol. 2010;37(3):301–9.

49. Beer TW, Drury P, Heenan PJ. Atypical fibroxanthoma: a histological and immunohistochemical review of 171 cases. Am J Dermatopathol. 2010;32(6):533–40.

50. Derre J, Lagace R, Nicolas A, Mairal A, Chibon F, Coindre JM, et al. Leiomyosarcomas and most malignant fibrous histiocytomas share very similar comparative genomic hybridization imbalances: an analysis of a series of 27 leiomyosarcomas. Lab Invest. 2001;81(2):211–5.

51. Fletcher CD. Solitary circumscribed neuroma of the skin (so-called palisaded, encapsulated neuroma). A clinicopathologic and immunohistochemical study. Am J Surg Pathol. 1989;13(7):574–80.

52. Reed RJ, Fine RM, Meltzer HD. Palisaded, encapsulated neuromas of the skin. Arch Dermatol. 1972;106(6):865–70.

53. Koutlas IG, Scheithauer BW. Palisaded encapsulated ("solitary circumscribed") neuroma of the oral cavity: a review of 55 cases. Head Neck Pathol. 2010;4(1):15–26.

54. Jokinen CH, Ragsdale BD, Argenyi ZB. Expanding the clinicopathologic spectrum of palisaded encapsulated neuroma. J Cutan Pathol. 2010;37(1):43–8.

55. Navarro M, Vilata J, Requena C, Aliaga A. Palisaded encapsulated neuroma (solitary circumscribed neuroma) of the glans penis. Br J Dermatol. 2000;142(5):1061–2.

56. Argenyi ZB, Cooper PH, Santa Cruz D. Plexiform and other unusual variants of palisaded encapsulated neuroma. J Cutan Pathol. 1993;20(1):34–9.

57. Argenyi ZB, Penick GD. Vascular variant of palisaded encapsulated neuroma. J Cutan Pathol. 1993;20(1):92–3.

58. Tsang WY, Chan JK. Epithelioid variant of solitary circumscribed neuroma of the skin. Histopathology. 1992;20(5):439–41.

59. Misago N, Inoue T, Narisawa Y. Unusual benign myxoid nerve sheath lesion: myxoid palisaded encapsulated neuroma (PEN) or nerve sheath myxoma with PEN/PEN-like features? Am J Dermatopathol. 2007;29(2):160–4.

60. Argenyi ZB. Immunohistochemical characterization of palisaded, encapsulated neuroma. J Cutan Pathol. 1990;17(6):329–35.

61. Gray MH, Rosenberg AE, Dickersin GR, Bhan AK. Glial fibrillary acidic protein and keratin expression by benign and malignant nerve sheath tumors. Hum Pathol. 1989;20(11):1089–96.

62. Kawahara E, Oda Y, Ooi A, Katsuda S, Nakanishi I, Umeda S. Expression of glial fibrillary acidic protein (GFAP) in peripheral nerve sheath tumors. A comparative study of immunoreactivity of GFAP, vimentin, S-100 protein, and neurofilament in 38 schwannomas and 18 neurofibromas. Am J Surg Pathol. 1988;12(2):115–20.

63. Memoli VA, Brown EF, Gould VE. Glial fibrillary acidic protein (GFAP) immunoreactivity in peripheral nerve sheath tumors. Ultrastruct Pathol. 1984;7(4):269–75.

64. Raue F, Frank-Raue K. Multiple endocrine neoplasia type 2: 2007 update. Horm Res. 2007;68 Suppl 5:101–4.

65. Argenyi ZB, Santa Cruz D, Bromley C. Comparative light-microscopic and immunohistochemical study of traumatic and palisaded encapsulated neuromas of the skin. Am J Dermatopathol. 1992;14(6): 504–10.

66. Fletcher CD, Theaker JM. Digital pacinian neuroma: a distinctive hyperplastic lesion. Histopathology. 1989;15(3):249–56.

67. Lassmann G, Lassmann H, Stockinger L. Morton's metatarsalgia. Light and electron microscopic observations and their relation to entrapment neuropathies. Virchows Arch A Pathol Anat Histol. 1976;370(4):307–21.

68. Riccardi VM. Mast-cell stabilization to decrease neurofibroma growth. Preliminary experience with ketotifen. Arch Dermatol. 1987;123(8):1011–6.

69. Gerber PA, Antal AS, Neumann NJ, Homey B, Matuschek C, Peiper M, et al. Neurofibromatosis. Eur J Med Res. 2009;14(3):102–5.

70. Ferner RE. Neurofibromatosis 1. Eur J Hum Genet. 2007;15(2):131–8.

71. Abbas O, Bhawan J. Cutaneous plexiform lesions. J Cutan Pathol. 2010;37(6):613–23.

72. Valeyrie-Allanore L, Ismaili N, Bastuji-Garin S, Zeller J, Wechsler J, Revuz J, et al. Symptoms associated with malignancy of peripheral nerve sheath tumours: a retrospective study of 69 patients with neurofibromatosis 1. Br J Dermatol. 2005;153(1):79–82.

73. Megahed M. Histopathological variants of neurofibroma. A study of 114 lesions. Am J Dermatopathol. 1994;16(5):486–95.

74. van Zuuren EJ, Posma AN. Diffuse neurofibroma on the lower back. J Am Acad Dermatol. 2003; 48(6):938–40.

75. Magro G, Amico P, Vecchio GM, Caltabiano R, Castaing M, Kacerovska D, et al. Multinucleated floret-like giant cells in sporadic and NF1-associated neurofibromas: a clinicopathologic study of 94 cases. Virchows Arch. 2010;456(1):71–6.

76. Puri PK, Tyler WB, Ferringer TC. Neurofibroma with clear cell change. Am J Dermatopathol. 2009; 31(5):453–6.

77. Nakashima K, Yamada N, Yoshida Y, Yamamoto O. Solitary sclerotic neurofibroma of the skin. Am J Dermatopathol. 2008;30(3):278–80.

78. Gonzalez-Vela MC, Val-Bernal JF, Gonzalez-Lopez MA, Drake M, Fernandez-Llaca JH. Pure sclerotic neurofibroma: a neurofibroma mimicking sclerotic fibroma. J Cutan Pathol. 2006;33(1):47–50.

79. Val-Bernal JF, Gonzalez-Vela MC. Cutaneous lipomatous neurofibroma: characterization and frequency. J Cutan Pathol. 2005;32(4):274–9.

80. Michal M, Fanburg-Smith JC, Mentzel T, Kutzner H, Requena L, Zamecnik M, et al. Dendritic cell neurofibroma with pseudorosettes: a report of 18 cases of a distinct and hitherto unrecognized neurofibroma variant. Am J Surg Pathol. 2001;25(5): 587–94.

81. Fisher DA, Chu P, McCalmont T. Solitary plexiform neurofibroma is not pathognomonic of von Recklinghausen's neurofibromatosis: a report of a case. Int J Dermatol. 1997;36(6):439–42.

82. Pizem J, Nicholson KM, Mraz J, Prieto VG. Melanocytic differentiation is present in a significant proportion of nonpigmented diffuse neurofibromas: a potential diagnostic pitfall. Am J Surg Pathol. 2013;37(8):1182–91.

83. Schaffer JV, Chang MW, Kovich OI, Kamino H, Orlow SJ. Pigmented plexiform neurofibroma: distinction from a large congenital melanocytic nevus. J Am Acad Dermatol. 2007;56(5):862–8.

84. Kazakov DV, Pitha J, Sima R, Vanecek T, Shelekhova K, Mukensnabl P, et al. Hybrid peripheral nerve sheath tumors: schwannoma-perineurioma and neurofibroma-perineurioma. A report of three cases in extradigital locations. Ann Diagn Pathol. 2005;9(1):16–23.

85. Zamecnik M, Michal M. Perineurial cell differentiation in neurofibromas. Report of eight cases including a case with composite perineurioma-neurofibroma features. Pathol Res Pract. 2001;197(8):537–44.

86. Feany MB, Anthony DC, Fletcher CD. Nerve sheath tumours with hybrid features of neurofibroma and schwannoma: a conceptual challenge. Histopathology. 1998;32(5):405–10.

87. Shelekhova KV, Danilova AB, Michal M, Kazakov DV. Hybrid neurofibroma-perineurioma: an additional example of an extradigital tumor. Ann Diagn Pathol. 2008;12(3):233–4.

88. Lin BT, Weiss LM, Medeiros LJ. Neurofibroma and cellular neurofibroma with atypia: a report of 14 tumors. Am J Surg Pathol. 1997;21(12):1443–9.

89. Chen Y, Klonowski PW, Lind AC, Lu D. Differentiating neurotized melanocytic nevi from neurofibromas using Melan-A (MART-1) immunohistochemical stain. Arch Pathol Lab Med. 2012;136(7):810–5.

90. Weiss SW, Langloss JM, Enzinger FM. Value of S-100 protein in the diagnosis of soft tissue tumors with particular reference to benign and malignant Schwann cell tumors. Lab Invest. 1983;49(3): 299–308.

91. Nonaka D, Chiriboga L, Rubin BP. Sox10: a pan-schwannian and melanocytic marker. Am J Surg Pathol. 2008;32(9):1291–8.

92. Karamchandani JR, Nielsen TO, van de Rijn M, West RB. Sox10 and S100 in the diagnosis of soft-tissue neoplasms. Appl Immunohistochem Mol Morphol. 2012;20(5):445–50.

93. Hirose T, Tani T, Shimada T, Ishizawa K, Shimada S, Sano T. Immunohistochemical demonstration of EMA/Glut1-positive perineurial cells and CD34-positive fibroblastic cells in peripheral nerve sheath tumors. Mod Pathol. 2003;16(4):293–8.

94. Yeh I, McCalmont TH. Distinguishing neurofibroma from desmoplastic melanoma: the value of the CD34 fingerprint. J Cutan Pathol. 2011;38(8):625–30.

95. Koga T, Iwasaki H, Ishiguro M, Matsuzaki A, Kikuchi M. Losses in chromosomes 17, 19, and 22q in neurofibromatosis type 1 and sporadic neurofibromas: a comparative genomic hybridization analysis. Cancer Genet Cytogenet. 2002;136(2):113–20.

96. Fetsch JF, Michal M, Miettinen M. Pigmented (melanotic) neurofibroma: a clinicopathologic and immunohistochemical analysis of 19 lesions from 17 patients. Am J Surg Pathol. 2000;24(3):331–43.

97. Fetsch JF, Miettinen M. Sclerosing perineurioma: a clinicopathologic study of 19 cases of a distinctive soft tissue lesion with a predilection for the fingers and palms of young adults. Am J Surg Pathol. 1997;21(12):1433–42.

98. Hornick JL, Fletcher CD. Soft tissue perineurioma: clinicopathologic analysis of 81 cases including those with atypical histologic features. Am J Surg Pathol. 2005;29(7):845–58.

99. Graadt van Roggen JF, McMenamin ME, Belchis DA, Nielsen GP, Rosenberg AE, Fletcher CD. Reticular perineurioma: a distinctive variant of soft tissue perineurioma. Am J Surg Pathol. 2001;25(4):485–93.

100. Hirose T, Scheithauer BW, Sano T. Perineurial malignant peripheral nerve sheath tumor (MPNST): a clinicopathologic, immunohistochemical, and ultrastructural study of seven cases. Am J Surg Pathol. 1998;22(11):1368–78.

101. Kaku Y, Fukumoto T, Louise Opada G, Anan T, Kimura T. A clinicopathologic and immunohisto-chemical study of 7 cases of sclerosing perineurioma. Am J Dermatopathol. 2014;37:122–8.

102. Folpe AL, Billings SD, McKenney JK, Walsh SV, Nusrat A, Weiss SW. Expression of claudin-1, a recently described tight junction-associated protein, distinguishes soft tissue perineurioma from potential mimics. Am J Surg Pathol. 2002;26(12):1620–6.

103. Fox MD, Gleason BC, Thomas AB, Victor TA, Cibull TL. Extra-acral cutaneous/soft tissue sclerosing perineurioma: an under-recognized entity in the differential of CD34-positive cutaneous neoplasms. J Cutan Pathol. 2010;37(10):1053–6.

104. Pina-Oviedo S, Ortiz-Hidalgo C. The normal and neoplastic perineurium: a review. Adv Anat Pathol. 2008;15(3):147–64.

105. Giannini C, Scheithauer BW, Jenkins RB, Erlandson RA, Perry A, Borell TJ, et al. Soft-tissue perineurioma. Evidence for an abnormality of chromosome 22, criteria for diagnosis, and review of the literature. Am J Surg Pathol. 1997;21(2):164–73.

106. Pitchford CW, Schwartz HS, Atkinson JB, Cates JM. Soft tissue perineurioma in a patient with neurofibromatosis type 2: a tumor not previously associated with the NF2 syndrome. Am J Surg Pathol. 2006;30(12):1624–9.

107. Lasota J, Fetsch JF, Wozniak A, Wasag B, Sciot R, Miettinen M. The neurofibromatosis type 2 gene is mutated in perineurial cell tumors: a molecular genetic study of eight cases. Am J Pathol. 2001;158(4):1223–9.

108. Sciot R, Dal Cin P, Hagemeijer A, De Smet L, Van Damme B, Van den Berghe H. Cutaneous sclerosing perineurioma with cryptic NF2 gene deletion. Am J Surg Pathol. 1999;23(7):849–53.

109. Mott RT, Goodman BK, Burchette JL, Cummings TJ. Loss of chromosome 13 in a case of soft tissue perineurioma. Clin Neuropathol. 2005;24(2):69–76.

110. Brock JE, Perez-Atayde AR, Kozakewich HP, Richkind KE, Fletcher JA, Vargas SO. Cytogenetic aberrations in perineurioma: variation with subtype. Am J Surg Pathol. 2005;29(9):1164–9.

111. Macarenco RS, Ellinger F, Oliveira AM. Perineurioma: a distinctive and underrecognized peripheral nerve sheath neoplasm. Arch Pathol Lab Med. 2007;131(4):625–36.

112. Thway K, Fisher C, Debiec-Rychter M, Calonje E. Claudin-1 is expressed in perineurioma-like low-grade fibromyxoid sarcoma. Hum Pathol. 2009;40(11):1586–90.

113. Ahrens WA, Ridenour III RV, Caron BL, Miller DV, Folpe AL. GLUT-1 expression in mesenchymal tumors: an immunohistochemical study of 247 soft tissue and bone neoplasms. Hum Pathol. 2008;39(10):1519–26.

114. Hornick JL, Bundock EA, Fletcher CD. Hybrid schwannoma/perineurioma: clinicopathologic analysis of 42 distinctive benign nerve sheath tumors. Am J Surg Pathol. 2009;33(10):1554–61.

115. Buscher CA, Izumi AK. A painful subcutaneous neurilemmoma attached to a peripheral nerve. J Am Acad Dermatol. 1998;38(1):122–4.

116. Rodriguez-Peralto JL, Riveiro-Falkenbach E, Carrillo R. Benign cutaneous neural tumors. Semin Diagn Pathol. 2013;30(1):45–57.

117. Parry DM, Eldridge R, Kaiser-Kupfer MI, Bouzas EA, Pikus A, Patronas N. Neurofibromatosis 2 (NF2): clinical characteristics of 63 affected individuals and clinical evidence for heterogeneity. Am J Med Genet. 1994;52(4):450–61.

118. Leverkus M, Kluwe L, Roll EM, Becker G, Brocker EB, Mautner VF, et al. Multiple unilateral schwannomas: segmental neurofibromatosis type 2 or schwannomatosis? Br J Dermatol. 2003;148(4):804–9.

119. Dahl I. Ancient neurilemmoma (schwannoma). Acta Pathol Microbiol Scand A. 1977;85(6):812–8.

120. Kurtkaya-Yapicier O, Scheithauer B, Woodruff JM. The pathobiologic spectrum of Schwannomas. Histol Histopathol. 2003;18(3):925–34.

121. Lisle A, Jokinen C, Argenyi Z. Cutaneous pseudoglandular schwannoma: a case report of an unusual histopathologic variant. Am J Dermatopathol. 2011;33(5):e63–5.

122. Kim YC, Park HJ, Cinn YW, Vandersteen DP. Benign glandular schwannoma. Br J Dermatol. 2001;145(5): 834–7.

123. Kang SK, Chang SE, Choi JH, Sung KJ, Moon KC, Koh JK. A case of cellular schwannoma of the skin presenting as a large ulcerated tumor on the ankle. J Dermatol. 2002;29(1):28–32.

124. Fletcher CD, Davies SE, McKee PH. Cellular schwannoma: a distinct pseudosarcomatous entity. Histopathology. 1987;11(1):21–35.

125. Woodruff JM, Godwin TA, Erlandson RA, Susin M, Martini N. Cellular schwannoma: a variety of schwannoma sometimes mistaken for a malignant tumor. Am J Surg Pathol. 1981;5(8):733–44.

126. Megahed M. Plexiform schwannoma. Am J Dermatopathol. 1994;16(3):288–93.

127. Punia RS, Dhingra N, Mohan H. Cutaneous plexiform schwannoma of the finger not associated with neurofibromatosis. Am J Clin Dermatol. 2008;9(2): 129–31.

128. Kao GF, Laskin WB, Olsen TG. Solitary cutaneous plexiform neurilemmoma (schwannoma): a clinicopathologic, immunohistochemical, and ultrastructural study of 11 cases. Mod Pathol. 1989;2(1): 20–6.

129. Fletcher CD, Davies SE. Benign plexiform (multinodular) schwannoma: a rare tumour unassociated with neurofibromatosis. Histopathology. 1986;10(9): 971–80.

130. Ko JY, Kim JE, Kim YH, Ro YS. Cutaneous plexiform schwannomas in a patient with neurofibromatosis type 2. Ann Dermatol. 2009;21(4):402–5.

131. Berg JC, Scheithauer BW, Spinner RJ, Allen CM, Koutlas IG. Plexiform schwannoma: a clinicopathologic overview with emphasis on the head and neck region. Hum Pathol. 2008;39(5):633–40.

132. Kaehler KC, Russo PA, Katenkamp D, Kreusch T, Neuber K, Schwarz T, et al. Melanocytic schwannoma of the cutaneous and subcutaneous tissues: three cases and a review of the literature. Melanoma Res. 2008;18(6):438–42.

133. Torres-Mora J, Dry S, Li X, Binder S, Amin M, Folpe AL. Malignant melanotic schwannian tumor: a clinicopathologic, immunohistochemical, and gene expression profiling study of 40 cases, with a proposal for the reclassification of "melanotic schwannoma". Am J Surg Pathol. 2014;38(1):94–105.

134. Zhang HY, Yang GH, Chen HJ, Wei B, Ke Q, Guo H, et al. Clinicopathological, immunohistochemical, and ultrastructural study of 13 cases of melanotic schwannoma. Chin Med J (Engl). 2005;118(17): 1451–61.

135. Carney JA. Psammomatous melanotic schwannoma. A distinctive, heritable tumor with special associations, including cardiac myxoma and the Cushing syndrome. Am J Surg Pathol. 1990;14(3):206–22.

136. Carney JA, Stratakis CA. Epithelioid blue nevus and psammomatous melanotic schwannoma: the unusual pigmented skin tumors of the Carney complex. Semin Diagn Pathol. 1998;15(3):216–24.

137. Utiger CA, Headington JT. Psammomatous melanotic schwannoma. A new cutaneous marker for Carney's complex. Arch Dermatol. 1993;129(2): 202–4.

138. Claessens N, Heymans O, Arrese JE, Garcia R, Oelbrandt B, Pierard GE. Cutaneous psammomatous melanotic schwannoma: non-recurrence with surgical excision. Am J Clin Dermatol. 2003;4(11): 799–802.

139. Thornton CM, Handley J, Bingham EA, Toner PG, Walsh MY. Psammomatous melanotic schwannoma arising in the dermis in a patient with Carney's complex. Histopathology. 1992;20(1):71–3.

140. Orosz Z. Cutaneous epithelioid schwannoma: an unusual benign neurogenic tumor. J Cutan Pathol. 1999;26(4):213–4.

141. Smith K, Mezebish D, Williams JP, Menon P, Rolfe A, Cobb M, et al. Cutaneous epithelioid schwannomas: a rare variant of a benign peripheral nerve sheath tumor. J Cutan Pathol. 1998;25(1):50–5.

142. Kindblom LG, Meis-Kindblom JM, Havel G, Busch C. Benign epithelioid schwannoma. Am J Surg Pathol. 1998;22(6):762–70.

143. Manganoni AM, Farisoglio C, Lonati A, Zorzi F, Tucci G, Pinton PG. Cutaneous epithelioid malignant schwannoma: review of the literature and case report. J Plast Reconstr Aesthet Surg. 2009;62(9): e318–21.

144. Woodruff JM, Selig AM, Crowley K, Allen PW. Schwannoma (neurilemoma) with malignant transformation. A rare, distinctive peripheral nerve tumor. Am J Surg Pathol. 1994;18(9):882–95.

145. Suchak R, Luzar B, Bacchi CE, Maguire B, Calonje E. Cutaneous neuroblastoma-like schwannoma: a report of two cases, one with a plexiform pattern, and a review of the literature. J Cutan Pathol. 2010;37(9):997–1001.

146. Fisher C, Chappell ME, Weiss SW. Neuroblastoma-like epithelioid schwannoma. Histopathology. 1995;26(2):193–4.

147. Lewis ZT, Geisinger KR, Pichardo R, Sangueza OP. Schwannoma with neuroblastoma-like rosettes: an unusual morphologic variant. Am J Dermatopathol. 2005;27(3):243–6.

148. Michal M, Kazakov DV, Belousova I, Bisceglia M, Zamecnik M, Mukensnabl P. A benign neoplasm with histopathological features of both schwannoma and retiform perineurioma (benign schwannoma-perineurioma): a report of six cases of a distinctive soft tissue tumor with a predilection for the fingers. Virchows Arch. 2004;445(4):347–53.

149. Macarenco AC, Macarenco RS. Intradermal monophasic hybrid schwannoma-perineurioma: a

diagnostic challenge. Am J Dermatopathol. 2010;32(5):526–8.

150. Phan DC, Gleason BC. Recent developments in benign peripheral nerve sheath tumors. J Cutan Pathol. 2008;35(12):1165–9.

151. Wechsler J, Lantieri L, Zeller J, Voisin MC, Martin-Garcia N, Wolkenstein P. Aberrant axon neurofilaments in schwannomas associated with phacomatoses. Virchows Arch. 2003;443(6):768–73.

152. Nascimento AF, Fletcher CD. The controversial nosology of benign nerve sheath tumors: neurofilament protein staining demonstrates intratumoral axons in many sporadic schwannomas. Am J Surg Pathol. 2007;31(9):1363–70.

153. Hamada Y, Iwaki T, Fukui M, Tateishi J. A comparative study of embedded nerve tissue in six NF2-associated schwannomas and 17 nonassociated NF2 schwannomas. Surg Neurol. 1997;48(4):395–400.

154. Selvanathan SK, Shenton A, Ferner R, Wallace AJ, Huson SM, Ramsden RT, et al. Further genotype–phenotype correlations in neurofibromatosis 2. Clin Genet. 2010;77(2):163–70.

155. Miyakawa T, Kamada N, Kobayashi T, Hirano K, Fujii K, Sasahara Y, et al. Neurofibromatosis type 2 in an infant with multiple plexiform schwannomas as first symptom. J Dermatol. 2007;34(1):60–4.

156. Mertens F, Dal Cin P, De Wever I, Fletcher CD, Mandahl N, Mitelman F, et al. Cytogenetic characterization of peripheral nerve sheath tumours: a report of the CHAMP study group. J Pathol. 2000;190(1):31–8.

157. Abo-Dalo B, Kutsche K, Mautner V, Kluwe L. Large intragenic deletions of the NF2 gene: breakpoints and associated phenotypes. Genes Chromosomes Cancer. 2010;49(2):171–5.

158. Wolff RK, Frazer KA, Jackler RK, Lanser MJ, Pitts LH, Cox DR. Analysis of chromosome 22 deletions in neurofibromatosis type 2-related tumors. Am J Hum Genet. 1992;51(3):478–85.

159. Hulsebos TJ, Plomp AS, Wolterman RA, Robanus-Maandag EC, Baas F, Wesseling P. Germline mutation of INI1/SMARCB1 in familial schwannomatosis. Am J Hum Genet. 2007;80(4):805–10.

160. Hulsebos TJ, Kenter SB, Jakobs ME, Baas F, Chong B, Delatycki MB. SMARCB1/INI1 maternal germ line mosaicism in schwannomatosis. Clin Genet. 2010;77(1):86–91.

161. Boyd C, Smith MJ, Kluwe L, Balogh A, Maccollin M, Plotkin SR. Alterations in the SMARCB1 (INI1) tumor suppressor gene in familial schwannomatosis. Clin Genet. 2008;74(4):358–66.

162. Hadfield KD, Newman WG, Bowers NL, Wallace A, Bolger C, Colley A, et al. Molecular characterisation of SMARCB1 and NF2 in familial and sporadic schwannomatosis. J Med Genet. 2008;45(6):332–9.

163. Sestini R, Bacci C, Provenzano A, Genuardi M, Papi L. Evidence of a four-hit mechanism involving SMARCB1 and NF2 in schwannomatosis-associated schwannomas. Hum Mutat. 2008;29(2):227–31.

164. Casey M, Vaughan CJ, He J, Hatcher CJ, Winter JM, Weremowicz S, et al. Mutations in the protein kinase A R1alpha regulatory subunit cause familial cardiac myxomas and Carney complex. J Clin Invest. 2000;106(5):R31–8.

165. Kirschner LS, Sandrini F, Monbo J, Lin JP, Carney JA, Stratakis CA. Genetic heterogeneity and spectrum of mutations of the PRKAR1A gene in patients with the Carney complex. Hum Mol Genet. 2000;9(20):3037–46.

166. Stratakis CA, Kirschner LS, Carney JA. Clinical and molecular features of the Carney complex: diagnostic criteria and recommendations for patient evaluation. J Clin Endocrinol Metab. 2001;86(9):4041–6.

167. Lespi PJ, Smit R. Verocay body-prominent cutaneous leiomyoma. Am J Dermatopathol. 1999;21(1):110–1.

168. Saad AG, Mutema GK, Mutasim DF. Benign cutaneous epithelioid Schwannoma: case report and review of the literature. Am J Dermatopathol. 2005;27(1):45–7.

169. Argenyi ZB, LeBoit PE, Santa Cruz D, Swanson PE, Kutzner H. Nerve sheath myxoma (neurothekeoma) of the skin: light microscopic and immunohistochemical reappraisal of the cellular variant. J Cutan Pathol. 1993;20(4):294–303.

170. Fetsch JF, Laskin WB, Hallman JR, Lupton GP, Miettinen M. Neurothekeoma: an analysis of 178 tumors with detailed immunohistochemical data and long-term patient follow-up information. Am J Surg Pathol. 2007;31(7):1103–14.

171. Barnhill RL, Dickersin GR, Nickeleit V, Bhan AK, Muhlbauer JE, Phillips ME, et al. Studies on the cellular origin of neurothekeoma: clinical, light microscopic, immunohistochemical, and ultrastructural observations. J Am Acad Dermatol. 1991;25(1 Pt 1):80–8.

172. Fetsch JF, Laskin WB, Miettinen M. Nerve sheath myxoma: a clinicopathologic and immunohistochemical analysis of 57 morphologically distinctive, S-100 protein- and GFAP-positive, myxoid peripheral nerve sheath tumors with a predilection for the extremities and a high local recurrence rate. Am J Surg Pathol. 2005;29(12):1615–24.

173. Hornick JL, Fletcher CD. Cellular neurothekeoma: detailed characterization in a series of 133 cases. Am J Surg Pathol. 2007;31(3):329–40.

174. Sheth S, Li X, Binder S, Dry SM. Differential gene expression profiles of neurothekeomas and nerve sheath myxomas by microarray analysis. Mod Pathol. 2011;24(3):343–54.

175. Goldstein J, Lifshitz T. Myxoma of the nerve sheath. Report of three cases, observations by light and electron microscopy and histochemical analysis. Am J Dermatopathol. 1985;7(5):423–9.

176. Fullen DR, Lowe L, Su LD. Antibody to S100a6 protein is a sensitive immunohistochemical marker for neurothekeoma. J Cutan Pathol. 2003;30(2):118–22.

177. Fried I, Sitthinamsuwan P, Muangsomboon S, Kaddu S, Cerroni L, McCalmont TH. SOX-10 and MiTF expression in cellular and 'mixed' neurothekeoma. J Cutan Pathol. 2014;41(8):640–5.

178. Rickert CH, Schwering EM, Siebers J, Hartmann C, von Deimling A, Paulus W. Chromosomal imbalances and NF2 mutational analysis in a series of 10 spinal nerve sheath myxomas. Histopathology. 2007;50(2):252–7.

179. Wang AR, May D, Bourne P, Scott G. PGP9.5: a marker for cellular neurothekeoma. Am J Surg Pathol. 1999;23(11):1401–7.

180. Plaza JA, Torres-Cabala C, Evans H, Diwan AH, Prieto VG. Immunohistochemical expression of S100A6 in cellular neurothekeoma: clinicopathologic and immunohistochemical analysis of 31 cases. Am J Dermatopathol. 2009;31(5):419–22.

181. Page RN, King R, Mihm Jr MC, Googe PB. Microphthalmia transcription factor and NKI/C3 expression in cellular neurothekeoma. Mod Pathol. 2004;17(2):230–4.

182. Kaddu S, Leinweber B. Podoplanin expression in fibrous histiocytomas and cellular neurothekeomas. Am J Dermatopathol. 2009;31(2):137–9.

183. Apisarnthanarax P. Granular cell tumor. An analysis of 16 cases and review of the literature. J Am Acad Dermatol. 1981;5(2):171–82.

184. Lack EE, Worsham GF, Callihan MD, Crawford BE, Klappenbach S, Rowden G, et al. Granular cell tumor: a clinicopathologic study of 110 patients. J Surg Oncol. 1980;13(4):301–16.

185. Fox MD, Billings SD, Gleason BC, Moore J, Thomas AB, Shea CR, et al. Expression of MiTF may be helpful in differentiating cellular neurothekeoma from plexiform fibrohistiocytic tumor (histiocytoid predominant) in a partial biopsy specimen. Am J Dermatopathol. 2012;34(2):157–60.

186. Suarez A, High WA. Immunohistochemical analysis of KBA.62 in 18 neurothekeomas: a potential marker for differentiating neurothekeoma, but a marker that may lead to confusion with melanocytic tumors. J Cutan Pathol. 2014;41(1):36–41.

187. Buley ID, Gatter KC, Kelly PM, Heryet A, Millard PR. Granular cell tumours revisited. An immunohistological and ultrastructural study. Histopathology. 1988;12(3):263–74.

188. Ordonez NG, Mackay B. Granular cell tumor: a review of the pathology and histogenesis. Ultrastruct Pathol. 1999;23(4):207–22.

189. Ordonez NG. Granular cell tumor: a review and update. Adv Anat Pathol. 1999;6(4):186–203.

190. Epstein DS, Pashaei S, Hunt Jr E, Fitzpatrick JE, Golitz LE. Pustulo-ovoid bodies of Milian in granular cell tumors. J Cutan Pathol. 2007;34(5):405–9.

191. Abu-Eid R, Landini G. Morphometrical differences between pseudo-epitheliomatous hyperplasia in granular cell tumours and squamous cell carcinomas. Histopathology. 2006;48(4):407–16.

192. Battistella M, Cribier B, Feugeas JP, Roux J, Le Pelletier F, Pinquier L, et al. Vascular invasion and other invasive features in granular cell tumours of the skin: a multicentre study of 119 cases. J Clin Pathol. 2014;67(1):19–25.

193. Zedek DC, Murphy BA, Shea CR, Hitchcock MG, Reutter JC, White WL. Cutaneous clear-cell granular cell tumors: the histologic description of an unusual variant. J Cutan Pathol. 2007;34(5):397–404.

194. Aldabagh B, Azmi F, Vadmal M, Neider S, Usmani AS. Plexiform pattern in cutaneous granular cell tumors. J Cutan Pathol. 2009;36(11):1174–6.

195. Lee J, Bhawan J, Wax F, Farber J. Plexiform granular cell tumor. A report of two cases. Am J Dermatopathol. 1994;16(5):537–41.

196. Matter A, Hewer E, Kappeler A, Fleischmann A, Vajtai I. Plexiform hybrid granular cell tumor/perineurioma: a novel variant of benign peripheral nerve sheath tumor with divergent differentiation. Pathol Res Pract. 2012;208(5):310–4.

197. Zarineh A, Costa ME, Rabkin MS. Multiple hybrid granular cell tumor-perineuriomas. Am J Surg Pathol. 2008;32(10):1572–7.

198. Zarineh A, Rabkin MS. Perineuriomas containing granular cells: 2 distinct variants? Am J Dermatopathol. 2008;30(6):636.

199. Heerema MG, Suurmeijer AJ. Sox10 immunohistochemistry allows the pathologist to differentiate between prototypical granular cell tumors and other granular cell lesions. Histopathology. 2012;61(5):997–9.

200. Raju GC, O'Reilly AP. Immunohistochemical study of granular cell tumour. Pathology. 1987;19(4):402–6.

201. Rekhi B, Jambhekar NA. Morphologic spectrum, immunohistochemical analysis, and clinical features of a series of granular cell tumors of soft tissues: a study from a tertiary referral cancer center. Ann Diagn Pathol. 2010;14(3):162–7.

202. Fine SW, Li M. Expression of calretinin and the alpha-subunit of inhibin in granular cell tumors. Am J Clin Pathol. 2003;119(2):259–64.

203. Hoshi N, Tsu-ura Y, Watanabe K, Suzuki T, Kasukawa R, Suzuki T. Expression of immunoreactivities to 75 kDa nerve growth factor receptor, trk gene product and phosphotyrosine in granular cell tumors. Pathol Int. 1995;45(10):748–56.

204. Le BH, Boyer PJ, Lewis JE, Kapadia SB. Granular cell tumor: immunohistochemical assessment of inhibin-alpha, protein gene product 9.5, S100 protein, CD68, and Ki-67 proliferative index with clinical correlation. Arch Pathol Lab Med. 2004;128(7):771–5.

205. Perosio PM, Brooks JJ. Expression of nerve growth factor receptor in paraffin-embedded soft tissue tumors. Am J Pathol. 1988;132(1):152–60.

206. Bellezza G, Colella R, Sidoni A, Del Sordo R, Ferri I, Cioccoloni C, et al. Immunohistochemical expression of Galectin-3 and HBME-1 in granular cell tumors: a new finding. Histol Histopathol. 2008;23(9):1127–30.

207. Gleason BC, Nascimento AF. HMB-45 and Melan-A are useful in the differential diagnosis between granular cell tumor and malignant melanoma. Am J Dermatopathol. 2007;29(1):22–7.

208. Mazur MT, Shultz JJ, Myers JL. Granular cell tumor. Immunohistochemical analysis of 21 benign tumors and one malignant tumor. Arch Pathol Lab Med. 1990;114(7):692–6.

209. Carinci F, Piattelli A, Rubini C, Fioroni M, Stabellini G, Palmieri A, et al. Genetic profiling of granular cell myoblastoma. J Craniofac Surg. 2004;15(5): 824–34.

210. Gomes CC, Fonseca-Silva T, Gomez RS. Evidence for loss of heterozygosity (LOH) at chromosomes 9p and 17p in oral granular cell tumors: a pilot study. Oral Surg Oral Med Oral Pathol Oral Radiol. 2013;115(2):249–53.

211. Nasser H, Danforth Jr RD, Sunbuli M, Dimitrijevic O. Malignant granular cell tumor: case report with a novel karyotype and review of the literature. Ann Diagn Pathol. 2010;14(4):273–8.

212. Papachristou DJ, Palekar A, Surti U, Cieply K, McGough RL, Rao UN. Malignant granular cell tumor of the ulnar nerve with novel cytogenetic and molecular genetic findings. Cancer Genet Cytogenet. 2009;191(1):46–50.

213. Di Tommaso L, Magrini E, Consales A, Poppi M, Pasquinelli G, Dorji T, et al. Malignant granular cell tumor of the lateral femoral cutaneous nerve: report of a case with cytogenetic analysis. Hum Pathol. 2002;33(12):1237–40.

214. Kanitakis J, Chouvet B. Granular-cell basal cell carcinoma of the skin. Eur J Dermatol. 2005;15(4): 301–3.

215. Maire G, Pedeutour F, Coindre JM. COL1A1-PDGFB gene fusion demonstrates a common histogenetic origin for dermatofibrosarcoma protuberans and its granular cell variant. Am J Surg Pathol. 2002;26(7):932–7.

216. Orosz Z. Atypical fibroxanthoma with granular cells. Histopathology. 1998;33(1):88–9.

217. Rhee DY, Lee HW, Chung WK, Chang SE, Lee MW, Choi JH, et al. Giant dermatofibroma with granular cell changes: side-effect of bee-venom acupuncture? Clin Exp Dermatol. 2009;34(5):e18–20.

218. Val-Bernal JF. Dermatofibroma with granular cells. Histopathology. 1997;31(5):481–2.

219. Wright NA, Thomas CG, Calame A, Cockerell CJ. Granular cell atypical fibroxanthoma: case report and review of the literature. J Cutan Pathol. 2010;37(3):380–5.

220. Beer TW. Keloidal and granular cell change in a series of 171 atypical fibroxanthomas. J Cutan Pathol. 2010;37(6):712–3.

221. Bhattacharyya I, Summerlin DJ, Cohen DM, Ellis GL, Bavitz JB, Gillham LL. Granular cell leiomyoma of the oral cavity. Oral Surg Oral Med Oral Pathol Oral Radiol Endod. 2006;102(3):353–9.

222. Jacyk WK, Rutten A, Requena L. Fibrous papule of the face with granular cells. Dermatology. 2008;216(1): 56–9.

223. Mentzel T, Wadden C, Fletcher CD. Granular cell change in smooth muscle tumours of skin and soft tissue. Histopathology. 1994;24(3):223–31.

224. Rios-Martin JJ, Delgado MD, Moreno-Ramirez D, Garcia-Escudero A, Gonzalez-Campora R. Granular cell atypical fibroxanthoma: report of two cases. Am J Dermatopathol. 2007;29(1):84–7.

225. Roncaroli F, Rossi R, Severi B, Martinelli GN, Eusebi V. Epithelioid leiomyoma of the breast with granular cell change: a case report. Hum Pathol. 1993;24(11):1260–3.

226. Shimokama T, Watanabe T. Leiomyoma exhibiting a marked granular change: granular cell leiomyoma versus granular cell schwannoma. Hum Pathol. 1992;23(3):327–31.

227. Lee AN, Stein SL, Cohen LM. Clear cell fibrous papule with NKI/C3 expression: clinical and histologic features in six cases. Am J Dermatopathol. 2005;27(4):296–300.

228. Rudisaile SN, Hurt MA, Santa Cruz DJ. Granular cell atypical fibroxanthoma. J Cutan Pathol. 2005;32(4):314–7.

229. Chaudhry IH, Calonje E. Dermal non-neural granular cell tumour (so-called primitive polypoid granular cell tumour): a distinctive entity further delineated in a clinicopathological study of 11 cases. Histopathology. 2005;47(2):179–85.

230. Habeeb AA, Salama S. Primitive nonneural granular cell tumor (so-called atypical polypoid granular cell tumor). Report of 2 cases with immunohistochemical and ultrastructural correlation. Am J Dermatopathol. 2008;30(2):156–9.

231. Lazar AJ, Fletcher CD. Primitive nonneural granular cell tumors of skin: clinicopathologic analysis of 13 cases. Am J Surg Pathol. 2005;29(7):927–34.

232. LeBoit PE, Barr RJ, Burall S, Metcalf JS, Yen TS, Wick MR. Primitive polypoid granular-cell tumor and other cutaneous granular-cell neoplasms of apparent nonneural origin. Am J Surg Pathol. 1991;15(1):48–58.

233. Lewin MR, Montgomery EA, Barrett TL. New or unusual dermatopathology tumors: a review. J Cutan Pathol. 2011;38(9):689–96.

234. Rabkin MS, Vukmer T. Granular cell variant of epithelioid cell histiocytoma. Am J Dermatopathol. 2012;34(7):766–9.

235. Lee J. Epithelioid cell histiocytoma with granular cells (another nonneural granular cell neoplasm). Am J Dermatopathol. 2007;29(5):475–6.

236. Conrad R, Perez MC. Congenital granular cell epulis. Arch Pathol Lab Med. 2014;138(1):128–31.

237. Vered M, Dobriyan A, Buchner A. Congenital granular cell epulis presents an immunohistochemical profile that distinguishes it from the granular cell tumor of the adult. Virchows Arch. 2009;454(3): 303–10.

238. Abo-Hager EA, Khater DS, Ahmed MM. Exploration of the histogenesis of congenital granular cell epulis: an immunohistochemical study. J Egypt Natl Canc Inst. 2009;21(2):77–83.

239. Childers EL, Fanburg-Smith JC. Congenital epulis of the newborn: 10 new cases of a rare oral tumor. Ann Diagn Pathol. 2011;15(3):157–61.

240. Fanburg-Smith JC, Meis-Kindblom JM, Fante R, Kindblom LG. Malignant granular cell tumor of soft tissue: diagnostic criteria and clinicopathologic correlation. Am J Surg Pathol. 1998;22(7):779–94.

241. Kapur P, Rakheja D, Balani JP, Roy LC, Amirkhan RH, Hoang MP. Phosphorylated histone H3, Ki-67, p21, fatty acid synthase, and cleaved caspase-3 expression in benign and atypical granular cell tumors. Arch Pathol Lab Med. 2007;131(1):57–64.

242. Nasser H, Ahmed Y, Szpunar SM, Kowalski PJ. Malignant granular cell tumor: a look into the diagnostic criteria. Pathol Res Pract. 2011;207(3):164–8.

243. Tang CK, Toker C. Trabecular carcinoma of the skin: an ultrastructural study. Cancer. 1978;42(5):2311–21.

244. Kroll MH, Toker C. Trabecular carcinoma of the skin: further clinicopathologic and morphologic study. Arch Pathol Lab Med. 1982;106(8):404–8.

245. Heath M, Jaimes N, Lemos B, Mostaghimi A, Wang LC, Penas PF, et al. Clinical characteristics of Merkel cell carcinoma at diagnosis in 195 patients: the AEIOU features. J Am Acad Dermatol. 2008;58(3):375–81.

246. Miller RW, Rabkin CS. Merkel cell carcinoma and melanoma: etiological similarities and differences. Cancer Epidemiol Biomarkers Prev. 1999;8(2):153–8.

247. Buell JF, Trofe J, Hanaway MJ, Beebe TM, Gross TG, Alloway RR, et al. Immunosuppression and Merkel cell cancer. Transplant Proc. 2002;34(5):1780–1.

248. Engels EA, Frisch M, Goedert JJ, Biggar RJ, Miller RW. Merkel cell carcinoma and HIV infection. Lancet. 2002;359(9305):497–8.

249. Feng H, Shuda M, Chang Y, Moore PS. Clonal integration of a polyomavirus in human Merkel cell carcinoma. Science. 2008;319(5866):1096–100.

250. Agelli M, Clegg LX. Epidemiology of primary Merkel cell carcinoma in the United States. J Am Acad Dermatol. 2003;49(5):832–41.

251. Mott RT, Smoller BR, Morgan MB. Merkel cell carcinoma: a clinicopathologic study with prognostic implications. J Cutan Pathol. 2004;31(3):217–23.

252. Albores-Saavedra J, Batich K, Chable-Montero F, Sagy N, Schwartz AM, Henson DE. Merkel cell carcinoma demographics, morphology, and survival based on 3870 cases: a population based study. J Cutan Pathol. 2010;37(1):20–7.

253. Al-Ahmadie HA, Mutasim DF, Mutema GK. A case of intraepidermal Merkel cell carcinoma within squamous cell carcinoma in-situ: Merkel cell carcinoma in-situ? Am J Dermatopathol. 2004;26(3):230–3.

254. Brown HA, Sawyer DM, Woo T. Intraepidermal Merkel cell carcinoma with no dermal involvement. Am J Dermatopathol. 2000;22(1):65–9.

255. Hashimoto K, Lee MW, D'Annunzio DR, Balle MR, Narisawa Y. Pagetoid Merkel cell carcinoma: epidermal origin of the tumor. J Cutan Pathol. 1998;25(10):572–9.

256. LeBoit PE, Crutcher WA, Shapiro PE. Pagetoid intraepidermal spread in Merkel cell (primary neuroendocrine) carcinoma of the skin. Am J Surg Pathol. 1992;16(6):584–92.

257. Rocamora A, Badia N, Vives R, Carrillo R, Ulloa J, Ledo A. Epidermotropic primary neuroendocrine (Merkel cell) carcinoma of the skin with Pautrierlike microabscesses. Report of three cases and review of the literature. J Am Acad Dermatol. 1987;16(6):1163–8.

258. Sirikanjanapong S, Melamed J, Patel RR. Intraepidermal and dermal Merkel cell carcinoma with squamous cell carcinoma in situ: a case report with review of literature. J Cutan Pathol. 2010;37(8):881–5.

259. Smith KJ, Skelton III HG, Holland TT, Morgan AM, Lupton GP. Neuroendocrine (Merkel cell) carcinoma with an intraepidermal component. Am J Dermatopathol. 1993;15(6):528–33.

260. Tan BH, Busam KJ, Pulitzer MP. Combined intraepidermal neuroendocrine (Merkel cell) and squamous cell carcinoma in situ with CM2B4 negativity and p53 overexpression(*). J Cutan Pathol. 2012;39(6):626–30.

261. Gillham SL, Morrison RG, Hurt MA. Epidermotropic neuroendocrine carcinoma. Immunohistochemical differentiation from simulators, including malignant melanoma. J Cutan Pathol. 1991;18(2):120–7.

262. Ferringer T, Rogers HC, Metcalf JS. Merkel cell carcinoma in situ. J Cutan Pathol. 2005;32(2):162–5.

263. Traest K, De Vos R, van den Oord JJ. Pagetoid Merkel cell carcinoma: speculations on its origin and the mechanism of epidermal spread. J Cutan Pathol. 1999;26(7):362–5.

264. Martin B, Poblet E, Rios JJ, Kazakov D, Kutzner H, Brenn T, et al. Merkel cell carcinoma with divergent differentiation: histopathological and immunohistochemical study of 15 cases with PCR analysis for Merkel cell polyomavirus. Histopathology. 2013;62(5):711–22.

265. Cerroni L, Kerl H. Primary cutaneous neuroendocrine (Merkel cell) carcinoma in association with squamous- and basal-cell carcinoma. Am J Dermatopathol. 1997;19(6):610–3.

266. Gomez LG, DiMaio S, Silva EG, Mackay B. Association between neuroendocrine (Merkel cell) carcinoma and squamous carcinoma of the skin. Am J Surg Pathol. 1983;7(2):171–7.

267. Iacocca MV, Abernethy JL, Stefanato CM, Allan AE, Bhawan J. Mixed Merkel cell carcinoma and squamous cell carcinoma of the skin. J Am Acad Dermatol. 1998;39(5 Pt 2):882–7.

268. Gould E, Albores-Saavedra J, Dubner B, Smith W, Payne CM. Eccrine and squamous differentiation in Merkel cell carcinoma. An immunohistochemical study. Am J Surg Pathol. 1988;12(10):768–72.

269. Fernandez-Figueras MT, Puig L, Gilaberte M, Gomez-Plaza Mdel C, Rex J, Ferrandiz C, et al. Merkel cell (primary neuroendocrine) carcinoma of the skin with nodal metastasis showing rhabdomyo-

sarcomatous differentiation. J Cutan Pathol. 2002; 29(10):619–22.

270. Isimbaldi G, Sironi M, Taccagni G, Declich P, Dell'Antonio A, Galli C. Tripartite differentiation (squamous, glandular, and melanocytic) of a primary cutaneous neuroendocrine carcinoma. An immunocytochemical and ultrastructural study. Am J Dermatopathol. 1993;15(3):260–4.

271. Hwang JH, Alanen K, Dabbs KD, Danyluk J, Silverman S. Merkel cell carcinoma with squamous and sarcomatous differentiation. J Cutan Pathol. 2008;35(10):955–9.

272. Rosso R, Paulli M, Carnevali L. Neuroendocrine carcinoma of the skin with lymphoepithelioma-like features. Am J Dermatopathol. 1998;20(5):483–6.

273. Vanchinathan V, Marinelli EC, Kartha RV, Uzieblo A, Ranchod M, Sundram UN. A malignant cutaneous neuroendocrine tumor with features of Merkel cell carcinoma and differentiating neuroblastoma. Am J Dermatopathol. 2009;31(2):193–6.

274. Boutilier R, Desormeau L, Cragg F, Roberts P, Walsh N. Merkel cell carcinoma: squamous and atypical fibroxanthoma-like differentiation in successive local tumor recurrences. Am J Dermatopathol. 2001;23(1):46–9.

275. Cooper L, Debono R, Alsanjari N, Al-Nafussi A. Merkel cell tumour with leiomyosarcomatous differentiation. Histopathology. 2000;36(6):540–3.

276. Skelton HG, Smith KJ, Hitchcock CL, McCarthy WF, Lupton GP, Graham JH. Merkel cell carcinoma: analysis of clinical, histologic, and immunohistologic features of 132 cases with relation to survival. J Am Acad Dermatol. 1997;37(5 Pt 1):734–9.

277. Andea AA, Coit DG, Amin B, Busam KJ. Merkel cell carcinoma: histologic features and prognosis. Cancer. 2008;113(9):2549–58.

278. Bichakjian CK, Olencki T, Alam M, Andersen JS, Berg D, Bowen GM, et al. Merkel cell carcinoma, version 1.2014. J Natl Compr Canc Netw. 2014;12(3):410–24.

279. Leong AS, Phillips GE, Pieterse AS, Milios J. Criteria for the diagnosis of primary endocrine carcinoma of the skin (Merkel cell carcinoma). A histological, immunohistochemical and ultrastructural study of 13 cases. Pathology. 1986;18(4):393–9.

280. Scott MP, Helm KF. Cytokeratin 20: a marker for diagnosing Merkel cell carcinoma. Am J Dermatopathol. 1999;21(1):16–20.

281. Chan JK, Suster S, Wenig BM, Tsang WY, Chan JB, Lau AL. Cytokeratin 20 immunoreactivity distinguishes Merkel cell (primary cutaneous neuroendocrine) carcinomas and salivary gland small cell carcinomas from small cell carcinomas of various sites. Am J Surg Pathol. 1997;21(2):226–34.

282. Schmidt U, Muller U, Metz KA, Leder LD. Cytokeratin and neurofilament protein staining in Merkel cell carcinoma of the small cell type and small cell carcinoma of the lung. Am J Dermatopathol. 1998;20(4):346–51.

283. Shah IA, Netto D, Schlageter MO, Muth C, Fox I, Manne RK. Neurofilament immunoreactivity in Merkel-cell tumors: a differentiating feature from small-cell carcinoma. Mod Pathol. 1993;6(1):3–9.

284. Pulitzer MP, Amin BD, Busam KJ. Merkel cell carcinoma: review. Adv Anat Pathol. 2009;16(3):135–44.

285. Cheuk W, Kwan MY, Suster S, Chan JK. Immunostaining for thyroid transcription factor 1 and cytokeratin 20 aids the distinction of small cell carcinoma from Merkel cell carcinoma, but not pulmonary from extrapulmonary small cell carcinomas. Arch Pathol Lab Med. 2001;125(2):228–31.

286. Leech SN, Kolar AJ, Barrett PD, Sinclair SA, Leonard N. Merkel cell carcinoma can be distinguished from metastatic small cell carcinoma using antibodies to cytokeratin 20 and thyroid transcription factor 1. J Clin Pathol. 2001;54(9):727–9.

287. Ralston J, Chiriboga L, Nonaka D. MASH1: a useful marker in differentiating pulmonary small cell carcinoma from Merkel cell carcinoma. Mod Pathol. 2008;21(11):1357–62.

288. Calder KB, Coplowitz S, Schlauder S, Morgan MB. A case series and immunophenotypic analysis of CK20−/CK7+ primary neuroendocrine carcinoma of the skin. J Cutan Pathol. 2007;34(12):918–23.

289. Reddi DM, Puri PK. Expression of focal TTF-1 expression in a case of CK7/CK20-positive Merkel cell carcinoma. J Cutan Pathol. 2013;40(4):431–3.

290. Acebo E, Vidaurrazaga N, Varas C, Burgos-Bretones JJ, Diaz-Perez JL. Merkel cell carcinoma: a clinicopathological study of 11 cases. J Eur Acad Dermatol Venereol. 2005;19(5):546–51.

291. Gu J, Polak JM, Van Noorden S, Pearse AG, Marangos PJ, Azzopardi JG. Immunostaining of neuron-specific enolase as a diagnostic tool for Merkel cell tumors. Cancer. 1983;52(6):1039–43.

292. McNiff JM, Cowper SE, Lazova R, Subtil A, Glusac EJ. CD56 staining in Merkel cell carcinoma and natural killer-cell lymphoma: magic bullet, diagnostic pitfall, or both? J Cutan Pathol. 2005;32(8):541–5.

293. Sur M, AlArdati H, Ross C, Alowami S. TdT expression in Merkel cell carcinoma: potential diagnostic pitfall with blastic hematological malignancies and expanded immunohistochemical analysis. Mod Pathol. 2007;20(11):1113–20.

294. Filtenborg-Barnkob BE, Bzorek M. Expression of anaplastic lymphoma kinase in Merkel cell carcinomas. Hum Pathol. 2013;44(8):1656–64.

295. Kolhe R, Reid MD, Lee JR, Cohen C, Ramalingam P. Immunohistochemical expression of PAX5 and TdT by Merkel cell carcinoma and pulmonary small cell carcinoma: a potential diagnostic pitfall but useful discriminatory marker. Int J Clin Exp Pathol. 2013;6(2):142–7.

296. Bernd HW, Krokowski M, Feller AC, Bartsch S, Thorns C. Expression of terminal desoxynucleotidyl transferase in Merkel cell carcinomas. Histopathology. 2007;50(5):676–8.

297. Buresh CJ, Oliai BR, Miller RT. Reactivity with TdT in Merkel cell carcinoma: a potential diagnostic pitfall. Am J Clin Pathol. 2008;129(6):894–8.

298. Sidiropoulos M, Hanna W, Raphael SJ, Ghorab Z. Expression of TdT in Merkel cell carcinoma and small cell lung carcinoma. Am J Clin Pathol. 2011;135(6):831–8.

299. Kennedy MM, Blessing K, King G, Kerr KM. Expression of bcl-2 and p53 in Merkel cell carcinoma. An immunohistochemical study. Am J Dermatopathol. 1996;18(3):273–7.

300. Zur Hausen A, Rennspiess D, Winnepenninckx V, Speel EJ, Kurz AK. Early B-cell differentiation in Merkel cell carcinomas: clues to cellular ancestry. Cancer Res. 2013;73(16):4982–7.

301. Sangoi AR, Cassarino DS. PAX-8 expression in primary and metastatic Merkel cell carcinoma: an immunohistochemical analysis. Am J Dermatopathol. 2013;35(4):448–51.

302. Dasgeb B, Mohammadi TM, Mehregan DR. Use of Ber-EP4 and epithelial specific antigen to differentiate clinical simulators of basal cell carcinoma. Biomark Cancer. 2013;5:7–11.

303. Mhawech-Fauceglia P, Herrmann FR, Bshara W, Odunsi K, Terracciano L, Sauter G, et al. Friend leukaemia integration-1 expression in malignant and benign tumours: a multiple tumour tissue microarray analysis using polyclonal antibody. J Clin Pathol. 2007;60(6):694–700.

304. Rossi S, Orvieto E, Furlanetto A, Laurino L, Ninfo V, Dei Tos AP. Utility of the immunohistochemical detection of FLI-1 expression in round cell and vascular neoplasm using a monoclonal antibody. Mod Pathol. 2004;17(5):547–52.

305. Llombart B, Monteagudo C, Lopez-Guerrero JA, Carda C, Jorda E, Sanmartin O, et al. Clinicopathological and immunohistochemical analysis of 20 cases of Merkel cell carcinoma in search of prognostic markers. Histopathology. 2005;46(6):622–34.

306. Nicholson SA, McDermott MB, Swanson PE, Wick MR. CD99 and cytokeratin-20 in small-cell and basaloid tumors of the skin. Appl Immunohistochem Mol Morphol. 2000;8(1):37–41.

307. Rajagopalan A, Browning D, Salama S. CD99 expression in Merkel cell carcinoma: a case series with an unusual paranuclear dot-like staining pattern. J Cutan Pathol. 2013;40(1):19–24.

308. Kontochristopoulos GJ, Stavropoulos PG, Krasagakis K, Goerdt S, Zouboulis CC. Differentiation between Merkel cell carcinoma and malignant melanoma: a immunohistochemical study. Dermatology. 2000;201(2):123–6.

309. Iwasaki T, Matsushita M, Kuwamoto S, Kato M, Murakami I, Higaki-Mori H, et al. Usefulness of significant morphologic characteristics in distinguishing between Merkel cell polyomavirus-positive and Merkel cell polyomavirus-negative Merkel cell carcinomas. Hum Pathol. 2013;44(9):1912–7.

310. Rodig SJ, Cheng J, Wardzala J, DoRosario A, Scanlon JJ, Laga AC, et al. Improved detection suggests all Merkel cell carcinomas harbor Merkel polyomavirus. J Clin Invest. 2012;122(12):4645–53.

311. Busam KJ, Jungbluth AA, Rekthman N, Coit D, Pulitzer M, Bini J, et al. Merkel cell polyomavirus expression in Merkel cell carcinomas and its absence in combined tumors and pulmonary neuroendocrine carcinomas. Am J Surg Pathol. 2009;33(9):1378–85.

312. Paik JY, Hall G, Clarkson A, Lee L, Toon C, Colebatch A, et al. Immunohistochemistry for Merkel cell polyomavirus is highly specific but not sensitive for the diagnosis of Merkel cell carcinoma in the Australian population. Hum Pathol. 2011;42(10):1385–90.

313. Matsushita M, Nonaka D, Iwasaki T, Kuwamoto S, Murakami I, Kato M, et al. A new in situ hybridization and immunohistochemistry with a novel antibody to detect small T-antigen expressions of Merkel cell polyomavirus (MCPyV). Diagn Pathol. 2014;9:65.

314. Scola N, Wieland U, Silling S, Altmeyer P, Stucker M, Kreuter A. Prevalence of human polyomaviruses in common and rare types of non-Merkel cell carcinoma skin cancer. Br J Dermatol. 2012;167(6):1315–20.

315. Hattori T, Takeuchi Y, Takenouchi T, Hirofuji A, Tsuchida T, Kabumoto T, et al. The prevalence of Merkel cell polyomavirus in Japanese patients with Merkel cell carcinoma. J Dermatol Sci. 2013;70(2):99–107.

316. Ota S, Ishikawa S, Takazawa Y, Goto A, Fujii T, Ohashi K, et al. Quantitative analysis of viral load per haploid genome revealed the different biological features of Merkel cell polyomavirus infection in skin tumor. PLoS One. 2012;7(6):e39954.

317. Dabner M, McClure RJ, Harvey NT, Budgeon CA, Beer TW, Amanuel B, et al. Merkel cell polyomavirus and p63 status in Merkel cell carcinoma by immunohistochemistry: Merkel cell polyomavirus positivity is inversely correlated with sun damage, but neither is correlated with outcome. Pathology. 2014;46(3):205–10.

318. Asioli S, Righi A, de Biase D, Morandi L, Caliendo V, Picciotto F, et al. Expression of p63 is the sole independent marker of aggressiveness in localised (stage I–II) Merkel cell carcinomas. Mod Pathol. 2011;24(11):1451–61.

319. Fleming KE, Ly TY, Pasternak S, Godlewski M, Doucette S, Walsh NM. Support for p63 expression as an adverse prognostic marker in Merkel cell carcinoma: report on a Canadian cohort. Hum Pathol. 2014;45(5):952–60.

320. Hall BJ, Pincus LB, Yu SS, Oh DH, Wilson AR, McCalmont TH. Immunohistochemical prognostication of Merkel cell carcinoma: p63 expression but not polyomavirus status correlates with outcome. J Cutan Pathol. 2012;39(10):911–7.

321. Koljonen V, Tukiainen E, Haglund C, Bohling T. Proliferative activity detected by Ki67 correlates with poor outcome in Merkel cell carcinoma. Histopathology. 2006;49(5):551–3.

322. Stetsenko GY, Malekirad J, Paulson KG, Iyer JG, Thibodeau RM, Nagase K, et al. p63 expression in Merkel cell carcinoma predicts poorer survival yet may have limited clinical utility. Am J Clin Pathol. 2013;140(6):838–44.

323. Vujic I, Marker M, Posch C, Muhlehner D, Monshi B, Breier F, et al. Merkel cell carcinoma: mitoses, expression of Ki-67 and bcl-2 correlate with disease progression. J Eur Acad Dermatol Venereol. 2015;29:542–8.

324. Fernandez-Figueras MT, Puig L, Musulen E, Gilaberte M, Ferrandiz C, Lerma E, et al. Prognostic significance of p27Kip1, p45Skp2 and Ki67 expression profiles in Merkel cell carcinoma, extracutaneous small cell carcinoma, and cutaneous squamous cell carcinoma. Histopathology. 2005;46(6):614–21.

325. Feinmesser M, Halpern M, Kaganovsky E, Brenner B, Fenig E, Hodak E, et al. C-Kit expression in primary and metastatic Merkel cell carcinoma. Am J Dermatopathol. 2004;26(6):458–62.

326. Samlowski WE, Moon J, Tuthill RJ, Heinrich MC, Balzer-Haas NS, Merl SA, et al. A phase II trial of imatinib mesylate in Merkel cell carcinoma (neuroendocrine carcinoma of the skin): a Southwest Oncology Group study (S0331). Am J Clin Oncol. 2010;33(5):495–9.

327. Su LD, Fullen DR, Lowe L, Uherova P, Schnitzer B, Valdez R. CD117 (KIT receptor) expression in Merkel cell carcinoma. Am J Dermatopathol. 2002;24(4):289–93.

328. Swick BL, Ravdel L, Fitzpatrick JE, Robinson WA. Merkel cell carcinoma: evaluation of KIT (CD117) expression and failure to demonstrate activating mutations in the C-KIT proto-oncogene—implications for treatment with imatinib mesylate. J Cutan Pathol. 2007;34(4):324–9.

329. Swick BL, Srikantha R, Messingham KN. Specific analysis of KIT and PDGFR-alpha expression and mutational status in Merkel cell carcinoma. J Cutan Pathol. 2013;40(7):623–30.

330. Allen PJ, Busam K, Hill AD, Stojadinovic A, Coit DG. Immunohistochemical analysis of sentinel lymph nodes from patients with Merkel cell carcinoma. Cancer. 2001;92(6):1650–5.

331. Su LD, Lowe L, Bradford CR, Yahanda AI, Johnson TM, Sondak VK. Immunostaining for cytokeratin 20 improves detection of micrometastatic Merkel cell carcinoma in sentinel lymph nodes. J Am Acad Dermatol. 2002;46(5):661–6.

332. Shalin SC, Cifarelli CP, Suen JY, Gao L. Loss of cytokeratin 20 and acquisition of thyroid transcription factor-1 expression in a Merkel cell carcinoma metastasis to the brain. Am J Dermatopathol. 2014;36(11):904–6.

333. Buck CB, Lowy DR. Getting stronger: the relationship between a newly identified virus and Merkel cell carcinoma. J Invest Dermatol. 2009;129(1):9–11.

334. Sastre-Garau X, Peter M, Avril MF, Laude H, Couturier J, Rozenberg F, et al. Merkel cell carcinoma of the skin: pathological and molecular evidence for a causative role of MCV in oncogenesis. J Pathol. 2009;218(1):48–56.

335. Bhatia K, Goedert JJ, Modali R, Preiss L, Ayers LW. Immunological detection of viral large T antigen identifies a subset of Merkel cell carcinoma tumors with higher viral abundance and better clinical outcome. Int J Cancer. 2010;127(6):1493–6.

336. Bhatia K, Goedert JJ, Modali R, Preiss L, Ayers LW. Merkel cell carcinoma subgroups by Merkel cell polyomavirus DNA relative abundance and oncogene expression. Int J Cancer. 2010;126(9):2240–6.

337. Sihto H, Kukko H, Koljonen V, Sankila R, Bohling T, Joensuu H. Clinical factors associated with Merkel cell polyomavirus infection in Merkel cell carcinoma. J Natl Cancer Inst. 2009;101(13):938–45.

338. Sihto H, Kukko H, Koljonen V, Sankila R, Bohling T, Joensuu H. Merkel cell polyomavirus infection, large T antigen, retinoblastoma protein and outcome in Merkel cell carcinoma. Clin Cancer Res. 2011;17(14):4806–13.

339. Schrama D, Peitsch WK, Zapatka M, Kneitz H, Houben R, Eib S, et al. Merkel cell polyomavirus status is not associated with clinical course of Merkel cell carcinoma. J Invest Dermatol. 2011;131(8):1631–8.

340. Martel-Jantin C, Pedergnana V, Nicol JT, Leblond V, Tregouet DA, Tortevoye P, et al. Merkel cell polyomavirus infection occurs during early childhood and is transmitted between siblings. J Clin Virol. 2013;58(1):288–91.

341. Andres C, Belloni B, Flaig MJ. Value of Merkel cell polyomavirus DNA detection in routine pathology. Am J Dermatopathol. 2011;33(3):329–30.

342. Laude HC, Jonchere B, Maubec E, Carlotti A, Marinho E, Couturaud B, et al. Distinct Merkel cell polyomavirus molecular features in tumour and non tumour specimens from patients with Merkel cell carcinoma. PLoS Pathog. 2010;6(8):e1001076.

343. Andres C, Ihrler S, Puchta U, Flaig MJ. Merkel cell polyomavirus is prevalent in a subset of small cell lung cancer: a study of 31 patients. Thorax. 2009;64(11):1007–8.

344. Hourdequin KC, Lefferts JA, Brennick JB, Ernstoff MS, Tsongalis GJ, Pipas JM. Merkel cell polyomavirus and extrapulmonary small cell carcinoma. Oncol Lett. 2013;6(4):1049–52.

345. Mertz KD, Paasinen A, Arnold A, Baumann M, Offner F, Willi N, et al. Merkel cell polyomavirus large T antigen is detected in rare cases of nonmelanoma skin cancer. J Cutan Pathol. 2013;40(6):543–9.

346. Ly TY, Walsh NM, Pasternak S. The spectrum of Merkel cell polyomavirus expression in Merkel cell carcinoma, in a variety of cutaneous neoplasms, and in neuroendocrine carcinomas from different anatomical sites. Hum Pathol. 2012;43(4):557–66.

347. Paulson KG, Lemos BD, Feng B, Jaimes N, Penas PF, Bi X, et al. Array-CGH reveals recurrent genomic changes in Merkel cell carcinoma including amplification of L-Myc. J Invest Dermatol. 2009;129(6):1547–55.

348. Van Gele M, Speleman F, Vandesompele J, Van Roy N, Leonard JH. Characteristic pattern of chromosomal gains and losses in Merkel cell carcinoma detected by comparative genomic hybridization. Cancer Res. 1998;58(7):1503–8.

349. Vortmeyer AO, Merino MJ, Boni R, Liotta LA, Cavazzana A, Zhuang Z. Genetic changes associated with primary Merkel cell carcinoma. Am J Clin Pathol. 1998;109(5):565–70.

350. Harnett PR, Kearsley JH, Hayward NK, Dracopoli NC, Kefford RF. Loss of allelic heterozygosity on distal chromosome 1p in Merkel cell carcinoma. A marker of neural crest origins? Cancer Genet Cytogenet. 1991;54(1):109–13.

351. Leonard JH, Cook AL, Nancarrow D, Hayward N, Van Gele M, Van Roy N, et al. Deletion mapping on the short arm of chromosome 1 in Merkel cell carcinoma. Cancer Detect Prev. 2000;24(6):620–7.

352. Van Gele M, Van Roy N, Ronan SG, Messiaen L, Vandesompele J, Geerts ML, et al. Molecular analysis of 1p36 breakpoints in two Merkel cell carcinomas. Genes Chromosomes Cancer. 1998;23(1):67–71.

353. Erstad DJ, Cusack Jr JC. Mutational analysis of Merkel cell carcinoma. Cancers (Basel). 2014;6(4):2116–36.

354. Houben R, Adam C, Baeurle A, Hesbacher S, Grimm J, Angermeyer S, et al. An intact retinoblastoma protein-binding site in Merkel cell polyomavirus large T antigen is required for promoting growth of Merkel cell carcinoma cells. Int J Cancer. 2012;130(4):847–56.

355. Cimino PJ, Robirds DH, Tripp SR, Pfeifer JD, Abel HJ, Duncavage EJ. Retinoblastoma gene mutations detected by whole exome sequencing of Merkel cell carcinoma. Mod Pathol. 2014;27(8):1073–87.

356. Sahi H, Savola S, Sihto H, Koljonen V, Bohling T, Knuutila S. RB1 gene in Merkel cell carcinoma: hypermethylation in all tumors and concurrent heterozygous deletions in the polyomavirus-negative subgroup. APMIS. 2014;122(12):1157–66.

357. Bobos M, Hytiroglou P, Kostopoulos I, Karkavelas G, Papadimitriou CS. Immunohistochemical distinction between Merkel cell carcinoma and small cell carcinoma of the lung. Am J Dermatopathol. 2006;28(2):99–104.

358. Hanly AJ, Elgart GW, Jorda M, Smith J, Nadji M. Analysis of thyroid transcription factor-1 and cytokeratin 20 separates Merkel cell carcinoma from small cell carcinoma of lung. J Cutan Pathol. 2000;27(3):118–20.

359. Knapp CF, Sayegh Z, Schell MJ, Rawal B, Ochoa T, Sondak VK, et al. Expression of CXCR4, E-cadherin, Bcl-2, and survivin in Merkel cell carcinoma: an immunohistochemical study using a tissue microarray. Am J Dermatopathol. 2012;34(6):592–6.

360. Elbashier SH, Nazarina AR, Looi LM. Cytokeratin immunoreactivity in Ewing sarcoma/primitive neuroectodermal tumour. Malays J Pathol. 2013;35(2):139–45.

361. Fernandez-Flores A, Suarez-Penaranda JM, Alonso S. Study of EWS/FLI-1 rearrangement in 18 cases of CK20+/CM2B4+ Merkel cell carcinoma using FISH and correlation to the differential diagnosis of Ewing sarcoma/peripheral neuroectodermal tumor. Appl Immunohistochem Mol Morphol. 2013;21(5):379–85.

362. Sahi H, Koljonen V, Kavola H, Haglund C, Tukiainen E, Sihto H, et al. Bcl-2 expression indicates better prognosis of Merkel cell carcinoma regardless of the presence of Merkel cell polyomavirus. Virchows Arch. 2012;461(5):553–9.

363. Terada T. Expression of NCAM (CD56), chromogranin A, synaptophysin, c-KIT (CD117) and PDGFRA in normal non-neoplastic skin and basal cell carcinoma: an immunohistochemical study of 66 consecutive cases. Med Oncol. 2013;30(1):444.

364. Daoud MA, Mete O, Al Habeeb A, Ghazarian D. Neuroendocrine carcinoma of the skin—an updated review. Semin Diagn Pathol. 2013;30(3):234–44.

365. Kikuchi A, Akiyama M, Han-Yaku H, Shimizu H, Naka W, Nishikawa T. Solitary cutaneous malignant schwannoma. Immunohistochemical and ultrastructural studies. Am J Dermatopathol. 1993;15(1):15–9.

366. Dabski C, Reiman Jr HM, Muller SA. Neurofibrosarcoma of skin and subcutaneous tissues. Mayo Clin Proc. 1990;65(2):164–72.

367. Woodruff JM. Pathology of tumors of the peripheral nerve sheath in type 1 neurofibromatosis. Am J Med Genet. 1999;89(1):23–30.

368. Stucky CC, Johnson KN, Gray RJ, Pockaj BA, Ocal IT, Rose PS, et al. Malignant peripheral nerve sheath tumors (MPNST): the Mayo Clinic experience. Ann Surg Oncol. 2012;19(3):878–85.

369. Tucker T, Wolkenstein P, Revuz J, Zeller J, Friedman JM. Association between benign and malignant peripheral nerve sheath tumors in NF1. Neurology. 2005;65(2):205–11.

370. Ducatman BS, Scheithauer BW. Malignant peripheral nerve sheath tumors with divergent differentiation. Cancer. 1984;54(6):1049–57.

371. Ducatman BS, Scheithauer BW, Piepgras DG, Reiman HM. Malignant peripheral nerve sheath tumors in childhood. J Neurooncol. 1984;2(3):241–8.

372. Ducatman BS, Scheithauer BW, Piepgras DG, Reiman HM, Ilstrup DM. Malignant peripheral

nerve sheath tumors. A clinicopathologic study of 120 cases. Cancer. 1986;57(10):2006–21.

373. George E, Swanson PE, Wick MR. Malignant peripheral nerve sheath tumors of the skin. Am J Dermatopathol. 1989;11(3):213–21.

374. Misago N, Ishii Y, Kohda H. Malignant peripheral nerve sheath tumor of the skin: a superficial form of this tumor. J Cutan Pathol. 1996;23(2):182–8.

375. Thomas C, Somani N, Owen LG, Malone JC, Billings SD. Cutaneous malignant peripheral nerve sheath tumors. J Cutan Pathol. 2009;36(8):896–900.

376. Takeuchi A, Ushigome S. Diverse differentiation in malignant peripheral nerve sheath tumours associated with neurofibromatosis-1: an immunohistochemical and ultrastructural study. Histopathology. 2001;39(3):298–309.

377. Woodruff JM, Christensen WN. Glandular peripheral nerve sheath tumors. Cancer. 1993;72(12): 3618–28.

378. Morphopoulos GD, Banerjee SS, Ali HH, Stewart M, Vasudev KS, Eyden BP, et al. Malignant peripheral nerve sheath tumour with vascular differentiation: a report of four cases. Histopathology. 1996; 28(5):401–10.

379. Rosenberg AS, Langee CL, Stevens GL, Morgan MB. Malignant peripheral nerve sheath tumor with perineurial differentiation: "malignant perineurioma". J Cutan Pathol. 2002;29(6):362–7.

380. Laskin WB, Weiss SW, Bratthauer GL. Epithelioid variant of malignant peripheral nerve sheath tumor (malignant epithelioid schwannoma). Am J Surg Pathol. 1991;15(12):1136–45.

381. Shimizu S, Teraki Y, Ishiko A, Shimizu H, Harada T, Mukai M, et al. Malignant epithelioid schwannoma of the skin showing partial HMB-45 positivity. Am J Dermatopathol. 1993;15(4):378–84.

382. McMenamin ME, Fletcher CD. Expanding the spectrum of malignant change in schwannomas: epithelioid malignant change, epithelioid malignant peripheral nerve sheath tumor, and epithelioid angiosarcoma: a study of 17 cases. Am J Surg Pathol. 2001;25(1):13–25.

383. Sangueza OP, Requena L. Neoplasms with neural differentiation: a review. Part II: Malignant neoplasms. Am J Dermatopathol. 1998;20(1):89–102.

384. Kang Y, Pekmezci M, Folpe AL, Ersen A, Horvai AE. Diagnostic utility of SOX10 to distinguish malignant peripheral nerve sheath tumor from synovial sarcoma, including intraneural synovial sarcoma. Mod Pathol. 2014;27(1):55–61.

385. Hirose T, Hasegawa T, Kudo E, Seki K, Sano T, Hizawa K. Malignant peripheral nerve sheath tumors: an immunohistochemical study in relation to ultrastructural features. Hum Pathol. 1992;23(8): 865–70.

386. Wick MR. Immunohistology of neuroendocrine and neuroectodermal tumors. Semin Diagn Pathol. 2000;17(3):194–203.

387. Chen WS, Chen PL, Lu D, Lind AC, Dehner LP. Growth-associated protein 43 in differentiating peripheral nerve sheath tumors from other non-neural spindle cell neoplasms. Mod Pathol. 2014; 27(2):184–93.

388. Pekmezci M, Reuss DE, Hirbe AC, Dahiya S, Gutmann DH, von Deimling A, et al. Morphologic and immunohistochemical features of malignant peripheral nerve sheath tumors and cellular schwannomas. Mod Pathol. 2015;28(2):187–200.

389. Hoshi N, Hiraki H, Yamaki T, Natsume T, Watanabe K, Suzuki T. Frequent expression of 75 kDa nerve growth factor receptor and phosphotyrosine in human peripheral nerve tumours: an immunohistochemical study on paraffin-embedded tissues. Virchows Arch. 1994;424(5):563–8.

390. Olsen SH, Thomas DG, Lucas DR. Cluster analysis of immunohistochemical profiles in synovial sarcoma, malignant peripheral nerve sheath tumor, and Ewing sarcoma. Mod Pathol. 2006;19(5):659–68.

391. Hoang MP, Sinkre P, Albores-Saavedra J. Expression of protein gene product 9.5 in epithelioid and conventional malignant peripheral nerve sheath tumors. Arch Pathol Lab Med. 2001;125(10):1321–5.

392. Wesche WA, Khare V, Rao BN, Bowman LC, Parham DM. Malignant peripheral nerve sheath tumor of bone in children and adolescents. Pediatr Dev Pathol. 1999;2(2):159–67.

393. Allison KH, Patel RM, Goldblum JR, Rubin BP. Superficial malignant peripheral nerve sheath tumor: a rare and challenging diagnosis. Am J Clin Pathol. 2005;124(5):685–92.

394. Matsunou H, Shimoda T, Kakimoto S, Yamashita H, Ishikawa E, Mukai M. Histopathologic and immunohistochemical study of malignant tumors of peripheral nerve sheath (malignant schwannoma). Cancer. 1985;56(9):2269–79.

395. Smith TA, Machen SK, Fisher C, Goldblum JR. Usefulness of cytokeratin subsets for distinguishing monophasic synovial sarcoma from malignant peripheral nerve sheath tumor. Am J Clin Pathol. 1999;112(5):641–8.

396. Daimaru Y, Hashimoto H, Enjoji M. Malignant "triton" tumors: a clinicopathologic and immunohistochemical study of nine cases. Hum Pathol. 1984;15(8):768–78.

397. Stasik CJ, Tawfik O. Malignant peripheral nerve sheath tumor with rhabdomyosarcomatous differentiation (malignant triton tumor). Arch Pathol Lab Med. 2006;130(12):1878–81.

398. Hirose T, Sumitomo M, Kudo E, Hasegawa T, Teramae T, Murase M, et al. Malignant peripheral nerve sheath tumor (MPNST) showing perineurial cell differentiation. Am J Surg Pathol. 1989;13(7):613–20.

399. Plaat BE, Molenaar WM, Mastik MF, Hoekstra HJ, te Meerman GJ, van den Berg E. Computer-assisted cytogenetic analysis of 51 malignant peripheral-nerve-sheath tumors: sporadic vs. neurofibromatosis-type-1-associated malignant schwannomas. Int J Cancer. 1999;83(2):171–8.

400. Thway K, Fisher C. Malignant peripheral nerve sheath tumor: pathology and genetics. Ann Diagn Pathol. 2014;18(2):109–16.

401. Brekke HR, Ribeiro FR, Kolberg M, Agesen TH, Lind GE, Eknaes M, et al. Genomic changes in chromosomes 10, 16, and X in malignant peripheral nerve sheath tumors identify a high-risk patient group. J Clin Oncol. 2010;28(9):1573–82.

402. Sabah M, Cummins R, Leader M, Kay E. Loss of p16 (INK4A) expression is associated with allelic imbalance/loss of heterozygosity of chromosome 9p21 in microdissected malignant peripheral nerve sheath tumors. Appl Immunohistochem Mol Morphol. 2006;14(1):97–102.

403. Mantripragada KK, Diaz de Stahl T, Patridge C, Menzel U, Andersson R, Chuzhanova N, et al. Genome-wide high-resolution analysis of DNA copy number alterations in NF1-associated malignant peripheral nerve sheath tumors using 32K BAC array. Genes Chromosomes Cancer. 2009;48(10): 897–907.

404. Bottillo I, Ahlquist T, Brekke H, Danielsen SA, van den Berg E, Mertens F, et al. Germline and somatic NF1 mutations in sporadic and NF1-associated malignant peripheral nerve sheath tumours. J Pathol. 2009;217(5):693–701.

405. Upadhyaya M, Kluwe L, Spurlock G, Monem B, Majounie E, Mantripragada K, et al. Germline and somatic NF1 gene mutation spectrum in NF1-associated malignant peripheral nerve sheath tumors (MPNSTs). Hum Mutat. 2008;29(1):74–82.

406. Bridge Jr RS, Bridge JA, Neff JR, Naumann S, Althof P, Bruch LA. Recurrent chromosomal imbalances and structurally abnormal breakpoints within complex karyotypes of malignant peripheral nerve sheath tumour and malignant triton tumour: a cytogenetic and molecular cytogenetic study. J Clin Pathol. 2004;57(11):1172–8.

407. Palla B, Su A, Binder S, Dry S. SOX10 expression distinguishes desmoplastic melanoma from its histologic mimics. Am J Dermatopathol. 2013;35(5): 576–81.

408. de Alava E. Transcripts, transcripts, everywhere. Adv Anat Pathol. 2001;8(5):264–72.

409. O'Sullivan MJ, Kyriakos M, Zhu X, Wick MR, Swanson PE, Dehner LP, et al. Malignant peripheral nerve sheath tumors with t(X;18). A pathologic and molecular genetic study. Mod Pathol. 2000;13(12): 1336–46.

New Insights in Vascular Lesions Development and Identification with Immunohistochemical Markers

8

Omar P. Sangüeza and Julio A. Diaz-Perez

Introduction

Vascular lesions include malformations, proliferations, and neoplasms, both benign and malignant. These lesions display a wide range of morphological appearances that makes their diagnosis and classification a challenge [1]. The introduction and use of immunohistochemical stains during the last decades has facilitated this task. Several endothelial cell markers have been developed; however a few of them have proved a true diagnostic value and clinical impact [2]. Initially, polyclonal anti-endothelial antibodies were developed [3]. The two more recognized members of this generation are: the antibody against von Willebrand factor (vWf), and the lectin Ulex Europaeus antigen (UEA) [4]. Both markers were broadly employed; however, soon it was realized that they were several limitations

for their use: low sensitivity for endothelial cells, large amounts of nonspecific "background" staining, and low specificity (mainly cross-reactions with epithelial cells) [2–4]. Using the monoclonal antibody technology, a second generation of antibodies was developed, providing higher specificity. These antibodies include: CD31, CD34, podoplanin (D2-40), and thrombomodulin and are the elite members of this generation. Later on, an antibody against the human erythrocyte-type glucose transporter protein (Glut-1) was developed, which showed accuracy in evaluating proliferative endothelium [2, 3]. These markers have achieved broad recognition, and currently they are accepted as the "conventional" endothelial cells markers [5].

CD31, is a type I transmembrane protein member of the immunoglobulin superfamily [5]. This molecule is expressed uniformly on the endothelium of blood vessels, and focally in lymphatic vessels, hematopoietic cells, and histiocytes [2, 5]. Other type I transmembrane protein, CD34, is also expressed on the endothelium of blood vessels; but shows insignificant value in the identification of vessels of lymphatic origin [6]. This molecule is also expressed in stem cells, and mature cells, including eccrine ducts, collagen bundles, and fibroblast [6]. Podoplanin is selectively and strongly expressed in lymphatic endothelium, showing lower expression in the endothelial cells of blood vessels [7]. The distinctive expression of CD34 and podoplanin is

O.P. Sangüeza, M.D. (✉)
Departments of Pathology and Dermatology,
Medical Center Boulevard, Wake Forest
University School of Medicine, Winston-Salem,
NC 27157, USA
e-mail: osanguez@wakehealth.edu

J.A. Diaz-Perez, M.D.
Division of Dermatopathology, Department of
Pathology, Wake Forest Baptist Medical Center,
4 Medical Center Blvd, Winston-Salem,
NC 27157, USA
e-mail: juliodiaz_82@yahoo.com

© Springer International Publishing Switzerland 2016
J.A. Plaza, V.G. Prieto (eds.), *Applied Immunohistochemistry in the Evaluation of Skin Neoplasms*, DOI 10.1007/978-3-319-30590-5_8

useful in the identification of the type of blood vessels, and their co-expression in vascular neoplasms is indicative of mixed blood and lymphatic endothelial differentiation, as seen in Kaposi's sarcoma (KS) [7, 8]. Thrombomodulin, a cell-surface glycoprotein, is similar to CD31 and capable of identifying almost all endothelial cells, in arteries, veins, capillaries, and lymphatic vessels [9]. However, thrombomodulin lacks the CD31 specificity and reacts also against mesothelium and keratinocytes [9]. Other putative endothelial markers including CD61, CD36, CD9, type IV collagen, and beta-integrins have a low-grade sensitivity and specificity.

During the last two decades, the use molecular genetics and biochemistry techniques have allowed to expand our knowledge on the pathogenesis of vascular lesions. This new information has facilitated the development of novel endothelial cell markers, which have help to identify the cell of origin for many vascular processes and also to determine the molecular mechanisms involved, which can be used for driven therapy. In this chapter, we will review these new advances.

New Insights in Vascular Lesions Development

The origin of vascular lesions has been a subject of debate since the late 1800s [10]. Virchow in 1863, postulated a relationship between hemangiomas and embryonic development, suggesting that remnants of the embryonic mesoderm were the cause of vascular lesions [11]. The current thought is that vascular alterations are the result of a lack of regulation of the proliferation rate of the endothelial cells and this will be the unifying pathological event for all vascular lesions [12]. Two hypothesis have been proposed to explain the lack of regulation of the endothelial cell proliferation seen in angiogenesis: the first hypothesis is based in the loss of regulation of the hematopoietic stem cells CD45+/CD117+/CD133+ that undergo differentiation to endothelial progenitor cells CD45−/CD117+/CD133+ (this is called the stem cell pathway or extrinsic

defect hypothesis); the second hypothesis postulated genetic mutations as the cause of endothelial cell neoplastic transformation (also known as genetic pathway or intrinsic defect hypothesis) [13, 14]. Furthermore, some authors have proposed that the cause is a complex network between these two mechanisms, highly regulated by pro and anti-angiogenic growth factors and inflammatory mediators [14].

The Stem Cell Pathway

This pathway has been generally related to external oncogenic causes as mechanical effects (chronic lymphedema) or chemotoxicity [13]. In the stem cell pathway, endothelial progenitor cells are liberated from the bone marrow due to the activation of metalloproteinase-9, resulting in migration of these cells from the bone marrow to blood vessels, when they lose the expression of CD133, and gain the expression of vascular endothelial growth factor receptor (VEGFR) 2, becoming CD45−/CD117+/CD133−/VEGFR-2+ cells [12]. This event is supported by the increased incidence of infantile hemangiomas after intrauterine procedures during pregnancy, like chorionic villous sampling which induces the liberation of stem cells [15, 16]. When the stem cells acquire this new phenotype they increase the autocrine liberation of VEGF-A [17]. The expression of VEGFR-2 is enhanced by VEGF-A after the decoy of VEGFR-1, initiating a potent pro-angiogenic stimuli [17]. Absence of VEGFR1 has proven to be lethal in mice, causing vascular obstructions due to uncontrollable proliferation of endothelial cells [17, 18]. Thus, with a decreased availability of VEGFR-1, more VEGF-A is liberated to bind and activate VEGFR-2. The abnormal activation of VEGFR-2 on the cell surface may also be beneficial to the survival of oncogenic cells as VEGF-A plays a critical role protecting against apoptosis [19]. Later on, these cells express CD31 and vWF. In this model the preservation of CD117 expression in neoplastic endothelial cells is an indicator of more aggressive behavior. The almost uniform expression of VEGFR-1, VEGFR-2, CD31, and vWf, with co-expression of CD117 in human angiosarcoma, and co-expression of CD32 a myeloid marker with lack of CD117 expression in human hemangioma supports this hypothesis [18]. Additionally, in vascular neoplasms is also observed the expression of pluripotential markers including CD34, SOX2, OCT4, and Nanog [20]. The occurrence of this event is associated with TP53 and NOTCH1 gene mutations, which are translated in increased expression of p53 and Notch proteins in angiosarcoma, and low expression of these markers in hemangioma [21]. In this model differences in expression in these markers will be secondary to tumor heterogeneity, which is supported by the co-expression of CD83 a dendritic cell marker inhuman infantile hemangioma, and the expression of CD14 in some human angiosarcomas [20].

The Genetic Pathway

This pathway is related with de novo mutations, rare genetic disorders, and previous irradiation [22]. This hypothesis entails that a somatic mutation in one or more genes controlling endothelial cell proliferation is responsible for tumor formation [22, 23]. Studies that show a typical location of hemangiomas in areas of developmental boundaries where fusion of embryonic cranium takes place support this hypothesis [23]. Furthermore, the observation of similar X-chromosome inactivation pattern in all hemangioma-derived endothelial cells and uniform immunoreactivity for glucose transporter-1 (Glut-1) in hemangiomas, which is not observed in normal skin or other vascular anomalies (including malformations) encourage this hypothesis [22]. However, is proved that stem cells can produce human glucose transporter-1 (GLUT-1) positive microvessels at 7–14 days [23]. Other studies have proved the presence of somatic mutations in VEGFR-2 and other proteins like tumor endothelial marker 8 (TEM8) in hemangiomas. Also the identification of WWTR1-CAMTA1 fusion as the genetic hallmark in epithelioid hemangioendothelioma has

provided an objective proof in the monoclonal origin. Other chromosomal aberrations and genetic mutations have been observed in hemangioma and angiosarcoma [24].

Cellular Regulators

Vascular lesions have a rich microenvironment [25]. Hemangiomas have an abundant number of inflammatory cells surrounding the proliferating vessels. One of these cells, the mast cells have been suggested that may act as initiators in the involution phase of hemangiomas, regulating proangiogenic and antiangiogenic factors [26]. Immunohistochemycal analyses have revealed also variations in the pericytes of hemangiomas that differ from other pericytes because lack of platelet-derived growth factor receptor-β (PDGFRβ) expression [27]. This could be secondary to high expression of JAGGED1, a ligand of the NOTCH signaling family in endothelial cell steam cells, which is required for pericyte differentiation [28].

Genetic Regulators

The heterogeneity seen in vascular neoplasms might be caused by intratumor clonal diversity, with secondary deregulation of different proteins [29]. The aberrant expression of transcription factors supports this regulatory mechanism. Alterations in angiopoietins/tyrosine kinase, fibroblast growth factor (FGF), stromal cell-derived factor-1α (SDF-1α), hepatocyte growth factor (HGF), Delta-like 1, -3, -4, Jagged-1 and -2 (the Notch ligands) have been documented [30]. Moreover, the participation of epigenetic regulators in the activation of nuclear factor-κB (NFκB), and the expression of selective micro-RNAs has also been observed [31].

This genetic heterogeneity, traduced in protein heterogeneity, might be the cause for the low response rates observed with molecular target therapy in vascular neoplasms [31]. For example, only 15 % of angiosarcomas respond to VEGFR-targeted agents in clinical trials [21].

These findings have provided a rationale for the development of a strategy of combination therapy with agents targeting multiple angiogenic growth factors, or agents that target common signaling pathways such as Akt, Notch, mTOR, angiopoietin/tie, or ERK (extracellular signal-regulated kinase) [18].

Specific Genetic Alterations in Angiosarcoma

Complex karyotypes and chromosomal instability are often observed in angiosarcomas. Activation of the oncogene *K-ras* through acquisition of specific point mutations is a common event in angiosarcoma [32]. The incidence of K-ras mutations seems to be highest in angiosarcomas associated with chemical agents [32]. Other common abnormalities observed in angiosarcoma are: TP53 mutations, deletions within the *CDKN2A* locus, Mdm-2 overexpression, and inactivation of p16^{INK4a}, p15^{INK4b}, and p14^{ARF} [32]. In whole genomic sequencing studies have been identified truncating mutations in the PTPRB (VE-PTP) gene, which encodes a tyrosine phosphatase that inhibits angiogenesis [32]. Mutations in PLCG1 with MYC amplification also have been identified and associated with secondary angiosarcoma [33]. Furthermore, in a whole-genome expression study identified involvement of RET, FLT4, CDKN2C, UNC5A, CTLA4, ISLR2, ICOS, RAB17, and RASGRP3 in secondary angiosarcoma [21]. Deregulation of MYC, RET, and CDKN2C were validated using immunohistochemistry [34]. In secondary angiosarcomas upregulation of RET creates induction of N-MYC and downregulation of CDKN2C [34].

Specific Genetic Alterations in Kaposi Sarcoma (KS) and Hemangioendothelioma

KS arises in individuals infected with human herpes virus 8 (HHV8) [35]. The HHV8 genome encodes viral homologs of cellular genes that promote the cell cycle and cellular immortalization, inhibit apoptosis, stimulate angiogenesis, and enable infected cells to evade the immune system [35]. TP53 mutations are rare in KS. But p53 protein function is suppressed through direct interaction with the HHV8-encoded latency-associated nuclear antigen (LANA). Chromosomal instability has been reported in hemangioendothelioma [36]. Furthermore, abnormalities in VEGF expression and p53 have also) been observed in hemangioendothelioma [36]. But the most relevant characteristic seen in epithelioid hemangioendothelioma is the presence of WWTR1-CAMTA1 fusion gene [24].

Specific Genetic Alterations in Infantile Hemangioma (IH)

In proliferating IHs increased expression of Jagged-1 and Notch-4 have been observed [36]. Also the transcription factor hypoxia inducible factor (HIF-1α), ang-1, and 2 are significantly upregulated in the IH endothelium. HIF-α is a major contributor to increase VEGF levels, and to disrupt autophagy. Other signaling pathways β-adrenergic mediated are de-regulated in IH [36, 37]. Alterations in genes implicated in cell adhesion (TIMP1, COL1A1, COL1A2, MMP1, MMP13, SERPINE2, COL4A6, LAMC2, MMP2, CD44, CAV1, CCL2, JAM3, CLDN11, LYVE-1), cell cycle (CCND2, CDKN2A, CCNA1, NCAPD2), and arachidonic acid production (ACSL5, FAP, LIPG, PLA2G4C) have also been observed [21]. Epigenetic alterations have been observed in conjunction with overexpression of CTAG2 [30].

Specific Genetic Alterations in Hemangioma

Chromosomal alterations including loss of heterozygosity at chromosome regions 5q, 13q14, and 17p13, as well as loss of the Y chromosome, and amplification of the cyclin-D1 gene on chromosome 11 have been documented in hemangiomas [23].

Specific Genetic Alterations in Congenital Malformations (CM)

In CM have been observed trysomies and particular mutations restricted to some groups as CCM1 (KRIT1), CCM2, and CCM3 mutations. These mutations seem to be highly regulated by epigenetic factors [18, 23]. Mutations in specific genes have been implicated thanks to sequencing analysis with particular syndromes or diseases such as: RASA1 in CM arterio venous malformation syndrome, GNAQ in port wine stains, AKT1 in Proteus syndrome, and PIK3CA in CLOVES syndrome, KTS, and megalencephaly-CM-polymicrogyria syndrome [38, 39].

New Endothelial Cell Immunohistochemical Markers

New Broad-Spectrum Endothelial Markers

Claudin-5

Claudins are a family of at least 24 proteins that are essential components of tight junctions [40]. These proteins participate in epithelial cellular barrier control and play a role in signal transduction [41]. A member of this family, Claudin-5, also known as TMDVCF (transmembrane protein deletion velocardiofacial syndrome), BEC1, and CPETRL1, is highly expressed in vascular endothelial cells of the lung, kidney, intestine, and dermis [40, 41]. In endothelium this protein plays an important role in the maintenance of the tight junction integrity. In normal tissues claudin-5 is also expressed in juxtaluminal, glandular, and ductal epithelial cells [42]. The gene CLDN5 located on chromosome 22q11.21 encodes for claudin-5 [40]. Deletion of this gene is found in patients with velocardiofacial syndrome or DiGeorge syndrome [42]. A study that used a polyclonal antibody showed that almost all angiosarcomas, KSs, kaposiform hemangioendotheliomas, epithelioid hemangioendotheliomas, hemangiomas (venous, intramuscular, capillary, and cavernous), and lymphangiomas expressed claudin-5 [42]. However, juvenile capillary hemangiomas are negative for claudin-5, probably reflecting immature endothelial phenotype. Biphasic synovial sarcoma is the only nonvascular stromal tumor that expresses claudin-5. The expression was also observed in carcinomas, especially those of the lung and pancreas; but not in mesotheliomas or melanomas [43]. Thus claudin-5 is useful in differentiate angiosarcoma, from hemangiopericytoma, epithelioid sarcoma, melanoma, and other mimickers [2]. Claudin-5 is no expressed in histiocytes and plasma cells, giving it a relevant specificity advantage in comparison with CD31. Claudin-5 has more sensitivity that ERG secondary to higher antigen preservation, and vWf. Currently are available two different antibodies, one polyclonal and another monoclonal, to be used in immunohistochemistry, both produce typically a strong and diffuse cytoplasmic staining with occasional membrane reactivity [40, 43].

ERG

ERG (avian v-ets erythroblastosis virus E26 oncogene homolog), also named as ERG-3 or p55, is a transcription factor of the ETS family whose members include FLI-1 and ETS-1. A gene located on chromosome 21q22.3 encodes for ERG [44]. This protein is involved in angiogenesis and endothelial apoptosis regulation [45]. In addition, ERG has been implicated in prostate carcinogenesis, as gene fusions involving androgen-regulated gene transmembrane protease serine 2 (TMPRSS2) and ERG are frequently observed in prostatic carcinoma [2, 44, 45]. It is also expressed in subsets of acute myeloid leukemia (including myeloid sarcomas), Ewing sarcoma meningioma, epithelioid sarcoma, and mesothelioma [46]. In addition, in human fetal tissue, ERG is expressed in subsets of primitive mesenchymal cells, and perichondrial mesenchyme, but not in mature cartilage, fibroblasts, or chondrosarcomas [44, 46]. In normal tissues the immunohistochemical expression of ERG is restricted to the nuclei of endothelial cells and immature myeloid cells in the bone marrow. In general, ERG is a highly

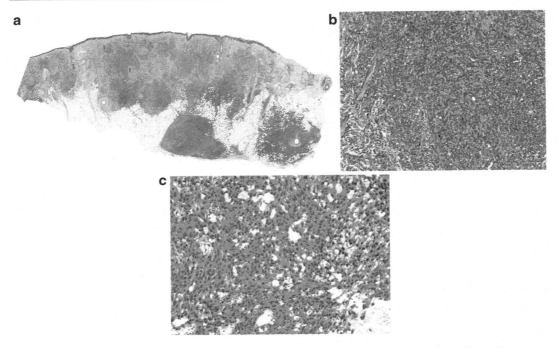

Fig. 8.1 (a) Scanning magnification of an epithelioid angiosarcoma (hematoxylin and eosin stain). (b) Higher magnification demonstrates epithelioid cells, some of them with vacuoles in their cytoplasm. No obvious vascular space noted (hematoxylin and eosin stain). (c) ERG stain confirms the vascular nature of the neoplasm

specific marker in human vascular lesions, been positive in hemangiomas, lymphangiomas, hemangioendotheliomas, Kaposi sarcomas and angiosarcomas [47] (Fig. 8.1). A higher expression in angiosarcomas (100%) has been reported, even better than CD31 (80–90%) [45, 47]. ERG is helpful in the distinction of hemorrhagic, poorly differentiated, and neuroendocrine carcinomas from angiosarcomas. Other non-endothelial vascular related tumors, such as glomus tumor, hemangiopericytoma/solitary fibrous tumor, and cerebellar hemangioblastoma, are uniformly negative for ERG [46, 48]. Additionally, ERG is not expressed in histiocytes, plasma cells, and platelets, which are positives for CD31 [49]. ERG is also valuable in identify lymphovascular invasion by other neoplasms, giving better results that podoplanin. Reasons why ERG is so called the most sensitive and specific marker for vascular differentiation [50]. Several polyclonal and monoclonal ERG antibodies are commercially available [2].

FLI-1

Friend leukemia integration 1 (FLI-1), also known as ESWR2, SIC-1 and transcription factor ERGB, is a member of the ETS family of transcription factors [51]. The ETS family consists in approximately 30 proteins that are characterized by a highly conserved helix-turn-helix DNA-binding domain [51, 52]. These proteins act as specific gene promoters. A gene located in chromosome 11q24 encodes FLI-1 [52, 53]. FLI-1 plays important physiological roles in blood vessels development, megakaryocytic differentiation, as well in myeloid and mononuclear cells development [52]. FLI-1 presents a strong nuclear staining that is very easy to evaluate. In normal tissues, FLI-1 is preferentially expressed in lymphocytes, endothelial cells, and in some hematopoietic cells, such as T lymphocytes and megakaryocytes, but it has also been reported in breast, prostate, colon, and squamous epithelium [51, 52]. FLI-1 is highly sensitive for endothelial derived neoplasms (94%), including hemangiomas, hemangioendotheliomas, KSs,

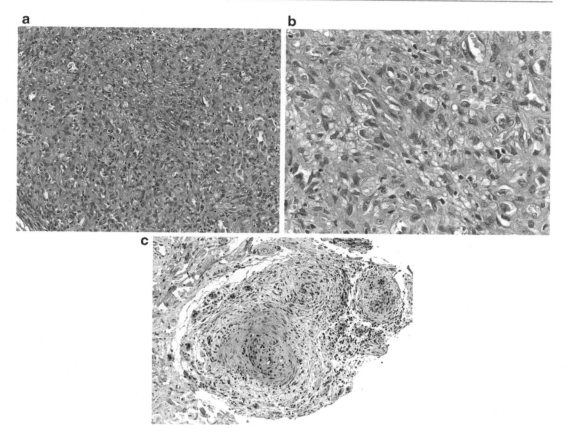

Fig. 8.2 (**a**) Epithelioid hemangioendothelioma showing a neoplasm composed of small vascular spaces some of them containing erythrocytes and admixed with cells with ample cytoplasm and centrally placed nuclei. (**b**) Most of the cells have cytoplasmic vacuoles (hematoxylin and eosin stain). (**c**) Fli-1 stain, please note the nuclear staining with this antibody

and angiosarcomas (Fig. 8.2). The expression of FLI-1 also well known in non-endothelial neoplasms as Ewing's sarcoma/primitive neuroectodermal tumors, which is the result of a specific translocation t(11;22)(q25;q12) that results in the expression of the EWS-FLI-1 oncogene [53, 54]. Other neoplasms that express FLI-1 are: Merkel cell carcinomas, neuroblastoma, lymphoblastic lymphoma, hemangiopericytoma, liposarcoma, medullary breast carcinoma, desmoplastic small round cell tumors, synovial sarcomas, aggressive lymphomas, melanomas, urothelial carcinoma, rhabdomyosarcoma, synovial sarcoma, and pulmonary adenocarcinoma [54, 55]. Several polyclonal and monoclonal antibodies are commercially available for immunohistochemistry [2].

LMO-2

LIM domain only 2 (LMO2), also named rhombotin-2, rhombotin-like-1, and T-cell transcription gene 2, is a small transcription cofactor composed by two cysteine-rich, zinc-binding LIM- domains required in angiogenesis and hematopoiesis [56]. This protein is encoded in a gene located on chromosome 11p13. The initial description of LMO2 was realized after the identification of the chromosomal translocation (t(11;14)(p13;q11) in T-cell acute leukemia [56, 57]. This protein is capable of interact with several genes activated in chromosomal translocations. In the presence of TAL-1/SCL1, LMO2 specifically activates transcription of cadherin in endothelial cells [58]. In normal tissues LMO2 is expressed in the nucleus of endothelial cells, breast myoepithelium, endometrium, germinal center B cells, erythroblast, myeloblasts, and megakaryocytes [58, 59]. LMO2 is expressed in vascular neoplasms such as: hemangiomas, lymphangiomas, hemangioendotheliomas, and 89 % of angiosarcomas [58, 59], but is negative in epithelioid hemangioendothelioma of bone and epithelioid angiosarcoma/epithelioid hemangioendothelioma of the pleura [58]. In nonvascular tumors, LMO2 expression is observed in T-cell lymphomas, giant cell tumors, juvenile xanthogranulomas, some gastrointestinal stromal tumors, small round blue cell tumors, and epithelial-myoepithelial neoplasms. LMO2 is typically negative in carcinomas [58, 59]. Furthermore, LMO2 expression is a favorable predictor in diffuse large B-cell lymphoma [60]. Several antibodies of LMO2 are commercially available [2].

VEGFR-2

VEGFR-2, also known as KDR (kinase insert domain receptor), Flk-1 (fetal liver kinase-1 in mice), and CD309, is a type V receptor tyrosine kinase encoded by the KDR gene located on chromosome 4q12 [61]. Physiologically, VEGFR-2 participates in the regulation of angiogenesis, and vascular permeability [61, 62]. In normal tissues, VEGFR-2 expression is observed

in endothelial and mesothelial cells. In vascular neoplasms VEGFR-2 is expressed in angiosarcoma, KS, and hemangiomas [62]. Spindle cell hemangiomas and retiform hemangioendothelioma present weak VEGFR-2 expression [63, 64]. Other nonvascular neoplasms that express VEGFR-2 are: epithelioid mesothelioma, lung adenocarcinomas, squamous cell carcinomas, chordomas, biphasic synovial sarcomas, and embryonal carcinomas [64, 65].

New Endothelial Markers Specifics for Blood Vessels

WT-1

Wilms tumor-1 (WT-1) is a tumor suppressor transcription factor protein encoded in the WT-1 gene located in chromosome 11p13 [66]. Physiologically, WT-1 plays an essential role in the development of the urogenital system, hematopoiesis, and angiogenesis. The angiogenic role of WT-1 is done thought VEGF regulation [67]. In vascular lesions WT-1 expression is observed in the nucleus of cells that compose pyogenic granulomas, arterio-venous malformations, infantile hemangiomas, noninvoluting congenital hemangiomas (Fig. 8.3), rapidly involuting congenital hemangiomas, hobnail hemangiomas,

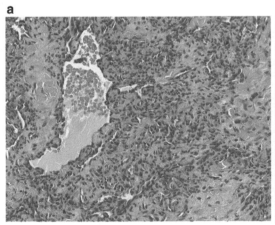
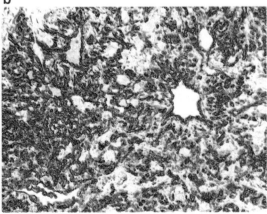

Fig. 8.3 (**a**) Infantile Hemangioma showing irregular vascular spaces, lined by prominent endothelial cells (hematoxylin and eosin stain). (**b**) These neoplasms are strongly positive when they are stained with WT-1. This antibody is negative in vascular malformations

spindle cell hemangiomas, epithelioid hemangio-endothelioma, and angiosarcomas [68]. Lymphatic and venous vascular malformations (port-wine stains, venous malformations, and lymphatic malformations) are uniformly negative for WT-1 [66, 68]. Nuclear WT-1 in also identified in tumors from different origin: Wilms' tumor, acute leukemia, ovarian tumors, and desmoplastic small round cell tumor [68]. WT-1 cytoplasmic staining is observed in tumors from gastrointestinal tract, lung, breast, uterus, prostate, urinary tract, melanoma, and several types of sarcoma [69, 70]. In immunohistochemistry, only nuclear staining is considered positive, and in vascular lesions is used to discriminate between arterial vascular neoplasms and non-arterial vascular malformations [68]. The cytoplasmic positivity of WT-1 in proliferative vascular lesions has been described in several studies [66].

New Endothelial Markers Specifics for Lymphatic Vessels

LYVE-1

Lymphatic vessel endothelial hyaluronan 1 (Lyve-1) is also known as lymphatic vessel endothelial hyaluronic acid receptor 1, hyaluronic acid receptor, XLKD1, and CRSBP-1 [71]. Lyve-1 is a type I membrane protein that acts as a major receptor for hyaluronan (extracellular matrix glycosamino-glycan hyaluronan), a component of the extracellular matrix. This protein is encoded in a gene located on chromosome 11p15 [72]. Physiologically, lyve-1 participates in cell migration during inflammation, and wound healing, through hyaluronan mediated transportation [73]. In normal tissues is uniformly expressed in lymphatic endothelial cells [73]. Sinusoidal endothelium of liver, spleen, and choroid bodies also express lyve-1, where hyaluronan is incorporated and degraded. Other organs where lyve-1 expression has been documented are: zona reticularis in the adrenal gland, Langerhans in the pancreas, tubular epithelium in the kidney [72]. Lyve-1 is also upregulated in macrophages by a variety of growth factors and cytokines in inflammatory conditions. Blood vascular endothelium and myoepithelial cells generally do not express lyve-1 [74]. Several studies have proved the participation of lyve-1 in cancer progression. In pathologic tissues, Lyve-1 is highly specific for proliferative lymphatic endothelium, including KSs, and lymphangioendotheliomatosis [71, 75]. Other neoplasms also express lyve-1 such as: pancreatic islet cells tumors, and gastrointestinal carcinoid tumors [75, 76]. The main relevance of this marker is lymphatic vessels identification, including cases of lymphovascular invasion. The overall performance of lyve-1 is similar to podoplanin [77]. Currently multiple anti-LYVE-1 antibodies are commercially available [2].

Prox-1

Prox1 is a nuclear transcription factor encoded in the homeobox gene PROX1 on chromosome 1q41. This protein induces the independent lymphatic development in several organs; it is also implicated in the development of neuroectodermal structures [78]. Knockout of PROX1 gene is usually fatal in mice secondary to lymphatics arrest and several other developmental defects [79]. Prox1 acts as regulator of podoplanin and differentiation factor in endothelial cells, crucial functions to archive the lymphatic endothelial cell phenotype. Prox-1 is expressed in the nucleus of lymphatic endothelial cells, with occasional nonspecific cytoplasmic expression. Blood vessels and pericytes do not express prox1 [80]. In non-endothelial tissues prox1 is expressed in: conjunctiva, lens, heart, liver, bile ducts, pancreas, retina, and nervous system [81]. Prox-1 is expressed in: lymphatic malformations, lymphangiomas, intralymphatic angioendothelioma (Dabska tumor), spindle cell hemangiomas, tufted hemangioma, kaposiform hemangioma, retiform hemangioendotheliomas, and KS [80–82]. In addition, some angiosarcomas and epithelioid hemangioendotheliomas also express prox-1 [81] (Fig. 8.4). The rest of vascular neoplasms are typically negative for prox-1 [80–83]. This marker is also positive in non-endothelial neoplasms such

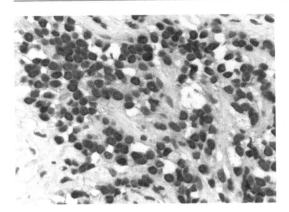

Fig. 8.4 Nuclear staining with Prox-1

as: colonic carcinoma, cholangiocarcinoma, synovial sarcoma, Ewings sarcoma, paraganglioma, neuroendocrine carcinoma, diffuse large B-cell lymphomas, and some adenocarcinomas [84] Prox-1 is generally negative in some mimics of angiosarcoma such as: metastatic melanoma, undifferentiated sarcomas, and sarcomatoid carcinomas [85, 86]. In comparison with podoplanin, prox-1 is less sensitive, but more specific lymphatic proliferations. Prox1 is commercially available [87].

VEGFR-3

VEGFR-3, also known as FLT4 and PCL, is a membrane-anchored tyrosine kinase encoded in chromosome 5q35.3. Physiologically, VEGFR-3 is essential in embryonic lymphangiogenesis [88]. In normal tissues VEGFR-3 is mainly expressed in lymphatic endothelial cells. The main use of this marker is in the identification of lymphatic endothelial cells [88, 89]. However, VEGFR-3 is also express in the endothelium of some blood vessels, myoepithelial cells, and even in non-endothelial cells [89]. VEGFR-3 is expressed in almost all KSs, kaposiform hemangioendotheliomas, papillary intralymphatic angioendotheliomas (Dabska tumor) and lymphangiomatosis [89, 90]. Furthermore is also observed in some angiosarcomas and capillary hemangiomas [91, 92]. VEGFR-3 antibodies for immunohistochemistry are commercially available [92].

New Markers to Evaluate Proliferative Endothelium

CAMTA1

Calmodulin-binding transcription activator 1 (CAMTA1) is a gene encoded on 1p36 chromosome, implicated with WWTR1 in t(1;3)(p36;q23-25) rearrangement seen in epithelioid hemangioendothelioma [93]. This translocation created the WWTR1-CAMTA1 fusion gene, which increases the expression of CAMTA1 inducing the development of epithelioid hemangioendothelioma and other vascular neoplasms [93, 94]. Genetic detection of WWTR1 or CAMTA1 fusion gene is highly sensitive and specific in the diagnosis of epithelioid hemangioendothelioma [94]. The immunohistochemical expression of CAMTA1 is observed in 83% of epithelioid hemangioendothelioma and other proliferative vascular neoplasms. However it is also expressed in several carcinomas, sarcomas with epithelioid characteristics (epithelioid sarcomas and rhabdoid tumors), mesothelioma and melanomas [93, 95]. Thus the relevance of CAMTA1 in diagnostic histopathology is minimal. CAMTA1 antibody to be used in routine immunohistochemistry is commercially available.

Endoglein

Endoglein (CD105), a 180-kDa homodimeric transmembrane glycoprotein, is a component of the transforming growth factor b-1 receptor complex [96]. Endoglein is highly upregulated on activated endothelial cells during angiogenesis, tumor angiogenesis, vascular homeostasis, cardiovascular development, and inflammation, but shows weak or negative expression on vascular endothelium of normal tissues [97]. In arteriovenous malformations (AVM) endoglein gene is mutated and has been implicated in the development of AVM's [98]. Several studies have shown that endoglein is a highly specific and more sensitive marker for angiogenesis than other commonly used endothelial antibodies [98, 99], showing a strong expression in the vasculature of solid tumors, while other markers such as CD31 and CD34 are weaker [98]. It is also highly expressed in growing or remodeling AVMs. In immunohistochemistry endoglein labeling is cytoplasmic and membranous [98]. Consequently, endoglein is a useful marker for neoplastic neovascularization and proliferating AVMs. Furthermore, recent data suggest that CD105 expression have prognostic value in various solid cancers [100].

HIF-1 Alpha (HIF-1a

HIF-1a is a nuclear protein that regulates the expression of more than 100 genes. These genes play roles in angiogenesis, metabolism, proliferation, and carcinogenesis (invasion, and metastasis) [101]. HIF-1a has been extensively)studied as a marker of hypoxia in pathological processes [102]. Hypoxia has been frequently observed in tumor development and progression, and is one of the most important stimuli for neovascularization. The effect of HIF-1a is mediated through transcriptional control of GLUT-1, pH regulators, glycolytic enzymes, and cell survival factors [101, 102]. In immunohistochemistry this marker is expressed in vascular malformations, pyogenic granuloma, and in the proliferative phase of hemangiomas [103]. In addition, HIF-1a has been documented as adverse prognostic factor in solid tumors, particularly head and neck tumors [102, 104].

TEMs

Human tumor endothelial markers (TEM) is a family of a transmembrane glycoproteins initially described after gene expression analysis in endothelial cells from human colorectal cancer. TEM1, also known as endosialin or CD248, is expressed on endothelial cells, pericytes, and fibroblasts [105]. The gene TEM1 encodes this protein induced by HIF-2a. TEM1 is implicated in vascular cell adhesion, migration, development, and neoangiogenesis [105]. Knockout mice for TEM1 are healthy and resistant to tumor growth, invasiveness, and metastasis [106]. This characteristic has been studied in order to develop new therapies for cancer. TEM1 is expressed in the vasculature of carcinomas, sarcomas, and brain tumors [107, 108]. Some studies have

associated its overexpression with poor survival [105]. TEM5 is involved in cell-cell and cell-matrix interactions during angiogenesis [108]. TEM5 is expressed on the surface of endothelial cells. Studies about its applicability in histopathology remains to be done. TEM7 is expressed in human tumor endothelium. This protein participates during the interaction between extracellular matrix and neoplastic cells. TEM-7 is also involved in angiogenesis [109]. TEM7 is also expressed in sarcomas, colorectal, breast, bladder, lung, gastric, kidney, liver, and lung cancer vasculature, where it has been proposed as a prognostic marker. Also the utility to target TEM-7 therapeutically is under investigation [109]. TEM8 is also expressed in areas with aberrant vascular formation of tumors. TEM8 is generally negative in normal tissues [110]. The physiologic function of TEM8 is unknown but it is thought to play a role in angiogenesis, cellular adhesion, cell migration, and extracellular matrix homeostasis. TEM8 is expressed in endothelial cells from multiple carcinomas including those of breast, colon, esophagus, lung, and bladder [111]. Several studies have analyzed TEM8 as target for cancer therapy [110, 111].

Myc

Myc is a transcription factor encoded by the gene MYC. Mutations in MYC, as t(8;14), have been described in several types of cancer. Upregulation of MYC causes over-expression in many genes; some of them are involved in cell proliferation, apoptosis, and angiogenesis [112]. MYC upregulation is seen in secondary angiosarcomas (radiotherapy related angiosarcoma), (Fig. 8.5) and is absent in atypical vascular proliferations secondary to radiotherapy [112, 113]. This upregulation have been validated with immunohistochemistry and in situ hybridization observing high expression of myc in radiation related breast angiosarcomas (55–100 %) [113–115]. Therefore, the immunohistochemical analysis of myc in atypical vascular proliferations related with radiotherapy will be useful distinguishing angiosarcoma from benign proliferations [113–117].

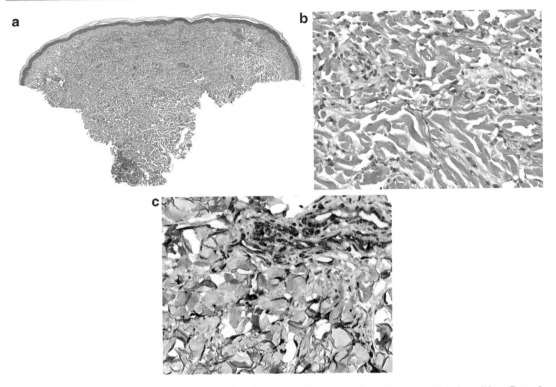

Fig. 8.5 Angiosarcoma of the breast post radiation ther- apy. (**a**) Scanning magnification showing numerous irreg- ular spaces in the dermis (hematoxylin and eosin stain). (**b**) These spaces are lined by prominent endothelial cells.

(**c**) The endothelial cells are positive for c-Myc. Cmyc is negative in benign vascular proliferations secondary to radiation therapy

Micro-RNAs

miRNAs are short ribonucleic acid molecules that usually have a size of 22 nucleotides [118]. These molecules act as epigenetic regulators in the post-transcriptional process of proteins. In the human genome, have been described more than 1000 miRNAs, which target around 60% of the encoded proteins [119]. Several miRNAs are rel- evant in angiogenesis regulation [119]. Low expression of mir-424 has been documented in the proliferative endothelium of senile hemangi- oma and infantile Hemangioma [120]. This alter- ation is not observed in normal blood vessels and vascular malformations [121] mir-424 acts down-regulating the expression of MEK1 and cyclin E1, both active inductors of cell prolifera- tion [119, 121, 122].

New Vascular Uses of Previously Developed Immunohistochemical Markers

CD30

CD30 is a transmembrane glycoprotein member of the tumor necrosis factor receptor super- fam- ily. CD30 mediates in the activation of NF-kB, playing functions in cellular proliferation and differentiation [123]. Classically, CD30 have been described as a marker of activated lymphoid cells, including T and B cells. The immunohisto- chemical membranous detection of this marker has established diagnostic relevance in Hodgkin lymphomas, large-cell anaplastic lymphoma, diffuse large B-cell lymphomas, lymphomatois papulosis, and T cell lymphomas [123, 124]. CD30 has been observed in variable degree expressed in endothelial cells proliferations and neoplasms, with high expression in angiosarcoma and hemangioendothelioma (30 %) [124]. Kaposi sarcoma, and hemangiomas are uniformly negative for this marker [123]. Other neoplasms that also express CD30 are: melanoma, embryonal carcinoma, and nasopharyngeal carcinoma [124, 125]. The roles of CD30 in malignant transformation of vascular endothelium need to be established. Also the applicability of specific anti-CD30 inhibitors (brentuximab vedotin and analogs) in driven molecular therapy for vascular lesions needs to be studied [123].

Desmoplakin

Desmoplakin is a desmosome-associated transmembrane glycoprotein expressed in lymphatic vessels but not in blood vessels [126]. This seems related to the presence of a continuous basement membrane in blood vessels, and a discontinuous or incomplete basement membrane in lymphatic vessels. Desmoplakin is combined with plakoglobin, desmocolin, and desmoglein, to form desmosomes [126]. Immunohistochemical studies using anti-desmoplakin have demonstrated strong reactivity with this antibody in human lymphatic vessels [126, 127]. Desmoplakin expression was observed at the junction of the lymphatic endothelial cell junction and cytoplasm. These results were validated with immunoelectron microscopy, showing better results than immunohistochemistry against anti-laminin and factor VIII [126]. Previous analyses in other mammals have shown similar results [128]. Antibodies against desmoplakin are easy to use and are commercially available [128].

PAL-E

Pathologische Anatomie Leiden-Endothelium (PAL-E) is a mouse monoclonal antibody of IgG2a targeted against plasmalemma vesicle-associated protein-1, a highly glycosylated, type II transmembrane glycoprotein expressed in endothelium involved in leukocyte trafficking [129]. PAL-E reacts strongly and specifically with blood vessel endothelial cells, but is absent in lymphatic endothelium and in brain blood vessels [130, 131]. Currently, PAL-E is the most specific marker available in immunohistochemistry to identify blood vessels, and differentiate them from lymphatic vessels [132–134]. This antibody is commercially available [129].

References

1. Rao P, Lahat G, Arnold C, Gavino AC, Lahat S, Hornick JL, et al. Angiosarcoma: a tissue microarray study with diagnostic implications. Am J Dermatopathol. 2013;35(4):432–7.
2. Ordóñez NG. Immunohistochemical endothelial markers: a review. Adv Anat Pathol. 2012;19(5): 281–95.
3. Millard PR, Heryet AR. An immunohistological study of factor VIII related antigen and Kaposi's sarcoma using polyclonal and monoclonal antibodies. J Pathol. 1985;146(1):31–8.
4. Ordóñez NG, Batsakis JG. Comparison of Ulex europaeus I lectin and factor VIII-related antigen in vascular lesions. Arch Pathol Lab Med. 1984;108(2): 129–32.
5. Vanchinathan V, Mizramani N, Kantipudi R, Schwartz EJ, Sundram UN. The vascular marker CD31 also highlights histiocytes and histiocyte-like cells within cutaneous tumors. Am J Clin Pathol. 2015;143(2):177–85.
6. Traweek ST, Kandalaft PL, Mehta P, Battifora H. The human hematopoietic progenitor cell antigen (CD34) in vascular neoplasia. Am J Clin Pathol. 1991;96(1):25–31.
7. Fukunaga M. Expression of D2-40 in lymphatic endothelium of normal tissues and in vascular tumours. Histopathology. 2005;46(4):396–402.
8. Kahn HJ, Bailey D, Marks A. Monoclonal antibody D2-40, a new marker of lymphatic endothelium, reacts with Kaposi's sarcoma and a subset of angiosarcomas. Mod Pathol. 2002;15(4):434–40.
9. Manning T, Smoller BR, Horn TD, El Darouti M, Marzouk S, Hadidi HE, et al. Evaluation of anti-thrombomodulin antibody as a tumor marker for vascular neoplasms. J Cutan Pathol. 2004;31(10):652–6.
10. Kleiman A, Keats EC, Chan NG, Khan ZA. Evolution of hemangioma endothelium. Exp Mol Pathol. 2012;93(2):264–72.
11. Pack GT, Miller TR. Hemangiomas; classification, diagnosis and treatment. Angiology. 1950;1(5): 405–26.

12. Boye E, Yu Y, Paranya G, Mulliken JB, Olsen BR, Bischoff J. Clonality and altered behavior of endothelial cells from hemangiomas. J Clin Invest. 2001;107(6):745–52.

13. Shon W, Ida CM, Boland-Froemming JM, Rose PS, Folpe A. Cutaneous angiosarcoma arising in massive localized lymphedema of the morbidly obese: a report of five cases and review of the literature. J Cutan Pathol. 2011;38(7):560–4.

14. Liu L, Kakiuchi-Kiyota S, Arnold LL, Johansson SL, Wert D, Cohen SM. Pathogenesis of human hemangiosarcomas and hemangiomas. Hum Pathol. 2013;44(10):2302–11.

15. Holmes LB. Chorionic villus sampling and hemangiomas. J Craniofac Surg. 2009;20 Suppl 1:675–7.

16. Bauland CG, Smit JM, Bartelink LR, Zondervan HA, Spauwen PH. Hemangioma in the newborn: increased incidence after chorionic villus sampling. Prenat Diagn. 2010;30(10):913–7.

17. Wen VW, MacKenzie KL. Modeling human endothelial cell transformation in vascular neoplasias. Dis Model Mech. 2013;6(5):1066–79.

18. Blatt J, Powell CM, Burkhart CN, Stavas J, Aylsworth AS. Genetics of hemangiomas, vascular malformations, and primary lymphedema. J Pediatr Hematol Oncol. 2014;36(8):587–93.

19. Wong WT, Huang NF, Botham CM, Sayed N, Cooke JP. Endothelial cells derived from nuclear reprogramming. Circ Res. 2012;111(10):1363–75.

20. Ritter MR, Reinisch J, Friedlander SF, Friedlander M. Myeloid cells in infantile hemangioma. Am J Pathol. 2006;168(2):621–8.

21. Behjati S, Tarpey PS, Sheldon H, Martincorena I, Van Loo P, Gundem G, et al. Recurrent PTPRB and PLCG1 mutations in angiosarcoma. Nat Genet. 2014;46(4):376–9.

22. Patiño-Seijas B, Lorenzo-Franco F, Rey-Sanjurjo JL, González-Cuesta M, López-Cedrún Cembranos JL. Vascular Lesions: GLUT-1 expression as a diagnostic tool to discriminate tumors from malformations. J Oral Maxillofac Surg. 2012;70(10):2333–42.

23. Ji Y, Chen S, Li K, Li L, Xu C, Xiang B. Signaling pathways in the development of infantile hemangioma. J Hematol Oncol. 2014;7:13.

24. Errani C, Sung YS, Zhang L, Healey JH, Antonescu CR. Monoclonality of multifocal epithelioid hemangioendothelioma of the liver by analysis of WWTR1-CAMTA1 breakpoints. Cancer Genet. 2012;205(1–2):12–7.

25. Stiles JM, Rowntree RK, Amaya C, Diaz D, Kokta V, Mitchell DC, et al. Gene expression analysis reveals marked differences in the transcriptome of infantile hemangioma endothelial cells compared to normal dermal microvascular endothelial cells. Vasc Cell. 2013;5(1):6.

26. Prey S, Leaute-Labreze C, Pain C, Moisan F, Vergnes P, Loot M, et al. Mast cells as possible targets of propranolol therapy: an immunohistological study of beta-adrenergic receptors in infantile haemangiomas. Histopathology. 2014;65(3):436–9.

27. Assaad AM, Kawut SM, Arcasoy SM, Rosenzweig EB, Wilt JS, Sonett JR, et al. Platelet-derived growth factor is increased in pulmonary capillary hemangiomatosis. Chest. 2007;131(3):850–5.

28. Boscolo E, Stewart CL, Greenberger S, Wu JK, Durham JT, Herman IM, et al. JAGGED1 signaling regulates hemangioma stem cell-to-pericyte/vascular smooth muscle cell differentiation. Arterioscler Thromb Vasc Biol. 2011;31(10):2181–92.

29. Koina ME, Baxter L, Adamson SJ, Arfuso F, Hu P, Madigan MC, et al. Evidence for lymphatics in the developing and adult human choroid. Invest Ophthalmol Vis Sci. 2015;56(2):1310–27.

30. Ji RC, Eshita Y, Xing L, Miura M. Multiple expressions of lymphatic markers and morphological evolution of newly formed lymphatics in lymphangioma and lymph node lymphangiogenesis. Microvasc Res. 2010;80(2):195–201.

31. Young RJ, Fernando M, Hughes D, Brown NJ, Woll PJ. Angiogenic growth factor expression in benign and malignant vascular tumours. Exp Mol Pathol. 2014;97(1):148–53.

32. Weihrauch M, Bader M, Lehnert G, Koch B, Wittekind C, Wrbitzky R, et al. Mutation analysis of K-ras-2 in liver angiosarcoma and adjacent nonneoplastic liver tissue from patients occupationally exposed to vinyl chloride. Environ Mol Mutagen. 2002;40(1):36–40.

33. Kunze K, Spieker T, Gamerdinger U, Nau K, Berger J, Dreyer T, et al. A recurrent activating PLCG1 mutation in cardiac angiosarcomas increases apoptosis resistance and invasiveness of endothelial cells. Cancer Res. 2014;74(21):6173–83.

34. Styring E, Seinen J, Dominguez-Valentin M, Domanski HA, Jönsson M, von Steyern FV, et al. Key roles for MYC, KIT and RET signaling in secondary angiosarcomas. Br J Cancer. 2014;111(2):407–12.

35. Gramolelli S, Schulz TF. The role of Kaposi sarcoma-associated herpesvirus in the pathogenesis of Kaposi sarcoma. J Pathol. 2015;235(2):368–80.

36. Janmohamed SR, Madern GC, de Laat PC, Oranje AP. Educational paper: pathogenesis of infantile haemangioma, an update 2014 (part I). Eur J Pediatr. 2015;174(1):97–103.

37. Melis M, Cau M, Corraine S, Secci S, Addis M, Melis M. Cerebral cavernous malformations and unilateral moyamoya in a patient with a new mutation in the KRIT-1 /CCM1 gene. Cerebrovasc Dis. 2014;38(4):311–2.

38. Kurek KC, Luks VL, Ayturk UM, Alomari AI, Fishman SJ, Spencer SA, et al. Somatic mosaic activating mutations in PIK3CA cause CLOVES syndrome. Am J Hum Genet. 2012;90(6):1108–15.

39. Lindhurst MJ, Sapp JC, Teer JK, Johnston JJ, Finn EM, Peters K, et al. A mosaic activating mutation in AKT1 associated with the proteus syndrome. N Engl J Med. 2011;365(7):611–9.

40. Miettinen M, Sarlomo-Rikala M, Wang ZF. Claudin-5 as an immunohistochemical marker for angiosarcoma and hemangioendotheliomas. Am J Surg Pathol. 2011;35(12):1848–56.

41. Hara H. Endoglin (CD105) and claudin-5 expression in cutaneous angiosarcoma. Am J Dermatopathol. 2012;34(7):779–82.

42. Yuan L, Le Bras A, Sacharidou A, Itagaki K, Zhan Y, Kondo M, et al. ETS-related gene (ERG) controls endothelial cell permeability via transcriptional regulation of the claudin 5 (CLDN5) gene. J Biol Chem. 2012;287(9):6582–91.

43. Jakab C, Halász J, Kiss A, Schaff Z, Rusvai M, Gálfi P, et al. Claudin-5 protein is a new differential marker for histopathological differential diagnosis of canine hemangiosarcoma. Histol Histopathol. 2009;24(7):801–13.

44. Miettinen M, Wang ZF, Paetau A, Tan SH, Dobi A, Srivastava S, et al. ERG transcription factor as an immunohistochemical marker for vascular endothelial tumors and prostatic carcinoma. Am J Surg Pathol. 2011;35(3):432–41.

45. Yaskiv O, Rubin BP, He H, Falzarano S, Magi-Galluzzi C, Zhou M. ERG protein expression in human tumors detected with a rabbit monoclonal antibody. Am J Clin Pathol. 2012;138(6):803–10.

46. Miettinen M, Wang Z, Sarlomo-Rikala M, Abdullaev Z, Pack SD, Fetsch JF. ERG expression in epithelioid sarcoma: a diagnostic pitfall. Am J Surg Pathol. 2013;37(10):1580–5.

47. Sullivan HC, Edgar MA, Cohen C, Kovach CK, HooKim K, Reid MD. The utility of ERG, CD31 and CD34 in the cytological diagnosis of angiosarcoma: an analysis of 25 cases. J Clin Pathol. 2015;68(1):44–50.

48. Stockman DL, Hornick JL, Deavers MT, Lev DC, Lazar AJ, Wang WL. ERG and FLI1 protein expression in epithelioid sarcoma. Mod Pathol. 2014;27(4):496–501.

49. McKay KM, Doyle LA, Lazar AJ, Hornick JL. Expression of ERG, an Ets family transcription factor, distinguishes cutaneous angiosarcoma from histological mimics. Histopathology. 2012;61(5):989–91.

50. Kim S, Park HK, Jung HY, Lee SY, Min KW, Kim WY, et al. ERG immunohistochemistry as an endothelial marker for assessing lymphovascular invasion. Korean J Pathol. 2013;47(4):355–64.

51. Rossi S, Orvieto E, Furlanetto A, Laurino L, Ninfo V, Dei Tos AP. Utility of the immunohistochemical detection of FLI-1 expression in round cell and vascular neoplasm using a monoclonal antibody. Mod Pathol. 2004;17(5):547–52.

52. Landry JR, Kinston S, Knezevic K, Donaldson IJ, Green AR, Göttgens B. Fli1, Elf1, and Ets1 regulate the proximal promoter of the LMO2 gene in endothelial cells. Blood. 2005;106(8):2680–7.

53. Folpe AL, Chand EM, Goldblum JR, Weiss SW. Expression of Fli-1, a nuclear transcription factor, distinguishes vascular neoplasms from potential mimics. Am J Surg Pathol. 2001;25(8):1061–6.

54. Cuda J, Mirzamani N, Kantipudi R, Robbins J, Welsch MJ, Sundram UN. Diagnostic utility of Fli-1 and D2-40 in distinguishing atypical fibroxanthoma from angiosarcoma. Am J Dermatopathol. 2013;35(3):316–8.

55. Rosado FG, Itani DM, Coffin CM, Cates JM. Utility of immunohistochemical staining with FLI1, D2-40, CD31, and CD34 in the diagnosis of acquired immunodeficiency syndrome-related and non-acquired immunodeficiency syndrome-related Kaposi sarcoma. Arch Pathol Lab Med. 2012;136(3):301–4.

56. Yamada Y, Pannell R, Forster A, Rabbitts TH. The LIM-domain protein Lmo2 is a key regulator of tumour angiogenesis: a new anti-angiogenesis drug target. Oncogene. 2002;21(9):1309–15.

57. Yamada Y, Pannell R, Forster A, Rabbitts TH. The oncogenic LIM-only transcription factor Lmo2 regulates angiogenesis but not vasculogenesis in mice. Proc Natl Acad Sci U S A. 2000;97(1):320–4.

58. Gratzinger D, Zhao S, West R, Rouse RV, Vogel H, Gil EC, et al. The transcription factor LMO2 is a robust marker of vascular endothelium and vascular neoplasms and selected other entities. Am J Clin Pathol. 2009;131(2):264–78.

59. Sun ZJ, Cai Y, Chen G, Wang R, Jia J, Chen XM, Zheng LW, Zhao YF. LMO2 promotes angiogenesis probably by up-regulation of bFGF in endothelial cells: an implication of its pathophysiological role in infantile haemangioma. Histopathology. 2010;57(4):622–32.

60. Lossos C, Bayraktar S, Weinzierl E, Younes SF, Hosein PJ, Tibshirani RJ, et al. LMO2 and BCL6 are associated with improved survival in primary central nervous system lymphoma. Br J Haematol. 2014;165(5):640–8.

61. Tokuyama W, Mikami T, Masuzawa M, Okayasu I. Autocrine and paracrine roles of VEGF/VEGFR-2 and VEGF-C/VEGFR-3 signaling in angiosarcomas of the scalp and face. Hum Pathol. 2010;41(3):407–14.

62. Jin Y, Liu Y, Lin Q, Li J, Druso JE, Antonyak MA, et al. Deletion of Cdc42 enhances ADAM17-mediated vascular endothelial growth factor receptor 2 shedding and impairs vascular endothelial cell survival and vasculogenesis. Mol Cell Biol. 2013;33(21):4181–97.

63. Miettinen M, Rikala MS, Rys J, Lasota J, Wang ZF. Vascular endothelial growth factor receptor 2 as a marker for malignant vascular tumors and mesothelioma: an immunohistochemical study of 262 vascular endothelial and 1640 nonvascular tumors. Am J Surg Pathol. 2012;36(4):629–39.

64. Lee YJ, Karl DL, Maduekwe UN, Rothrock C, Ryeom S, D'Amore PA, et al. Differential effects of VEGFR-1 and VEGFR-2 inhibition on tumor metastases based on host organ environment. Cancer Res. 2010;70(21):8357–67.

65. Yonemori K, Tsuta K, Ando M, Hirakawa A, Hatanaka Y, Matsuno Y, et al. Contrasting prognostic implications of platelet-derived growth factor receptor-β and vascular endothelial growth factor receptor-2 in patients with angiosarcoma. Ann Surg Oncol. 2011;18(10):2841–50.

66. Galfione SK, Ro JY, Ayala AG, Ge Y. Diagnostic utility of WT-1 cytoplasmic stain in variety of vascular lesions. Int J Clin Exp Pathol. 2014;7(5): 2536–43.

67. Fernandez-Flores A, Fierro S, Larralde M. Expression of WT-1 by the vascular component of acral pseudolymphomatous angiokeratoma of children. J Cutan Pathol. 2015;42(1):50–5.

68. Fernandez-Flores A, Saeb-Lima M. Correct evaluation and interpretation of WT-1 immunostaining in vascular lesions. J Cutan Pathol. 2014;41(9):754–5.

69. Garrido-Ruiz MC, Rodriguez-Pinilla SM, Pérez-Gómez B, Rodriguez-Peralto JL. WT 1 expression in nevi and melanomas: a marker of melanocytic invasion into the dermis. J Cutan Pathol. 2010;37(5): 542–8.

70. McCluggage WG. WT-1 immunohistochemical expression in small round blue cell tumours. Histopathology. 2008;52(5):631–2.

71. Akishima Y, Ito K, Zhang L, Ishikawa Y, Orikasa H, Kiguchi H, et al. Immunohistochemical detection of human small lymphatic vessels under normal and pathological conditions using the LYVE-1 antibody. Virchows Arch. 2004;444(2):153–7.

72. Platonova N, Miquel G, Regenfuss B, Taouji S, Cursiefen C, Chevet E, et al. Evidence for the interaction of fibroblast growth factor-2 with the lymphatic endothelial cell marker LYVE-1. Blood. 2013;121(7):1229–37.

73. Noda Y, Amano I, Hata M, Kojima H, Sawa Y. Immunohistochemical examination on the distribution of cells expressed lymphatic endothelial marker podoplanin and LYVE-1 in the mouse tongue tissue. Acta Histochem Cytochem. 2010; 43(2):61–8.

74. Boettcher MC, Eivazi B, Roessler M, Bette M, Cai C, Wiegand S, et al. Involvement of LYVE-1-positive endothelial cells in the formation of non-lymphatic vascular malformations. Histopathology. 2010;57(5):764–8.

75. Hata H, Aoyagi S, Homma E, Muramatsu R, Shimizu H. Lymphangiosarcoma with strong positivity of D2-40 and LYVE-1 presenting different clinical features from angiosarcoma. J Dermatol. 2014;41(7):656–7.

76. Florez-Vargas A, Vargas SO, Debelenko LV, Perez-Atayde AR, Archibald T, Kozakewich HP, et al. Comparative analysis of D2-40 and LYVE-1 immunostaining in lymphatic malformations. Lymphology. 2008;41(3):103–10.

77. Heinzelbecker J, Kempf KM, Kurz K, Steidler A, Weiss C, Jackson DG, et al. Lymph vessel density in seminomatous testicular cancer assessed with the specific lymphatic endothelium cell markers D2-40 and LYVE-1: correlation with pathologic parameters and clinical outcome. Urol Oncol. 2013;31(7):1386–94.

78. Wilting J, Papoutsi M, Christ B, Nicolaides KH, von Kaisenberg CS, Borges J, et al. The transcription factor Prox1 is a marker for lymphatic endothelial cells in normal and diseased human tissues. FASEB J. 2002;16(10):1271–3.

79. Dadras SS, Skrzypek A, Nguyen L, Shin JW, Schulz MM, Arbiser J, et al. Prox-1 promotes invasion of kaposiform hemangioendotheliomas. J Invest Dermatol. 2008;128(12):2798–806.

80. Miettinen M, Wang ZF. Prox1 transcription factor as a marker for vascular tumors-evaluation of 314 vascular endothelial and 1086 nonvascular tumors. Am J Surg Pathol. 2012;36(3):351–9.

81. Le Huu AR, Jokinen CH, Rubin BP, Mihm MC, Weiss SW, North PE, et al. Expression of prox1, lymphatic endothelial nuclear transcription factor, in Kaposiform hemangioendothelioma and tufted angioma. Am J Surg Pathol. 2010;34(11):1563–73.

82. Wang L, Gao T, Wang G. Expression of Prox, 1, D2-40, and WT1 in spindle cell hemangioma. J Cutan Pathol. 2014;41(5):447–50.

83. Benevenuto de Andrade BA, Ramírez-Amador V, Anaya-Saavedra G, Martínez-Mata G, Fonseca FP, Graner E, et al. Expression of PROX-1 in oral Kaposi's sarcoma spindle cells. J Oral Pathol Med. 2014;43(2):132–6.

84. Reis RM, Reis-Filho JS, Longatto Filho A, Tomarev S, Silva P, Lopes JM. Differential Prox-1 and CD 31 expression in mucousae, cutaneous and soft tissue vascular lesions and tumors. Pathol Res Pract. 2005;201(12):771–6.

85. Cimpean AM, Poenaru Sava M, Raica M, Ribatti D. Preliminary evidence of the presence of lymphatic vessels immunoreactive for D2-40 and Prox-1 in human pterygium. Oncol Rep. 2011;26(5):1111–3.

86. Sultan A, Dadras SS, Bay JM, Teng NN. Prox-1, Podoplanin and HPV staining assists in identification of lymphangioma circumscriptum of the vulva and discrimination from vulvar warts. Histopathology. 2011;59(6):1274–7.

87. da Cunha Castro EC, Galambos C. Prox-1: a specific and sensitive marker for lymphatic endothelium in normal and diseased human tissues. Ann Thorac Surg. 2011;92(1):407.

88. Folpe AL, Veikkola T, Valtola R, Weiss SW. Vascular endothelial growth factor receptor-3 (VEGFR-3): a marker of vascular tumors with presumed lymphatic differentiation, including Kaposi's sarcoma, kaposiform and Dabska-type hemangioendotheliomas, and a subset of angiosarcomas. Mod Pathol. 2000;13(2): 180–5.

89. Petrova TV, Bono P, Holnthoner W, Chesnes J, Pytowski B, Sihto H, et al. VEGFR-3 expression is restricted to blood and lymphatic vessels in solid tumors. Cancer Cell. 2008;13(6):554–6.

90. Parsons A, Sheehan DJ, Sangueza OP. Retiform hemangioendotheliomas usually do not express D2-40 and VEGFR-3. Am J Dermatopathol. 2008; 30(1):31–3.

91. Kilvaer TK, Valkov A, Sorbye S, Smeland E, Bremnes RM, Busund LT, et al. Profiling of VEGFs and VEGFRs as prognostic factors in soft tissue sarcoma: VEGFR-3 is an independent predictor of poor prognosis. PLoS One. 2010;5(12):e15368.

92. Itakura E, Yamamoto H, Oda Y, Furue M. Tsuneyoshi M. VEGF-C and VEGFR-3 in a series of lymphangiomas: is superficial lymphangioma a true lymphangioma? Virchows Arch. 2009;454(3):317–25.

93. Yusıflı Z, Kösemehmetoğlu K. CAMTA1 immunostaining is not useful in differentiating epithelioid hemangioendothelioma from its potential mimickers. Turk Patoloji Derg. 2014;30(3):159–65.

94. Anderson T, Zhang L, Hameed M, Rusch V, Travis WD, Antonescu CR. Thoracic epithelioid malignant vascular tumors: a clinicopathologic study of 52 cases with emphasis on pathologic grading and molecular studies of WWTR1-CAMTA1 fusions. Am J Surg Pathol. 2015;39(1):132–9.

95. Boudousquie AC, Lawce HJ, Sherman R, Olson S, Magenis RE, Corless CL. Complex translocation [7;22] identified in an epithelioid hemangioendothelioma. Cancer Genet Cytogenet. 1996;92(2): 116–21.

96. Wang JJ, Sun XC, Hu L, Liu ZF, Yu HP, Li H, et al. Endoglin (CD105) expression on microvessel endothelial cells in juvenile nasopharyngeal angiofibroma: tissue microarray analysis and association with prognostic significance. Head Neck. 2013;35(12):1719–25.

97. López-Novoa JM, Bernabeu C. The physiological role of endoglin in the cardiovascular system. Am J Physiol Heart Circ Physiol. 2010;299(4): H959–74.

98. Hou F, Dai Y, Dornhoffer JR, Suen JY, Fan CY, Saad AG, et al. Expression of endoglin (CD105) and endothelial nitric oxide synthase in head and neck arteriovenous malformations. JAMA Otolaryngol Head Neck Surg. 2013;139(3):237–43.

99. Mahmoud M, Allinson KR, Zhai Z, Oakenfull R, Ghandi P, Adams RH, et al. Pathogenesis of arteriovenous malformations in the absence of endoglin. Circ Res. 2010;106(8):1425–33.

100. Miyata Y, Mitsunari K, Asai A, Takehara K, Mochizuki Y, Sakai H. Pathological significance and prognostic role of microvessel density, evaluated using CD31, CD34, and CD105 in prostate cancer patients after radical prostatectomy with neoadjuvant therapy. Prostate. 2015;75(1):84–91.

101. de Oliveira DH, da Silveira EJ, de Medeiros AM, Alves PM, Queiroz LM. Study of the etiopathogenesis and differential diagnosis of oral vascular lesions by immunoexpression of GLUT-1 and HIF-1α. J Oral Pathol Med. 2014;43(1):76–80.

102. Shibaji T, Nagao M, Ikeda N, Kanehiro H, Hisanaga M, Ko S, et al. Prognostic significance of HIF-1 alpha overexpression in human pancreatic cancer. Anticancer Res. 2003;23(6C):4721–7.

103. Medici D, Olsen BR. Rapamycin inhibits proliferation of hemangioma endothelial cells by reducing HIF-1-dependent expression of VEGF. PLoS One. 2012;7(8):e42913.

104. Tan HH, Ge ZZ, Gao YJ, Chen HM, Fang JY, Chen HY, et al. The role of HIF-1, angiopoietin-2, Dll4 and Notch1 in bleeding gastrointestinal vascular malformations and thalidomide-associated actions: a pilot in vivo study. J Dig Dis. 2011;12(5):349–56.

105. Mehran R, Nilsson M, Khajavi M, Du Z, Cascone T, Wu HK, et al. Tumor endothelial markers define novel subsets of cancer-specific circulating endothelial cells associated with antitumor efficacy. Cancer Res. 2014;74(10):2731–41.

106. Facciponte JG, Ugel S, De Sanctis F, Li C, Wang L, Nair G, et al. Tumor endothelial marker 1-specific DNA vaccination targets tumor vasculature. J Clin Invest. 2014;124(4):1497–511.

107. Bagley RG, Rouleau C, St Martin T, Boutin P, Weber W, Ruzek M, et al. Human endothelial precursor cells express tumor endothelial marker 1/endosialin/CD248. Mol Cancer Ther. 2008;7(8):2536–46.

108. Vallon M, Essler M. Proteolytically processed soluble tumor endothelial marker (TEM) 5 mediates endothelial cell survival during angiogenesis by linking integrin alpha(v)beta3 to glycosaminoglycans. J Biol Chem. 2006;281(45):34179–88.

109. Bagley RG, Rouleau C, Weber W, Mehraein K, Smale R, Curiel M, et al. Tumor endothelial marker 7 (TEM-7): a novel target for antiangiogenic therapy. Microvasc Res. 2011;82(3):253–62.

110. Verma K, Gu J, Werner E. Tumor endothelial marker 8 amplifies canonical Wnt signaling in blood vessels. PLoS One. 2011;6(8):e22334.

111. Gutwein LG, Al-Quran SZ, Fernando S, Fletcher BS, Copeland EM, Grobmyer SR. Tumor endothelial marker 8 expression in triple-negative breast cancer. Anticancer Res. 2011;31(10):3417–22.

112. Ginter PS, Mosquera JM, MacDonald TY, D'Alfonso TM, Rubin MA, Shin SJ. Diagnostic utility of MYC amplification and anti-MYC immunohistochemistry in atypical vascular lesions, primary or radiation-induced mammary angiosarcomas, and primary angiosarcomas of other sites. Hum Pathol. 2014; 45(4):709–16.

113. Manner J, Radlwimmer B, Hohenberger P, Mössinger K, Küffer S, Sauer C, et al. MYC high level gene amplification is a distinctive feature of angiosarcomas after irradiation or chronic lymphedema. Am J Pathol. 2010;176(1):34–9.

114. Shon W, Sukov WR, Jenkins SM, Folpe AL. MYC amplification and overexpression in primary cutaneous angiosarcoma: a fluorescence in-situ hybridization and immunohistochemical study. Mod Pathol. 2014;27(4):509–15.

115. Fernandez AP, Sun Y, Tubbs RR, Goldblum JR, Billings SD. FISH for MYC amplification and anti-MYC immunohistochemistry: useful diagnostic tools in the assessment of secondary angiosarcoma and atypical vascular proliferations. J Cutan Pathol. 2012;39(2):234–42.

116. Mentzel T, Schildhaus HU, Palmedo G, Büttner R, Kutzner H. Postradiation cutaneous angiosarcoma after treatment of breast carcinoma is characterized by MYC amplification in contrast to atypical vascular lesions after radiotherapy and control cases: clinicopathological, immunohistochemical and molecular analysis of 66 cases. Mod Pathol. 2012; 25(1):75–85.

117. Ko JS, Billings SD, Lanigan CP, Buehler D, Fernandez AP, Tubbs RR. Fully automated dual-color dual-hapten silver in situ hybridization staining for MYC amplification: a diagnostic tool for discriminating secondary angiosarcoma. J Cutan Pathol. 2014;41(3):286–92.

118. Kuehbacher A, Urbich C, Dimmeler S. Targeting microRNA expression to regulate angiogenesis. Trends Pharmacol Sci. 2008;29(1):12–5.

119. Urbich C, Kuehbacher A, Dimmeler S. Role of microRNAs in vascular diseases, inflammation, and angiogenesis. Cardiovasc Res. 2008;79(4):581–8.

120. Bonauer A, Boon RA, Dimmeler S. Vascular microRNAs. Curr Drug Targets. 2010;11(8):943–9.

121. Nakashima T, Jinnin M, Etoh T, Fukushima S, Masuguchi S, Maruo K, et al. Down-regulation of mir-424 contributes to the abnormal angiogenesis via MEK1 and cyclin E1 in senile hemangioma: its implications to therapy. PLoS One. 2010;5(12): e14334.

122. Zhang D, Shi Z, Li M, Mi J. Hypoxia-induced miR-424 decreases tumor sensitivity to chemotherapy by inhibiting apoptosis. Cell Death Dis. 2014;5:e1301.

123. Alimchandani M, Wang ZF, Miettinen M. CD30 expression in malignant vascular tumors and its diagnostic and clinical implications: a study of 146 cases. Appl Immunohistochem Mol Morphol. 2014;22(5):358–62.

124. Weed BR, Folpe AL. Cutaneous CD30-positive epithelioid angiosarcoma following breast-conserving therapy and irradiation: a potential diagnostic pitfall. Am J Dermatopathol. 2008;30(4):370–2.

125. Aggerholm-Pedersen N, Bærentzen S, Holmberg Jørgensen JP, Safwat A. A rare case of CD30(+), radiation-induced cutaneous angiosarcoma misdiagnosed as T-cell lymphoma. J Clin Oncol. 2011;29(13):e362–4.

126. Ebata N, Nodasaka Y, Sawa Y, Yamaoka Y, Makino S, Totsuka Y, et al. Desmoplakin as a specific marker of lymphatic vessels. Microvasc Res. 2001;61(1):40–8.

127. Kowalczyk AP, Navarro P, Dejana E, Bornslaeger EA, Green KJ, Kopp DS, et al. VE-cadherin and desmoplakin are assembled into dermal microvascular endothelial intercellular junctions: a pivotal role for plakoglobin in the recruitment of desmoplakin to intercellular junctions. J Cell Sci. 1998;111(Pt 20):3045–57.

128. Fedele C, Berens D, Rautenfeld V, Pabst R. Desmoplakin and Plakoglobin—specific markers of lymphatic vessels in the skin? Anat Histol Embryol. 2004;33(3):168–71.

129. Niemelä H, Elima K, Henttinen T, Irjala H, Salmi M, Jalkanen S. Molecular identification of PAL-E, a widely used endothelial-cell marker. Blood. 2005; 106(10):3405–9.

130. Schlingemann RO, Dingjan GM, Emeis JJ, Blok J, Warnaar SO, Ruiter DJ. Monoclonal antibody PAL-E specific for endothelium. Lab Invest. 1985; 52(1):71–6.

131. Keuschnigg J, Tvorogov D, Elima K, Salmi M, Alitalo K, Salminen T, et al. PV-1 is recognized by the PAL-E antibody and forms complexes with NRP-1. Blood. 2012;120(1):232–5.

132. Jaalouk DE, Ozawa MG, Sun J, Lahdenranta J, Schlingemann RO, Pasqualini R, et al. The original Pathologische Anatomie Leiden-Endothelium monoclonal antibody recognizes a vascular endothelial growth factor binding site within neuropilin-1. Cancer Res. 2007;67(20):9623–9.

133. Keuschnigg J, Henttinen T, Auvinen K, Karikoski M, Salmi M, Jalkanen S. The prototype endothelial marker PAL-E is a leukocyte trafficking molecule. Blood. 2009;114(2):478–84.

134. Xu B, deWaal RM, Mor-Vaknin N, Hibbard C, Markovitz DM, Kahn ML. The endothelial cell-specific antibody PAL-E identifies a secreted form of vimentin in the blood vasculature. Mol Cell Biol. 2004;24(20):9198–206.

Part V

Immunohistology of Cutaneous Lymphoma

Immunohistology and Molecular Studies of Cutaneous B-Cell Lymphomas

9

Juan F. García

Overview

Cutaneous lymphomas represent a unique group of lymphomas and are the second most frequent extranodal lymphomas [1]. They can be defined as lymphoproliferative skin infiltrates of T-cell, B-cell, or natural killer cell lineage, which primarily occur in and remain confined to the skin in most patients, and by definition, without detectable extracutaneous manifestations at diagnosis.

Although B-cell lymphomas account for the majority of nodal lymphomas, primary cutaneous B-cell lymphomas (PCBCL) only represent around 20–25 % of all cutaneous lymphomas, and the large majority of primary lymphomas in the skin correspond to mature T-cell neoplasms [2, 3]. The frequency of cutaneous lymphomas is 0.3 case per 100,000 population per year, with 10 % (in the United States) to 20 % (in Europe), mostly represented by marginal zone lymphomas, or follicle center lymphomas [4, 5].

Moreover, they cannot be considered just as "cutaneous manifestations" of lymph-node counterpart lymphomas. Although the skin can be secondary involved by oncologic hematologic proliferations, some of the morphologic criteria which are applied in the diagnosis of lymphoma in the lymph nodes, do not work in the same way in the skin. An example of this is primary cutaneous follicle center lymphoma, which, in many occasions, has no follicular formation, especially at early stages [6].

Molecular studies also contribute to remark these differences among cutaneous lymphomas and their homonymous lymph node entities. In large B-cell lymphoma, for instance, the translocation t(14; 18) is frequently found in the lymph node, while rare in the skin [6, 7]. While the translocation t(14;18) is not found in primary cutaneous follicular lymphoma, it is usually present when the skin is secondary involved by this type of lymphoma.

Because most of these neoplasms have an overall favorable prognosis [4, 8, 9], proper recognition is vital for appropriate therapy and to avoid overtreatment in most cases. The 5-year overall survival rate for most cases of PCBCL is greater than 90 %, except in diffuse large B-cell lymphoma, for which the 5-year survival rate is 20–50 % [8, 10, 11]. The tumor type and the extent of cutaneous involvement are the most relevant prognostic factors in PCBCL [9, 12]. Therapy may include surgical excision, antibiotics, and radiotherapy, depending on whether the patient has solitary or multiple lesions. Likewise, cases of primary PCBCL associated with a poorer prognosis, such as primary cutaneous diffuse

J.F. García, M.D., Ph.D. (✉)
Department of Pathology, MD Anderson Cancer Center Madrid, C/ Arturo Soria, 270,
Madrid 28033, Spain
e-mail: jfgarcia@mdanderson.es

© Springer International Publishing Switzerland 2016
J.A. Plaza, V.G. Prieto (eds.), *Applied Immunohistochemistry in the Evaluation of Skin Neoplasms*, DOI 10.1007/978-3-319-30590-5_9

large B-cell lymphoma, leg-type and intravascular large B-cell lymphoma, treatment is different for isolated or grouped lesions than for multiple lesions [13, 14]. Although cutaneous T-cell lymphomas can be stratified in prognostically relevant clinical stages [15], no generally accepted staging classification exists for PCBCL.

In the differential diagnosis of PCBCL, it is also relevant some considerations about some entities which are mainly extracutaneous lymphomas but which frequently involve the skin as a secondary site, such as lymphomatoid granulomatosis [16], chronic lymphocytic leukemia [11], mantle cell lymphoma [17], and Burkitt lymphoma [18].

On the other hand, the distinction between reactive and malignant conditions can be sometimes very difficult in hematoxylin-eosin, so that terms as pseudolymphoma or lymphocytoma [19, 20] were at some point coined in skin pathology, remarking this lack of accuracy in predicting their behavior.

The diagnosis of PCBCL is established by analysis of skin biopsy specimen, and is based on histomorphological features and immunohistochemistry in many cases. PCBCL exhibits a typical growth pattern, referred to as a B-cell pattern [5] (Fig. 9.1). It is characterized by a nodular

Table 9.1 WHO-EORTC classification for primary cutaneous B-cell lymphomas

Indolent clinical behavior
Primary cutaneous marginal-zone B-cell lymphoma
Primary cutaneous follicle-center lymphoma
Intermediate-aggressive clinical behavior
Primary cutaneous diffuse large B-cell lymphoma, leg-type
Primary cutaneous diffuse large B-cell lymphoma, other
Primary cutaneous intravascular large B-cell lymphoma

infiltrate (often well demarcated) of densely packed lymphoid cells in the dermis with convex margins, without significant interstitial infiltration and without epidermotropism. The subepidermal grenz zone is free of lymphoid cells. In some instances, also genotyping and cytogenetic studies could be useful for diagnosis [21].

The World Health Organization (WHO) published in 2008 the last revision of the Classification of Tumors of Haematopoietic and Lymphoid Tissues [22]. Table 9.1 shows the current classification for primary cutaneous B-cell lymphomas. This scheme is based on the previous works made by the European Organization for Research and Treatment of Cancer (EORTC)—Cutaneous Lymphomas Task Force [23], and subsequent revisions [3].

The development of cutaneous lymphoma is only partially understood. Most probably represents a multifactorial process, with various etiologic factors intervening over a long period. In many PCBCL types, the disease begins as a hyperreactive inflammatory process [8, 24]. Subsequently, inadequate regulation of cell proliferation and defective oncogene and/or suppressor gene expression will promote the transition from preneoplastic conditions to neoplasia [25]. The precise classification of this initial manifestations and the transition from "pseudo" and "pre" malignancies to "early" tumors will represent a major goal for research.

Some important factors initiating PCBCL are related with modifications of the local immune milieu, due to immunodeficiency disorders or, in many cases, infections with oncogenic bacteria

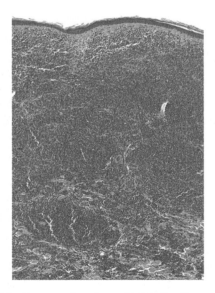

Fig. 9.1 Cuatenous lymphoma (H&E): B-cell pattern

(e.g., *Borrelia burgdorferi* in cutaneous B-cell lymphomas similarly to the situation of Helicobacter pylori in mucosa-associated lymphoid tissue [MALT] lymphomas) [26–28]. The precise role of the lymphoma microenvironment and the many interactions between tumor cells and reactive immune cells is still unknown.

This chapter will cover the main histopathological and immunohistochemical features useful for diagnosis of these challenging conditions, and also the main indications for molecular techniques and clonality studies.

Immunohistochemistry Studies in the Evaluation of Cutaneous B-Cell Lymphomas

Immunohistochemistry (IHC) have been stabilized as the gold standard for immunophenotyping the different lymphoid subpopulations in Pathology, and as an aid in the differential diagnosis and classification of most cancers.

There are many factors that influence the immunohistochemical staining, therefore precise immunoassays must be performed only with a high degree of technical rigor and validated protocols.

Since many of the clinical features of cutaneous lymphomas are similar, and also the histomorphological characteristics of the skin infiltrates can be analogous in the most common forms of PCBCL [11, 29], the immunophenotypical patterns are the most important support in the differentiation of the various entities (Table 9.2).

Common IHC Markers for B-Cell Phenotyping

CD20 is a transmembrane, nonglycosylated protein expressed on B-cell precursors and mature B cells, but is lost following differentiation into plasma cells. The antibody reacts with an intracytoplasmic epitope localized on the CD20 antigen and labels cells of the B-cell lineage. It is a useful tool for the classification of neoplasms of B-cell derivation.

In addition, CD20 is also a target for therapy. Rituximab, a chimeric monoclonal antibody targeted against CD20, was the first monoclonal antibody to be approved for therapeutic use.

CD10 is a cell surface metallopeptidase, expressed on early lymphoid progenitor cells and on a small subset of immature B cells in bone marrow, but is lost as the cells reach maturation. CD10 is, however, re-expressed on proliferating B cells. The antibody is useful for the identification of follicular lymphoma [21, 30] (in particular nodal follicular lymphoma), Burkitt's lymphoma, and precursor B-cell acute lymphoblastic leukemia.

CD23 is primarily expressed on B cells and monocytes, including a strong expression on Epstein-Barr Virus-transformed B lymphoblasts. Together with a panel of other antibodies, CD23 is particularly useful for differentiation between CD23-positive B-cell chronic lymphocytic leukemia/small lymphocytic lymphoma and CD23-negative mantle cell lymphoma [17, 31]. This antigen is also expressed by follicular dendritic cells in normal conditions, providing a useful

Table 9.2 Typical differential IHC features between common cutaneous B-cell proliferations

	Bcl-2	Bcl-6	CD10	MUM1/IRF4	Ig light chains
MZL	+	−	−	−	Monotypic (restricted) expression
Primary cutaneous FCL	−	+	+/−	−	
Secondary FCL	+	+	+	−	
DLBCL, leg-type	++	+	−	+	
PSL	−	+	+	−	Polytypic expression

MZL marginal zone B-cell lymphoma, *FCL* follicle center lymphoma, *DCBCL* diffuse large B-cell lymphoma, *PSL* B-cell pseudolymphoma pattern for recognizing normal follicles and follicular lymphoma.

CD5 antibody reacts with CD5 expressed on B and T cells and may be useful for the identification of B and T-cell malignancies. This includes B-cell chronic lymphoid leukemia, B-cell small lymphocytic lymphoma, and mantle cell lymphoma [17].

CD43 is a transmembrane cell surface protein that in humans is encoded by the SPN (sialophorin). CD43 is a major sialoglycoprotein on the surface of human T lymphocytes, monocytes, granulocytes, and some B lymphocytes, which appears to be important for immune function and may be part of a physiologic ligand–receptor complex involved in T-cell activation. CD43 can be demonstrated in the normal T-cells and it is also positive in a range of lymphoid and myeloid tumors. It is commonly expressed in B-cell, chronic lymphocytic leukemia/small lymphocytic lymphoma and mantle cell lymphoma [17]. This antigen is also expressed by the malignant cells in primary cutaneous marginal-zone B-cell lymphoma [32].

BCL2 is the founding member of the Bcl-2 family of regulator proteins that regulate cell death (apoptosis), by either inducing (pro-apoptotic) it or inhibiting it (anti-apoptotic). BCL2 is specifically considered as an important anti-apoptotic protein and is thus classified as an oncogene. The overexpression of the BCL2 protein is common in most B-cell lymphomas, including cutaneous marginal-zone B-cell lymphoma, primary cutaneous diffuse large B-cell lymphoma, leg-type, and other diffuse large B-cell lymphomas [11]. In nodal (systemic) follicular lymphoma, a chromosomal translocation commonly occurs, t(14;18), which places the BCL2 gene next to the immunoglobulin heavy chain locus [6, 7]. This fusion gene is deregulated, leading to the transcription of excessively high levels of BCL2 protein. In contrast, BCL2 expression and BCL2 translocation are both negative in primary cutaneous follicle-center lymphoma [6].

Proliferative marker MIB1/Ki-67. The protein is encoded by the MKI67 gene (antigen identified by monoclonal antibody Ki-67). It is strictly associated with cell proliferation. Ki-67 is a cellular marker for proliferation, and is often correlated with the clinical course of cancer. High proliferation index is commonly found in aggressive lymphomas [12, 33, 34].

Immunoglobulin Light and Heavy Chain Expression

A common useful marker for clonality is the demonstration of restricted expression of immunoglobulin light chains [35]. In most mature B-cell lymphomas the neoplastic B-lymphocytes will express cytoplasmic immunoglobulins. The mature form of the receptor is made of two heavy chains (γ, α, μ, δ, and ε for the different isotypes IgA, IgD, IgG, IgM, and IgE, respectively), and of two light chains (kappa and lambda). In normal conditions, the process of allele exclusion and immunoglobulin maturation will select the expression of a unique form of light chain in each B lymphocyte (physiologically, 60 % of kappa and 40 % lambda B-cells). The immunohistochemical detection of selective (or dominant) light chain expression in a B-cell population is highly suggestive of clonality (light chain restriction) [19].

Even though it has been currently adopted as a common technique in most pathology laboratories, the immunohistochemical protocol needs to be well optimized. In tissue sections, however, reliable detection of light chain expression is often difficult to assess due to soluble Ig molecules in extracellular tissues, sometimes overlaying the cellular Ig expression. It is recommended the use of high dilutions of polyclonal antibodies recognizing the different light chains, coupled with epitope retrieval techniques buffered with low pH.

On the other hand, intense expression of heavy chains can be detected in some lymphomas with plasmocellular differentiation [32] and also in plasma cell neoplasms [32, 36, 37]. Some variable expression of immunoglobulins can be detected in most B-cell lymphomas, as a standard marker of B-cell derivation. Thus, the great majority of lymphomas will express variable amounts of IgM and IgD. Also, IgG expression is useful to distinguish primary cutaneous marginal-zone B-cell lymphomas [38].

Transcription Factors

Transcription factors are DNA-binding proteins capable of activating or repressing gene regulation. In the last years several new monoclonal antibodies have been incorporated to routine, directed against a wide variety of transcription factors and other proteins involved in transcriptional regulation [36].

Because these proteins are important regulators of development and cell cycle control, they represent markers for lineage and also provide functional information. The strong nuclear expression and the low extracellular background is an additional advantage for immunophenotyping in tissue sections.

Some antibodies commonly used are:

PAX5

The gene is a member of the paired box (PAX) family of transcription factors. The PAX proteins are important regulators in early development, and alterations in the expression of their genes are thought to contribute to neoplastic transformation. The PAX5 gene encodes the B-cell lineage-specific activator protein (BSAP) that is expressed at early, but not late stages of B-cell differentiation (terminal plasma cells are PAX5 negative) [36]. Its expression has also been detected in developing CNS and testis.

PAX5 expression is useful to establish the B-cell lineage in cases with null or aberrant expression of common B-cell markers.

IRF4/MUM-1

Multiple myeloma oncogene-1 (MUM-1), belongs to the interferon regulatory factor (IRF4) family of transcription factors. The IRFs are important in the regulation of interferons in response to viral infections, and in the regulation of interferon-inducible genes. This family member is lymphocyte specific, involved in the maturation of B- and T-cells, and in plasma cell differentiation [33, 36].

MUM-1 expression is particularly useful for the diagnosis of primary cutaneous diffuse large B-cell lymphoma, leg-type, and its distinction from other diffuse large B-cell lymphomas [39].

MNDA

The myeloid cell nuclear differentiation antigen (MNDA) is detected only in nuclei of cells of the granulocyte-monocyte lineage and a subset of the marginal B-cells. In recent studies, MNDA was especially expressed by lymphomas derived from the marginal zone, such as mucosa-associated lymphoid-tissue lymphoma, splenic marginal-zone lymphoma, and NMZL [40]. MNDA expression was rarely observed in FL, a characteristic that is of potential value in distinguishing between NMZL and FL [41].

BCL6

BCL6 (B-Cell Lymphoma 6 Protein) is a zinc finger transcription factor. The encoded protein acts as a sequence-specific repressor of transcription. It has been shown to modulate IL-4 responses of B-cells, and BCL6 expression is mainly required for germinal center (GC) formation and antibody affinity maturation. Also, BCL6 down regulation is essential for plasma cell differentiation [6].

BCL6 nuclear expression is particularly useful for the differential diagnosis of follicular center lymphomas, both in cutaneous and extracutaneous localizations, and also for the diagnosis of cutaneous diffuse large B-cell lymphoma and Burkitt lymphomas [25].

Molecular Studies in the Evaluation of Cutaneous B-Cell Lymphomas

Molecular techniques in skin biopsies of suspected lymphoproliferative disorders are increasingly demanded in routine. They are mainly aimed to detection of B- and T-cell clonality, and identification of specific cytogenetic alterations.

Detection of Clonality

The analysis of the antigen receptors of B- and T-cells, the B-cell receptor (BCR, immunoglobulin) and T-cell receptor (TCR), represents a crucial challenge for the study of the adaptive immune response in normal and disease-related situations. The expressed BCR and TCR repertoires represent a potential of 2×10^{12} combinations per individual [42, 43]. This huge diversity results from mechanisms that occur at the DNA level during the immunoglobublin and TCR molecular synthesis. These mechanisms include the combinatorial rearrangements of the variable (V), diversity (D), and joining (J) genes, the N-diversity (deletion and addition at random of nucleotides during the V-(D)-J rearrangement) and, for BCR, somatic hypermutations (induced by the AID enzyme) [32]. Clonality detection in human samples is based on the detection of the patterns of rearrangements in the B- and T-cell receptor genes, and has been demonstrated as a reliable tool for clonality assessment [44].

Detection of clonality in a suspected lymphoproliferation is a valuable diagnostic criterion in many B-cell proliferations when morphology and immunophenotyping are not conclusive [44, 45]. This is particularly true in all suspect T-cell proliferations, in lymphoproliferations in immunodeficient patients, including post-transplant patients, and for monitoring and clinical follow-up in most lymphoma types. These techniques are also particularly useful for analyzing small biopsies, such as skin samples that in many cases present patchy and indistinct lymphoid infiltrations. Finally, the detection of clonality by molecular techniques is mandatory in the presence of discordances between clinical and pathological features [45].

Molecular techniques are broadly applicable for the detection of clonally rearranged Ig/TCR genes and certain chromosome aberrations. This previously concerned complex methods of Southern blot analysis, which has gradually been replaced by PCR techniques. Currently, the most commonly used method for clonality detection is the Multiplex PCR, electrophoresis, and fragment analysis (gene-scan analyses,

Fig. 9.2). Previous publications have implemented and standardized the use of multiplex PCR for diagnostic clonality studies as well as for the identification of PCR targets suitable for the detection of clonality in small formalin-fixed paraffin-embedded (FFPE) tissue samples [44, 46].

Clonality studies can be highly informative, but several limitations and potential pitfalls might hamper the interpretation of the results. First, limited sensitivity, related to normal polyclonal background (the detection limit varies between 1 and 10 %, dependent on the applied techniques and on the relative size of the "background" of polyclonal B- and T-lymphocytes) [47]. Second, the detection of clonality does not always imply the presence of a malignancy, and some clinically benign proliferations may show clonal results [45]. This implies that results of molecular clonality studies should always be interpreted in the context of the clinical, morphological, and immunophenotypic features.

Finally, false-negative results can be obtained by PCR analysis of Ig and TCR genes because of improper annealing of the applied PCR primers to the rearranged gene segments, or due to the occurrence of somatic hypermutations in rearranged Ig genes of germinal center and postgerminal center B-cell malignancies. In practice, the combined application of IGH (VH–JH and DH–JH) and IGK probes can detect virtually all clonal B-cell proliferations, even in B-cell malignancies with high levels of somatic mutations.

Molecular Cytogenetic Techniques

Fluorescence in situ hybridization (FISH) has become the main tool for detection of common cytogenetic abnormalities in routine, mainly gene translocations [48]. This technique allows the detection of specific DNA sequences using fluorescence-labeled probes. Thus, numeric and / or structural alterations can be easily analyzed. Different variants of FISH have overcome the limitations of previous PCR or RT-PCR based techniques for the identification of chromosomal alterations in lymphoma [49].

Fig. 9.2 Clonality analysis using gene-scan: polyclonal pattern (*top*) and monoclonal pattern (*bottom*)

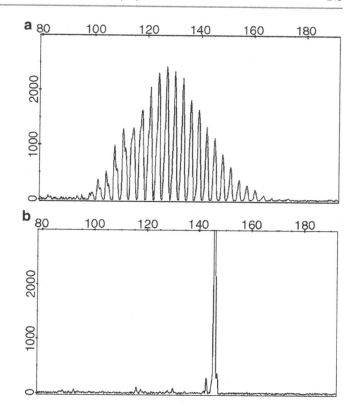

This technique is suitable for many different types of diagnostic samples, including cell suspensions, blood, bone marrow aspirations, and also FFPE tissue samples [50]. This recent availability of FISH techniques for direct evaluation of chromosomal alterations (interphase nuclei) on tissue sections has allowed the integration of genomics with functional and structural features. For efficiency, it is also important the control of some variables that could interfere with the hybridization, such as the time of formalin fixation, thickness of tissue sections. Also, the correlation with morphological characteristics and distribution of the lymphoid infiltrations may avoid many false negative results.

Dual color dual fusion probes: based in the use of specific probes for each of the gen loci involved in a given chromosomal rearrangement, marked with different fluorofores [50]. The presence of the gene translocation will result in the juxtaposition of signals. In general, this kind of probes gives higher rates of false positive results, due to common overlapping of nuclei in tissue sections. Some common examples of these probes:

- LSI t(14;18)(q32;q21) [IGH-BCL2]. It can be detected in approximately 80–90 % of nodal folicular lymphomas, and also in 30 % of diffuse large B-cell lymphomas (nodal). The detection of IGH-BCL2 gene rearrangement is an useful marker for the differential diagnosis between primary cutaneous follicle-center lymphoma and secondary involvement of the skin by systemic follicular lymphoma.
- LSI t(8;14)(q24;q32) [IgH-MYC], detected in approximately 80 % of Burkitt lymphomas.
- LSI t(11;18)(q21;q21) [API2-MALT]. Is the most frequent gene rearrangement in extranodal marginal zone lymphomas, in particular in gastric and lung MALT lymphomas.
- LSI t(11;14)(q13;q32) [IGH-CCND1]. Is the characteristic marker for mantle cell lymphoma.

Break apart probes: or "split" probes. In this approach the two probes are design to hybridize contiguous genetic regions of a given gene participating in a chromosomal translocation, flanking the breakpoint. Thus, the presence of the)translocation will be identified by the split of the two signals, juxtaposed in normal cells. Most of these probes allow the identification of oncogene rearrangements, independently of the different partner genes that can be implicated in the translocation [48, 50]. Common examples of these probes commercially available: BCL2, MYC, BCL6, ALK, MALT, IGH, etc.

Primary Cutaneous Marginal Zone B-Cell Lymphoma (MALT-Type)

Marginal zone B-cell lymphoma (MALT-type) is an indolent cutaneous lymphoma, accounting for approximately 7–10 % of all cutaneous lymphomas [51, 52]. A number of synonyms are used based on previous and current classification [3, 22]:

- WHO classification (2008)—Extranodal marginal zone lymphoma of mucosa-associated lymphoid tissue (MALT lymphoma).
- WHO/EORTC classification (2005)—Primary cutaneous marginal zone lymphoma (MZL).
- WHO classification (2001)—Extranodal marginal zone lymphoma of MALT-type.
- Revised European American Lymphoma (REAL) classification (1997)—Extranodal MZL.
- EORTC classification (1997)—Primary cutaneous MZL.

Other (confusing) terms include immunocytoma and primary cutaneous plasmacytoma.

Although it has been reported in children, it is most commonly seen in patients in their fourth decade [46, 53]. Clinically, MZL manifests as solitary or multiple reddish, dome-shaped papules, nodules, or erythematous plaques, frequently located on the trunk and extremities and,

to a lesser extent, on the head and neck area [32, 53]. Lesions could be single or multiple, and they can follow a long clinical course, with several regressions and recurrences along the years. Some cases with spontaneous regression has been related with anetodermia.

Extranodal MZL may develop from reactive infiltrates that represent immune responses to external factors or autoantigens. An etiopathological relationship to Borrelia burgdorferi has been demonstrated in some cases [8, 26].

Histologic findings of primary cutaneous MZL include a nodular or diffuse non-epidermotropic infiltrate composed of small to medium-sized lymphoid cells with indented nuclei and abundant, pale cytoplasm (marginal zone cells, monocytoid B-cells) or lymphoplasmacytoid cells [32]. Darker chromatin-rich cells are surrounded by pale-staining cells, resulting in a characteristic inverse pattern. Remnants of reactive germinal centers are present, sometimes colonized by tumor cells and reactive T cells (Fig. 9.3).

The tumor cells express an unspecific B-cell immunophenotype, CD19+, CD20+, CD22+, CD79a+. Most cases are CD43+ and BCL2+ (although reactive germinal centers, when present, are BCL2 negative). Tumor cells are negative for CD5, CD10, CD23, and BCL6, thus allowing their separation from other small B-cell lymphomas [8, 30].

Plasma cells, often located at the periphery of the infiltrates, show monotypic expression of immunoglobulin light chain kappa more frequently than lambda [54]. Plasmacytoid cells may be present in confluent aggregates.

A variable number of reactive CD3+ T cells are present. In many cases this T-cell rich microenvironment cause overlapping features with T-cell lymphomas, in particular cutaneous CD4+ small-medium T-cell lymphoma. Moreover, primary cutaneous marginal zone lymphoma and primary cutaneous CD4+ small/medium-sized pleomorphic T-cell lymphoma may show some overlapping clinical, morphological, and immunophenotypical features [55]. Both lesions can present as solitary nodules or tumors in the face

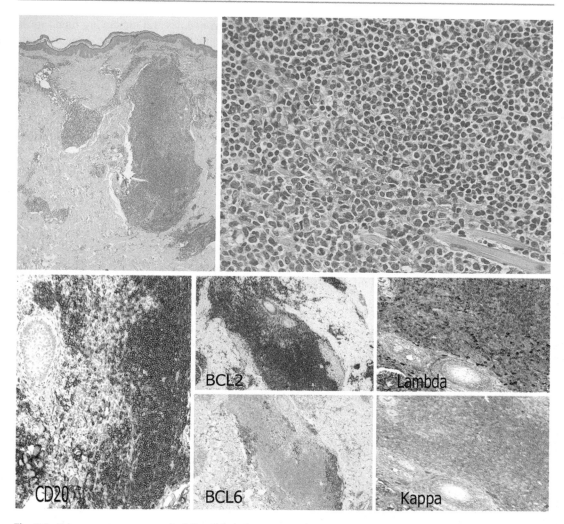

Fig. 9.3 Primary cutaneous marginal B-cell lymphoma. Low- and high-power views (*top panels*) showing nodular dermal infiltrate composed by small- and medium-sized lymphoid cells with marginal zone differentiation. IHC analyses show B-cell immunophenotype (BCL2+, BCL6−), with residual germinal centers (BCL2−, BCL6+) and monotypic Ig light chain expression

or the upper trunk, composed by a polymorphous infiltration of small lymphocytes without significant atypical features. Some cases of marginal zone lymphoma may also show an enriched microenvironment of T_{FH} cells (PD-1+). In complex cases, molecular analyses by PCR can demonstrate the presence of B- or T-cell clonality,

Clusters of CD123-positive plasmacytoid dendritic cells are present in MZL, but they are found to a lesser extent in other cutaneous B-cell lymphoma forms [56].

Primary cutaneous MZL with high numbers of monotypic plasma cells and lymphoplasmacytoid cells showing intranuclear periodic acid-Schiff–positive globular inclusions (Dutcher bodies) was previously referred to as cutaneous immunocytoma [32, 46].

Molecular analysis has shown that IgH genes are clonally rearranged in most cases [52]. The translocation t(11;18), as is seen in the nodal counterpart, is usually not found in primary cutaneous MZL [49].

Based on the configuration of the IgH locus, two different molecular subtypes can be recognized [11, 29]:

- With Ig class switch and associated with expression of IgG, mainly IgG4; This form is characterized by the scarcity of neoplastic B-cells, and used to be accompanied by high number of reactive T-lymphocytes, with TFH2 phenotype (CD4+, PD1+) [55].
- Without Ig class switch; these cases express IgM, are characterized by diffuse sheets of neoplastic B-cells, CXCR3 expression, and association with B. burgdorferi infection [8].

The prognosis of MZL (MALT-type) is excellent [5, 11], with a 5-year survival rate of greater than 95%. First-line treatments for solitary lesions include surgical excision, antibiotics, and radiotherapy. Antibiotics and radiotherapy, but not surgical excision, are also first-line treatments for multiple lesions.

Primary Cutaneous Follicle Center Lymphoma

Primary cutaneous follicle center lymphoma (FCL) is an indolent lymphoma of follicle center cells (predominantly centrocytes with an admixture of centroblasts). The prevalence rate is approximately 12% [57].

Synonyms based on previous classification systems are as follows:

- WHO classification (2008)—Primary cutaneous FCL.
- WHO/EORTC classification (2005)—Primary cutaneous FCL.
- WHO classification (2001)—Cutaneous FCL.
- REAL classification (1997)—FCL, follicular.
- EORTC classification (1997)—Primary cutaneous follicle center cell lymphoma.

Reticulohistiocytoma of the back, or Crosti lymphoma, is a variant of cutaneous FCL [21, 31].

Clinically, nodules and tumors are found most frequently in the head and neck area, but they are also found in other locations of the body [2]. A firm consistency without ulceration is very typical.

Histologically, three growth patterns can be differentiated: follicular, follicular and diffuse, and diffuse [31]. The diffuse pattern is, in fact, the most common seen in primary cutaneous FCL (Fig. 9.4). The infiltrates are composed mainly of centrocyte-like cells with intermingled centroblasts and immunoblasts. A subepidermal grenz zone is present in most cases. Mitoses, tingible body macrophages, and starry-sky features, typically found in reactive lymph follicles [21], are rare or absent in FCL.

Immunophenotypically, the cells in FCL express CD19+, CD20+, CD22+, CD43+, CD79a+, CD5−, and BCL6+. Characteristically, BCL2 protein expression is negative [6, 49] (Fig. 9.4). CD10+ is expressed in some cases with a follicular growth pattern [6, 31]. Follicular dendritic cells (CD23+/CD21+) are arranged in an irregular network. The MUM/IRF4 antigen, which is positive in DLBCL, is not expressed in FCL and may be helpful in differentiating FCL with a diffuse growth pattern from DLBCL [33]. Rare cases may express CD30 [58].

Molecular analysis shows clonal rearrangement of immunoglobulin genes [21]. In contrast to secondary skin involvement in FCL, chromosomal translocation of t(14;18), and BCL2 gene rearrangement are absent in most cases of primary cutaneous FCL [6, 59] (Fig. 9.5). Although rare, when chromosomal abnormalities do exist, mostly of BCL2 or MALT1, there appears to be no change in prognosis [7]. A reciprocal translocation between the long arms of chromosomes 12 and 21, t(12;21)(q13;q22), has been found in a patient with primary cutaneous FCL [60].

Primary cutaneous FCL has an excellent prognosis, with a 5-year survival rate of greater than 90%, and it recurs in up to 40% of patients [4, 10]. Extracutaneous spread occurs very rarely. Primary cutaneous FCL arising at the legs, multiple lesions, and those cases with expression of FOX-P1 appear to have a worse prognosis and should be treated more aggressively, similar to diffuse large B-cell lymphoma (DLBCL), leg-type [4, 34].

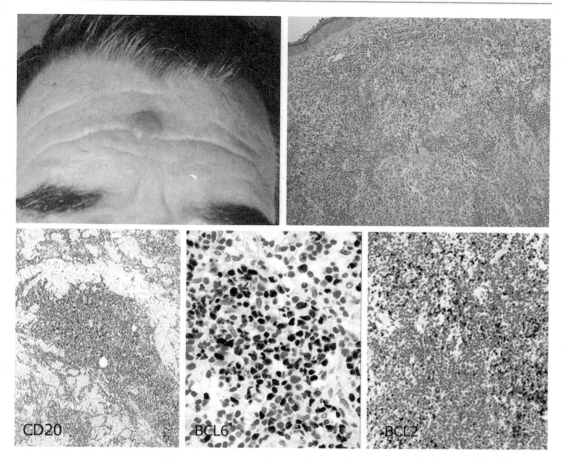

Fig. 9.4 Primary cutaneous follicle center lymphoma. Characteristic clinical presentation; dermal nodular/follicular infiltrate of BCL2–/BCL6+ centrocytic B-cells

A bone marrow biopsy should be performed in patients with FCL and DLBCL, in order to confirm the primary cutaneous origin and to exclude extracutaneous origin of the lymphoproliferative disorder [4].

Primary Cutaneous Diffuse Large B-Cell Lymphoma, Leg-Type

Primary cutaneous diffuse large B-cell lymphoma (DLBCL) is an aggressive cutaneous B-cell lymphoma that accounts for approximately 6 % of all cutaneous lymphomas. It is associated with a relatively poor prognosis compared with other PCBCLs, with a 5-year survival rate of 20–55 %, and it tends to spread to lymph nodes and extracutaneous sites [33, 39].

Two groups of primary cutaneous DLBCL have been differentiated: leg-type and DLBCL, other [61]. The leg type usually occurs on the lower legs of elderly women. The term is similar to terms used in the classification of other extranodal lymphomas (e.g., nasal-type). It manifests with a distinct phenotype and can also be present in other locations of the body, such as the face and neck (15–20 % of cases, with a similar poor prognosis) [34, 62]. DLBCL, other includes T-cell/histiocyte-rich DLBCL, plasmablastic lymphoma, intravascular large B-cell lymphoma, and other types that do not fulfill the criteria for a DLBCL, leg-type [29, 34].

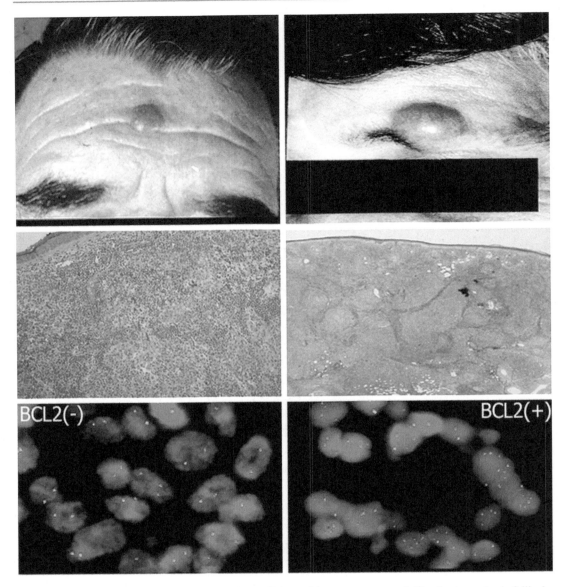

Fig. 9.5 Primary cutaneous follicle center lymphoma (*left panels*) versus cutaneous infiltration by systemic follicular lymphoma. BCL2 gene rearrangement is the main differential feature

Synonyms based on previous classification are as follows:

- WHO classification (2008)—Primary cutaneous DLBCL, leg-type.
- WHO/EORTC classification (2005)—Primary cutaneous DLBCL (including [1] DLBCL, leg-type; and [2] DLBCL, other).
- WHO classification (2001)—DLBCL.

- REAL classification (1997)—DLBCL.
- EORTC classification (1997)—Primary cutaneous large B-cell lymphoma of the leg.

Clinically, these lymphomas usually manifest as a solitary nodule or as multiple tumors restricted to one anatomic area (Fig. 9.6). They have a strong tendency for extracutaneous spread into regional lymph nodes and other extracutane-

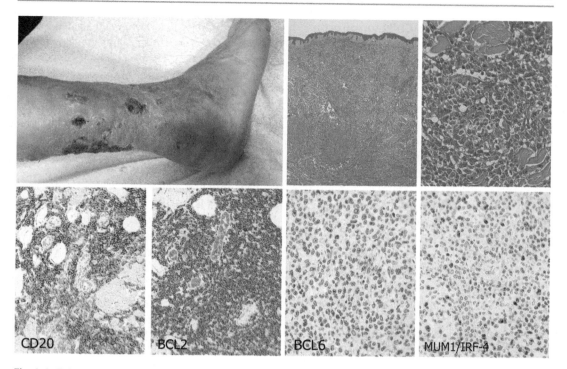

Fig. 9.6 Primary cutaneous diffuse large B-cell lymphoma, leg-type. Ulcerated nodules and tumors in the leg, composed by a diffuse dermal infiltration of large B-cells with typical immunophenotype (BCL2+/BCL6+/MUM1+)

ous sites. Primary cutaneous DLBCL, leg-type, seems to have a worse prognosis when located to the leg than when involving other areas, like the head and neck [9, 62].

The histological features are characterized by a diffuse infiltrate sparing a thin subepidermal grenz zone in most cases, covering the entire dermis, destroying adnexal structures, and extending into the subcutaneous tissue (Fig. 9.6). The tumor cells are large B cells, centroblasts, and immunoblasts. Centrocytes, which are typically seen in FCL, are minimal or absent in DLBCL [39].

The immunophenotype of the neoplastic cells is CD19+, CD20+, CD22+, CD5−, CD10−, CD79a+, BCL2+, BCL6−/+, MUM1+, FOXP1+, CD138−, cyclin D1−. The strong positivity for BCL2 protein and MUM1/IRF-4 allows differentiation of FCL with a diffuse growth pattern from DLBCL [29]. Characteristically, tumor cells are IgM+ [11]. Networks of CD21-positive follicular dendritic cells are not found in DLBCL [4].

Reactive T-cells are rare, in contrast with primary cutaneous FCL and MZL [12].

Molecular analysis shows clonal rearrangement of immunoglobulin genes. In primary cutaneous DLBCL, t(14; 18) and the bcl-2/JH translocation cannot be detected [62]. There is a high prevalence of MYD88 L265P mutation (a leucine to proline mutation at codon 265 [L265P] (33–61 %) of cases, which has also been linked to a worse prognosis [63]. Finally, gene expression profiles of DLBCL and FCL with a diffuse growth pattern are different [33].

Primary Cutaneous Diffuse Large B-Cell Lymphoma, Other

This category includes intravascular large B-cell lymphoma, cutaneous lymphomatoid granulomatosis, T-cell/histiocyte-rich DLBCL, plasmablastic lymphoma, and other types that do not fulfill the criteria for a DLBCL, leg-type [25, 34].

Intravascular Large B-Cell Lymphoma

Intravascular lymphoma (IVL) is a rare subtype of extranodal diffuse large B-cell lymphoma with a distinct presentation. The disease is characterized by the proliferation of clonal lymphocytes within small vessels with relative sparing of the surrounding tissue [64]. The clinical symptoms of the disease are dependent on the specific organ involvement, which most often includes the central nervous system and skin. The diagnosis is almost exclusively made by surgical biopsy of a suspected site of involvement [13].

It has been described in patients ranging from 34 to 90 years of age, with a median age of 70 years [65]. It occurs equally in women and men. Because this disease is quite rare, only one retrospective series has reported a substantial number of patients [13].

The predilection of the tumor cells for capillary endothelium is likely related to the expression of molecules on the surface of lymphocytes that allows for preferential binding within the vascular channel. Two alternative theories have been suggested. Aberrant expression of CD11a and CD49d (VLA-4) on IVL cells has been proposed as a possible mechanism because these adhesion molecules would enable tumor cells to home to CD54 (CD11a ligand) and CD106 (CD49d ligand), which are expressed on endothelial cell surfaces [66]. Alternatively, some study showed that IVL cells were consistently lacking in CD29 (β1 integrin) and CD54 (ICAM-1), both of which are regarded as essential for lymphocyte homing and transvascular migration [67].

IVL is extremely heterogeneous in its clinical presentation and has been described in the small vessels of nearly every organ. The majority of cases can be grouped into a few discrete presentations: (a) central nervous system (CNS) involvement, (b) cutaneous involvement, (c) fever of unknown origin, and (d) hemophagocytic syndrome [68].

IVL involvement of the skin was seen as a predominant feature in 15 of 38 patients in the largest series, with 10 of 38 patients presenting with skin lesions alone [13]. Of these 15 patients,

four had a solitary skin lesion and 11 had multiple lesions. Lesions can appear as maculopapular eruptions, nodules, plaques, tumors, hyperpigmented patches, palpable purpura, ulcers, and infiltrative "peau d'orange." These clinical manifestations have been misdiagnosed as cellulitis, gangrene, vasculitis, squamous cell carcinoma, and Kaposi's sarcoma. The skin lesions tend to favor the proximal extremities, lower abdomen, and submammary areas.

The immunophenotype of the malignant lymphocytes is usually B, positive for common B-cell antigens, CD19+, CD20+, CD79a+ (Fig. 9.7), although cases with T-cell receptor rearrangements have been reported [8]. Several cases have been reported to express CD5 [69]. Natural killer cell phenotype were reported in a single case [70]. One study of genetic alterations in IVL describes chromosomal abnormalities in 1p (4 of 6 cases) and trisomy 18 (4 of 6 cases) [71].

Most cases of IVL are associated with a poor prognosis and should be treated systemically. There are examples in the literature of long-term remissions with the use of combination chemotherapy such as R-CHOP [72]. Patients with disease limited to the skin (26 % of cases) were invariably females, and exhibited a significantly better outcome than the remaining patients [13].

Lymphomatoid Granulomatosis

Lymphomatoid granulomatosis is a rare multisystemic, angiocentric, and angiodestructive B-cell lymphoproliferative disease that involves extranodal sites, especially the lungs, skin, and nervous system. It is associated with Epstein-Barr virus (EBV) infection and may progress to DLBCL [73].

Patients are usually adults, although some cases have been observed in children. The clinical presentation is characterized by multiple erythematous papules, plaques, or tumors, commonly ulcerated, with predilection for the trunk and extremities [22].

Cutaneous manifestations usually coincide (sometimes may precede) to lung involvement.

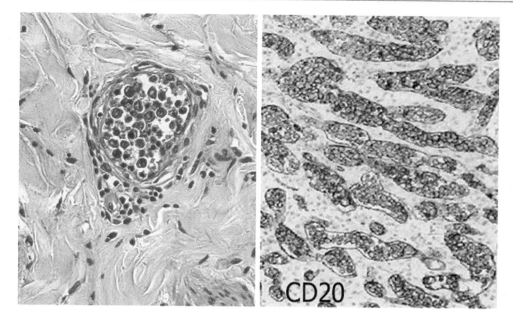

Fig. 9.7 Intravascular large B-cell lymphoma

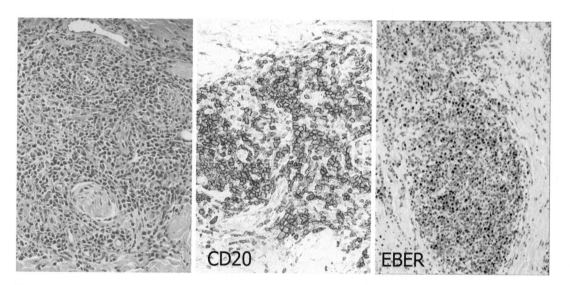

Fig. 9.8 Lymphomatoid granulomatosis. EBV can be demonstrated in large B-cells by EBER in situ hybridization

In fact, the existence of true primary cutaneous cases is still controversial, and always must be ruled out other EBV-associated entities that can occur in the skin [74].

The histopathological features include diffuse and angiocentric infiltrates with large areas of necrosis, sometimes with granulomatous features, and with variable number of large B-cells (Fig. 9.8), EBV+ (EBER in situ hybridization is needed for EBV demonstration in most cases) [75, 76].

Three different histopathological grades have been defined: (a) grade 1 lesions correspond to polymorphous infiltrates without significant atypia; EBV+ cells are very few; (b) grade 2 correspond to polymorphous infiltrates with scattered large cells or small clusters; and (c) grade 3 lesions are characterized by sheets of large atypical B-cells (Fig. 9.8), frequently with areas of necrosis [3, 22]. Some cases may present vascular occlusion and necrosis, with fibrinoid changes ("lymphocytic vasculitis").

Immunohistochemistry may show a predominance of T-cells, mostly of helper (CD4+) phenotype. However, the large atypical cells express B-cell markers (CD20, CD79a), and usually CD30+ and MUM1+. EBER in situ hybridization is positive in tumor cells in almost all cases (Fig. 9.8).

In the differential diagnosis it must be considered other EBV-related aggressive lymphomas that can present in the skin, usually associated with immunodeficiency [75, 77]. Also, EBV-positive diffuse large B-cell lymphoma of the elderly must be ruled out [48], in particular in cases without the typical lung involvement.

The prognosis is usually poor, and depends of the degree of systemic involvement. Systemic chemotherapy with Rituximab is used in grade 3 lesions; no clear guidelines are available for grades 1 and 2.

Other Cutaneous Diffuse Large B-Cell Lymphomas

Besides the specific primary cutaneous DLBCL subtypes described, several clinical and histopathological variants of DLBCL have been described, mainly T-cell/histiocyte-rich DLBCL, plasmablastic lymphoma, and other (rare) subtypes.

In general, these lesions correspond to primarily tumors of older adults, with histomorphological and phenotypical features similar to their nodal counterparts. Prognosis is generally poor [25].

Secondary Involvement of the Skin by Systemic B-Cell Lymphomas

Variants of systemic B-cell lymphomas that are not primarily cutaneous, may present with secondary skin involvement. The most common forms are precursor B-cell lymphoblastic lymphoma, mantle cell lymphoma, chronic lymphocytic leukemia (CLL), or Burkitt lymphoma.

The skin is a common site of involvement in precursor B-cell lymphoblastic lymphoma [2], along with bone, soft tissues, and lymph nodes. It is predominantly a disease of children and young adults. Although in some cases the disease can be aggressive, there is a relatively high remission rate with standard chemotherapy.

Microscopically; there is diffuse dermic infiltration by a monomorphous population of medium size lymphoid cells with immature/blastic features and high mitotic activity. Common phenotype include expression of CD19, CD20, and CD79a, CD10, and TdT [22].

Skin involvement in mantle cell lymphoma is rare and usually secondary [17]. The most common extranodal sites are gastrointestinal tract and Waldeyer's ring. Tumor cells have a mature B phenotype, CD20+, CD5+, CD43+, BCL2+. In addition, Cyclin D1 overexpression as a consequence of the translocation t(11;14) is the most useful marker for the tumor cells.

Cutaneous lesions arising during the course of B-cell CLL are relatively frequent, and may occur in up to 25 % of patients [78]. Skin infiltration by neoplastic B-lymphocytes manifests as solitary, grouped, or generalized papules, plaques, nodules, or large tumors [79, 80]. Prognosis in CLL patients with cutaneous infiltration is rather good and it does not significantly affect patients' survival. Secondary cutaneous malignancies are also frequent complications in patients with CL. Nonspecific, secondary cutaneous lesions are also frequently observed in CLL patients, including infectious or hemorrhagic lesions, vasculitis, purpura, generalized pruritus, exfoliative erythroderma, and paraneoplastic pemphigus [81, 82]. An exaggerated reaction to an insect bite and insect bite-like reactions have been also observed [83].

Burkitt lymphoma is an aggressive tumor of germinal center origin, with a well-known morphology characterized by medium-sized mature lymphoid cells, with GC phenotype: CD20+, CD10+, BCL6+, BCL2− (in almost all cases), and very high proliferation index (with ki67 index near 100 %) [25]. In rare cases of cutaneous presentation, the differential diagnosis of Burkitt lymphoma must include B-cell lymphoblastic lymphoma, and diffuse large B-cell lymphoma. In addition, the overexpression of nuclear MYC protein can be detected by IHC as a surrogate of MYC gene rearrangements [84, 85]. Burkitt lymphoma occurs endemically in children in Central Africa, where is associated with EBV infection in most cases. Sporadic EBV-negative cases may be seen in association with HIV-induced immunodeficiency.

Differential Diagnosis of Primary Cutaneous B-Cell Lymphomas

Cutaneous B-cell lymphoma must be differentiated from cutaneous T-cell lymphoma (CTCL) and B-cell pseudolymphoma. In addition, various types of PCBCL must be differentiated.

Differentiation of PCBCL from CTCL

Most CTCLs show typical clinical features. The history in CTCL usually involves a prediagnostic-preneoplastic phase over several years, during which differentiation from dermatitis may be challenging or even impossible. In contrast, CBCL lesions evolve quickly, usually within a few weeks [15].

The most significant discriminating histological feature between T- and B-cell lymphomas of the skin is the growth pattern, which is horizontal and epidermotropic in CTCL and is spherical and nonepidermotropic in most PCBCL [86]. Moreover, infiltrating cells in CTCL tend to be small and irregularly shaped, with convoluted and indented nuclei. Cells in cutaneous B-cell lymphoma usually are oval or roundish, reflecting the shapes of large follicular center cells, immunoblasts, or plasma cells. The immunophenotypical features are clearly different and will correspond to the T- or B-cell lineage.

Noteworthy, in some instances, primary cutaneous marginal zone lymphoma and primary cutaneous CD4+ small/medium-sized pleomorphic T-cell lymphoma may show some overlapping clinical, morphological, and immunophenotypical

features [55]. Both lesions can present as solitary nodules or tumors in the face or the upper trunk, and can be composed by a polymorphous infiltration of small lymphocytes without significant atypical features. This cell infiltration is mostly composed by T-cells with T_{FH} phenotype (PD-1+), but some cases of marginal zone lymphoma may also show an enriched microenvironment of T_{FH} cells. In difficult cases, molecular analyses by PCR can demonstrate the presence of B- or T-cell clonality, respectively [55].

Differentiation of CBCL and B-Cell Pseudolymphoma

In many cases, the most important differential diagnosis of PCBCL is from B-cell pseudolymphoma (PSL) (lymphoid hyperplasia) of the skin [19, 87]. Clinically, PSL is usually located as a single nodule on the face, neck, mammillae, or scrotum following B. burgdorferi infection through a tick bite, tattooing, or other mechanical or infectious irritants [88].

Histologically, the infiltrate in PCBCL is usually dome shaped with a convex border of infiltrative nodules. In PSL, it is wedge shaped, showing concave borders of the infiltrate. The latter may show regular germinal center formation, as is seen in reactive lymph nodes. Eosinophils, polyclonal plasma cells, and many T cells are present in the periphery and within the follicular area [87].

Immunophenotypically, the polytypic expression of both kappa and lambda light chains in the infiltrate argues in favor of PSL. In PSL, the networks of CD21+ dendritic cells are regular, round, or oval; in many PCBCL they are irregular, if present at all.

Genotyping reveals clonal rearrangement of immunoglobulin genes in most cases of PCBCL and lacks clonality in PSL [89].

Differentiation of Cutaneous B-Cell Lymphoma Subtypes

In many cases, the various types of PCBCL appear clinically quite similar. However, a few criteria are seen more frequently in one or another type. Nodules and tumors of MZL and of FCL demonstrate a hard consistency. Nodules occur more frequently in the head and neck area in FCL and on the trunk or arms in MZL, whereas single or grouped tumors on the lower legs typically appear in DLBCL, leg-type, in elderly patients.

The histological growth pattern is nodular in MZL, nodular or diffuse in FCL, and usually diffuse in DLBCL, leg-type. The infiltrating cells correspond in morphology to their normal counterparts, which are small lymphocytes and large follicle center cells, immunoblasts, and smaller mantle cells or marginal zone monocytoid or plasmacytoid B cells.

Table 9.2 illustrates the main differential IHC features between common cutaneous B-cell proliferations.

Gene rearrangement studies are helpful adjunctive diagnostic markers in the differentiation of CBCL from CTCL and B-cell PSL, but they do not allow discrimination between CBCL subtypes [57].

References

1. Newton R, Ferlay J, Beral V, Devesa SS. The epidemiology of non-Hodgkin's lymphoma: comparison of nodal and extra-nodal sites. Int J Cancer. 1997; 72(6):923–30.
2. Burg G, Kaudewitz P, Klepzig K, Przybilla B, Braun-Falco O. Cutaneous B-cell lymphoma. Dermatol Clin. 1985;3(4):689–704.
3. Willemze R, Jaffe ES, Burg G, et al. WHO-EORTC classification for cutaneous lymphomas. Blood. 2005;105(10):3768–85.
4. Golling P, Cozzio A, Dummer R, French L, Kempf W. Primary cutaneous B-cell lymphomas—clinicopathological, prognostic and therapeutic characterisation of 54 cases according to the WHO-EORTC classification and the ISCL/EORTC TNM classification system for primary cutaneous lymphomas other than mycosis fungoides and Sezary syndrome. Leuk Lymphoma. 2008;49(6):1094–103.
5. Jenni D, Karpova MB, Seifert B, et al. Primary cutaneous lymphoma: two-decade comparison in a population of 263 cases from a Swiss tertiary referral centre. Br J Dermatol. 2011;164(5):1071–7.
6. Franco R, Fernández-Vázquez A, Mollejo M, et al. Cutaneous presentation of follicular lymphomas. Mod Pathol. 2001;14(9):913–9.
7. Abdul-Wahab A, Tang SY, Robson A, et al. Chromosomal anomalies in primary cutaneous follicle center cell lymphoma do not portend a poor prognosis. J Am Acad Dermatol. 2014;70(6): 1010–20.
8. Kempf W, Kazakov DV, Mitteldorf C. Cutaneous lymphomas: an update. Part 2: B-cell lymphomas and related conditions. Am J Dermatopathol. 2014;36(3):197–208. quiz 209-110.
9. Kodama K, Massone C, Chott A, Metze D, Kerl H, Cerroni L. Primary cutaneous large B-cell lymphomas: clinicopathologic features, classification, and prognostic factors in a large series of patients. Blood. 2005;106(7):2491–7.
10. Sarris AH, Braunschweig I, Medeiros LJ, et al. Primary cutaneous non-Hodgkin's lymphoma of Ann Arbor stage I: preferential cutaneous relapses but high cure rate with doxorubicin-based therapy. J Clin Oncol. 2001;19(2):398–405.
11. Wilcox RA. Cutaneous B-cell lymphomas: 2015 update on diagnosis, risk-stratification, and management. Am J Hematol. 2015;90(1):73–6.
12. Zinzani PL, Quaglino P, Pimpinelli N, et al. Prognostic factors in primary cutaneous B-cell lymphoma: the Italian Study Group for Cutaneous Lymphomas. J Clin Oncol. 2006;24(9):1376–82.
13. Ferreri AJ, Campo E, Seymour JF, et al. Intravascular lymphoma: clinical presentation, natural history, management and prognostic factors in a series of 38 cases, with special emphasis on the "cutaneous variant". Br J Haematol. 2004;127(2):173–83.
14. Grange F, Joly P, Barbe C, et al. Improvement of survival in patients with primary cutaneous diffuse large B-cell lymphoma, leg type, in France. JAMA Dermatol. 2014;150(5):535–41.
15. Olsen E, Vonderheid E, Pimpinelli N, et al. Revisions to the staging and classification of mycosis fungoides and Sezary syndrome: a proposal of the International Society for Cutaneous Lymphomas (ISCL) and the cutaneous lymphoma task force of the European Organization of Research and Treatment of Cancer (EORTC). Blood. 2007;110(6):1713–22.
16. De Unamuno Bustos B, Zaragoza Ninet V, Ballester Sánchez R, García Rabasco A, Alegre de Miquel V. Epstein-Barr virus-positive diffuse large B-cell lymphoma in an elderly patient. Clin Exp Dermatol. 2014;39(4):484–7.
17. Motegi S, Okada E, Nagai Y, Tamura A, Ishikawa O. Skin manifestation of mantle cell lymphoma. Eur J Dermatol. 2006;16(4):435–8.
18. Jacobson MA, Hutcheson AC, Hurray DH, Metcalf JS, Thiers BH. Cutaneous involvement by Burkitt lymphoma. J Am Acad Dermatol. 2006;54(6): 1111–3.
19. Burg G, Schmid MH, Küng E, Dommann S, Dummer R. Semimalignant ("pseudolymphomatous") cutaneous B-cell lymphomas. Dermatol Clin. 1994;12(2):399–407.
20. Cerroni L, Volkenandt M, Rieger E, Soyer HP, Kerl H. bcl-2 protein expression and correlation with the interchromosomal 14;18 translocation in cutaneous

lymphomas and pseudolymphomas. J Invest Dermatol. 1994;102(2):231–5.

21. Mirza I, Macpherson N, Paproski S, et al. Primary cutaneous follicular lymphoma: an assessment of clinical, histopathologic, immunophenotypic, and molecular features. J Clin Oncol. 2002;20(3): 647–55.

22. Swerdlow SH, Campo E, Harris NL et al. WHO classification of tumours of haematopoietic and lymphoid tissues. Lyon, France: IARC Press; 2008.

23. Willemze R, Kerl H, Sterry W, et al. EORTC classification for primary cutaneous lymphomas: a proposal from the Cutaneous Lymphoma Study Group of the European Organization for Research and Treatment of Cancer. Blood. 1997;90(1):354–71.

24. Michaelis S, Kazakov DV, Schmid M, Dummer R, Burg G, Kempf W. Hepatitis C and G viruses in B-cell lymphomas of the skin. J Cutan Pathol. 2003;30(6):369–72.

25. Jaffe ES. The 2008 WHO classification of lymphomas: implications for clinical practice and translational research. Hematology Am Soc Hematol Educ Program. 2009:523–31

26. Cerroni L, Zöchling N, Pütz B, Kerl H. Infection by Borrelia burgdorferi and cutaneous B-cell lymphoma. J Cutan Pathol. 1997;24(8):457–61.

27. Garbe C, Stein H, Dienemann D, Orfanos CE. Borrelia burgdorferi-associated cutaneous B cell lymphoma: clinical and immunohistologic characterization of four cases. J Am Acad Dermatol. 1991;24(4): 584–90.

28. Kütting B, Bonsmann G, Metze D, Luger TA, Cerroni L. Borrelia burgdorferi-associated primary cutaneous B cell lymphoma: complete clearing of skin lesions after antibiotic pulse therapy or intralesional injection of interferon alfa-2a. J Am Acad Dermatol. 1997;36(2 Pt 2):311–4.

29. Swerdlow SH, Quintanilla-Martinez L, Willemze R, Kinney MC. Cutaneous B-cell lymphoproliferative disorders: report of the 2011 Society for Hematopathology/European Association for Haematopathology workshop. Am J Clin Pathol. 2013;139(4):515–35.

30. Hoefnagel JJ, Vermeer MH, Jansen PM, Fleuren GJ, Meijer CJ, Willemze R. Bcl-2, Bcl-6 and CD10 expression in cutaneous B-cell lymphoma: further support for a follicle centre cell origin and differential diagnostic significance. Br J Dermatol. 2003; 149(6):1183–91.

31. Cerroni L, Arzberger E, Pütz B, et al. Primary cutaneous follicle center cell lymphoma with follicular growth pattern. Blood. 2000;95(12):3922–8.

32. Tomaszewski MM, Abbondanzo SL, Lupton GP. Extranodal marginal zone B-cell lymphoma of the skin: a morphologic and immunophenotypic study of 11 cases. Am J Dermatopathol. 2000;22(3): 205–11.

33. Hoefnagel JJ, Dijkman R, Basso K, et al. Distinct types of primary cutaneous large B-cell lymphoma identified by gene expression profiling. Blood. 2005;105(9):3671–8.

34. Paulli M, Lucioni M, Maffi A, Croci GA, Nicola M, Berti E. Primary cutaneous diffuse large B-cell lymphoma (PCDLBCL), leg-type and other: an update on morphology and treatment. G Ital Dermatol Venereol. 2012;147(6):589–602.

35. Rijlaarsdam U, Bakels V, van Oostveen JW, et al. Demonstration of clonal immunoglobulin gene rearrangements in cutaneous B-cell lymphomas and pseudo-B-cell lymphomas: differential diagnostic and pathogenetic aspects. J Invest Dermatol. 1992;99(6): 749–54.

36. Hoefnagel JJ, Mulder MM, Dreef E, et al. Expression of B-cell transcription factors in primary cutaneous B-cell lymphoma. Mod Pathol. 2006;19(9):1270–6.

37. Morgan GJ, Walker BA, Davies FE. The genetic architecture of multiple myeloma. Nat Rev Cancer. 2012;12(5):335–48.

38. Aarts WM, Willemze R, Bende RJ, Meijer CJ, Pals ST, van Noesel CJ. VH gene analysis of primary cutaneous B-cell lymphomas: evidence for ongoing somatic hypermutation and isotype switching. Blood. 1998;92(10):3857–64.

39. Paulli M, Viglio A, Vivenza D, et al. Primary cutaneous large B-cell lymphoma of the leg: histogenetic analysis of a controversial clinicopathologic entity. Hum Pathol. 2002;33(9):937–43.

40. Kanellis G, Roncador G, Arribas A, et al. Identification of MNDA as a new marker for nodal marginal zone lymphoma. Leukemia. 2009;23(10):1847–57.

41. Metcalf RA, Monabati A, Vyas M, et al. Myeloid cell nuclear differentiation antigen is expressed in a subset of marginal zone lymphomas and is useful in the differential diagnosis with follicular lymphoma. Hum Pathol. 2014;45(8):1730–6.

42. Child FJ, Woolford AJ, Calonje E, Russell-Jones R, Whittaker SJ. Molecular analysis of the immunoglobulin heavy chain gene in the diagnosis of primary cutaneous B cell lymphoma. J Invest Dermatol. 2001;117(4):984–9.

43. Bahler DW, Kim BK, Gao A, Swerdlow SH. Analysis of immunoglobulin V genes suggests cutaneous marginal zone B-cell lymphomas recognise similar antigens. Br J Haematol. 2006;132(5):571–5.

44. Evans PA, Pott C, Groenen PJ, et al. Significantly improved PCR-based clonality testing in B-cell malignancies by use of multiple immunoglobulin gene targets. Report of the BIOMED-2 Concerted Action BHM4-CT98-3936. Leukemia. 2007;21(2):207–14.

45. Langerak AW, Groenen PJ, Brüggemann M, et al. EuroClonality/BIOMED-2 guidelines for interpretation and reporting of Ig/TCR clonality testing in suspected lymphoproliferations. Leukemia. 2012;26(10): 2159–71.

46. Kempf W, Kazakov DV, Buechner SA, et al. Primary cutaneous marginal zone lymphoma in children: a

report of 3 cases and review of the literature. Am J Dermatopathol. 2014;36(8):661–6.

47. Fraga M, Sánchez-Verde L, Forteza J, García-Rivero A, Piris MA. T-cell/histiocyte-rich large B-cell lymphoma is a disseminated aggressive neoplasm: differential diagnosis from Hodgkin's lymphoma. Histopathology. 2002;41(3):216–29.

48. Montes-Moreno S, Odqvist L, Diaz-Perez JA, et al. EBV-positive diffuse large B-cell lymphoma of the elderly is an aggressive post-germinal center B-cell neoplasm characterized by prominent nuclear factor-kB activation. Mod Pathol. 2012;25(7):968–82.

49. de la Fouchardiere A, Gazzo S, Balme B, et al. Cytogenetic and molecular analysis of 12 cases of primary cutaneous marginal zone lymphomas. Am J Dermatopathol. 2006;28(4):287–92.

50. van Rijk A, Mason D, Jones M, et al. Translocation detection in lymphoma diagnosis by split-signal FISH: a standardised approach. J Hematop. 2008; 1(2):119–26.

51. Bailey EM, Ferry JA, Harris NL, Mihm MC, Jacobson JO, Duncan LM. Marginal zone lymphoma (low-grade B-cell lymphoma of mucosa-associated lymphoid tissue type) of skin and subcutaneous tissue: a study of 15 patients. Am J Surg Pathol. 1996;20(8): 1011–23.

52. Cerroni L, Signoretti S, Höfler G, et al. Primary cutaneous marginal zone B-cell lymphoma: a recently described entity of low-grade malignant cutaneous B-cell lymphoma. Am J Surg Pathol. 1997;21(11): 1307–15.

53. Grønbaek K, Møller PH, Nedergaard T, et al. Primary cutaneous B-cell lymphoma: a clinical, histological, phenotypic and genotypic study of 21 cases. Br J Dermatol. 2000;142(5):913–23.

54. Takino H, Li C, Hu S, et al. Primary cutaneous marginal zone B-cell lymphoma: a molecular and clinicopathological study of cases from Asia, Germany, and the United States. Mod Pathol. 2008;21(12): 1517–26.

55. Rodríguez Pinilla SM, Roncador G, Rodríguez-Peralto JL, et al. Primary cutaneous CD4+ small/medium-sized pleomorphic T-cell lymphoma expresses follicular T-cell markers. Am J Surg Pathol. 2009;33(1):81–90.

56. Kutzner H, Kerl H, Pfaltz MC, Kempf W. CD123-positive plasmacytoid dendritic cells in primary cutaneous marginal zone B-cell lymphoma: diagnostic and pathogenetic implications. Am J Surg Pathol. 2009;33(9):1307–13.

57. Burg G, Kempf W, Cozzio A, et al. WHO/EORTC classification of cutaneous lymphomas 2005: histological and molecular aspects. J Cutan Pathol. 2005;32(10):647–74.

58. Kempf W, Kazakov DV, Rütten A, et al. Primary cutaneous follicle center lymphoma with diffuse CD30 expression: a report of 4 cases of a rare variant. J Am Acad Dermatol. 2014;71(3):548–54.

59. Child FJ, Russell-Jones R, Woolford AJ, et al. Absence of the t(14;18) chromosomal translocation in primary cutaneous B-cell lymphoma. Br J Dermatol. 2001;144(4):735–44.

60. Jelic TM, Berry PK, Jubelirer SJ, et al. Primary cutaneous follicle center lymphoma of the arm with a novel chromosomal translocation t(12;21) (q13;q22): a case report. Am J Hematol. 2006;81(6):448–53.

61. Senff NJ, Hoefnagel JJ, Jansen PM, et al. Reclassification of 300 primary cutaneous B-Cell lymphomas according to the new WHO-EORTC classification for cutaneous lymphomas: comparison with previous classifications and identification of prognostic markers. J Clin Oncol. 2007; 25(12):1581–7.

62. Grange F, Beylot-Barry M, Courville P, et al. Primary cutaneous diffuse large B-cell lymphoma, leg type: clinicopathologic features and prognostic analysis in 60 cases. Arch Dermatol. 2007;143(9):1144–50.

63. Pham-Ledard A, Beylot-Barry M, Barbe C, et al. High frequency and clinical prognostic value of MYD88 L265P mutation in primary cutaneous diffuse large B-cell lymphoma, leg-type. JAMA Dermatol. 2014;150(11):1173–9.

64. Perniciaro C, Winkelmann RK, Daoud MS, Su WP. Malignant angioendotheliomatosis is an angiotropic intravascular lymphoma. Immunohistochemical, ultrastructural, and molecular genetics studies. Am J Dermatopathol. 1995;17(3):242–8.

65. Ferreri AJ, Dognini GP, Campo E, et al. Variations in clinical presentation, frequency of hemophagocytosis and clinical behavior of intravascular lymphoma diagnosed in different geographical regions. Haematologica. 2007;92(4):486–92.

66. Kanda M, Suzumiya J, Ohshima K, Tamura K, Kikuchi M. Intravascular large cell lymphoma: clinicopathological, immuno-histochemical and molecular genetic studies. Leuk Lymphoma. 1999;34(5–6):569–80.

67. Ponzoni M, Arrigoni G, Gould VE, et al. Lack of CD 29 (beta1 integrin) and CD 54 (ICAM-1) adhesion molecules in intravascular lymphomatosis. Hum Pathol. 2000;31(2):220–6.

68. Zuckerman D, Seliem R, Hochberg E. Intravascular lymphoma: the oncologist's "great imitator". Oncologist. 2006;11(5):496–502.

69. Estalilla OC, Koo CH, Brynes RK, Medeiros LJ. Intravascular large B-cell lymphoma. A report of five cases initially diagnosed by bone marrow biopsy. Am J Clin Pathol. 1999;112(2):248–55.

70. Wu H, Said JW, Ames ED, et al. First reported cases of intravascular large cell lymphoma of the NK cell type: clinical, histologic, immunophenotypic, and molecular features. Am J Clin Pathol. 2005;123(4): 603–11.

71. Tsukadaira A, Okubo Y, Ogasawara H, et al. Chromosomal aberrations in intravascular lymphomatosis. Am J Clin Oncol. 2002;25(2):178–81.

72. Ferreri AJ, Campo E, Ambrosetti A, et al. Anthracycline-based chemotherapy as primary treatment for intravascular lymphoma. Ann Oncol. 2004; 15(8):1215–21.

73. McNiff JM, Cooper D, Howe G, et al. Lymphomatoid granulomatosis of the skin and lung. An angiocentric T-cell-rich B-cell lymphoproliferative disorder. Arch Dermatol. 1996;132(12):1464–70.

74. Quéreux G, Brocard A, Peuvrel L, Knol AC, Renaut JJ, Dréno B. Lymphomatoid granulomatosis revealed by cutaneous lesions. Ann Dermatol Venereol. 2011;138(8–9):591–6.

75. Sebire NJ, Haselden S, Malone M, Davies EG, Ramsay AD. Isolated EBV lymphoproliferative disease in a child with Wiskott-Aldrich syndrome manifesting as cutaneous lymphomatoid granulomatosis and responsive to anti-CD20 immunotherapy. J Clin Pathol. 2003;56(7):555–7.

76. Saruta H, Tsuruta D, Hashikawa K, et al. Old-aged case of indolent grade III lymphomatoid granulomatosis successfully treated only with oral prednisolone. J Dermatol. 2013;40(11):942–3.

77. Kwon EJ, Katz KA, Draft KS, et al. Posttransplantation lymphoproliferative disease with features of lymphomatoid granulomatosis in a lung transplant patient. J Am Acad Dermatol. 2006;54(4):657–63.

78. Plaza JA, Comfere NI, Gibson LE, et al. Unusual cutaneous manifestations of B-cell chronic lymphocytic leukemia. J Am Acad Dermatol. 2009;60(5):772–80.

79. Rosman IS, Nunley KS, Lu D. Leukemia cutis in B-cell chronic lymphocytic leukemia presenting as an episodic papulovesicular eruption. Dermatol Online J. 2011;17(9):7.

80. Maughan C, Kolker S, Markus B, Young J. Leukemia cutis coexisting with dermatofibroma as the initial presentation of B-cell chronic lymphocytic leukemia/small lymphocytic lymphoma. Am J Dermatopathol. 2014;36(1):e14–5.

81. di Meo N, Stinco G, Trevisan G. Cutaneous B-cell chronic lymphocytic leukaemia resembling a granulomatous rosacea. Dermatol Online J. 2013;19(10):20033.

82. Robak E, Robak T. Skin lesions in chronic lymphocytic leukemia. Leuk Lymphoma. 2007;48(5):855–65.

83. Blum RR, Phelps RG, Wei H. Arthropod bites manifesting as recurrent bullae in a patient with chronic lymphocytic leukemia. J Cutan Med Surg. 2001;5(4):312–4.

84. Eberle FC, Salaverria I, Steidl C, et al. Gray zone lymphoma: chromosomal aberrations with immunophenotypic and clinical correlations. Mod Pathol. 2011;24(12):1586–97.

85. Lin P, Dickason TJ, Fayad LE, et al. Prognostic value of MYC rearrangement in cases of B-cell lymphoma, unclassifiable, with features intermediate between diffuse large B-cell lymphoma and Burkitt lymphoma. Cancer. 2012;118(6):1566–73.

86. Willemze R, Meijer CJ. EORTC classification for primary cutaneous lymphomas: the best guide to good clinical management. European Organization for Research and Treatment of Cancer. Am J Dermatopathol. 1999;21(3):265–73.

87. Hussein MR. Cutaneous pseudolymphomas: inflammatory reactive proliferations. Expert Rev Hematol. 2013;6(6):713–33.

88. Levy E, Godet J, Cribier B, Lipsker D. Pseudolymphoma of the skin: ambiguous terminology: a survey among dermatologists and pathologists. Ann Dermatol Venereol. 2013;140(2):105–11.

89. Bergman R. Pseudolymphoma and cutaneous lymphoma: facts and controversies. Clin Dermatol. 2010;28(5):568–74.

Immunohistology and Molecular Studies of Cutaneous T-Cell Lymphomas and Mimics

Carlos A. Torres-Cabala, Phyu P. Aung, Roberto N. Miranda, and Jonathan L. Curry

Introduction

Cutaneous lymphomas comprise a diverse group of tumors characterized by primary involvement of the skin without obvious clinical, radiologic, or laboratory evidence of extracutaneous spread. After some attempts for an adequate systematic approach to lymphomas primary to the skin, the World Health Organization (WHO) and European Organization for Research and Treatment of Cancer (EORTC) classification seems to have reached final consensus [1]. Cutaneous T-cell lymphomas (CTCL) are the most common pri-

mary lymphomas of the skin [2]. The diagnosis of these cases is based on histomorphology, clinical presentation, and, in many circumstances, immunohistochemical and/or molecular testing. A panel of markers is often needed for immunohistochemical analysis. This panel includes antibodies against T-cell-specific antigens and other molecules that may help in the correct characterization of the process.

Antibodies Commonly Used for the Immunohistochemical Evaluation of T-Cell Lymphomas Involving the Skin

Markers of T-Cell Lineage

Demonstration of T-cell lineage of a lymphoid proliferation is based on the expression of certain cell surface molecules designated as cluster of differentiation (CD) antigens. The rationale for using these markers is that neoplastic lymphoid proliferations recapitulate the pattern of expression of surface molecules that occurs in the stages of maturation of normal T lymphocytes. Thus, early in the maturation process of T cells in the thymus, cortical thymocytes display an "immature" phenotype, characterized by the expression of terminal deoxynucleotidyl transferase (TdT), CD1a, CD2, CD3, CD5, and CD7. The last four are considered pan-T cell markers, since they are essentially present in all the maturation stages of

C.A. Torres-Cabala, M.D. (✉) • J.L. Curry, M.D.
Department of Dermatology, The University of Texas MD Anderson Cancer Center, Houston, TX, USA

Department of Pathology, The University of Texas MD Anderson Cancer Center,
1515 Holcombe Blvd., Unit 85, Houston, TX 77030, USA
e-mail: ctcabala@mdanderson.org

P.P. Aung, M.D., Ph.D.
Department of Pathology, The University of Texas MD Anderson Cancer Center,
1515 Holcombe Blvd., Unit 85, Houston, TX 77030, USA
e-mail: paung@mdanderson.org

R.N. Miranda, M.D.
Department of Hematopathology, The University of Texas MD Anderson Cancer Center,
Houston, TX, USA
e-mail: roberto.miranda@mdanderson.org

© Springer International Publishing Switzerland 2016
J.A. Plaza, V.G. Prieto (eds.), *Applied Immunohistochemistry in the Evaluation of Skin Neoplasms*, DOI 10.1007/978-3-319-30590-5_10

T-cells. As the maturation process proceeds, cortical thymocytes that initially are double negative for CD4 and CD8 become double positive and finally, the more mature cells express only CD4 or CD8.

The T-cell receptor (TCR) is the surface molecule that recognizes antigens and is the central actor within the adaptive immune response. The *TCR* genes are designated as α, β, γ, and δ. These genes undergo sequential rearrangements and deletions to give rise to two main populations of T lymphocytes with TCRs composed of either αβ or γδ chains. βF-1 is an antibody that recognizes the αβ TCR. TCRgamma is a recently developed antibody directed against γδ TCR. These two markers are useful to determine whether a lymphoma displays αβ or γδ phenotype, which might have profound consequences in diagnosis and therapy.

The diagnosis of T-cell lymphomas is based, most of the times, on the expression of pan-T cell antigens by the tumor cells, the frank predominance of either CD4 or CD8-positive tumor cells (indicative of clonal expansion), and/or the complete or partial lack of reactivity for one or more pan T-cell markers, interpreted as aberrant loss of the antigen and therefore supportive of a neoplastic nature of the cells in question.

Markers of Activation

CD30 is the prototypic marker of activation of T-cells, B-cells, and monocytes. CD30 is a transmembrane protein that shows homology with members of the tumor necrosis factor (TNF) receptor superfamily [3]. Although the exact function of CD30 is not fully understood, it activates a number of signaling pathways and apoptosis, as seen in anaplastic large cell lymphoma (ALCL) [4].

CD25 is also expressed in activated B and T cells and detects the α chain of the interleukin-2 receptor. It has been reported that high CD25 expression is associated with advanced cutaneous T cell lymphoma [5].

Cytotoxic Protein Markers

Perforin and granzyme B are involved in the pore-forming activity of cytotoxic lymphocytes

[6]. T-cell intracellular antigen-1 (TIA-1) is another granule-associated cytotoxic protein that is detected in cytotoxic T and NK cells, regardless of their activation status. Perforin and granzyme B, however, are inducible after activation in all cytotoxic cells [7].

Markers of Proliferation

Ki67 detects a nuclear protein associated with tumor cell proliferation. The antigen is expressed in all phases of the proliferating cell cycle except G0 [8]. High proliferation rate is usually indicative of a high grade lymphoma.

Tumor-Associated Oncogene and Translocation Products

Translocations involving the anaplastic lymphoma kinase (*ALK*) gene on chromosome 2p23 and the nucleophosmin (*NPM*) gene on chromosome 5q35 are found in anaplastic large cell lymphoma (ALCL) [9]. Two categories of ALCL, based on the presence or absence of translocations involving *ALK* are currently recognized. The detection of ALK protein is highly indicative of chromosomal rearrangement involving *ALK*, and therefore immunohistochemistry is the preferred method for determination of status of *ALK* translocations [10].

p53 is a tumor suppressor gene mutated in over half of human malignant tumors, although rarely found in peripheral T cell lymphomas. Its homolog *p63* is even less frequently mutated and its function not very well understood [11]. *p63* rearrangements, however, have been described in subtypes of T-cell lymphomas, specifically cutaneous lymphomas with aggressive clinical behavior [12, 13].

Molecular Studies in the Evaluation of Cutaneous T-Cell Lymphomas

Many different molecular techniques can be applied for the study of T-cell proliferations in the skin. Polymerase chain reaction (PCR), fluorescence in situ hybridization (FISH), comparative genomic hybridization (CGH), gene arrays, and proteomics are some of the tests available for the evaluation of skin specimens involved by T-cell processes.

The utility of molecular testing mainly rests on the identification of clonal populations of lymphocytes. Identification of clonal rearrangements of the *TCR* gene in general supports a diagnosis of lymphoma while polyclonal cell populations usually indicate a reactive process. It is important to keep in mind, however, that fully integration of clinical, pathological, and molecular findings is required to render a definitive diagnosis.

T-Cell Receptor Gene Rearrangement Analysis

The analysis of clonal rearrangements of the *TCR* gene has long been used to characterize a lymphoid population as monoclonal or polyclonal [14]. As it was mentioned above, the TCR is composed of α, β, γ, and δ chains. The large majority of mature T lymphocytes express the α/β TCR. Regardless what TCR (α/β or γ/δ) is expressed, the most frequent gene rearrangement detected in the T cells is the one that involves the γ gene [15]. The *TCR* gene rearrangements occur in the following sequence: δ, α, γ, β. Of note, the δ receptor locus is located within the α gene, and therefore deletion of the δ locus has most likely occurred when the α gene is rearranged [16]. Rearrangements of the δ, γ, and β chains can be detected by PCR-based methods [17]. Fewer primers are required for PCR amplification of the γ chain gene, due to its lesser variation of sequences compared to the δ and β chains [18]. It is important to emphasize that *TCR* γ gene rearrangements are found in both γ/δ and α/β T cell lymphomas, although α/β T lymphoma cells do not express the rearrangement [17]. This is the reason why the *TCR* γ gene rearrangement detection test is the most popular when dealing with a suspicious T cell proliferation. Evaluation of *TCR* β gene rearrangement is useful to discriminate a monoclonal population in a background of polyclonal reactive cells [19], which in theory makes it a more specific test. Although γ and β chains gene rearrangement analyses cover most of the situations where clonality needs to be confirmed, rare cases of T-cell lymphomas may present rearrangements of the δ chain as the only evidence of clonality [20].

High resolution capillary electrophoresis is used to separate the products of PCR and electropherograms are analyzed. The number and height of the resulting peaks are evaluated to interpret the lymphoid proliferation as clonal or polyclonal. Overall, more than five peaks are considered evidence of polyclonal proliferations while one or two dominant peaks whose height exceeds that of the polyclonal background by a ratio of 2:1 to 3:1 are regarded as indicative of a monoclonal T-cell lymphoid proliferation [21].

TCR gene rearrangements tests are very sensitive. The minimum percentage of detectable clonal cells by these methods is around 1 % [22]. Although the sensitivity and specificity of the test depends on the type of sample analyzed along with technical issues, it is generally accepted that the method is about 70 % sensitive and 97 % specific, in the case of mycosis fungoides (MF) [23] Low numbers of malignant T-cells or real absence of *TCR* gene rearrangement in the lymphoma cells may render false negative (for clonality) results [24]. Pseudoclonality or false positive tests are often attributed to the presence of very few T-cells in a sparse and reactive infiltrate [25]. In these cases it is recommended to run duplicate analyses of the sample since the dominant peaks detected in reactive conditions are not reproducible, as opposite to those seen in clonal proliferations [26].

A fairly common practice in dermatopathology is to demonstrate identical T-cell clones at different anatomical sites (the so-called stable clonal pattern [25]) as a way to support a neoplastic origin of the process. This has been regarded as a highly specific tool in discriminating between MF and inflammatory conditions [27]. As in any other molecular test, the identification of identical T-cell clones in different anatomical locations needs to be interpreted in the context of clinical and histopathological (and immunohistochemical) findings. This pattern has been reported in some inflammatory and "borderline" processes [28]. Moreover, the occurrence of subclones has been described in T-cell lymphomas [29], along with the presence of clonal heterogeneity in MF lesions from distinct anatomical sites [30, 31].

In Situ Hybridization Studies

Primary cutaneous ALCL rarely demonstrates the t(2;5)(p23;q35)*ALK/NPM,* as opposite to ALK-positive systemic ALCL [32, 33]. FISH can be used to investigate *ALK* gene rearrangements [34], although immunohistochemical methods are widely utilized. Investigation of other translocations, such as those that involve *IRF4* may be useful in the diagnosis of primary cutaneous ALCL [35].

Latent Epstein-Barr virus (EBV) infection is often diagnosed by the demonstration of Epstein-Barr virus-encoded mRNA (EBER) in the nuclei of infected cells by FISH [36].

Immunohistochemical and Molecular Profile of Cutaneous T-Cell Lymphomas

Table 10.1 shows the most common immunohistochemical studies utilized in the evaluation of cutaneous T-cell lymphomas and their typical expression pattern.

Mycosis Fungoides

Mycosis fungoides (MF) is the most common type of CTCL [1]. The disease poses considerable diagnostic difficulties, especially in its early stages. Clinical findings are extremely important for a correct interpretation of the skin biopsy. It is generally accepted that a diagnosis of MF requires adequate clinical pathological correlation. MF is mostly a disease of middle-aged or elderly individuals; however, cases in young adult and children are well documented. Initially, the disease presents with flat scaly patches located, in the classic MF, on sun-protected areas such as the buttocks, groins, lower abdomen, and thighs. Women may present with involvement of the breasts. Sometimes the lesions exhibit erythema, hypo, or hyperpigmentation. The initial lesions can be very subtle and persist for long time before calling the patient and physician's

attention. Most of patients with small lesions of MF in patch stage have an indolent course, even without any therapy. Some cases, however, present with disseminated patches that evolve to plaques, defined as indurated, raised, and flat lesions. These lesions then progress to tumors. Patients in this stage (third or tumor stage) present with ulcerated large nodules that may involve sun-exposed skin. Extracutaneous dissemination such as to the lymph nodes, liver, spleen, or any other organ can be documented as the disease progresses. Immunodeficiency occurs in late stages of the disease and it is the main cause of death [37].

The histopathological changes in MF usually correlate with the clinical appearance of the lesions. Biopsies from early patch-stage MF patients are probably the most difficult to interpret. The changes may be extremely subtle and therefore easy to miss. Typical cases reveal psoriasiform hyperplasia of the epidermis. A mild to moderate lymphocytic infiltrate is usually present involving the papillary dermis and adopting a perivascular distribution. In many cases, the infiltrate is composed of small lymphocytes with mild or minimal cytologic atypia. Migration of the lymphocytes to the epidermis (epidermotropism) is generally considered a diagnostic finding. However, epidermotropism may be only focal and therefore additional biopsies may be necessary if clinical suspicion of MF persists. The dermis usually shows changes associated to chronicity, such as fibrosis. With progression the cytologic atypia becomes more pronounced and the typical cerebriform appearance of the neoplastic lymphocytes is more evident. Epidermotropism may also increase and Pautrier's microabscesses can be present. The dermal infiltrate may adopt a lichenoid appearance; the combination of psoriasiform hyperplasia and lichenoid infiltrate ("psoriasiform lichenoid pattern") is common in classic MF. In plaque and tumor lesions the dermal infiltrate is denser and extends into the reticular dermis. Tumor lesions in particular may involve the subcutaneous adipose tissue. The lymphocytes in tumor stage MF may display large cell (large cell transformation) and even anaplastic features that make them indistinguishable from ALCL.

Table 10.1 Immunophenotypic profile of primary cutaneous T-cell lymphomas

	CD3	CD4	CD8	CD7	CD5	CD2	CD30	βF1	TCRγ	CD56	TIA-1	Granzyme B	Perforin	PD-1	CXCL13	CD20	EBER ISH
Mycosis fungoides	+	+ (Most) Negative (in CD8+ and double negative variants)	Negative (most) + (Hypo/hyperpigmented variants) Double positive CD4+CD8+ exist	-/+	+/-	+/-	Can be + (usually with large cell transformation)	+ (Most)	Negative (some cases reported as positive)	-/+	-/+	-/+	-/+	Rarely+	NA	Rarely +	Negative
Sézary syndrome	+	+	Negative	+/-	+/-	+/-	Can be +	+	Negative	-/+	-/+	-/+	-/+	+	NA	NA	Negative
CD30+ T-cell lymphoproliferative disorders	+/- (ALCL often negative)	+ (Most of ALCL and LyP types A, B, C)	+ (LyP type D, E?, and rarely ALCL)	+/-	+/-	+/-	+ (Except some cases of LyP type B)	+ (Most)	Negative (some cases reported as positive)	-/+	-/+	-/+	-/+	NA	NA	Rarely +	Negative
Subcutaneous panniculitis-like T-cell lymphoma	+	Negative	+	+/-	+/-	+/-	Negative	+	Negative	Negative	+/-	+/-	+/-	NA	NA	NA	Negative
Peripheral T-cell lymphoma, unspecified	+	+ (Most) Negative (in CD8+ and double positive CD4+CD8+variants)	Negative (most) + (in CD8+ and double positive CD4+CD8+variants)	-/+	+/-	+/-	Can be +	+	Negative	-/+	-/+	-/+	-/+	NA	NA	Rarely +	Rarely +
Aggressive epidermotropic CD8+ cytotoxic T-cell lymphoma	+	Negative	+	-/+	Negative	-/+	Negative	+	Negative	+/-	+/-	+/-	+/-	NA	NA	Negative	Negative
γ/δ T cell lymphoma	+	Negative	Negative (most) + (some cases)	+/-	Negative	-/+	Can be +	Negative	+	+/-	+	+	+	NA	NA	NA	Negative (rare cases reported as +)
CD4+ small/medium-sized T-cell lymphoma/proliferation	+	+	Negative ("CD8+ variants" reported)	+/-	+/-	+/-	Negative	+	Negative	Negative	+/-	+/-	+/-	+	+	NA	Negative
Extranodal NK/T-cell lymphoma, nasal type	Negative (surface), + (cytoplasmic and T-cell variants)	Negative	Negative (+ in T cell lineage tumors)	-/+	Negative	+	-/+	Negative (except in T cell lineage tumors)	Negative (except in T cell lineage tumors)	+	+	+	+	NA	NA	NA	+ (Rare cases reported as negative)
Hydroa vacciniforme-like cutaneous T-cell lymphoma	+	Negative	+	+/-	+/-	+/-	-/+	+	Negative	+/-	+/-	+/-	+/-	NA	NA	NA	+
Adult T-cell leukemia/lymphoma	+	+	Negative	Negative	+/-	+/-	-/+ CD25 +	+	Negative	Negative	-/+	-/+	-/+	NA	NA	NA	Negative
Angioimmunoblastic T-cell lymphoma	+	+	Negative	+/-	+/-	+/-	-/+	+	Negative	Negative	-/+	-/+	-/+	+	+	NA	Negative

EBER Epstein-Barr virus-encoded mRNA, *ISH* in situ hybridization, *ALCL* anaplastic large cell lymphoma, *LyP* lymphomatoid papulosis

Besides the classic clinical and histopathological presentations of MF, a number of variants have been described in the literature [38]. These variegated clinical and histopathological presentations make the diagnosis of early stage MF sometimes a difficult task. Again, integration of clinical, histopathological, immunophenotypic, and molecular findings is strongly recommended for diagnosis, and scoring systems based on these characteristics, such as the one proposed by Pimpinelli et al. [39] are widely utilized. Staging of MF, based on clinical and histopathological findings, correlates with prognosis [40].

Immunohistochemical studies are often performed in early and advanced stages of MF. The role of immunohistochemistry in the diagnosis of early lesions of MF has been subject of some controversy since it appears that it is not associated with prognosis [41] and the findings may overlap with inflammatory conditions [42]. Most of the MF cases display a T helper CD3+, CD4+, CD8−, βF1+ phenotype. Demonstration of loss of CD2, CD5, or CD7 may help in the diagnosis [22] (Fig. 10.1).

Immunophenotypic variants are well documented. CD8+ mycosis fungoides was first described as having two different clinical presentations: one aggressive, associated with a CD2−, CD7+ phenotype, and another more chronic, similar to typical MF, displaying a CD2+, CD7− profile [43]. The conventional, less aggressive CD8+ MF appears to be more frequent in children and young adults and to have a CD3+, CD8+, CD4−, CD2+, TIA-1+, CD56−/+ phenotype [44, 45]. Clinically, hypopigmented and/or hyperpigmented patches, and plaques are often seen, especially in dark-skinned individuals [46–48]. Unusual presentations, such as bullous [49] and poikilodermatous [50] have been reported in the literature.

Double positive CD4+CD8+ and double negative CD4−CD8− MF are other rarely seen immunophenotypic variants. Double positive CD4+CD8+ MF may present with lesions similar to morphea [51] while double negative CD4−CD8− MF may range from typical MF lesions to hypopigmented, ichthyosiform, purpuric [52],

and erythema gyratum-like [53] presentations (Fig. 10.2). The double negative CD4−CD8− MF must be distinguished from γ/δ T cell lymphoma, although cases clinically compatible with MF have been reported to display a γ/δ phenotype [52]. Expression of PD-1 has been reported in a case of CD4−CD8− MF, suggesting a possible follicular T-cell helper origin [54].

Rare cases of clinical and histological typical MF with γ/δ phenotype have been documented in the literature [55]. Some controversy still exists to whether these cases should be considered within the γ/δ T cell lymphoma category [56] or they represent phenotypic variants of MF.

Other antibodies sometimes used in the immunohistochemical evaluation of MF cases in the clinical practice are CD30, TIA-1, granzyme B, CD25, and cutaneous lymphocyte antigen (CLA). CD30 expression has been linked to large cell transformation of MF [57]. It is useful to remember, however, that large cell transformation is primarily a morphological concept, defined as more than 25 % of the MF cells being large. CD30 positivity, although usually present, may not be detected in an otherwise large cell transformed MF. Cytotoxic markers have been well described in MF, especially associated with progression to tumor stage [58]. CD25 is essentially tested for purposes of therapy with denileukin diftitox [59]. CLA has been reported as extensively expressed in early stages of MF and lost in tumor lesions [60]. Expression of CD20 is a rare phenomenon seen in MF [61].

Immunohistochemical analysis of MF biopsies is routinely performed in our institution. The information obtained from immunophenotyping is used not only for diagnosis but also as a baseline profile. This is especially useful when subsequent skin biopsies or other organs are involved. Immunophenotype switch with progression, however, has been documented and may be a not uncommon phenomenon [62].

Molecular studies are usually performed in those cases of MF that cannot be reliably diagnosed on clinical and histopathological grounds alone. The goal is to demonstrate a clonal population of T-cells that would support a

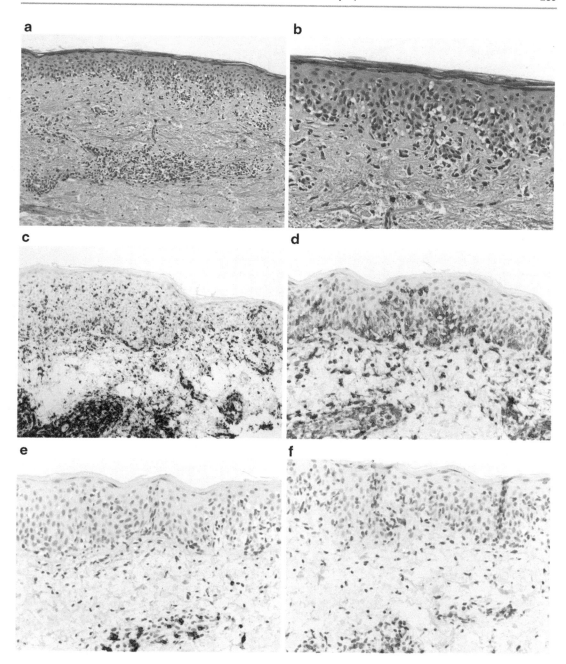

Fig. 10.1 (a) At low magnification, patch lesions of mycosis fungoides (MF) frequently reveal a mild perivascular lymphocytic infiltrate with involvement of the epidermis (H&E, 10×). (b) Notice the typical epidermotropism by hyperchromatic lymphocytes, many of them showing perinuclear clear haloes (H&E, 20×). (c) A CD3 immunohistochemical study demonstrates the perivascular and epidermotropic lymphocytes to be predominantly CD3+ T cells. The atypical cells are distributed along the dermal/epidermal junction ("string of pearls" sign) (immunoperoxidase, 10×). (d) The atypical lymphocytes both intraepidermal and dermal are positive for CD4. Intraepidermal Langerhans cells and dermal histiocytic cells are also positive for this marker (immunoperoxidase, 20×). (e) The epidermotropic lymphocytes are negative for CD8 in this typical example of patch lesion of MF. Only scattered small reactive CD8+ lymphocytes are present within the dermis (immunoperoxidase, 20×). (f) Complete loss of expression of CD7 by the epidermotropic atypical lymphocytes and most of the dermal lymphocytes is noted, supporting an abnormal phenotype of this T-cell process, interpreted as MF, patch stage (immunoperoxidase, 20×)

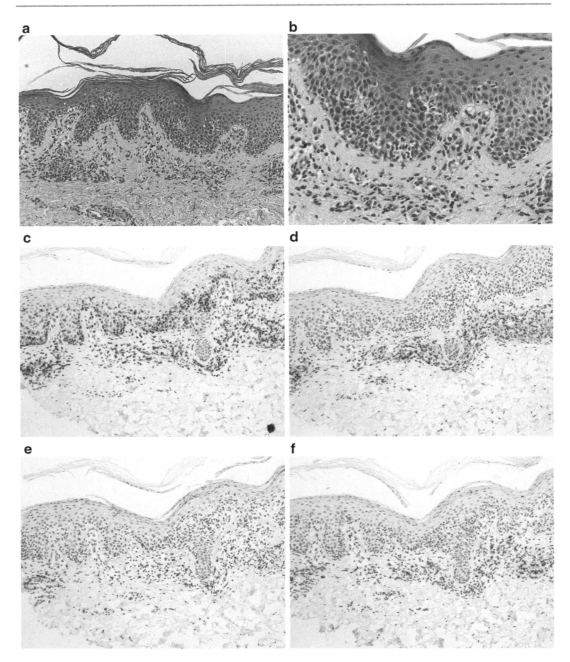

Fig. 10.2 (**a**) An immunophenotypic variant of mycosis fungoides (MF). The histopathological findings are very similar to those seen in Fig. 10.1. Prominent epidermotropism and fibrosis of the papillary dermis are seen (H&E, 20×). (**b**) The numerous epidermotropic lymphocytes are small and display mild cytologic atypia (H&E, 40×). (**c**) An immunohistochemical study for CD3 highlights the epidermotropic and dermal lymphocytes (immunoperoxidase, 20×). (**d**) CD4 is negative in the epidermotropic lymphocytes. Some dermal lymphocytes and histiocytes are labeled with the marker (immunoperoxidase, 20×). (**e**) Very rare intraepidermal lymphocytes, most likely reactive, are positive for CD8. Most of the intraepidermal and dermal lymphocytes are negative for CD8 (immunoperoxidase, 20×). (**f**) A number of intraepidermal lymphocytes reveal weak labeling with CD7, interpreted as partial loss of expression of the marker, compared to CD3. The immunophenotype seen in this case is compatible with double negative CD4-CD8– MF. The patient presented with typical lesions of MF (immunoperoxidase, 20×)

neoplastic nature of the process [63]. The most popular tests are based on PCR methods, although Southern blot is still considered the gold standard [64]. TCR-γ and β chains gene rearrangements are the most commonly tested in practice, as previously discussed [65, 66].

It should be emphasized that a positive result for *TCR* gene rearrangement is not diagnostic by itself. Molecular results need to be correlated with clinical, histological, and immunohistochemical findings. One situation where a false positive test is possible is when the lymphocytic infiltrate is minimal or mild [67]. Running duplicate analyses is recommended to rule out pseudoclonality [25]. False negative tests can be obtained as a result of limited sensitivity of the PCR-based methods used for *TCR* gene rearrangement determination [25]. In situations where the clinical and histopathological settings are supportive of MF, negative or oligoclonal *TCR* gene rearrangement results do not rule out the diagnosis.

Among the many mimickers of MF, drug reactions are especially notorious. Drug reactions may show atypical lymphocytes and exocytosis making them difficult to distinguish from mycosis fungoides on histopathological grounds. Clinical information is critical in these cases since a temporal relationship between initiation of therapy and cutaneous lesions is often noted. Discontinuation of the offending drug usually results in resolution of the lesions. Common drugs associated with pseudolymphomatous infiltrates are anticonvulsants such as carbamazepine [68], phenytoin, sodium valproate; antihypertensives such as angiotensin-converting enzyme inhibitors and β-blockers, among many others [69]. It seems that drug induced pseudolymphomas often present as solitary lesions, as opposite to MF. Immunohistochemical studies may be useful in the differential diagnosis if the infiltrate demonstrate lack of clear predominance of either CD4 or CD8 and no loss of pan-T cell markers is identified [70]. Most of the cases of drug induced MF-like reactions are polyclonal by PCR-based *TCR* gene rearrangement testing, although clonal proliferations may be detected [71]. Inflammatory conditions may simulate MF on clinical and histopathological grounds. The

list of conditions that may mimic MF includes persistent nodular arthropod bite reactions, secondary syphilis, lymphomatoid dermatitis, nodular scabies, actinic reticuloid, fungal infections, lichen sclerosus et atrophicus, lichen striatus, lichenoid keratosis, pigmented purpuric dermatosis, allergic contact dermatitis, connective tissue disease, and inflamed vitiligo [70, 72]. In general, the demonstration of a mixture of CD4+ and CD8+ cells without clear predominance of either one, the retained expression of pan-T cell markers, and the polyclonal pattern of TCR gene rearrangement by PCR, all support the reactive nature of these processes. However, clinical pathological correlation cannot be overemphasized when evaluating these cases.

Sézary Syndrome

Sézary syndrome (SS) is clinically characterized by erythroderma and lymphadenopathy, along with the presence of the so-called Sézary cells in peripheral blood. SS has been long considered as the leukemic counterpart of MF. However, it seems that some differences exist between erythrodermic MF and SS [73]. It appears that SS and MF constitute malignancies of thymic memory T cells and skin resident effector memory T cells, respectively [74]. Frequent clinical overlapping exists between these two entities and therefore a diagnosis of SS is made using strict criteria that include the demonstration of a T-cell clone in peripheral blood, peripheral blood lymphocytosis with a CD4+/CD8+ ratio greater than 10, and circulating Sézary cells greater than 1×10^9/L.

The histopathological features of SS are largely identical to those seen in MF. Lack of epidermotropism and low grade cytologic atypia are commonly seen in SS and therefore may be useful in its distinction from MF [75]. The majority of cases exhibit a CD3+, CD4+, CD8– phenotype. It appears that SS expresses PD-1 more frequently than erythrodermic MF [76].

As mentioned above, clonal *TCR* gene rearrangements are demonstrated in peripheral blood of patients with SS [14]. These clonal peaks can be identical to the monoclonal *TCR* gene rearrangements detected in skin samples [77], giving further support to a common neoplastic process involving different anatomical sites. In some instances, however, different clonal peaks are identified in peripheral blood and skin, suggesting clonal heterogeneity in at least a number of cases [25, 30]. False positive results in peripheral blood have been associated with autoimmune disorders [28], advanced age [78], and other noncutaneous lymphomas and inflammatory skin conditions [14]. In rare cases, SS cases may fail to demonstrate T cell clones in peripheral blood [79].

Primary Cutaneous CD30-Positive T-Cell Lymphoproliferative Disorders

Primary cutaneous CD30-positive T-cell lymphoproliferative disorders (CD30+ LPD) constitute the second most common cutaneous T cell lymphoma/lymphoid proliferations. The category comprises a spectrum of diseases ranging from lymphomatoid papulosis (LyP) to primary cutaneous anaplastic large cell lymphoma (C-ALCL). Borderline lesions are also recognized. Clinically LyP presents as a benign eruption of papulonodular lesions that recur and regress spontaneously. Patients with C-ALCL, on the other hand, usually present with one or multiple localized ulcerated nodules that may regress [80]. Clinical workup is mandatory to distinguish C-ALCL from systemic ALCL with secondary involvement of the skin. Of note, other cutaneous lymphomas, such as mycosis fungoides with large cell transformation, may show CD30 expression, as mentioned above [81].

LyP is characterized by a polymorphous dermal infiltrate of small and large lymphocytes, admixed with variable numbers of neutrophils, eosinophils, and histiocytes. The infiltrate spares the subcutis. LyP demonstrates a spectrum of histologic appearances, classified as A, B, and C

types [82] (Fig. 10.3). The most common presentation is the type A, that shows aggregates of large Reed-Sternberg-like CD30+ cells in a background of inflammatory cells, and therefore resembling Hodgkin lymphoma. Type B LyP can be histologically indistinguishable from MF, and reportedly it can lack expression of CD30. Because of the clinical presentation, typical of LyP, this subtype is best regarded as a type of LyP although papular mycosis fungoides is difficult to rule out without good clinical pathological correlation. Type C histologically resembles ALCL since it is composed of large CD30-positive cells arranged in sheets with minimal inflammatory background. New types of LyP have been recently described. The "type D" LyP is characterized by a proliferation of lymphoid cells with only scattered or absent other inflammatory cells. The proliferating lymphoid cells express CD8, as opposed to the other types, which show a CD4+ phenotype [83] (Fig. 10.4). LyP type D mimics primary cutaneous aggressive epidermotropic CD8+ cytotoxic T-cell lymphoma but it differs clinically and immunophenotypically, since the latter is usually negative for CD30 [84]. Angiocentric and angioinvasive distribution of the cells in LyP ("type E") may constitute a confounding factor in the differential diagnosis of LyP with other angiocentric lymphomas, such as NK/T lymphomas [85, 86]. Folliculocentrism and folliculotropism have been long described in LyP [87], and proposed to be characteristic of the "type F" LyP [88]. Intermediate or hybrid forms, especially between LyP A and B types, have been described.

C-ALCL exhibits abundant large pleomorphic cells involving dermis and extending into the subcutis. In most cases, the accompanying inflammatory infiltrate (seen in most of the cases of LyP) is scarse or absent. A rare variant, however, the neutrophil-rich ALCL, can be difficult to diagnose due to the presence of an abscess-like infiltrate [89] (Fig. 10.5). Borderline lesions with features of both LyP

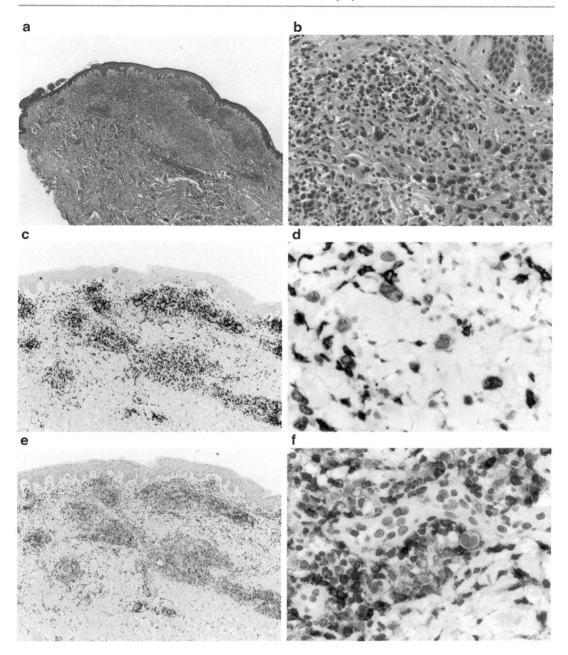

Fig. 10.3 (a) Lymphomatoid papulosis (LyP) presents as a nodular/perivascular infiltrate, often showing a wedge shape, infiltrating dermis (H&E, 4×). (b) The infiltrate is composed of a mixture of large cells in a background of small lymphocytes, rare neutrophils, and plasma cells, in a Hodgkin-like pattern (LyP type A) (H&E, 20×). (c) The infiltrate is predominantly composed of CD3+ cells (immunoperoxidase, 10×). (d) The large cells are mostly positive for CD3 although variable intensity of the label-ing can occur (immunoperoxidase, 40×). (e) The T-cells are predominantly CD4+. Scattered CD8-positive small lymphocytes are present (not shown) (immunoperoxidase, 10×). (f) The large atypical cells are weakly positive for CD4 (immunoperoxidase, 40×). (g) CD30 labels the large atypical cells, some of them arranged in clusters (immu-noperoxidase, 10×). (h) The large cells reveal typical membranous and perinuclear Golgi-like pattern of expres-sion of CD30 (immunoperoxidase, 40×)

g h

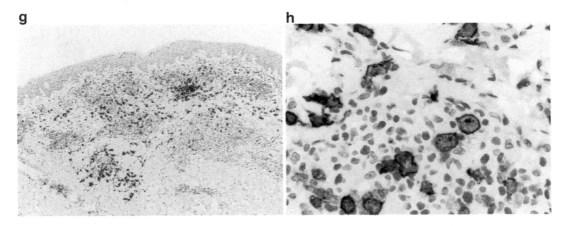

Fig. 10.3 (continued)

and ALCL may support the postulate of these lesions being a continuum.

The large cells present in CD30+ LPD are usually positive for CD4 and the activation markers CD30 and CD25. In our experience, LyP cells often express CD3 while C-ALCL frequently shows loss of one or more panT-cell antigens such as CD3, CD2, CD5, and CD7 (Fig. 10.5). As already mentioned, cases of CD8+ LyP and C-ALCL are well recognized. Many cases of CD30+LPD express cytotoxic proteins such as perforin, granzyme B, and TIA-1. Most cases are TCR α/β but cases of γ/δ phenotype, especially CD8+, have been reported [90, 91]. C-ALCL is usually negative for ALK, in contrary to its systemic counterpart [92, 93]. Expression of EMA is sometimes used in the distinction between C-ALCL and systemic ALCL, since the latter is usually positive for EMA [94].

Clonal rearrangements of *TCR* in CD30+ LPD have been variably reported [95, 96]. Identical clones can be detected in CD30+ LPD lesions occurring in different anatomical sites [97] and in LyP and concomitant lesions of mycosis fungoides [96, 98]. C-ALCL cases usually lack t(2;5) and ALK expression by immunohistochemistry [99]. Translocations involving *IRF4* (interferon

regulatory factor-4), detected in C-ALCL but not in systemic ALCL, have been reported as useful in this differential diagnosis [35]. Recently, chromosomal rearrangements of the DUSP22-IRF4 locus have been identified in cases of LyP [100].

Subcutaneous Panniculitis-Like T Cell Lymphoma

Subcutaneous panniculitis-like T-cell lymphomas (SPTCL) present with subcutaneous nodules or plaques on lower extremities with or without systemic symptoms. Hemophagocytic syndrome may be present; however it appears to be not as common as initially reported [101]. Examination of skin biopsies in these cases shows a lobular panniculitis with minimal or only mild dermal involvement. Epidermotropism is rare. The tumor is composed of an admixture of small, medium, or large cells with variable numbers of histiocytes. The lymphoma cells arrange around adipocyte spaces in a rimming pattern. Erythrophagocytosis, fat necrosis, and karyorrhexis are variably seen.

The immunophenotype of these tumors is typically CD3+, CD8+, and CD4−. The current definition of SPTCL includes only tumors

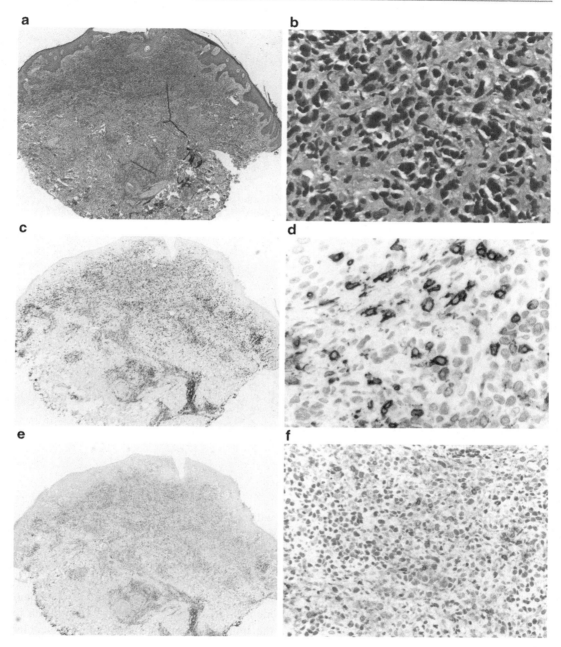

Fig. 10.4 (a) Lymphomatoid papulosis, CD8+ ("type D"). The low magnification appearance of this lesion is very similar to that seen in Fig. 10.3 (H&E, 4×). (b) The composition of the infiltrate, however, differs from typical LyP. Scattered large cells in a monomorphic background of small lymphocytes are seen. Eosinophils or neutrophils are not identified (H&E, 40×). (c) CD3 labels most of the cells composing the infiltrate (immunoperoxidase, 4×). (d) In this case, some of the large cells are negative for CD3 while some of the smaller cells are only weakly positive for the marker (immunoperoxidase, 40×). (e) The infiltrate shows numerous cells expressing CD4 (immunoperoxidase, 4×). (f) At higher magnification it is evident that only small reactive lymphocytes and histiocytes are positive for CD4 (immunoperoxidase, 20×). (g) Strong and diffuse expression of CD8 is noted in the lesion (immunoperoxidase, 4×). (h) The large and most of the small lymphocytes composing the lesion are positive for CD8 (immunoperoxidase, 20×). (i) CD30 labels numerous cells arranged in small and large clusters (immunoperoxidase, 4×). (j) The large cells are predominantly positive for CD30, although variations in labeling intensity are observed (immunoperoxidase, 20×)

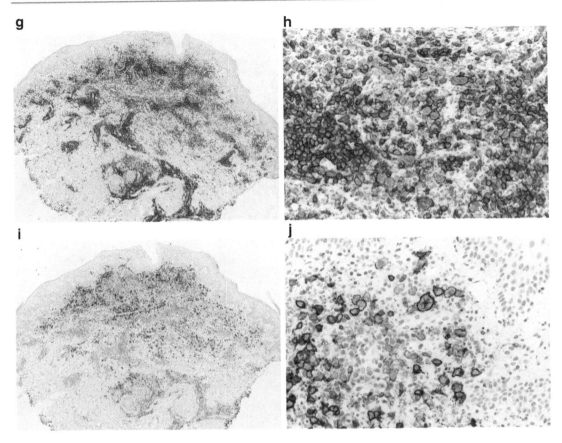

Fig. 10.4 (continued)

with α/β phenotype [1]. Cytotoxic markers are usually positive and CD30 is generally negative (Fig. 10.6).

The differential diagnosis is wide and includes inflammatory and neoplastic lymphoid processes. Other lymphomas with involvement of subcutis such as primary cutaneous γ/δ T-cell lymphoma should be suspected in cases with marked dermal or epidermal involvement and/or usunual phenotype, such as double negative CD4– CD8–. Extensive angiocentrism with necrosis along

with a CD4–, CD8–, CD56+, EBER+ phenotype are diagnostic of extranodal NK/T lymphoma. Inflammatory conditions that may show similar findings are lupus erythematosus profundus, Weber-Christian disease, histiocytic cytophagic panniculitis, and reactive panniculitis to drugs or injections. In addition to the immunohistochemical findings, molecular analysis for *TCR* gene rearrangements may help in the distinction between inflammatory conditions and SPTCL, since most cases of SPTCL are monoclonal [102].

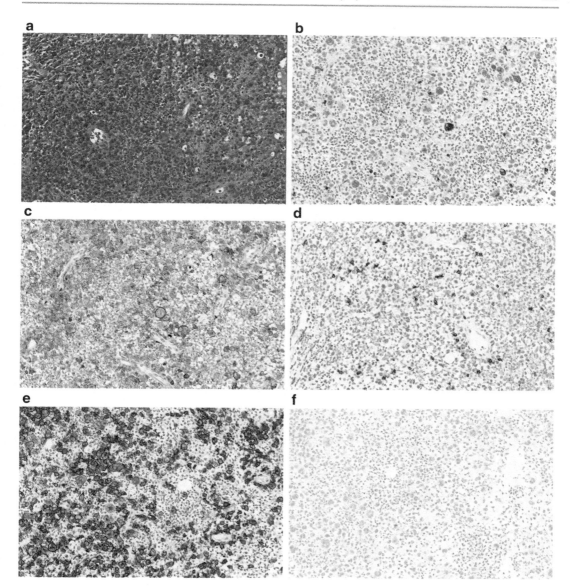

Fig. 10.5 (a) Primary cutaneous anaplastic large cell lymphoma (C-ALCL), neutrophil-rich. Large pleomorphic cells admixed with cells displaying horseshoe-like nuclei (hallmark cells) are seen. Numerous neutrophils and scattered small lymphocytes are also present (H&E, 20×). (b) The atypical cells show variable labeling with CD3, ranging from negative to strongly positive. This is not an uncommon finding in C-ALCL (immunoperoxi- dase, 20×). (c) Most of the atypical cells are positive for CD4, the most common phenotype in C-ALCL (immuno- peroxidase, 20×). (d) Only rare small reactive lympho- cytes are positive for CD8 (immunoperoxidase, 20×). (e) There is strong and diffuse expression of CD30 by the atypical cells (immunoperoxidase, 20×). (f) ALK is nega- tive by immunohistochemistry, a common finding in C-ALCL (immunoperoxidase, 20×)

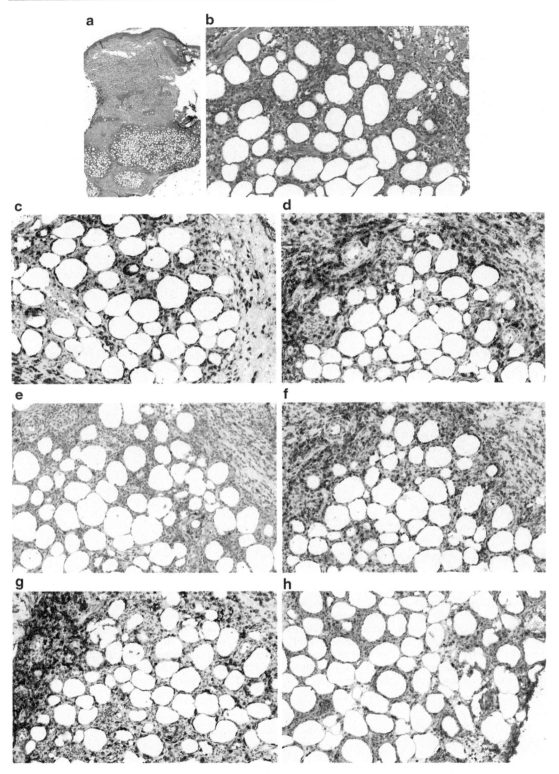

Fig. 10.6 (a) Subcutaneous panniculitis-like T-cell lymphoma (SPTCL). The tumor cells primarily involve subcutaneous adipose tissue in a lobular panniculitis-like pattern (H&E, 2×). (b) The lymphocytes show cytologic atypia. Rimming of the atypical around the adipocytes is partially seen (H&E, 20×). (c) CD3 labels most of the infiltrating

Primary Cutaneous Peripheral T-Cell Lymphoma (PTL), Unspecified

This group emcompasses heterogeneous cutaneous T-cell lymphomas that do not fit in any of the well recognized types. In the WHO/EORTC classification, three provisional categories are included within this group: primary cutaneous aggressive epidermotropic CD8-positive cytotoxic T-cell lymphoma, cutaneous gamma/delta-positive T-cell lymphoma, and primary cutaneous small/medium CD4-positive T-cell lymphoma/proliferation. Lymphomas that do not fit in any of these provisional categories are designated as PTL, unspecified.

The immunophenotype of PTL, unspecified, is variable but most of the cases are CD3+, CD4+,CD8– (with a subset of CD8+CD4–, CD4–CD8–, or CD4+CD8+ cases) [103], βF1+, TCRγ–. CD30 may be expressed by the tumor cells, and some cases are CD20+ [104] or EBER+ [105].

These tumors are frequently clonal by TCR gene rearrangement analysis. It appears that a considerable number of cases show clonal or oligoclonal immunoglobulin heavy-chain gene rearrangements, explained by either EBV+ B cells or presence of a concomitant clonal B-cell population [106].

Primary Cutaneous Aggressive Epidermotropic CD8-Positive Cytotoxic T-Cell Lymphoma

Also known as Berti's lymphoma [107], this is a very rare tumor clinically characterized by eruptive multiple skin nodules that rapidly disseminate to other organs, although lymph nodes are generally spared [107]. The prognosis is usually poor.

The histological picture of the tumor is characterized by striking epidermotropism by atypi-

cal cells that range from small to large. Ulceration and blister formation can be seen. Angiocentric distribution with angioinvasion can be identified.

Immunophenotypically, these tumors are CD3+, CD8+, CD4–, CD5–, TCR α/β+. They usually express cytotoxic markers such as TIA-1, granzyme B, and perforin. Loss of other panT-cell markers such as CD7 and CD2 can be seen. CD30 is usually not expressed by the tumor cells, a useful clue in the differential diagnosis.

Monoclonal TCR gene rearrangement has been reported in most of the reported cases [108, 109]. The differential diagnosis includes CD8+ mycosis fungoides, especially the pagetoid reticulosis variant. Clinical presentation as a solitary lesion favors pagetoid reticulosis.

CD30+ LPD with CD8+ phenotype (type D LyP, CD8+ C-ALCL) can be distinguished by their diffuse expression of CD30 and clinical manifestations. Primary cutaneous γ/δ T cell lymphoma, although clinically similar, displays a different immunophenotype.

Primary Cutaneous γ/δ-Positive T-Cell Lymphoma

Primary cutaneous γ/δ T cell lymphoma (PCGDTCL) is another aggressive tumor that appears to originate from the skin activated cytotoxic γ/δ T cells. It typically occurs in young adults, more females that males, and presents with multiple lesions, commonly on proximal lower extremities, with frequent mucosal involvement [110]. The tumor has a poor prognosis [111].

PCGDTCL displays a variety of histologic presentations, sometimes seen in the same biopsy: epidermotropic, dermal, and subcutaneous [110, 112]. Combinations of these patterns are often present. The tumor may show

Fig. 10.6 (continued) cells and highlights their arrangement around the adipocytes (immunoperoxidase, 20×). (**d**) The atypical lymphocytes are positive for CD8 (immunoperoxidase, 20×). (**e**) CD4 labels only scattered small lymphocytes and histiocytic cells (immunoperoxidase, 20×). (**f**) The tumor cells are positive for TIA-1, with a character-

istic granular pattern of expression (immunoperoxidase, 20×). (**g**) Most of the infiltrating atypical lymphocytes are positive for βF1, including the cells around adipocytic cells (immunoperoxidase, 20×). (**h**) In contrast, only scattered cells are positive for TCRγ, supporting an α/β phenotype of this lymphoma (immunoperoxidase, 20×)

rimming of adipocytes, similar to that seen in SPTCL [112].

The tumor cells are CD3+, CD5−, CD7−, and usually double negative for CD4 and CD8 [113], although may express CD8. CD56 is often positive. A cytotoxic phenotype, with strong expression of granzyme B, TIA-1, and perforin, is usually seen [56]. Demonstration of γ/δ phenotype by the tumor cells is done by immunohistochemistry; the tumor cells are positive TCRγ and TCRδ (the last requires frozen tissue) and negative for βF1 (Fig. 10.7). Some cases have been reported as positive for EBV (EBER) [56]; it is still unclear whether these should be considered as extranodal NK/T cell lymphomas with γ/δ phenotype. Similarly, cases displaying clinical and histological features of MF have been reported to harbor a γ/δ phenotype. While some consider these cases as examples of "indolent" γ/δ T cell lymphoma [114], others interpret them as MF with γ/δ phenotype [55].

TCR gene rearrangement analysis by PCR reveals a clonal population in most of the cases [56, 110].

reported. The tumors have an indolent course; however, rare cases demonstrating more aggressive behavior are documented [116].

The histological appearance of PCSMTCL is that of a dense dermal infiltrate composed of small to medium-sized T cells. Focal epidermotropism can be seen. Most of the lymphocytes are positive for CD3, CD4, and βF1. These lymphocytes are negative for TCRγ and CD30. Loss of panT-cell markers is rare. Numerous CD20+ B cells are often present. A reactive infiltrate composed of variable number of CD8+ T cells, plasma cells, eosinophils, and histiocytes, is present. It seems that at least some cases have a follicular T helper phenotype, expressing BCL-6, PD-1, and CXCL13 [117] (Fig. 10.8).

Some authors require the identification of clonal *TCR* gene rearrangements for diagnosis of PCSMTCL, reserving the designation of atypical lymphoid proliferation to those cases clinically and histologically compatible with PCSMTCL but polyclonal by PCR analysis. In fact, about 60 % of cases in a series of PCSMTCL were found to have a monoclonal rearrangement of the TCR γ [115].

Primary Cutaneous Small/Medium CD4-Positive T-Cell Lymphoma/ Proliferation

Primary cutaneous (pleomorphic) CD4-positive small/medium-sized T-cell lymphoma/proliferation (PCSMTCL) is another provisional category in the 2008 WHO/EORTC classification. Controversy still exists about whether this entity truly represents a malignant proliferation or it should be better regarded as an atypical lymphoid proliferation of undetermined significance [115]. Clinically, PCSMTCL usually presents as a single lesion on the head and neck or trunk area. Cases presenting with multiple lesions have been

Primary Cutaneous Extranodal NK/T-Cell Lymphoma, Nasal Type

The category of primary cutaneous extranodal NK/T-cell lymphoma, nasal type (ENKTL) comprises lymphomas of natural killer (NK) and cytotoxic T-cells, along with some lymphomas with indeterminate lineage (NK/T) [118]. The vast majority of cases are associated with EBV infection [119] and therefore more common in Asian and Latin American countries [120–122]. These lymphomas are less common than their nasal counterparts. Patients with ENKTL present with multiple ulcerated nodules with necrotic centers. The prognosis is poor [123].

Fig. 10.7 (**a**) Primary cutaneous γ/δ T cell lymphoma (PCGDTCL), epidermotropic variant. The epidermis is involved by medium- and large-sized atypical lymphocytes. Scattered dyskeratotic keratinocytes and extravasated red blood cells are seen (H&E, 10×) (**b**) The atypical lymphocytes are diffusely positive for CD3 (immunoperoxidase, 4×). (**c**) The epidermotropic atypical lymphocytes are negative for CD4. Numerous small dermal lymphocytes and intraepidermal Langerhans cells are positive for CD4

(immunoperoxidase, 4×). (**d**) The tumor cells are negative or weakly positive for CD8 (immunoperoxidase, 4×). (**e**) The atypical lymphocytes are negative for βF1. Most of the small reactive dermal lymphocytes express βF1 (immunoperoxidase, 10×). (**f**) Strong and diffuse expression of TCRγ is seen in the atypical, intraepidermal lymphocytes (immunoperoxidase, 10×). The lymphoma cells are positive for the cytotoxic markers TIA-1 (**g**) and Granzyme B (**h**) (immunoperoxidase, 4×)

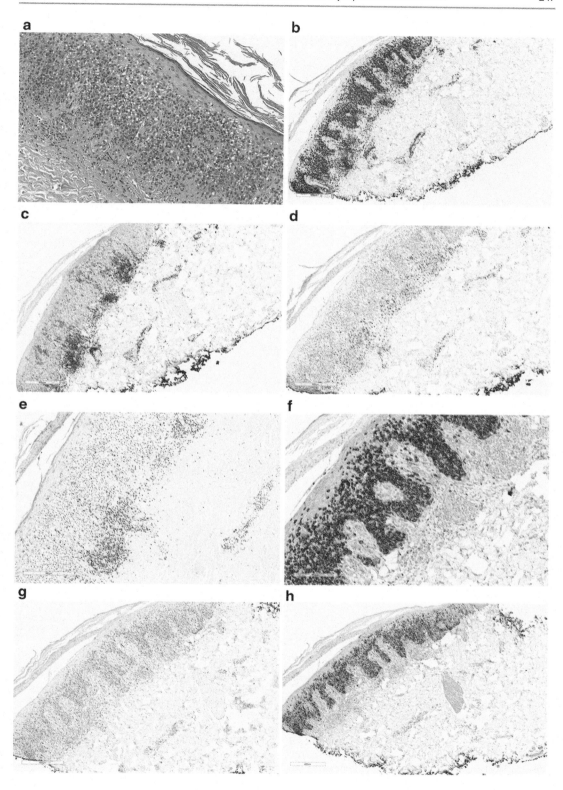

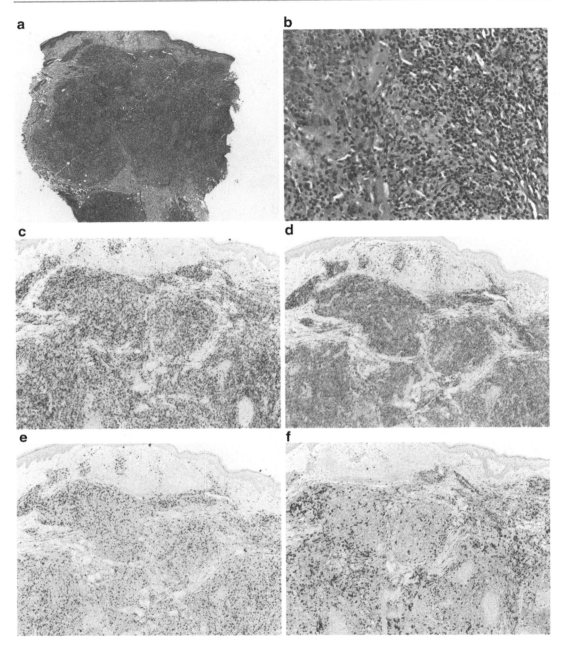

Fig. 10.8 Primary cutaneous (pleomorphic) CD4-positive small/medium-sized T-cell lymphoma/proliferation (PCSMTCL). (**a**) Low magnification reveals a dense infiltrate occupying superficial and deep dermis. The infiltrate is polymorphous and spares the epidermis (H&E, 2×). (**b**) The infiltrate is composed of a mixture of small to medium size lymphocytes, histiocytes, and scattered plasma cells. Notice the focal adnexotropism (H&E, 20×). (**c**) CD3 labels most of the lymphocytes composing the infiltrate (immunoperoxidase, 10×). (**d**) CD4 is diffusely positive throughout the infiltrate. Histiocytes account for the larger number of CD4+ cells detected in relation to the CD3+ lymphocytes (immunoperoxidase, 10×). (**e**) A considerable number of CD8+ lymphocytes are present within the infiltrate (immunoperoxidase, 10×). (**f**) CD20+ B lymphocytes are also present admixed with the T cells (immunoperoxidase, 10×). (**g**) Scattered cells are positive for CXCL-13 (immunoperoxidase, 20×). (**h**) Numerous cells, some of them in small clusters, express PD-1, a finding interpreted as evidence of follicular T-helper phenotype (immunoperoxidase, 20×)

g   h

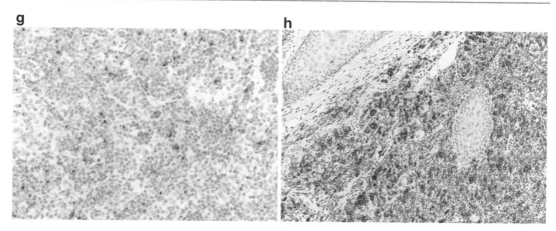

Fig. 10.8 (continued)

Histologically, the tumor cells arrange in a dense dermal infiltrate showing angiocentrism and necrosis [124]. The lymphoma cells vary in size and many mitotic figures are seen. The tumor may infiltrate the subcutis, mimicking SPTCL. The classical phenotype of this tumor is CD2+, CD56+, cytoplasmic CD3+, and surface CD3–. CD7 may be positive but other T-cell markers such as CD5, CD4, and CD8 are usually negative, except in the cases of T-cell lineage (Fig. 10.9). The NK lymphomas are negative for βF1 and TCRγ. Cytotoxic markers are usually positive, along with Fas and Fas ligand [125].

Almost all the cases are positive for EBV by EBER ISH. However, rare cases of EBV-negative ENKTL have been reported [126]. The tumors of NK lineage are negative for *TCR* gene rearrangements while the T-cell lymphomas almost invariably show monoclonal populations [127, 128]. NK-cell killer immunoglobulin-like receptor (KIR) analysis through reverse transcriptase PCR can be used to demonstrate monoclonality in tumors of NK lineage [129].

Hydroa Vacciniforme-Like Cutaneous T-Cell Lymphoma

A variant of ENKTL, according to the WHO/EORTC classification, hydroa vacciniforme-like cutaneous T-cell lymphoma (HVTL) is also closely associated with EBV infection [130]. The

disease has a particular clinical presentation and predilection for children and young adults living in regions of Latin America and Asia [131, 132]. Multiple vesicles and papules on sun-exposed areas that leave scars, clinically resembling hydroa vacciniforme, are characteristic of this tumor. The patients usually have a history of hypersensitivity to mosquito bites. The current thinking is that HVTL belongs to a spectrum of EBV-related T-cell lymphoid proliferations of the skin that include typical hydroa vacciniforme and aggressive lymphomas [133].

HVTL cells display a CD3+, CD2+, CD8+ phenotype, with frequent expression of cytotoxic markers. *TCR* gene rearrangement is identified in variable proportion of cases [134, 135]. EBER ISH is positive, usually in large numbers of lymphocytes (Fig. 10.10). Analysis of skin crusts and scales for EBER-1 and *Bam*HI A rightward transcripts (BARTs) by real time PCR has been reported as highly sensitive and specific [136].

Cutaneous Adult T-Cell Leukemia/Lymphoma

Adult T-cell leukemia/lymphoma (ATLL) is caused by the human T-cell leukemia virus type I (HTLV-1). The disease has a specific geographic distribution, being endemic in Japan, the Caribbean islands, South America, and regions of Central Africa. It affects lymph nodes and bone

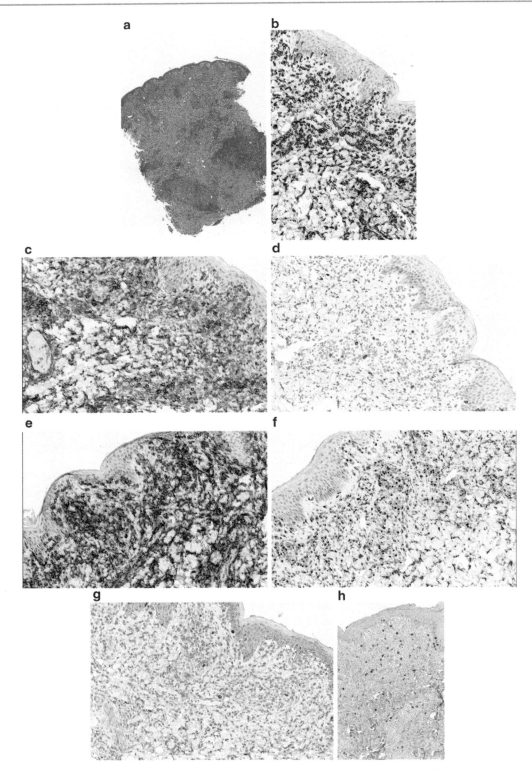

Fig. 10.9 Primary cutaneous extranodal NK/T-cell lymphoma, nasal type (ENKTL). (**a**) A dense nodular infiltrate involving superficial and deep dermis is seen. The lymphocytes show angiocentric distribution. Interface changes are present (H&E, 2×). (**b**) The tumor cells are positive for CD3, indicating a T-cell lineage of

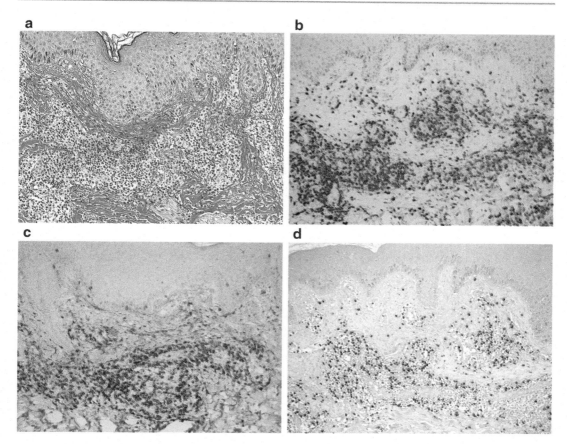

Fig. 10.10 Hydroa vacciniforme-like cutaneous T-cell lymphoma (HVTL). (**a**) Small and medium size atypical lymphocytes involve the dermis in a nodular pattern of distribution (H&E, 10×). (**b**) The atypical cells are posi- tive for CD3 (immunoperoxidase, 10×). (**c**) Most of the atypical lymphocytes are CD8+ (immunoperoxidase, 10×). (**d**) EBER is positive in most of the atypical cells (in situ hybridization, 10×)

marrow and it can involve the skin in a secondary fashion. Cutaneous ATLL presents with purely cutaneous involvement, without evidence of systemic disease [137, 138].

Cutaneous ATLL reveals a predominantly perivascular distribution of the tumor cells. The cells may demonstrate mild to severe epidermotropism. The classical immunoprolife is CD3+, CD4+, CD8−, CD7−, CD25+ (Fig. 10.11) [139]. Demonstration of monoclonal integration of HTLV-1 proviral DNA can be done by Southern blot analysis [140]. It seems that extraordinary integration patterns of HTLV-1 proviral DNA are associated with distinct clinical and pathological subtypes and prognosis [141]. The differential diagnosis includes MF, from which many cases are histologically indistinguishable. Clinical characteristics of the disease and HTLV-1 positive serology should guide to the correct diagnosis.

Fig. 10.9 (continued) the cells in this particular case (immunoperoxidase, 10×). (**c**) The atypical cells are negative for CD4. Small lymphocytes and histiocytes express CD4 (immunoperoxidase, 20×). (**d**) The lymphoma cells are negative for CD8 (immunoperoxidase, 20×). (**e**) Strong expression of CD56 is noted in the tumor cells (immunoperoxidase, 20×). (**f**) The tumor cells are positive for TIA-1, indicating a cytotoxic phenotype (immunoperoxidase, 20×). (**g**) The atypical lymphocytes are negative for TCRγ, ruling out a γ/δ T-cell lymphoma (immunoperoxidase, 20×). (**h**) The tumor cells are positive for EBER (in situ hybridization, 20×)

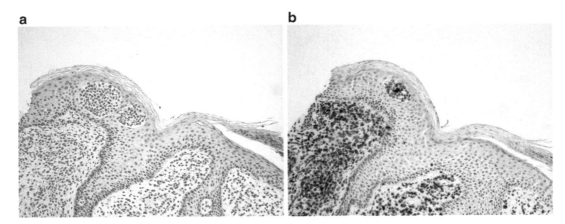

Fig. 10.11 Cutaneous adult T-cell leukemia/lymphoma (ATLL). (**a**) The morphological appearance of ATLL can be indistinguishable from MF. Notice the presence of Pautrier's microabscesses in this case. The tumor cells display irregular convoluted nuclei (H&E, 10×). (**b**) The lymphoma cells are positive for CD25 (immunoperoxidase, 10×)

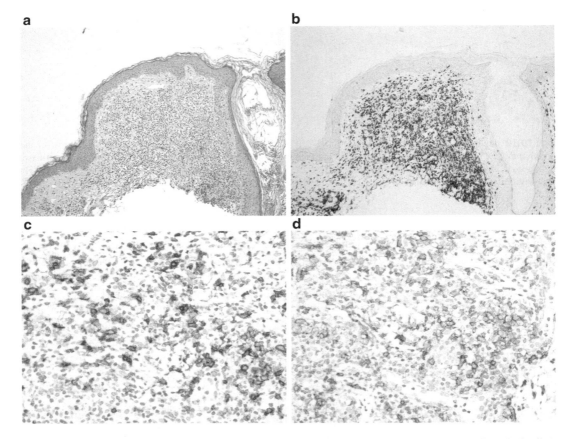

Fig. 10.12 Angioimmunoblastic T-cell lymphoma (AITL). (**a**) Involvement of the skin by AITL in this case is characterized by a polymorphous lymphoid infiltrate (H&E, 10×). (**b**) The lymphocytes are positive for CD3 (immunoperoxidase, 10×). (**c**) A subset of atypical cells is positive for CD10 (immunoperoxidase, 40×). (**d**) Expression of PD-1 by the atypical cells is also noted (immunoperoxidase, 40×)

Angioimmunoblastic T-Cell Lymphoma

Angioimmunoblastic T-cell lymphoma (AITL) is a peripheral T-cell lymphoma of follicular helper T cell postulated origin and associated with EBV-infected B cells in a large number of cases [142, 143]. Patients present with systemic symptoms such as fever and weight loss along with lymphadenopathy and hepatosplenomegaly. Cutaneous lesions are common and manifest as macular, papular, and/or plaque-like/nodular eruptions [144]. It is still not clear whether these skin lesions are reactive or lymphomatous in nature.

The histological appearance of AITL involving skin is variegated. It can range from a very mild superficial perivascular infiltrate with lymphocytes and eosinophils to dense superficial and deep infiltrates of atypical lymphocytes [145]. Vascular changes such as hyperplasia or vasculitis are frequent. It is accepted that the neoplastic cells are CD3+, CD4+, with rare loss of pan-T cell markers. Follicular helper T cell markers such as CD10, PD-1, CXCL13, and bcl-6 are reported to be useful for diagnosis (Fig. 10.12) [146]. Contrary to nodal AITL, cutaneous AITL is only occasionally positive for EBV [147]. Interestingly, while most of the cases are demonstrated to be clonal by *TCR* gene rearrangement analysis, a high proportion of cases are also positive for *IgH* gene rearrangements [148].

References

1. Willemze R, Jaffe ES, Burg G, Cerroni L, Berti E, Swerdlow SH, et al. WHO-EORTC classification for cutaneous lymphomas. Blood. 2005;105(10):3768–85.
2. Willemze R, Meijer CJ. Rationale of a new classification for the group of primary cutaneous lymphomas. Semin Cutan Med Surg. 2000;19(2):71–7.
3. Younes A, Kadin ME. Emerging applications of the tumor necrosis factor family of ligands and receptors in cancer therapy. J Clin Oncol. 2003;21(18):3526–34.
4. Gause A, Pohl C, Tschiersch A, Da Costa L, Jung W, Diehl V, et al. Clinical significance of soluble CD30 antigen in the sera of patients with untreated Hodgkin's disease. Blood. 1991;77(9):1983–8.
5. Talpur R, Jones DM, Alencar AJ, Apisarnthanarax N, Herne KL, Yang Y, et al. CD25 expression is correlated with histological grade and response to denileukin diftitox in cutaneous T-cell lymphoma. J Invest Dermatol. 2006;126(3):575–83.
6. Berke G. PELs and the perforin and granzyme independent mechanism of CTL-mediated lysis. Immunol Rev. 1995;146:21–31.
7. Kanavaros P, Boulland ML, Petit B, Arnulf B, Gaulard P. Expression of cytotoxic proteins in peripheral T-cell and natural killer-cell (NK) lymphomas: association with extranodal site, NK or Tgammadelta phenotype, anaplastic morphology and CD30 expression. Leuk Lymphoma. 2000;38(3-4):317–26.
8. Pich A, Ponti R, Valente G, Chiusa L, Geuna M, Novero D, et al. MIB-1, Ki67, and PCNA scores and DNA flow cytometry in intermediate grade malignant lymphomas. J Clin Pathol. 1994;47(1):18–22. Pubmed Central PMCID: 501749.
9. Morris SW, Kirstein MN, Valentine MB, Dittmer K, Shapiro DN, Look AT, et al. Fusion of a kinase gene, ALK, to a nucleolar protein gene, NPM, in non-Hodgkin's lymphoma. Science. 1995;267(5196):316–7.
10. Hapgood G, Savage KJ. The biology and management of systemic anaplastic large cell lymphoma. Blood. 2015;126(1):17–25.
11. Alexandrova EM, Moll UM. Role of p53 family members p73 and p63 in human hematological malignancies. Leuk Lymphoma. 2012;53(11):2116–29.
12. Vasmatzis G, Johnson SH, Knudson RA, Ketterling RP, Braggio E, Fonseca R, et al. Genome-wide analysis reveals recurrent structural abnormalities of TP63 and other p53-related genes in peripheral T-cell lymphomas. Blood. 2012;120(11):2280–9.
13. Chavan RN, Bridges AG, Knudson RA, Ketterling RP, Comfere N, Wada DA, et al. Somatic rearrangement of the TP63 gene preceding development of mycosis fungoides with aggressive clinical course. Blood Cancer J. 2014;4:e253. Pubmed Central PMCID: 4220651.
14. Sandberg Y, Heule F, Lam K, Lugtenburg PJ, Wolvers-Tettero IL, van Dongen JJ, et al. Molecular immunoglobulin/T- cell receptor clonality analysis in cutaneous lymphoproliferations. Experience with the BIOMED-2 standardized polymerase chain reaction protocol. Haematologica. 2003;88(6):659–70.
15. Theodorou I, Raphael M, Bigorgne C, Fourcade C, Lahet C, Cochet G, et al. Recombination pattern of the TCR gamma locus in human peripheral T-cell lymphomas. J Pathol. 1994;174(4):233–42. Epub 1994/12/01. eng.
16. Baer R, Boehm T, Yssel H, Spits H, Rabbitts TH. Complex rearrangements within the human J delta-C delta/J alpha-C alpha locus and aberrant recombination between J alpha segments. EMBO J. 1988;7(6):1661–8. Pubmed Central PMCID: 457150, Epub 1988/06/01. eng.

17. van Dongen JJ, Langerak AW, Bruggemann M, Evans PA, Hummel M, Lavender FL, et al. Design and standardization of PCR primers and protocols for detection of clonal immunoglobulin and T-cell receptor gene recombinations in suspect lymphoproliferations: report of the BIOMED-2 Concerted Action BMH4-CT98-3936. Leukemia. 2003;17(12): 2257–317. Epub 2003/12/13. eng.

18. Trainor KJ, Brisco MJ, Wan JH, Neoh S, Grist S, Morley AA. Gene rearrangement in B- and T-lymphoproliferative disease detected by the polymerase chain reaction. Blood. 1991;78(1):192–6. Epub 1991/07/01. eng.

19. Assaf C, Hummel M, Steinhoff M, Geilen CC, Orawa H, Stein H, et al. Early TCR-beta and TCR-gamma PCR detection of T-cell clonality indicates minimal tumor disease in lymph nodes of cutaneous T-cell lymphoma: diagnostic and prognostic implications. Blood. 2005;105(2):503–10.

20. van Krieken JH, Elwood L, Andrade RE, Jaffe ES, Cossman J, Medeiros LJ. Rearrangement of the T-cell receptor delta chain gene in T-cell lymphomas with a mature phenotype. Am J Pathol. 1991;139(1):161–8. Pubmed Central PMCID: 1886140, Epub 1991/07/01. eng.

21. Sprouse JT, Werling R, Hanke D, Lakey C, McDonnel L, Wood BL, et al. T-cell clonality determination using polymerase chain reaction (PCR) amplification of the T-cell receptor gamma-chain gene and capillary electrophoresis of fluorescently labeled PCR products. Am J Clin Pathol. 2000;113(6):838–50. Epub 2000/06/30. eng.

22. Wood GS, Greenberg HL. Diagnosis, staging, and monitoring of cutaneous T-cell lymphoma. Dermatol Ther. 2003;16(4):269–75.

23. Meyerson HJ. Flow cytometry for the diagnosis of mycosis fungoides. G Ital Dermatol Venereol. 2008;143(1):21–41.

24. Weiss LM, Picker LJ, Grogan TM, Warnke RA, Sklar J. Absence of clonal beta and gamma T-cell receptor gene rearrangements in a subset of peripheral T-cell lymphomas. Am J Pathol. 1988;130(3):436–42. Pubmed Central PMCID: 1880671, Epub 1988/03/01. eng.

25. Ponti R, Fierro MT, Quaglino P, Lisa B, Paola FC, Michela O, et al. TCRgamma-chain gene rearrangement by PCR-based GeneScan: diagnostic accuracy improvement and clonal heterogeneity analysis in multiple cutaneous T-cell lymphoma samples. J Invest Dermatol. 2008;128(4):1030–8. Epub 2007/11/09. eng.

26. Klemke CD, Poenitz N, Dippel E, Hummel M, Stein H, Goerdt S. T-cell clonality of undetermined significance. Arch Dermatol. 2006;142(3):393–4. Epub 2006/03/22. eng.

27. Thurber SE, Zhang B, Kim YH, Schrijver I, Zehnder J, Kohler S. T-cell clonality analysis in biopsy specimens from two different skin sites shows high specificity in the diagnosis of patients with suggested mycosis fungoides. J Am Acad Dermatol. 2007;57(5):782–90.

28. Guitart J, Magro C. Cutaneous T-cell lymphoid dyscrasia: a unifying term for idiopathic chronic dermatoses with persistent T-cell clones. Arch Dermatol. 2007;143(7):921–32.

29. Rubben A, Kempf W, Kadin ME, Zimmermann DR, Burg G. Multilineage progression of genetically unstable tumor subclones in cutaneous T-cell lymphoma. Exp Dermatol. 2004;13(8):472–83. Epub 2004/07/22. eng.

30. Bignon YJ, Souteyrand P, Roger H, Fonck Y, Bernard D, Chassagne J, et al. Clonotypic heterogeneity in cutaneous T-cell lymphomas. Cancer Res. 1990;50(20):6620–5.

31. Vega F, Luthra R, Medeiros LJ, Dunmire V, Lee SJ, Duvic M, et al. Clonal heterogeneity in mycosis fungoides and its relationship to clinical course. Blood. 2002;100(9):3369–73.

32. Morris SW, Kirstein MN, Valentine MB, Dittmer KG, Shapiro DN, Saltman DL, et al. Fusion of a kinase gene, ALK, to a nucleolar protein gene, NPM, in non-Hodgkin's lymphoma. Science. 1994;263(5151):1281–4.

33. Gould JW, Eppes RB, Gilliam AC, Goldstein JA, Mikkola DL, Zaim MT, et al. Solitary primary cutaneous CD30+ large cell lymphoma of natural killer cell phenotype bearing the t(2;5)(p23;q35) translocation and presenting in a child. Am J Dermatopathol. 2000;22(5):422–8.

34. Chuang SS, Hsieh YC, Ye H, Hwang WS. Lymphohistiocytic anaplastic large cell lymphoma involving skin: a diagnostic challenge. Pathol Res Pract. 2009;205(4):283–7.

35. Wada DA, Law ME, Hsi ED, Dicaudo DJ, Ma L, Lim MS, et al. Specificity of IRF4 translocations for primary cutaneous anaplastic large cell lymphoma: a multicenter study of 204 skin biopsies. Mod Pathol. 2011;24(4):596–605. Pubmed Central PMCID: 3122134, Epub 2010/12/21. eng.

36. Herbst H, Steinbrecher E, Niedobitek G, Young LS, Brooks L, Muller-Lantzsch N, et al. Distribution and phenotype of Epstein-Barr virus-harboring cells in Hodgkin's disease. Blood. 1992;80(2):484–91. Epub 1992/07/15. eng.

37. Kim YH, Liu HL, Mraz-Gernhard S, Varghese A, Hoppe RT. Long-term outcome of 525 patients with mycosis fungoides and Sezary syndrome: clinical prognostic factors and risk for disease progression. Arch Dermatol. 2003;139(7):857–66.

38. Ahn CS, ALSayyah A, Sangueza OP. Mycosis fungoides: an updated review of clinicopathologic variants. Am J Dermatopathol. 2014;36(12):933–48. quiz 49–51.

39. Pimpinelli N, Olsen EA, Santucci M, Vonderheid E, Haeffner AC, Stevens S, et al. Defining early mycosis fungoides. J Am Acad Dermatol. 2005;53(6):1053–63.

40. Zinzani PL, Ferreri AJ, Cerroni L. Mycosis fungoides. Crit Rev Oncol Hematol. 2008;65(2):172–82.

41. Massone C, Crisman G, Kerl H, Cerroni L. The prognosis of early mycosis fungoides is not influ-

enced by phenotype and T-cell clonality. Br J Dermatol. 2008;159(4):881–6.

42. Murphy M, Fullen D, Carlson JA. Low CD7 expression in benign and malignant cutaneous lymphocytic infiltrates: experience with an antibody reactive with paraffin-embedded tissue. Am J Dermatopathol. 2002;24(1):6–16.

43. Agnarsson BA, Vonderheid EC, Kadin ME. Cutaneous T cell lymphoma with suppressor/cytotoxic (CD8) phenotype: identification of rapidly progressive and chronic subtypes. J Am Acad Dermatol. 1990;22(4):569–77.

44. Whittam LR, Calonje E, Orchard G, Fraser-Andrews EA, Woolford A, Russell-Jones R. CD8-positive juvenile onset mycosis fungoides: an immunohistochemical and genotypic analysis of six cases. Br J Dermatol. 2000;143(6):1199–204.

45. Sawada Y, Sugita K, Kabashima R, Hino R, Nakamura M, Koga C, et al. CD8+ CD56+ mycosis fungoides with an indolent clinical behaviour: case report and literature review. Acta Derm Venereol. 2010;90(5):525–6.

46. El-Shabrawi-Caelen L, Cerroni L, Medeiros LJ, McCalmont TH. Hypopigmented mycosis fungoides: frequent expression of a CD8+ T-cell phenotype. Am J Surg Pathol. 2002;26(4):450–7.

47. Pavlovsky L, Mimouni D, Amitay-Laish I, Feinmesser M, David M, Hodak E. Hyperpigmented mycosis fungoides: an unusual variant of cutaneous T-cell lymphoma with a frequent CD8+ phenotype. J Am Acad Dermatol. 2012;67(1):69–75.

48. Dummer R, Kamarashev J, Kempf W, Haffner AC, Hess-Schmid M, Burg G. Junctional CD8+ cutaneous lymphomas with nonaggressive clinical behavior: a CD8+ variant of mycosis fungoides? Arch Dermatol. 2002;138(2):199–203.

49. Kasugai K, Yanagishita T, Takeo T, Takahashi E, Tamada Y, Matsumoto Y, et al. CD8-positive mycosis fungoides bullosa. Eur J Dermatol. 2012;22(4):563–4.

50. Ada S, Gulec AT. CD8+ poikilodermatous mycosis fungoides with a nonaggressive clinical behaviour and a good response to psoralen plus ultraviolet A treatment. Br J Dermatol. 2007;157(5):1064–6.

51. Knapp CF, Mathew R, Messina JL, Lien MH. CD4/CD8 dual-positive mycosis fungoides: a previously unrecognized variant. Am J Dermatopathol. 2012;34(3):e37–9.

52. Hodak E, David M, Maron L, Aviram A, Kaganovsky E, Feinmesser M. CD4/CD8 double-negative epidermotropic cutaneous T-cell lymphoma: an immunohistochemical variant of mycosis fungoides. J Am Acad Dermatol. 2006;55(2):276–84.

53. Nagase K, Shirai R, Okawa T, Inoue T, Misago N, Narisawa Y. CD4/CD8 double-negative mycosis fungoides mimicking erythema gyratum repens in a patient with underlying lung cancer. Acta Derm Venereol. 2014;94(1):89–90.

54. Kempf W, Kazakov DV, Cipolat C, Kutzner H, Roncador G, Tomasini D. CD4/CD8 double negative mycosis fungoides with PD-1 (CD279) expression—

a disease of follicular helper T-cells? Am J Dermatopathol. 2012;34(7):757–61.

55. Barzilai A, Goldberg I, Shibi R, Kopolovic J, Trau H. Mycosis fungoides expressing gamma/delta T-cell receptors. J Am Acad Dermatol. 1996;34(2 Pt 1):301–2.

56. Guitart J, Weisenburger DD, Subtil A, Kim E, Wood G, Duvic M, et al. Cutaneous gammadelta T-cell lymphomas: a spectrum of presentations with overlap with other cytotoxic lymphomas. Am J Surg Pathol. 2012;36(11):1656–65.

57. Wood GS, Bahler DW, Hoppe RT, Warnke RA, Sklar JL, Levy R. Transformation of mycosis fungoides: T-cell receptor beta gene analysis demonstrates a common clonal origin for plaque-type mycosis fungoides and CD30+ large-cell lymphoma. J Invest Dermatol. 1993;101(3):296–300.

58. Vermeer MH, Geelen FA, Kummer JA, Meijer CJ, Willemze R. Expression of cytotoxic proteins by neoplastic T cells in mycosis fungoides increases with progression from plaque stage to tumor stage disease. Am J Pathol. 1999;154(4):1203–10. Pubmed Central PMCID: 1866574.

59. Prince HM, Martin AG, Olsen EA, Fivenson DP, Duvic M. Denileukin diftitox for the treatment of CD25 low-expression mycosis fungoides and Sezary syndrome. Leuk Lymphoma. 2013;54(1):69–75. Pubmed Central PMCID: 3523809.

60. Magro CM, Dyrsen ME. Cutaneous lymphocyte antigen expression in benign and neoplastic cutaneous B- and T-cell lymphoid infiltrates. J Cutan Pathol. 2008;35(11):1040–9.

61. Martin B, Stefanato C, Whittaker S, Robson A. Primary cutaneous CD20-positive T-cell lymphoma. J Cutan Pathol. 2011;38(8):663–9.

62. Aung PP, Climent F, Muzzafar T, Curry JL, Patel KP, Servitje O, et al. Immunophenotypic shift of CD4 and CD8 antigen expression in primary cutaneous T-cell lymphomas: a clinicopathologic study of three cases. J Cutan Pathol. 2014;41(1):51–7.

63. Liebmann RD, Anderson B, McCarthy KP, Chow JW. The polymerase chain reaction in the diagnosis of early mycosis fungoides. J Pathol. 1997;182(3):282–7.

64. Guitart J, Camisa C, Ehrlich M, Bergfeld WF. Long-term implications of T-cell receptor gene rearrangement analysis by Southern blot in patients with cutaneous T-cell lymphoma. J Am Acad Dermatol. 2003;48(5):775–9.

65. Signoretti S, Murphy M, Cangi MG, Puddu P, Kadin ME, Loda M. Detection of clonal T-cell receptor gamma gene rearrangements in paraffin-embedded tissue by polymerase chain reaction and nonradioactive single-strand conformational polymorphism analysis. Am J Pathol. 1999;154(1):67–75. Pubmed Central PMCID: 1853445.

66. Li N, Bhawan J. New insights into the applicability of T-cell receptor gamma gene rearrangement analysis in cutaneous T-cell lymphoma. J Cutan Pathol. 2001;28(8):412–8.

67. Groenen PJ, Langerak AW, van Dongen JJ, van Krieken JH. Pitfalls in TCR gene clonality testing: teaching cases. J Hematop. 2008;1(2):97–109. Pubmed Central PMCID: 2713482, Epub 2009/08/12. eng.

68. Rijlaarsdam U, Scheffer E, Meijer CJ, Kruyswijk MR, Willemze R. Mycosis fungoides-like lesions associated with phenytoin and carbamazepine therapy. J Am Acad Dermatol. 1991;24(2 Pt 1): 216–20.

69. Ploysangam T, Breneman DL, Mutasim DF. Cutaneous pseudolymphomas. J Am Acad Dermatol. 1998;38(6 Pt 1):877–95. quiz 96-7.

70. Arps DP, Chen S, Fullen DR, Hristov AC. Selected inflammatory imitators of mycosis fungoides: histologic features and utility of ancillary studies. Arch Pathol Lab Med. 2014;138(10):1319–27.

71. Magro CM, Crowson AN, Kovatich AJ, Burns F. Drug-induced reversible lymphoid dyscrasia: a clonal lymphomatoid dermatitis of memory and activated T cells. Hum Pathol. 2003;34(2):119–29.

72. Reddy K, Bhawan J. Histologic mimickers of mycosis fungoides: a review. J Cutan Pathol. 2007;34(7):519–25.

73. Olsen EA, Rook AH, Zic J, Kim Y, Porcu P, Querfeld C, et al. Sezary syndrome: immunopathogenesis, literature review of therapeutic options, and recommendations for therapy by the United States Cutaneous Lymphoma Consortium (USCLC). J Am Acad Dermatol. 2011;64(2):352–404. Epub 2010/12/15. eng.

74. Campbell JJ, Clark RA, Watanabe R, Kupper TS. Sezary syndrome and mycosis fungoides arise from distinct T-cell subsets: a biologic rationale for their distinct clinical behaviors. Blood. 2010;116(5):767–71. Pubmed Central PMCID: 2918332.

75. Diwan AH, Prieto VG, Herling M, Duvic M, Jone D. Primary Sezary syndrome commonly shows low-grade cytologic atypia and an absence of epidermotropism. Am J Clin Pathol. 2005;123(4):510–5.

76. Cetinozman F, Jansen PM, Vermeer MH, Willemze R. Differential expression of programmed death-1 (PD-1) in Sezary syndrome and mycosis fungoides. Arch Dermatol. 2012;148(12):1379–85.

77. Beylot-Barry M, Sibaud V, Thiebaut R, Vergier B, Beylot C, Delaunay M, et al. Evidence that an identical T cell clone in skin and peripheral blood lymphocytes is an independent prognostic factor in primary cutaneous T cell lymphomas. J Invest Dermatol. 2001;117(4):920–6.

78. Delfau-Larue MH, Laroche L, Wechsler J, Lepage E, Lahet C, Asso-Bonnet M, et al. Diagnostic value of dominant T-cell clones in peripheral blood in 363 patients presenting consecutively with a clinical suspicion of cutaneous lymphoma. Blood. 2000;96(9):2987–92.

79. Dereure O, Balavoine M, Salles MT, Candon-Kerlau S, Clot J, Guilhou JJ, et al. Correlations between clinical, histologic, blood, and skin polymerase chain reaction outcome in patients treated for mycosis fungoides. J Invest Dermatol. 2003;121(3):614–7.

80. Willemze R, Beljaards RC. Spectrum of primary cutaneous CD30 (Ki-1)-positive lymphoproliferative disorders. A proposal for classification and guidelines for management and treatment. J Am Acad Dermatol. 1993;28(6):973–80.

81. Bekkenk MW, Geelen FA, van Voorst Vader PC, Heule F, Geerts ML, van Vloten WA, et al. Primary and secondary cutaneous CD30(+) lymphoproliferative disorders: a report from the Dutch Cutaneous Lymphoma Group on the long-term follow-up data of 219 patients and guidelines for diagnosis and treatment. Blood. 2000;95(12):3653–61.

82. Willemze R, Kerl H, Sterry W, Berti E, Cerroni L, Chimenti S, et al. EORTC classification for primary cutaneous lymphomas: a proposal from the Cutaneous Lymphoma Study Group of the European Organization for Research and Treatment of Cancer. Blood. 1997;90(1):354–71.

83. Saggini A, Gulia A, Argenyi Z, Fink-Puches R, Lissia A, Magana M, et al. A variant of lymphomatoid papulosis simulating primary cutaneous aggressive epidermotropic CD8+ cytotoxic T-cell lymphoma. Description of 9 cases. Am J Surg Pathol. 2010;34(8):1168–75.

84. McQuitty E, Curry JL, Tetzlaff MT, Prieto VG, Duvic M, Torres-Cabala C. The differential diagnosis of CD8-positive ("type D") lymphomatoid papulosis. J Cutan Pathol. 2014;41(2):88–100.

85. Wu WM, Tsai HJ. Lymphomatoid papulosis histopathologically simulating angiocentric and cytotoxic T-cell lymphoma: a case report. Am J Dermatopathol. 2004;26(2):133–5.

86. Kempf W, Kazakov DV, Scharer L, Rutten A, Mentzel T, Paredes BE, et al. Angioinvasive lymphomatoid papulosis: a new variant simulating aggressive lymphomas. Am J Surg Pathol. 2013;37(1):1–13.

87. Pierard GE, Ackerman AB, Lapiere CM. Follicular lymphomatoid papulosis. Am J Dermatopathol. 1980;2(2):173–80.

88. Kempf W, Kazakov DV, Baumgartner HP, Kutzner H. Follicular lymphomatoid papulosis revisited: a study of 11 cases, with new histopathological findings. J Am Acad Dermatol. 2013;68(5):809–16.

89. Mann KP, Hall B, Kamino H, Borowitz MJ, Ratech H. Neutrophil-rich, Ki-1-positive anaplastic large-cell malignant lymphoma. Am J Surg Pathol. 1995;19(4):407–16.

90. Cardoso J, Duhra P, Thway Y, Calonje E. Lymphomatoid papulosis type D: a newly described variant easily confused with cutaneous aggressive CD8-positive cytotoxic T-cell lymphoma. Am J Dermatopathol. 2012;34(7):762–5.

91. Martinez-Escala ME, Sidiropoulos M, Deonizio J, Gerami P, Kadin ME, Guitart J. gammadelta T-cell-rich variants of pityriasis lichenoides and lymphomatoid papulosis: benign cutaneous disorders to be distinguished from aggressive cutaneous gammad-

elta T-cell lymphomas. Br J Dermatol. 2015;172(2):372–9.

92. de Bruin PC, Beljaards RC, van Heerde P, Van Der Valk P, Noorduyn LA, Van Krieken JH, et al. Differences in clinical behaviour and immunophenotype between primary cutaneous and primary nodal anaplastic large cell lymphoma of T-cell or null cell phenotype. Histopathology. 1993;23(2):127–35.

93. ten Berge RL, Oudejans JJ, Ossenkoppele GJ, Pulford K, Willemze R, Falini B, et al. ALK expression in extranodal anaplastic large cell lymphoma favours systemic disease with (primary) nodal involvement and a good prognosis and occurs before dissemination. J Clin Pathol. 2000;53(6):445–50. Pubmed Central PMCID: 1731216.

94. ten Berge RL, Snijdewint FG, von Mensdorff-Pouilly S, Poort-Keesom RJ, Oudejans JJ, Meijer JW, et al. MUC1 (EMA) is preferentially expressed by ALK positive anaplastic large cell lymphoma, in the normally glycosylated or only partly hypoglycosylated form. J Clin Pathol. 2001;54(12):933–9. Pubmed Central PMCID: 1731330.

95. Greisser J, Palmedo G, Sander C, Kutzner H, Kazakov DV, Roos M, et al. Detection of clonal rearrangement of T-cell receptor genes in the diagnosis of primary cutaneous CD30 lymphoproliferative disorders. J Cutan Pathol. 2006;33(11):711–5.

96. Zackheim HS, Jones C, Leboit PE, Kashani-Sabet M, McCalmont TH, Zehnder J. Lymphomatoid papulosis associated with mycosis fungoides: a study of 21 patients including analyses for clonality. J Am Acad Dermatol. 2003;49(4):620–3.

97. Chott A, Vonderheid EC, Olbricht S, Miao NN, Balk SP, Kadin ME. The dominant T cell clone is present in multiple regressing skin lesions and associated T cell lymphomas of patients with lymphomatoid papulosis. J Invest Dermatol. 1996;106(4):696–700.

98. de la Garza Bravo MM, Patel KP, Loghavi S, Curry JL, Torres Cabala CA, Cason RC, et al. Shared clonality in distinctive lesions of lymphomatoid papulosis and mycosis fungoides occurring in the same patients suggests a common origin. Hum Pathol. 2015;46(4):558–69.

99. DeCoteau JF, Butmarc JR, Kinney MC, Kadin ME. The t(2;5) chromosomal translocation is not a common feature of primary cutaneous CD30+ lymphoproliferative disorders: comparison with anaplastic large-cell lymphoma of nodal origin. Blood. 1996;87(8):3437–41.

100. Karai LJ, Kadin ME, Hsi ED, Sluzevich JC, Ketterling RP, Knudson RA, et al. Chromosomal rearrangements of 6p25.3 define a new subtype of lymphomatoid papulosis. Am J Surg Pathol. 2013;37(8):1173–81.

101. Gonzalez CL, Medeiros LJ, Braziel RM, Jaffe ES. T-cell lymphoma involving subcutaneous tissue. A clinicopathologic entity commonly associated with hemophagocytic syndrome. Am J Surg Pathol. 1991;15(1):17–27.

102. Willemze R, Jansen PM, Cerroni L, Berti E, Santucci M, Assaf C, et al. Subcutaneous panniculitis-like T-cell lymphoma: definition, classification, and prognostic factors: an EORTC Cutaneous Lymphoma Group Study of 83 cases. Blood. 2008;111(2):838–45. Epub 2007/10/16. eng.

103. Hastrup N, Ralfkiaer E, Pallesen G. Aberrant phenotypes in peripheral T cell lymphomas. J Clin Pathol. 1989;42(4):398–402. Pubmed Central PMCID: 1141912.

104. Yao X, Teruya-Feldstein J, Raffeld M, Sorbara L, Jaffe ES. Peripheral T-cell lymphoma with aberrant expression of CD79a and CD20: a diagnostic pitfall. Mod Pathol. 2001;14(2):105–10.

105. Quintanilla-Martinez L, Fend F, Moguel LR, Spilove L, Beaty MW, Kingma DW, et al. Peripheral T-cell lymphoma with Reed-Sternberg-like cells of B-cell phenotype and genotype associated with Epstein-Barr virus infection. Am J Surg Pathol. 1999;23(10):1233–40.

106. Tan BT, Warnke RA, Arber DA. The frequency of B- and T-cell gene rearrangements and epstein-barr virus in T-cell lymphomas: a comparison between angioimmunoblastic T-cell lymphoma and peripheral T-cell lymphoma, unspecified with and without associated B-cell proliferations. J Mol Diagn. 2006;8(4):466–75. Pubmed Central PMCID: 1867616, quiz 527.

107. Berti E, Tomasini D, Vermeer MH, Meijer CJ, Alessi E, Willemze R. Primary cutaneous CD8-positive epidermotropic cytotoxic T cell lymphomas. A distinct clinicopathological entity with an aggressive clinical behavior. Am J Pathol. 1999;155(2):483–92. Pubmed Central PMCID: 1866866.

108. Introcaso CE, Kim EJ, Gardner J, Junkins-Hopkins JM, Vittorio CC, Rook AH. CD8+ epidermotropic cytotoxic T-cell lymphoma with peripheral blood and central nervous system involvement. Arch Dermatol. 2008;144(8):1027–9.

109. Santucci M, Pimpinelli N, Massi D, Kadin ME, Meijer CJ, Muller-Hermelink HK, et al. Cytotoxic/natural killer cell cutaneous lymphomas. Report of EORTC Cutaneous Lymphoma Task Force Workshop. Cancer. 2003;97(3):610–27.

110. Toro JR, Beaty M, Sorbara L, Turner ML, White J, Kingma DW, et al. gamma delta T-cell lymphoma of the skin: a clinical, microscopic, and molecular study. Arch Dermatol. 2000;136(8):1024–32.

111. Toro JR, Liewehr DJ, Pabby N, Sorbara L, Raffeld M, Steinberg SM, et al. Gamma-delta T-cell phenotype is associated with significantly decreased survival in cutaneous T-cell lymphoma. Blood. 2003;101(9):3407–12.

112. Massone C, Chott A, Metze D, Kerl K, Citarella L, Vale E, et al. Subcutaneous, blastic natural killer (NK), NK/T-cell, and other cytotoxic lymphomas of the skin: a morphologic, immunophenotypic, and molecular study of 50 patients. Am J Surg Pathol. 2004;28(6):719–35.

113. Jones D, Vega F, Sarris AH, Medeiros LJ. CD4-CD8-"Double-negative" cutaneous T-cell lymphomas share common histologic features and an aggressive clinical course. Am J Surg Pathol. 2002;26(2):225–31.

114. Kempf W, Kazakov DV, Scheidegger PE, Schlaak M, Tantcheva-Poor I. Two cases of primary cutaneous lymphoma with a gamma/delta+ phenotype and an indolent course: further evidence of heterogeneity of cutaneous gamma/delta+ T-cell lymphomas. Am J Dermatopathol. 2014;36(7):570–7.

115. Beltraminelli H, Leinweber B, Kerl H, Cerroni L. Primary cutaneous CD4+ small-/medium-sized pleomorphic T-cell lymphoma: a cutaneous nodular proliferation of pleomorphic T lymphocytes of undetermined significance? A study of 136 cases. Am J Dermatopathol. 2009;31(4):317–22.

116. Garcia-Herrera A, Colomo L, Camos M, Carreras J, Balague O, Martinez A, et al. Primary cutaneous small/medium CD4+ T-cell lymphomas: a heterogeneous group of tumors with different clinicopathologic features and outcome. J Clin Oncol. 2008;26(20):3364–71.

117. Rodriguez Pinilla SM, Roncador G, Rodriguez-Peralto JL, Mollejo M, Garcia JF, Montes-Moreno S, et al. Primary cutaneous CD4+ small/medium-sized pleomorphic T-cell lymphoma expresses follicular T-cell markers. Am J Surg Pathol. 2009;33(1):81–90.

118. Chan JKCQ-ML, Ferry JA, Peh SC. Extranodal NK/T-cell lymphoma, nasal-type. In: Swerdlow SHCE, Harris NL, et al., editors. WHO classification of tumours of haematopoietic and lymphoid tissues. Lyon: IARC Press; 2008. p. 285–8.

119. Jaffe ES. Nasal and nasal-type T/NK cell lymphoma: a unique form of lymphoma associated with the Epstein-Barr virus. Histopathology. 1995;27(6):581–3.

120. Arber DA, Weiss LM, Albujar PF, Chen YY, Jaffe ES. Nasal lymphomas in Peru. High incidence of T-cell immunophenotype and Epstein-Barr virus infection. Am J Surg Pathol. 1993;17(4):392–9. Epub 1993/04/01. eng.

121. Chan JK. Natural killer cell neoplasms. Anat Pathol. 1998;3:77–145. Epub 1999/07/02. eng.

122. Au WY, Weisenburger DD, Intragumtornchai T, Nakamura S, Kim WS, Sng I, et al. Clinical differences between nasal and extranasal natural killer/T-cell lymphoma: a study of 136 cases from the International Peripheral T-Cell Lymphoma Project. Blood. 2009;113(17):3931–7. Epub 2008/11/26. eng.

123. Liao JB, Chuang SS, Chen HC, Tseng HH, Wang JS, Hsieh PP. Clinicopathologic analysis of cutaneous lymphoma in Taiwan: a high frequency of extranodal natural killer/t-cell lymphoma, nasal type, with an extremely poor prognosis. Arch Pathol Lab Med. 2010;134(7):996–1002.

124. Jaffe ES, Chan JK, Su IJ, Frizzera G, Mori S, Feller AC, et al. Report of the Workshop on Nasal and Related Extranodal Angiocentric T/Natural Killer Cell Lymphomas. Definitions, differential diagnosis, and epidemiology. Am J Surg Pathol. 1996;20(1):103–11.

125. Ohshima K, Suzumiya J, Shimazaki K, Kato A, Tanaka T, Kanda M, et al. Nasal T/NK cell lymphomas commonly express perforin and Fas ligand: important mediators of tissue damage. Histopathology. 1997;31(5):444–50.

126. Natkunam Y, Smoller BR, Zehnder JL, Dorfman RF, Warnke RA. Aggressive cutaneous NK and NK-like T-cell lymphomas: clinicopathologic, immunohistochemical, and molecular analyses of 12 cases. Am J Surg Pathol. 1999;23(5):571–81.

127. Rodriguez J, Romaguera JE, Manning J, Ordonez N, Ha C, Ravandi F, et al. Nasal-type T/NK lymphomas: a clinicopathologic study of 13 cases. Leuk Lymphoma. 2000;39(1-2):139–44.

128. Gaal K, Sun NC, Hernandez AM, Arber DA. Sinonasal NK/T-cell lymphomas in the United States. Am J Surg Pathol. 2000;24(11):1511–7. Epub 2000/11/15. eng.

129. Lin CW, Lee WH, Chang CL, Yang JY, Hsu SM. Restricted killer cell immunoglobulin-like receptor repertoire without T-cell receptor gamma rearrangement supports a true natural killer-cell lineage in a subset of sinonasal lymphomas. Am J Pathol. 2001;159(5):1671–9. Pubmed Central PMCID: 1867044, Epub 2001/11/07. eng.

130. Kohler S, Iwatsuki K, Jaffe ES, Chan JKC. Extranodal NK/T-cell lymphoma, nasal type. In: LeBoit PEBG, Weedon D, Sarasin A, editors. Pathology and genetics of skin tumors. Lyon: IARC Press; 2006. p. 191–2.

131. Barrionuevo C, Anderson VM, Zevallos-Giampietri E, Zaharia M, Misad O, Bravo F, et al. Hydroa-like cutaneous T-cell lymphoma: a clinicopathologic and molecular genetic study of 16 pediatric cases from Peru. Appl Immunohistochem Mol Morphol. 2002;10(1):7–14.

132. Iwatsuki K, Ohtsuka M, Akiba H, Kaneko F. Atypical hydroa vacciniforme in childhood: from a smoldering stage to Epstein-Barr virus-associated lymphoid malignancy. J Am Acad Dermatol. 1999;40(2 Pt 1):283–4. Epub 1999/02/20. eng.

133. Iwatsuki K, Satoh M, Yamamoto T, Oono T, Morizane S, Ohtsuka M, et al. Pathogenic link between hydroa vacciniforme and Epstein-Barr virus-associated hematologic disorders. Arch Dermatol. 2006;142(5):587–95. Epub 2006/05/17. eng.

134. Rodriguez-Pinilla SM, Barrionuevo C, Garcia J, Martinez MT, Pajares R, Montes-Moreno S, et al. EBV-associated cutaneous NK/T-cell lymphoma: review of a series of 14 cases from peru in children and young adults. Am J Surg Pathol. 2010;34(12):1773–82.

135. Magana M, Sangueza P, Gil-Beristain J, Sanchez-Sosa S, Salgado A, Ramon G, et al. Angiocentric cutaneous T-cell lymphoma of childhood (hydroa-like lymphoma): a distinctive type of cutaneous T-cell lymphoma. J Am Acad Dermatol. 1998;38(4):574–9.

136. Yamamoto T, Tsuji K, Suzuki D, Morizane S, Iwatsuki K. A novel, noninvasive diagnostic probe for hydroa vacciniforme and related disorders: detection of latency-associated Epstein-Barr virus transcripts in the crusts. J Microbiol Methods. 2007;68(2):403–7.

137. Tokura YJE, Sander CA. Cutaneous adult T-cell leukaemia/lymphoma. In: LeBoit PE, Burg G, Weedon D, Sarasin A, editors. Pathology and genetics of skin tumors. Lyon: IARC Press; 2006. p. 189–90.

138. Yagi H, Takigawa M, Hashizume H. Cutaneous type of adult T cell leukemia/lymphoma: a new entity among cutaneous lymphomas. J Dermatol. 2003;30(9):641–3.

139. Shimoyama M. Diagnostic criteria and classification of clinical subtypes of adult T-cell leukaemia-lymphoma. A report from the Lymphoma Study Group (1984-87). Br J Haematol. 1991;79(3):428–37.

140. Tsukasaki K, Hermine O, Bazarbachi A, Ratner L, Ramos JC, Harrington Jr W, et al. Definition, prognostic factors, treatment, and response criteria of adult T-cell leukemia-lymphoma: a proposal from an international consensus meeting. J Clin Oncol. 2009;27(3):453–9. Pubmed Central PMCID: 2737379, Epub 2008/12/10. eng.

141. Chuang SS. Cutaneous non-MF T-cell and NK-cell lymphoproliferative disorders. In: Murphy MJ, editor. Molecular diagnostics in dermatology and dermatopathology. New York: Humana Press; 2011. p. 241–2.

142. Weiss LM, Jaffe ES, Liu XF, Chen YY, Shibata D, Medeiros LJ. Detection and localization of Epstein-Barr viral genomes in angioimmunoblastic lymphadenopathy and angioimmunoblastic lymphadenopathy-like lymphoma. Blood. 1992;79(7):1789–95.

143. Wagner HJ, Bein G, Bitsch A, Kirchner H. Detection and quantification of latently infected B lymphocytes in Epstein-Barr virus-seropositive, healthy individuals by polymerase chain reaction. J Clin Microbiol. 1992;30(11):2826–9. Pubmed Central PMCID: 270536.

144. Botros N, Cerroni L, Shawwa A, Green PJ, Greer W, Pasternak S, et al. Cutaneous manifestations of angioimmunoblastic T-cell lymphoma: clinical and pathological characteristics. Am J Dermatopathol. 2015;37(4):274–83.

145. Martel P, Laroche L, Courville P, Larroche C, Wechsler J, Lenormand B, et al. Cutaneous involvement in patients with angioimmunoblastic lymphadenopathy with dysproteinemia: a clinical, immunohistological, and molecular analysis. Arch Dermatol. 2000;136(7):881–6.

146. Dupuis J, Boye K, Martin N, Copie-Bergman C, Plonquet A, Fabiani B, et al. Expression of CXCL13 by neoplastic cells in angioimmunoblastic T-cell lymphoma (AITL): a new diagnostic marker providing evidence that AITL derives from follicular helper T cells. Am J Surg Pathol. 2006;30(4):490–4.

147. Brown HA, Macon WR, Kurtin PJ, Gibson LE. Cutaneous involvement by angioimmunoblastic T-cell lymphoma with remarkable heterogeneous Epstein-Barr virus expression. J Cutan Pathol. 2001;28(8):432–8.

148. Balaraman B, Conley JA, Sheinbein DM. Evaluation of cutaneous angioimmunoblastic T-cell lymphoma. J Am Acad Dermatol. 2011;65(4):855–62.

Immunohistology of Leukemia Cutis and Histiocytic Tumors

Maria Teresa Fernández Figueras, Gustavo Tapia, José Luis Mate, and Aurelio Ariza

Introduction

The diseases studied in this chapter constitute a heterogeneous group of lesions that range from reactive conditions to highly aggressive neoplasms. These entities have been grouped into two main sections. The first one deals with myeloproliferative neoplasms and includes mastocytosis as well, since even in cases of mastocytosis with clinical symptoms seemingly limited to the skin a potential systemic involvement should be investigated. Also in the first section, leukemia cutis and myeloid sarcoma have been put together due to the considerable overlap of these two entities. The second group includes conditions caused by proliferation of dendritic cells such as Langerhans cell histiocytosis, Langerhans cell sarcoma, and indeterminate dendritic cell tumor. Then, the chapter deals with macrophage-related diseases, including juvenile xanthogranuloma and related diseases, hemophagocytic lymphohistiocytosis, multicentric reticulohistiocytosis, reticulohistiocytoma, Rosai-Dorfman disease, cutaneous Kikuchi-Fujimoto disease, and cutaneous intralymphatic histiocytosis. Multicentric reticulohistiocytosis and solitary reticulohistiocytoma, also known as solitary epithelioid histiocytoma, have been considered separately since despite their sharing many microscopical and immunohistochemical features they are distinct entities with striking clinical differences. Multicentric reticulohistiocytosis can involve extracutaneous locations and is frequently associated with a rheumatological disease, whereas solitary reticulohistiocytoma seems to be tumoral in nature. Finally, the malignant histiocytic and dendritic cell sarcomas include histiocytic sarcoma, follicular dendritic cell sarcoma, and interdigitating dendritic cell sarcoma. During the elaboration of this book, a revised classification of histiocytoses and neoplasms of the macrophage-dendritic cell lineages has been proposed (Blood 2016;127:2672–81). The authors divide the histiocytosis into five groups: (1) Langerhans-related histiocytosis, (2) cutaneous and muco-cutaneous histiocytosis, (3) malignant histiocytoses, (4) Rosai-Dorfman disease, and (5) haemophagocytic lymphohistiocytosis and macrophage activation syndrome. In addition, they include Erdheim–Chester disease among the group of Langerhans cell histiocytosis. This recent proposal of a new paradigm shows how dynamic this field continues to be.

M.T.F. Figueras, M.D. (✉) • G. Tapia, M.D.
J.L. Mate, M.D. • A. Ariza, M.D.
Department of Pathology, Hospital Universitari Germans Trias i Pujol, Universitat Autònoma de Barcelona, Badalona, Barcelona 08916, Spain
e-mail: maiteffig@gmail.com

© Springer International Publishing Switzerland 2016
J.A. Plaza, V.G. Prieto (eds.), *Applied Immunohistochemistry in the Evaluation of Skin Neoplasms*, DOI 10.1007/978-3-319-30590-5_11

Myeloproliferative Neoplasms and Leukemic Infiltrates

Leukemia Cutis/Myeloid Sarcoma

Leukemia cutis (LC) is defined as skin infiltration by lymphoid or myeloid malignant cells [1]. According to the World Health Organization (WHO), the term myeloid sarcoma (MS) is used when the infiltrate consists of myeloid blasts, with or without maturation, and the lesion presents as a tumor mass effacing normal tissue architecture [2]. MS has also been designated as granulocytic sarcoma and chloroma. In this chapter, we will focus on myeloid LC (MLC) and MS.

Regarding lymphocytic leukemias, the percentage of LC largely depends on the leukemia subtype. Skin involvement is frequent in T-cell prolymphocytic leukemia and adult T-cell leukemia/lymphoma, often as the first manifestation of the disease [3, 4]. In contrast, B-cell chronic lymphocytic leukemia, the most common form of leukemia in adults, seldom involves the skin, although LC may be the first manifestation in rare instances [5–7].

With regard to myeloid leukemias, skin infiltration occurs in 2–20 % overall. Most cases correspond to acute myeloid leukemias (AMLs), especially those with monocytic differentiation (M4 and M5 subtypes of the FAB classification), followed by chronic myelomonocytic leukemia (CMML) [8–10]. Myelodysplastic neoplasms (MDNs) and myeloproliferative neoplasms (MPNs) rarely infiltrate the skin and, when they do, it is often a reflection of disease progression [11, 12]. MLC is more frequent in pediatric than adult leukemias and may also develop in association with congenital leukemia [13].

In regard to the underlying hematologic disease, three main onset forms of skin infiltration have been described. MLC develops in patients with a known hematologic malignancy in about 65 % of cases, in some of which it represents disease progression or relapse. In up to 28 % of cases MLC appears at the time the myeloid disorder is diagnosed and the cutaneous lesions may be the initial sign leading to the leukemia diagnosis. Finally, in about 7 % of patients MLC is found in the absence of any underlying hematologic malignancy, the terms "aleukemic LC" and "aleukemic MS" having been used in these cases [1, 8, 14].

Clinically, MLC usually presents as multiple, infiltrated plaques and/or nodules of red-brown or violaceous appearance. Solitary lesions account for less than one-third of cases. Distribution of lesions varies among different reports, the regions more often involved being the scalp, trunk, and extremities (Fig. 11.1).

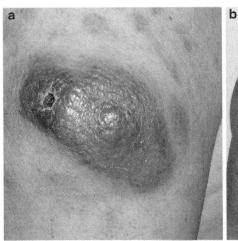 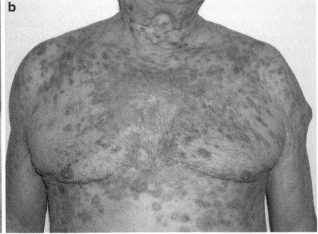

Fig. 11.1 (a) Violaceous, tumoral nodule surrounded by erythematous macules in the arm of a patient with acute myeloid leukemia. (b) Multiple brown, infiltrated macules in the trunk of a patient with leukemia cutis (Courtesy of Dr. JM Carrascosa, Dpt. of Dermatology, Hospital Germans Trias i Pujol, Badalona, Spain)

Leukemic gingival hyperplasia and oral lesions are particularly frequent in AML with monocytic differentiation [1, 8]. Unusual presentations include hyperpigmentation [15], fingertip hypertrophy [16], facial erythema [17], vasculitis [18], and drug-like eruption [19]. Nonleukemic cutaneous manifestations, referred to as "leukemids," are frequent and may be due to drug reaction, opportunistic infection, or cytopenias [8].

Morphologic evaluation of skin biopsies shows a dermal, nodular or diffuse, interstitial infiltration of immature myeloid cells, often with perivascular and periadnexal accentuation. The infiltrate density is very variable (Figs. 11.2 and 11.3). In some cases, an "Indian-file"-like pattern between collagen bundles may be seen (Fig. 11.4). The subcutaneous fat is frequently infiltrated. A Grenz zone is appreciated between the lesion and the typically uninvolved epidermis, although epidermal ulceration may be seen in some cases. Mitotic figures and apoptotic bodies are frequent [1, 8–10]. The myeloid cell infiltrate composition depends largely on the leukemia subtype, there being a morphologic correlation between bone marrow and peripheral blood findings. Thus, in FAB AML M1 and M2 subtypes, myeloblasts and immature myeloid cells are the predominant cell components; in FAB M4 and M5 subtypes, the infiltrate shows a monocytic morphology, with oval- or kidney-shaped blast cells; and in CMML, MDS, and MPN the infiltrate is heterogeneous, with blast cells intermingled with mature granulocytes, eosinophils, and mast cells [1, 8]. Aleukemic forms of LC are associated with an aggressive histology including high mitotic indeces, apoptotic bodies, and highly dense, diffuse patterns of infiltration (Fig. 11.5) [8].

Vasculitis [18], abundant giant cells [20], granuloma annulare-like [8], and Sweet-like patterns [21] are among the rare morphologic manifestations described in LC.

Immunohistochemistry

Even though several studies have found some bone marrow and skin discrepancies concerning myeloid neoplastic cells immunophenotypes, immunohistochemistry plays a pivotal role in the diagnosis of myeloid LC. The most sensitive markers are CD68, lysozyme, CD43, and CD33, which are expressed in nearly all LC instances. Myeloperoxidase, found in just half of the cases, is less useful. CD34 and CD117, both immature myeloid cell markers, are immunoreactive in less than one-third of cases, in contrast to their common positivity in the bone marrow. Importantly, CD4, CD56, and C123 may be positive in some cases, raising the possibility of a blastic plasmacytoid dendritic cell neoplasm (BPDCN). Other immunohistochemical stains found in a variable proportion of cases include CD163, CD14, CD11c, CD45, and CD15. B-cell (CD20, PAX5, CD79) and T-cell (CD2, CD3, CD5) markers are negative [8, 10, 22–25].

Molecular Biology

Molecular biology techniques play an important role in the diagnosis, differential diagnosis, and prognostic evaluation of MLC. Molecular or chromosomal alterations may be demonstrated in about 50 % of cases, and closely mirror those found in their leukemic counterpart [26–28]. An increased incidence of aneuploidy of chromosome 8 has been repeatedly reported [29, 30].

Differential Diagnosis

Differential diagnosis of MLC includes B-cell lymphomas (especially diffuse large B-cell lymphoma), T-cell lymphomas (especially anaplastic large cell lymphoma and lymphomatoid papulosis), Merkel cell carcinoma, metastatic carcinoma, melanoma, and BPDCN. B-cell and T-cell malignancies express B-cell (CD20, CD79 and PAX5) or T-cell (CD2, CD3, and CD5) lineage-specific markers, frequently show clonal immunoglobulin or T-cell receptor genes, and are negative for myeloid markers. Merkel cell carcinoma and metastatic carcinoma may be excluded with the aid of cytokeratin and S100-protein immunostains, respectively.

Distinction between BPDCN and MLC may be very difficult, as both diseases share morphological and immunohistochemical properties. Moreover, the presence of blastic plasmacytic cells has been described in MLC lesions. Differential diagnosis between these entities is

Fig. 11.2 Two examples of leukemia cutis. (**a–c**) A case showing mild perivascular infiltration (**a**, Hematoxilin-Eosin; 40×) of blastic leukemic cells (**c**, Hematoxilin-eosin; 400×). (**b–d**) In this case the infiltration is more dense, with perivascular nodules of neoplastic cells (**b**, Hematoxilin-eosin; 40× and 100×)

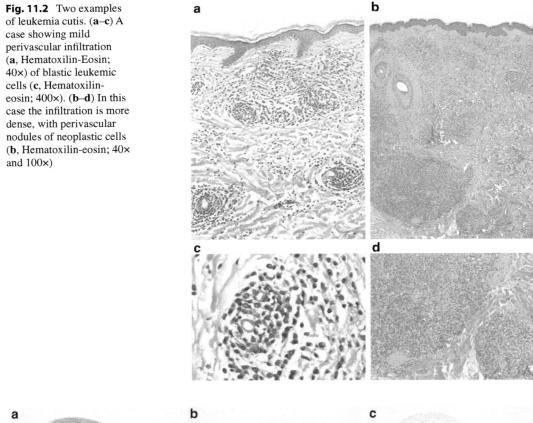

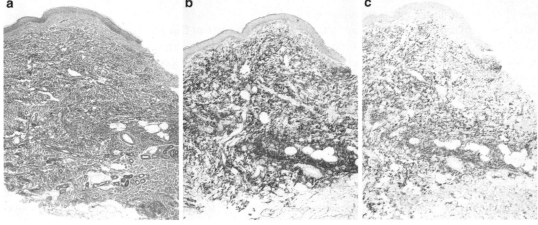

Fig. 11.3 Myeloid leukemia cutis showing interstitial and perivascular infiltration (**a**, Hematoxilin-eosin; 40×). Neoplastic cells are positive for lysozyme (**b**; 40×) and CD68 (**c**, 40×)

further *discussed* in the description of BPDCN [24, 25].

Immunohistochemistry-based diagnostic algorithms have been proposed [1, 23].

Clues and Pitfalls

- Consider the diagnosis of MLC in any infil-trate of blast-appearing cells, even in patients with unknown hematologic malignancy. The

Fig. 11.4 Infiltration by leukemic cells among collagen bundles with an "Indian-file"-like pattern [Hematoxilin-eosin (**a**) and CD68 immunostain (**b**); 200×]

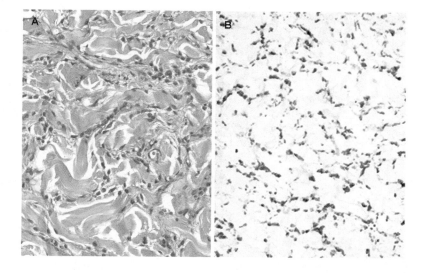

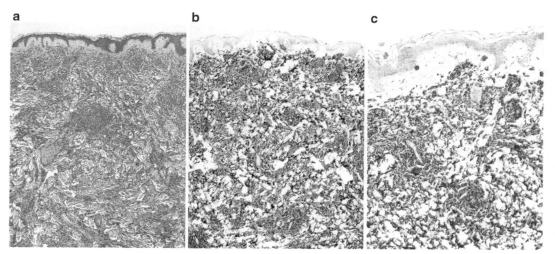

Fig. 11.5 Myeloid sarcoma showing a dense, diffuse infiltrate of leukemic cells in the dermis without epidermal involvement (**a**) (Hematoxilin-eosin; 40×). The cells are positive for CD33 (**b**; 40×) and myeloperoxidase (**c**; 100×)

initial immunohistochemical panel should include CD68, lysozyme, or CD43.

- Expression of CD4, CD56, CD123, or other blastic plasmacytoid dendritic cell-associated markers may be seen in a variable proportion of MLC cases. Consider the differential diagnosis with BPDCN.
- MLC has been seen in patients with suspected diagnosis of Sweet syndrome, especially the histiocytoid variant described by Requena et al. Thus, when a diagnosis of histiocytoid Sweet syndrome is being considered, addi-

tional immunohistochemical and /or molecular studies should be performed in order to exclude MLC [21, 31].

Blastic Plasmacytoid Dendritic Cell Neoplasm

Blastic plasmacytoid dendritic cell neoplasm (BPDCN) is an aggressive hematological tumor produced by the clonal proliferation of immature plasmacytoid dendritic cells (PDCs) (professional

Fig. 11.6 Erythematous macule on the scalp with a nodular, hyperkeratotic area

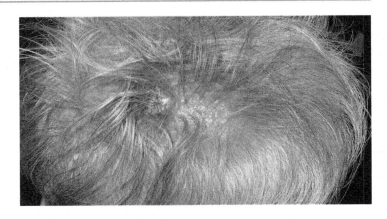

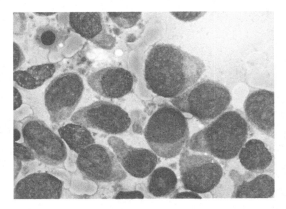

Fig. 11.7 Bone marrow aspirate shows infiltration by blast cells with fine chromatin and abundant, peripheral cytoplasm (May-Grünwald-Giemsa, 1000×)

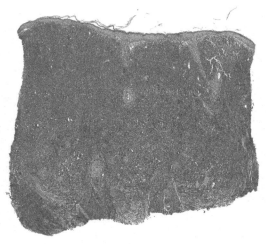

Fig. 11.8 Panoramic view of a nodular skin lesion. Blast cells diffusely infiltrate the dermis, without epidermal involvement (Hematoxilin-eosin, 20×)

type-1 interferon-producing cells) [32]. The uncertainties about BPDCN histogenesis had for the last 20 years are reflected in the variety of terms used to define this entity, including "agranular CD4+ natural killer (NK) cell leukemia" [33], "blastic NK cell leukemia/lymphoma" [34] and "CD4+ CD56+ hematodermic neoplasm/tumor" [35]. BPDCN is classified as an acute myeloid leukemia in the current 2008 World Health Organization (WHO) classification of tumors of hematopoietic and lymphoid tissues [32].

BPDCN shows a male/female ratio of 2–3:1. Most patients are older adults, with a mean age between 60 and 70 years, although BPDCN may occur at any age [36]. Patients usually show localized or disseminated cutaneous manifestations, such as nodules, bruise-like lesions, or erythematous plaques (Fig. 11.6). Lymphadenopathies, bone marrow, and peripheral blood involvement is

common at diagnosis, and it invariably develops during disease's progression (Fig. 11.7) [36, 37]. A relationship with myeloid and myelomonocytic leukemia has been reported in 10–20 % of cases [38, 39].

Skin lesions typically show a monomorphic infiltration of medium-sized blast cells with irregular nuclei, fine chromatin, one to three small nucleoli, and scanty cytoplasm devoid of granulation. The infiltration is diffuse and dense in nodular lesions and perivascular with scattered nodules in bruise-like and plaque lesions. The epidermis is uninvolved, with a Grenz zone, and the subcutaneous fat may be infiltrated as the neoplasm progresses (Figs. 11.8 and 11.9). Angioinvasion/

angiodestruction and coagulative necrosis are absent. Mitotic activity is variable, but usually not prominent [36–38].

Immunohistochemistry

Neoplastic cells coexpress CD4, CD56, CD45RA, CD43, and PDC-related antigens such as CD123, T-cell leukemia-1 (TCL1) [40], cutaneous lymphocyte-associated antigen (CLA) [41], interferon α-dependent molecule MxA, blood dendritic cell antigen 2 (BDCA2/CD303) [42], Spi-B transcription factor [43], CD2-associated protein (CD2AP) and BCL11A, among others [44]. However, up to 50 % of cases show an incomplete dendritic cell phenotype (Fig. 11.10) [36].

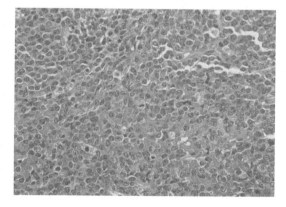

Fig. 11.9 The blasts are medium-sized, with fine chromatin, small nucleoli, and moderate cytoplasm without granulation (Hematoxilin-eosin, 200×)

BPDCN is negative for lineage-specific markers of B cells (CD20, CD79, and CD19), T cells (CD3 and CD5), myeloid and monocytic cells (myeloperoxidase, CD15, CD13, CD14, and lysozyme), with the exception of CD33 and CD7. Interestingly, terminal deoxynucleotidyl transferase (TdT) is positive in up to one third of cases while the hematopoietic precursor cell markers CD34 and CD117 are consistently negative. Epstein–Barr virus-encoded small RNAs (EBERs) are negative [36, 39, 42, 44].

Although this neoplasm definition was based on CD4 and CD56 positivity, negativity for CD4 or CD56 has been reported in rare instances [36]. This negative result does not exclude the diagnosis of BPDCN, if the remaining characteristics and phenotype are present. According to the WHO 2008 criteria, cases that share some, but not all, immunophenotypic markers with PDCs should be better classified as "acute leukemia of ambiguous lineage" [32].

Molecular Biology

T-cell and B-cell receptor genes are usually germline in most cases [6]. Karyotypic analysis and array-based comparative genomic hybridization have shown multiple genetic alterations in two-thirds of cases, mostly deletions on chromosomes 5q, 12p, 13q, 6q, 15q, 7p 9p, and 9q [45, 46]. Gene-expression profiling studies have found canonical activation of NFkB pathway [47] and

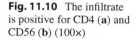

Fig. 11.10 The infiltrate is positive for CD4 (**a**) and CD56 (**b**) (100×)

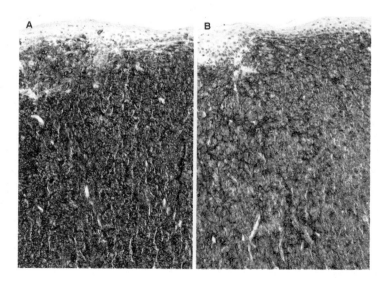

next-generation sequencing approaches have evidenced mutations in several genes including TET2, IKZF3, and ZEB2 [48, 49]. However, none of these genetic abnormalities are specific for BPDCN and may be detected in other hematological malignancies.

Differential Diagnosis

The differential diagnosis of BPDCN is broad and includes T acute lymphoblastic leukemia/lymphoma (T-ALL), acute myeloid leukemia/myeloid sarcoma (AML/MS), cutaneous T/NK cell nasal-type lymphoma and Langerhans cell histiocytosis. Careful clinical evaluation and extensive immunophenotypic analysis is required, as immunophenotypic overlap with these neoplasms is frequent.

Expression of cytoplasmic CD3 and CD34 and T-cell receptor clonal rearrangement are helpful features to differentiate T-ALL from BPDCN, while TdT is not useful in this setting. T/NK cell nasal-type lymphomas are CD56+ and may occasionally express CD4, but neoplastic cells are rather pleomorphic, angioinvasion and necrosis are frequent, cells express cytoplasmic CD3 and TIA-1 and, importantly, are EBER positive, which excludes BPDCN [50]. Langerhans cell histiocytosis may exhibit a blastic morphology, expresses CD4 and CD56 and may be CD123-positive, but the correct diagnosis must be made with the aid of appropriate markers (S100, CD1a, and langerin) [51]. Differential diagnosis with AML/MS may be challenging, since cases with monocytic differentiation may show positivity for CD4, CD56, and CD123. Moreover, some PDC-related antigens may be expressed in AML/MS. Consequently, a broad panel of immunohistochemical markers is mandatory to make an accurate diagnosis. Findings indicative of AML/MS are the presence of granulated myeloid cells on close inspection, positivity for myeloperoxidase or lysozyme, CD13, CD14, CD34, or CD117, and negativity for MxA, TCL1, and TdT. Immunohistochemistry for BDCA2 and CLA is not useful in this context [24, 25, 52].

Clues and Pitfalls

- Consider BPDCN in any monomorphic and diffuse blast cell infiltration of the dermis, especially in elderly patients.

- CD4 and CD56 positivity strongly suggests BPDCN, but may be found in several other entities. In the presence of CD4+CD56+ infiltrates, a complete immunohistochemical panel must be performed, including antibodies for B-cell, T-cell, myelo-monocytic, and PDC-related antigens.
- Negativity for CD4, CD56, or PDC-related antigens does not rule out the diagnosis of BPDCN if other features of this condition are present.
- Non-neoplastic aggregates of PDC may be seen in association with myeloid disorders [22].

Precursor Lymphoblastic Leukemia/Lymphoma

Lymphoblastic lymphoma (LBL) is the tumor form of lymphoblastic leukemia. Both LBL and lymphoblastic leukemia consist of precursor cells (lymphoblasts) that may show a B-cell or T-cell phenotype. The leukemic presentation form predominates among B-cell neoplasms, in which it accounts for 90 % of cases. In contrast, T-cell neoplasms present as lymphomas in 85–90 % of cases [53, 54].

Bone marrow infiltration by over 25 % lymphoblasts is the criterion to be met for the diagnosis of leukemia. B lymphoblastic lymphoma (B-LBL) usually involves the skin, soft tissue, bone, and lymph nodes and may coexist with a certain degree of leukemic expression [55–57]. T lymphoblastic lymphoma (T-LBL) usually presents as a large mediastinal mass, enlarged lymph nodes, or involvement of organs such as the skin, tonsils, spleen, liver, testes, or central nervous system [58].

Skin involvement takes place more often in LBL than in lymphoblastic leukemia, its frequency being higher in B-LBL (15–20 %) than in T-LBL (<5 %). Lesions appear as reddish or purple subcutaneous nodules which usually are solitary and involve the head and neck of children in B-LBL, whereas in T-LBL they are often multiple and involve the chest wall, legs, and back of adolescent or young adults [59, 60]. A dermal lesion may be the first manifestation of disease of the cellular infiltrate in both B-LBL

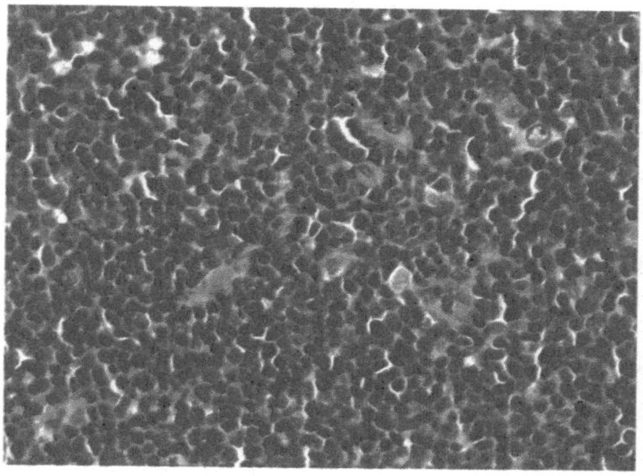

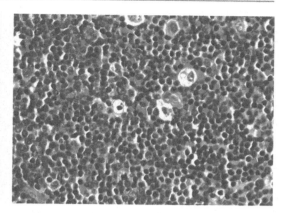

Fig. 11.11 Lymphoblastic leukemia. Dermal infiltrate in a patient diagnosed with T-cell lymphoblastic lymphoma. Note the marked monotony of the cellular infiltrate

Fig. 11.12 Lymphoblastic leukemia. Focal starry-sky pattern

and T-LBL, so that at times a biopsy is performed when pertinent clinical information and peripheral blood and bone marrow study results are still unavailable.

Histologically, there is a diffuse monotonous infiltration of the dermis by intermediate-sized atypical lymphoid elements with scanty cytoplasms and round or convoluted nuclei showing finely particulated chromatin and visible nucleoli. Mitotic figures are common and areas with a "starry-sky" pattern are often seen. The epidermis is spared and it is uncommon for the neoplasm to destroy annexial structures (Figs. 11.11 and 11.12).

Immunohistochemistry

B-LBL is characterized by the expression of precursor cell markers (such as terminal deoxynucleotidyl transferase, TdT), CD99 or, less often, CD34 [61] (Fig. 11.13). B-cell marker expression is variable. Among the latter, the more useful are CD20, CD79a, and, particularly, PAX5. There may be positivity for CD10. In some cases, myeloid lineage cell markers such as CD13 or CD33 may be positive. Therefore, a too restricted immunohistochemical study may cause problems of diagnostic interpretation.

T-LBL usually expresses TdT, CD99, and, less commonly, CD34. T-cell markers (CD1a, CD2, CD3, CD4, CD5, and CD8) are variably expressed [62] (Fig. 11.14). Coexpression of

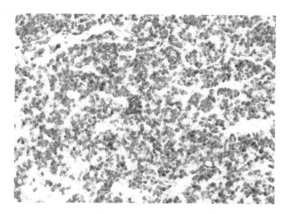

Fig. 11.13 Lymphoblastic leukemia. TdT nuclear immunostain of tumor cells

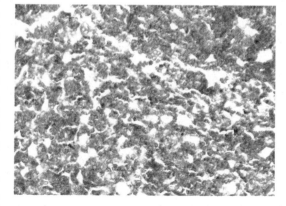

Fig. 11.14 Lymphoblastic lymphoma. Cells strongly positive for CD3 in lymphoblastic T-cell lymphoma

CD4 and CD8 is frequent and CD10 is positive in a high number of cases. Similarly to B-LBL, there may be expression of CD13 or CD33.

Molecular Biology

IGH DJ rearrangement is present in most B-ALL cases. TCR rearrangement may coexist with IGH DJ rearrangement in up to 70 % of B-ALL cases. TCR may be clonal in T-LBL, but up to 20 % of cases may show IgH clonality. Therefore, the utility of IGH DJ and TCR rearrangement studies to confirm B-cell or T-cell lineage is limited.

Some B-LBL cases are associated with characteristic cytogenetic alterations (*BCR-ABL1* translocation, *MLL* rearrangement, etc) that identify specific clinicopathological entities [53].

Differential Diagnosis

LBL diagnosis should pose no problems if appropriate clinical information is available and a complete immunohistochemical study is performed. Major difficulties may arise when clinical information is incomplete or the disease starts as a skin lesion. In these settings monotony and immaturity of the cell infiltrate and patient age are of great help in suggesting the correct diagnosis. When in doubt, immunohistochemistry may confirm the diagnosis by showing combined positivity for precursor cell markers (TdT and CD99), CD10, and B-cell markers (in B-LBL) or T-cell markers (in T-LBL). Obviously, the hematologist should be contacted so that a comprehensive study of the patient is carried out [63].

The cell infiltrate monotony could induce confusion with skin involvement by blastoid mantle cell lymphoma. However, the problem is solved by knowledge of relevant clinical features in conjunction with a complete immunohistochemical study including cyclin D1 or SOX11 [64–66]. Combined positivity for T-cell markers and CD10 may suggest angioimmunoblastic lymphoma with cutaneous involvement. Again, clinical information and immunohistochemical study of TdT and other markers greatly help.

Expression of CD34 and myeloid lineage markers may be reminiscent of myeloid sarcoma in some cases, but a more extensive immunophenotypic study may solve the problem.

Blastic plasmacytoid dendritic cell neoplasm (BPDCN), although mostly seen in old patients, may present at any age and usually causes dermal lesions, which are histopathologically similar to T-LBL. The CD3−, CD4+, CD123+, and CD56+ immunophenotype is very characteristic of this entity. Nonetheless, it should be kept in mind that up to a third of BPDCN cases may express TdT. Usually, T-LBL will be positive for other T-cell antigens such as CD2, CD3, CD5, and CD7. A complete hematologic study is necessary to establish the diagnosis in some cases [67].

Nonhematologic small round-cell tumors such as Ewing's sarcoma, neuroblastoma, malignant rhabdoid tumors, and Merkel cell carcinoma may present with skin lesions. These tumors should be ruled out with the aid of appropriate immunohistochemical panels when there is negativity for lymphoblastic lymphoma markers [68]. It should be noted that positivity for TdT and PAX5 has been observed in nearly 80 % of cases of Merkel cell carcinoma [69, 70].

Clues and Pitfalls

- The immunohistochemical study should include TdT and CD99 when confronted with a difficult-to-classify dermal lymphoproliferative lesion, particularly in children, adolescents, or young adults.
- Expression of myeloid lineage markers such as CD13 or CD33 does not exclude LBL.
- Angioimmunoblastic lymphoma may coexpress T-cell markers and CD10, but is negative for precursor cell markers (TdT).
- BPDCN should be ruled out when a dermal lesion is positive for CD4 and CD56, even in the presence of TdT immunoreactivity.

Mastocytosis

Mastocytosis comprises a heterogeneous group of diseases characterized by proliferation and accumulation of clonal mast cells in one or more organs. The World Health Organization (WHO) variants of mastocytosis are shown in Table 11.1. Skin is the organ most commonly involved in mastocytosis, and three main clinical-pathological subtypes are recognized: (1) urticaria pigmentosa (UP)/maculopapular cutaneous mastocytosis (MPCM), (2) diffuse cutaneous mastocytosis (DCM), and (3) mastocytoma of skin (nodular mastocytosis) [71]. Cutaneous infiltration in mast cell leukemia and mast cell sarcoma is extremely rare.

Table 11.1 World Health Organization classification of mastocytosis[a]

	Skin lesions
Cutaneous mastocytosis (CM)	+
Urticaria pigmentosa (UP)/	−
maculopapular CM (MPCM)	−
Diffuse CM	
Mastocytoma of skin	
Indolent systemic mastocytosis (SM)	+
Smoldering SM	+
Isolated bone marrow mastocytosis	−/+
Systemic mastocytosis with associated clonal hematological non-mast cell lineage disease (SM-AHNMD)	−
Aggressive systemic mastocytosis (ASM)	−/+
Lymphadenopathic mastocytosis with eosinophilia	
Mast cell leukemia (MCL)	−
Aleukemic MCL	
Mast cell sarcoma (MCS)	−
Extracutaneous mastocytoma	−

[a]Horny HP, Metcalfe DD, Bennett JM, Bain BJ. Mastocytosis. In: Swerdlow SH, Campo E, Harris NL, Jaffe ES, Pileri SA, Stein H et al. eds. WHO Classification of Tumours of Haematopoietic and Lymphoid Tissues. 4th ed. Lyon France: IARC Press; 2008:54–63

UP is the most common variant of cutaneous mastocytosis (CM), accounting for 70–90 % of patients, and up to 75 % onset in the first years of life. Adult-onset UP is in most cases indicative of systemic mastocytosis (SM), and appropriate investigation of bone marrow and serum tryptase should be performed (Fig. 11.15) [72–74]. Telangiectasia macularis eruptiva perstans (TMEP) is considered a rare form of MPCM. DCM (1–3 % of patients) and mastocytoma of skin (10–30 % of patients) are almost exclusive of childhood [75].

Lesions of CM vary in the different clinical-pathological subtypes. The Darier's sign is useful in clinical diagnosis. UP/MPCM generally presents with an eruption of multiple hyperpigmented macules or, less frequently, papules. The trunk is the most common localization of lesions, followed by the extremities. The rare TMEP variant is characterized by slightly pigmented macules with telangiectasia. In DCM, skin is diffusely thickened and erythematous and blistering is common. Mastocytoma presents as solitary nodular lesions of the trunk, head, or wrists (Fig. 11.16).

The histopathological findings of CM are characterized by cutaneous infiltration of mast cells, predominantly in the upper third of the dermis; the number of mast cells varies in the clinical subtypes (Fig. 11.17). In the usual UP/MPCM lesions, fusiform mast cells are found mostly around blood vessels, with some eosinophils and superficial edema. Nodular aggregates of mast cells are rarely found. Basal hyperpigmentation

Fig. 11.15 Bone marrow infiltration by mast cells in a case of systemic mastocytosis (**a**, Hematoxilin-eosin, 200×). CD117 immunostain highlight the mast cells (inset). Bone marrow aspirate shows elongated mast cells (**b**, May-Grünwald-Giemsa, 1000×)

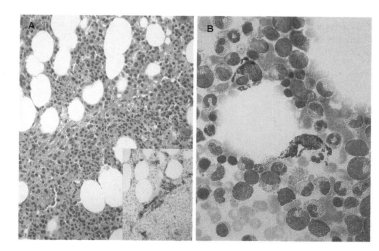

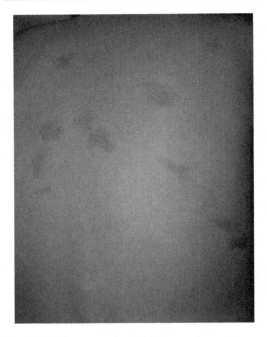

Fig. 11.16 Presence of multiple hyperpigmented macules on the back of a child with cutaneous mastocytosis (Courtesy of Dr. JM Carrascosa, Dpt. Of Dermatology, Hospital Germans Trias I Pujol, Badalona, Spain)

of the epidermis is a diagnostic clue. The rare TMEP is characterized by dilated vessels and a slight increase in perivascular mast cells that can be undetectable without appropriate immunohistochemical stains. In DCM, a band-like or dermal diffuse, sheet-like infiltrate of round mast cells is found (Fig. 11.18a, b). Subepidermal edema with vesiculobullous changes is frequent in infants. Mastocytoma of the skin is characterized by dense aggregates of round mast cells that infiltrate diffusely the papillary and reticular dermis, sometimes extending to subcutaneous tissues (Fig. 11.18c, d). The overlying epidermis is often elevated but uninfiltrated [76, 77].

Immunohistochemistry

Mast cells are positive for CD45, CD68, CD33, CD43, HLA-DR, CD117 (CKIT), and Tryptase. Of these, Tryptase is the most lineage-specific marker. Both CD117 and tryptase are commonly used to highlight mast cells in tissue samples. Aberrant expression of CD2 and/or CD25 in cutaneous mast cells may be indicative of SM

Fig. 11.17 A case of cutaneous mastocytosis with weak infiltration. Panoramic view shows a dermal superficial infiltration of mast cells (**a**, Hematoxilin-eosin; 40×). High power examination shows the interstitial and perivascular distribution of the infiltrate (**c**, Hematoxilin-eosin; 200×). Tryptase stain highlights the mast cell infiltrate (**b**; 40×, **d**; 200×)

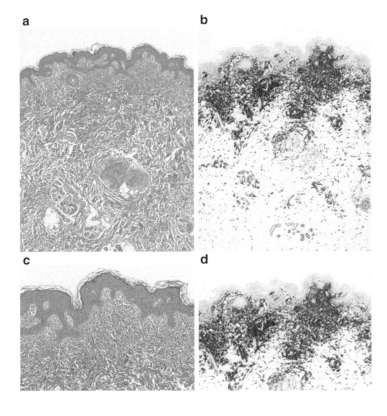

Fig. 11.18 Two representative cases of cutaneous mastocytosis. (**a, b**) Superficial, band-like infiltrate of mast cells in the dermis, without epidermal involvement (**a**, Hematoxilin-eosin, 40×; **b**, CD117, 40×). (**c, d**) Dense infiltration of papillary and reticular dermis by mast cells (**c**, Hematoxilin-eosin, 40×), positive for CD117 (**d**, Hematoxilin-eosin, 40×)

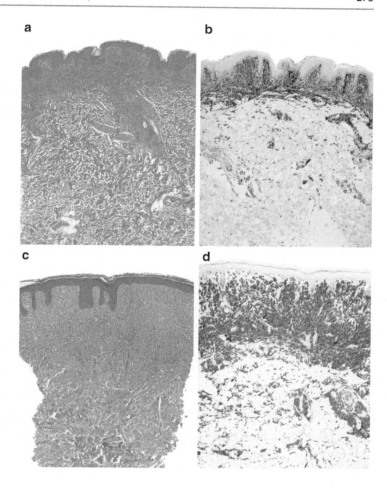

with secondary cutaneous involvement [78–80]. Recently, CD30 expression has been demonstrated in SM, including indolent and aggressive forms, and could be a potential target-based therapy [81, 82]. One case of CD30 positive CM has been reported, although it probably represented a secondary skin infiltration by SM [83].

Molecular Biology

Activating point mutations in KIT gene (especially D816V) are present in almost all patients with SM (Fig. 11.19). Early reports suggested that KIT mutations were not present in CM cases, but recent data show activating point mutations in 67–83 % of CM both in infants and adults. Interestingly, alternative mutations (other than D816V) are frequently found in CM [84–86].

Differential Diagnosis

The histopathological and clinical features of CM, including Darier's sign, are characteristic enough as to provide the correct diagnosis in almost all patients. Lesions with subtle infiltration by mast cells could be missed without suitable clinical information and special stains that highlight mast cells.

Clues and Pitfalls

- CD117 and/or tryptase positivity must be necessary to highlight mast cells in CM with scarce infiltration. CD117 is also positive in hematopoietic progenitor cells and tryptase in basophils, which eventually can lead to a misdiagnosis.
- Diagnosis of CM requires appropriate investi-

Wild type

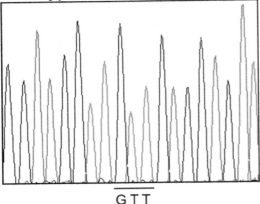

GTT

c.1679T>G:p.V560G

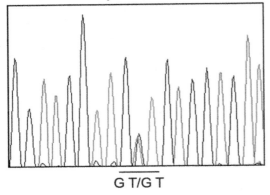

G T/G T

Fig. 11.19 Identification of V560G mutation in the c-Kit gene by PCR

gation in order to exclude SM, especially in adult-onset instances or in cases with CD25 expression.

Histiocytic and Dendritic Cell Disorders

Langerhans Cell Histiocytosis/ Langerhans Cell Sarcoma

Langerhans cell histiocytosis (LCH) is a rare disease more commonly seen in children, although it may present at any age. For more than 50 years it has been much debated whether LCH is an inflammatory, infectious, immunologic, or neoplastic condition. Recently, demonstration of

clonality and *BRAF* mutations in LCH has lent support to the neoplastic character of this peculiar disorder [87].

LCH localized form with involvement of only one site (classic eosinophilic granuloma) shows very few symptoms and a strong trend towards spontaneous resolution [88, 89]. An osteolytic lesion with spread to the adjacent soft tissue is more commonly observed, but lymph nodes, lung, or skin may be alternatively involved. Multifocal forms combine simultaneous lesions in several of these locations. Skull and mandible involvement is quite common. Skull lesions may be associated with diabetes insipidus (Hand-Schülller-Christian). The more severe disseminated form (Abt-Letterer-Siwe) is seen in children, who add liver and spleen involvement to skin and bone lesions [88, 89].

Independently of clinical presentation and aggressiveness, LCH diagnosis is based on the identification of characteristic Langerhans cells (LCs). LCs show a peculiar elongated folded nucleus with little atypia, finely particulated chromatin, a discrete nucleolus, and variable proliferative activity. Cytoplasms are eosinophilic and moderately abundant. LCH lesions show an inflammatory/granulomatous appearance and consist of numerous LCs intermingled with eosinophils, histiocytes, multinucleated cells, neutrophils, and lymphocytes (Fig. 11.20). LCs relative density diminishes as the lesions mature and LCs are replaced by foamy histiocytes and fibrous tissue. The first structural evidence leading to the grouping of the various LCH forms was the observation of Birbeck granules. Subsequently, immunohistochemical techniques have greatly facilitated the study of these conditions [87, 88].

Langerhans cell sarcoma (LCS) is the obviously malignant counterpart of LCH. LCS usually presents in adults in a multiorganic fashion, with common infiltration of the skin and neighboring tissues. Histologically, LCS shows marked atypia, pleomorphism, and a high mitotic index, with no features suggestive of LC differentiation. Consequently, LCS diagnosis is mostly based on immunohistochemical findings and/or ultrastructural demonstration of Birbeck granules [89, 90].

Immunohistochemistry

LCH diagnosis requires evidence of CD1a and langerin (CD207) expression in LCs (Figs. 11.21 and 11.22) [88, 91]. Although S-100 protein is usually positive, its diagnostic usefulness is not as robust as that of CD1a and langerin owing to its low specificity [92]. In contrast, CD1a and langerin are highly specific for LCH and very useful for the differential diagnosis with other histiocytosis [93]. Additionally, CD68, CD4, and vimentin are often immunoreactive in LCH, although as happens with S-100 protein their low specificity makes their use unpractical.

There is a good correlation between the presence of *BRAF* mutations and immunoreactivity with specific antibodies against mutant BRAF-V600E protein. Although not all cases with the mutant protein are immunohistochemically posi-

tive, discrepancies are few [94, 95]. Even so, we believe that the diagnostic usefulness of anti-BRAF antibodies is limited, since a positive immunoreaction is obtained in just 60 % of LCH cases. That notwithstanding, the screening use of this antibody for detection of potentially mutated cases susceptible of treatment with specific inhibitors is very promising.

LCS usually expresses LC markers. Nevertheless, expression is focal and irregular in some cases, in which ultrastructural evidence of Birbeck granules may be extremely helpful (Fig. 11.23) [96].

Molecular Biology

In the last few years proof has accrued on the existence of a constitutive activation of the RAS-

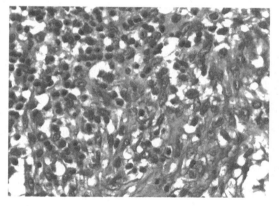

Fig. 11.20 Langerhans cell histiocytosis. Dermal infiltrate of granulomatous appearance containing numerous Langerhans cells and eosinophils

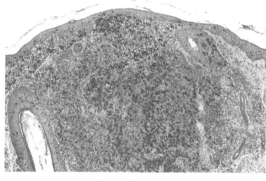

Fig. 11.22 Langerhans cell histiocytosis. Langerin (CD207) is the most specific immunohistochemical marker of Langerhans cell histiocytosis (courtesy of Dr. L. Requena, Dept of Dermatology, Fundación Jiménez Díaz, Madrid, Spain)

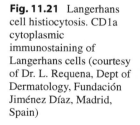

Fig. 11.21 Langerhans cell histiocytosis. CD1a cytoplasmic immunostaining of Langerhans cells (courtesy of Dr. L. Requena, Dept of Dermatology, Fundación Jiménez Díaz, Madrid, Spain)

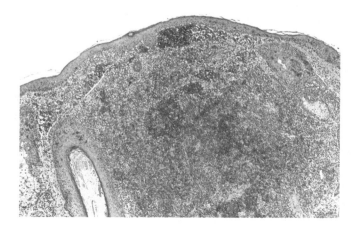

Fig. 11.23 Langerhans cell histiocytosis. Birbeck granules are the ultrastructural hallmark of Langerhans cells. They can appear in the typical tennis-racquet shape (**a**) or as trilaminate structures (**b**)

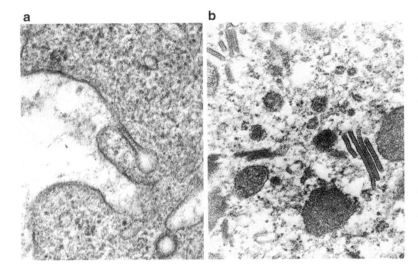

RAF-MAPK-ERK pathway in LCH. In about 60 % of LCH cases, activation of extracellular signal-regulated kinase (ERK) is caused by BRAF exon 15 V600D mutation. A similar biologic effect is achieved by somatic MAP2K1 mutations in approximately 27 % of LCH cases. Interestingly, both mechanisms are mutually exclusive. In rare LCH cases other mutations, such as those of ARAF, may induce ERK activation in the absence of BRAF mutations. These alterations, which ultimately result in ERK activation, take place in both unifocal and multifocal LCH cases, and even in congenital instances of the disease [97–101].

Probably, molecular determination of the aforesaid alterations will play a more important role in the selection of specific therapeutic targets than as diagnostic tools. In this context, the results recently obtained with specific inhibitors are highly promising. Most likely, the design of powerful specific inhibitors will soon provide efficient therapeutic weapons for the management of LCH [102, 103].

Differential Diagnosis

Generally speaking, LCH differential diagnosis includes inflammatory conditions totally or partially constituted by histiocytes (non-Langerhans cell histiocytosis).

The latter include juvenile xantogranuloma, a morphologically different lesion with foamy histiocytes and Touton giant cells. Lack of positivity for CD1a and langerin provides the diagnosis in doubtful cases [104].

Rosai-Dorfman disease occasionally involves the skin and may mimic LCH. The presence of foamy histiocytes with emperipolesis and, again, CD1a and langerin negative immunostaing are key features in support of this condition.

Erdheim-Chester disease is a systemic disease that at times involves the skin. Collections of enlarged histiocytes with clear cytoplasm are characteristic. Immunohistochemical studies including langerin and CD1a are diagnostically very helpful.

Usually, the differential diagnosis with dendritic cell tumors is not problematic, since their high tumor cell density and negativity for LC markers lead to their identification. Indeterminate dendritic cell tumor, a rare tumor of dendritic cells, may express CD1a and S-100 protein. Nevertheless, their negative langerin immunostaining and lack of Birbeck granules point to the correct diagnosis [105].

Mast cell proliferations, histiocytic sarcoma, myelomonocytic leukemia, and anaplastic large cell lymphoma may give rise to cutaneous lesions that occasionally cause diagnostic problems.

Clinical data and a complete immunophenotypic study are essential for the diagnosis.

Clues and Pitfalls

- When confronted with an inflammatory/histiocytic lesion, CD1a and langerin expression should be investigated to rule out LCH. Other less-specific markers, such as S-100 protein and CD4, must be cautiously evaluated, since other histiocytic conditions may create diagnostic confusion.
- Indeterminate dendritic cell tumor may give rise to differential diagnosis problems, since it may be positive for S-100 protein and CD1a. Absence of langerin and Birbeck granules are helpful diagnostic clues.
- Immunoreactivity for BRAF may be useful for selecting treatments with specific inhibitors.
- LCS may show partial expression of LCH markers. In these cases, electron microscopic study may solve the issue.

Indeterminate Dendritic Cell Tumor

Indeterminate dendritic cell tumor, also known as indeterminate cell histiocytosis (ICT), is an uncommon entity of unclear histogenesis. Its ill-defined morphologic features are intermediate between those of Langerhans cell hitiocytosis and other histiocytic conditions [106]. Clinically, ICT is characterized by solitary or multiple dermal papulonodular lesions involving the trunk, neck, face, and limbs. These lesions are usually asymptomatic and show a benign behavior. Spontaneous regression, at least partial, is a common outcome [107, 108].

There are ICT cases with extracutaneous osseous or corneal involvement and systemic symptoms, but they are exceptional [109, 110]. It is quite intriguing that this rare disease is occasionally associated with malignant hematologic conditions such as follicular lymphoma, acute myeloid leukemia, and lymphoblastic lymphoma [105, 106, 111, 112].

Histologically, ICT shows a dense dermal infiltrate that may reach the subcutis and rarely exhibits

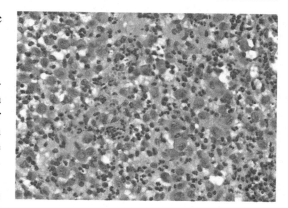

Fig. 11.24 Indeterminate dendritic cell tumor. Inflammatory appearance, with histiocyte-like cells, polymorphonuclear leukocytes and eosinophils (Courtesy of Dr. C. Barranco, Hospital del Mar, Barcelona, Spain)

its epidermotropism. The infiltrate consists of a mixture of lymphocytes, eosinophils, and large-sized cells with wide cytoplasms and oval folded or indented nuclei showing fine chromatin, inconspicuous nuclei, and delicate membranes (Fig. 11.24). Multinucleated giant cells may be seen as well. Cell atypia is generally absent and mitoses are either very scanty or not present.

Immunohistochemistry

ICT has a distinctive immunohistochemical profile. Similarly to what happens in LCH, dendritic cells are positive for S-100 protein and CD1a in ICT, but the latter lacks Birbeck granules and, consequently, shows negativity for langerin (CD207) (Figs. 11.25 and 11.26). It should be kept in mind, however, that positive immunostainings for S-100 protein and CD1a are irregularly distributed in some ICT cases [105, 110].

CD45 and histiocytic markers (CD68 and CD4) may be positive. CD30 and other B or T lymphoid markers are negative, as are follicular dendritic cell markers such as CD21, CD23, and CD35.

Molecular Biology

No much knowledge is available of the molecular changes related to this condition. Occasional cases associated with neoplastic hematologic disease have shown a clonal relationship

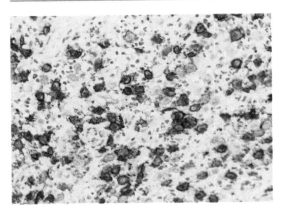

Fig. 11.25 Indeterminate dendritic cell tumor. Positive CD1a immunostaining of dendritic cells (Courtesy of Dr. C. Barranco, Hospital del Mar, Barcelona, Spain)

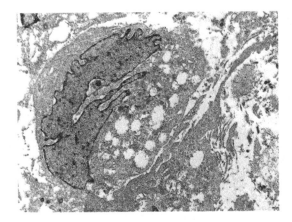

Fig. 11.26 Indeterminate dendritic cell tumor. There is no ultrastructural evidence of Birbeck granules (Courtesy of Dr. J Lloreta, Hospital del Mar, Barcelona, Spain)

between ICT and the accompanying lymphoid neoplasm. Specifically, t(14:18) has been identified in both ICT lesions and associated follicular lymphoma cells. Possibly, divergent differentiation from a common cell precursor is the underlying mechanism in some of these instances. Clonality has not been detected in ICT cases unrelated to hematologic neoplasms [105, 112]. Understanding of ICT molecular mechanisms is in need of much study and there is no proof that it shares the molecular alterations recently described in LCH.

Differential Diagnosis

ICT differential diagnosis includes genuinely histiocytic conditions and LCH. The combination of positive immunoreactivity for CD1a and S-100 protein and negative immunostaining for langerin is characteristic of this entity [106].

Juvenile xanthogranuloma and reticulohistiocytoma may partially mimic ICT, but their negativity for both S-100 protein and CD1a is very helpful. Other genuinely histiocytic conditions, such as Rosai-Dorfman disease, show distinctive morphologic features that allow their distinction, although recourse to immunohistochemistry greatly helps to clarify doubtful cases.

Dendritic cell tumors may express S-100 protein, but their densely cellular appearance and lack of CD1a expression are very useful diagnostic clues.

LCH may be morphologically very similar to ICT and then poses significant differential diagnostic problems. In this setting immunohistochemistry for CD1 and langerin is essential, langerin negativity being very suspicious for ICT. Electron microscopic demonstration of lack of Birbeck granules is also recommended to confirm de diagnosis of ICT.

Clues and Pitfalls

- When confronted with a lesion suspicious for LCH, langerin expression should be investigated. Langerin negativity is very suggestive of ICT.
- When ICT is associated with a malignant hematologic condition, there may be a clonal relationship between both. Investigation of clonality is advised in these circumstances.

Xanthogranuloma and Related Disorders

Juvenile xanthogranuloma (JXG) is a non-Langerhans dendritic cell histiocytic disorder that usually appears in the first two decades of life [113]. Most JXGs are solitary dermal nodules measuring from a few millimeters to 1–2 cm, although giant forms (often 4–5 cm in diameter) have also been described [114]. A high proportion of cases occur on the face or trunk and are skin colored, yellowish, or erythematous. Less frequently, patients present with multiple lesions, exhibit a lichenoid appearance [115] or show involvement of deep-seated cutaneous locations [116]. Visceral or systemic involvement is rare but, when present, it may be the cause of death, especially in neonates [113]. Nevertheless, the clinical course of most JXGs is self-limited.

Microscopically, JXG consists of an intradermal proliferation of spindle cells, mononuclear

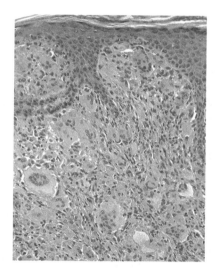

Fig. 11.27 Juvenile xanthogranuloma consisting of an intradermal proliferation of histiocytes, most of them multinucleated. Foamy cytoplasms, a result of xanthomization, tend to occupy the periphery, whereas nuclei are centrally located forming a ring

histiocytes, and multinucleated giant cells, some of them Touton type. Touton cells are characterized by multiple nuclei in a ring disposition around an area of dense pink cytoplasm, which is surrounded by a rim of foamy cytoplasm (Fig. 11.27). Touton cells are less frequent in JXG in extracutaneous locations [113]. The epidermis is usually separated from the proliferation by a thin band, but periadnexal involvement is quite common (Fig. 11.28a, b). Lymphocytes and eosinophils can also be present within the histiocytic infiltrate. Nonlipidized [117] and mitotically active cases can simulate malignant mesenchymal neoplasms [118].

The association of JXG and neurofibromatosis types 1 and 2 (NF1 and NF2) [119, 120] is well recognized and may form a triad with juvenile chronic myelogenous leukemia (JCML) [121, 122]. The combination of JXG and Langerhans cell histiocytosis (LCH) in the same patient has been interpreted as an argument in favor of their common histogenesis [123].

JXG is one of the conditions in a group of related disorders including cephalic histiocytosis, spindle cell xanthogranuloma, disseminated juvenile xanthogranuloma, progressive nodular histiocytosis (PNH), generalized eruptive histiocytosis, xanthoma disseminatum, and Erdheim-Chester disease (ECD) (Fig. 11.29). Among these disorders, some are more frequent in adults [124–126], some are multifocal and/or show extracutaneous

Fig. 11.28 Juvenile xanthogranuloma separated from the epidermis by a thin layer of dermal collagen but extending downward surrounding a follicle. The histiocytes are positive for both CD68 (**a**) and factor XIIIa (**b**)

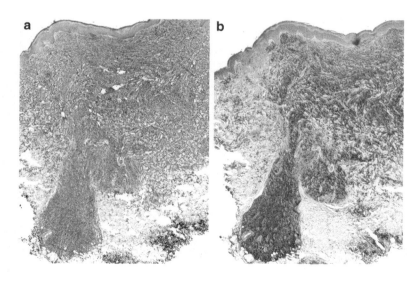

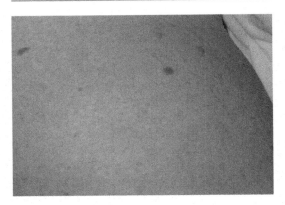

Fig. 11.29 Patient with Erdheim-Chester disease under study for neurological symptoms. Until the dermatological examination, these inconspicuous cutaneous papules had been clinically missed (Courtesy of Dr. I. Bielsa, Dept. of Dermatology, Hospital Germans Trias i Pujol, Badalona, Spain)

involvement and some have important impact on the quality of life, causing serious illness or even death.

The diagnosis of JXG-related disorders can be challenging. First, because cutaneous lesions are often microscopically and immunophenotypically indistinguishable from solitary JXG. Second, because of the rarity of most of these entities, which makes difficult to achieve a general agreement on their classification and the establishment of clear-cut diagnostic criteria.

Patients with PNH are adults that develop multiple xanthomatous papules and pedunculated or deep-seated nodules. The lesions, which measure 1-3 cm in diameter, may be disfiguring. Some patients also present systemic symptoms and visceral involvement [124, 125].

Worse still is ECD, characterized by the involvement of internal organs, especially bone and lung. Symmetrical osteosclerosis of long bones is a frequent manifestation. Heart, retroperitoneum, and periaortic spaces are other common sites in this condition, as is the central nervous system, whose involvement may cause diabetes insipidus [126]. ECD patients often complain of systemic symptoms such as fever, weakness, and weight loss. ECD cutaneous lesions tend to be periocular [124]. The clinical course varies considerably and depends to a great extent on the extension of the disease, some cases being paucisymptomatic, whereas others are rapidly fatal [126].

Immunohistochemistry

All JXGs are positive for usual histiocytic markers [113, 128] such as CD68 (KP1 and PG-M1) (Fig. 11.28a), CD31 [129], CD163 [130] and fascin [128], often with a coarse granular pattern. JXG also immunostains for factor XIIIa (a marker of dermal dendrocytes) (Fig. 11.28b), LCA, CD4, CD14, HLA-DR, and vimentin [113, 128]. Although most cases are negative for S100 protein, there are some reports of positivity [131] mainly in the first months of life [132], with loss of expression in parallel with maturation [133]. All JXG cases are negative for langerin, CD1a, CD3, CD21, CD34, and CD35 [128].

Molecular Biology

The cellular origin and causes of proliferation in JXG and related entities are not well known. Nevertheless, molecular biology studies are providing the basis to better understand the complex mechanisms underlying JXG pathogenesis. The roles of proinflammatory cytokines and several oncogenic pathways have been invoked in this regard. A clonal T-cell receptor gamma (TCR-γ) rearrangement was demonstrated in the cells of a JXG associated with acute lymphoblastic leukemia, with both conditions presenting an identical bi-allelic rearrangement [134]. Clonal mutations have also been demonstrated in Erdheim-Chester disease [135], which similarly to Langerhans cell histiocytosis (LCH) also shows a high prevalence of *BRAF(V600E)* mutations (>50 % of patients) [136–139]. The latter phenomenon has never been reported in JXG [143].

The demonstration of *BRAF (V600E)* mutation has provided new insights on the pathogenesis of these diseases. It has been hypothesized that mutated *BRAF* might trigger a process of oncogene-induced senescence, with cell-cycle arrest and induction of pro-inflammatory molecules that would be responsible for the inflammatory local and systemic infiltrates [139].

Differential Diagnosis

With the exception of *BRAF*-mutated ECD cases, there are no reliable microscopic or immunohistochemical clues to differentiate a JXG cutaneous lesion from one associated with some other JXG-related disorder (Fig. 11.30) [136–139]. Consequently, the differential diagnosis among the various entities in this group should be based on their clinical features. CD4 and LCA expression in JXG may be used to distinguish it from dermatofibroma when the latter is heavily lipidized or the former is not [128]. JXG distinction from reticulohistiocytoma is usually based on histopathological criteria, but frequent factor XIIIa expression in the former and usual lack thereof in the latter help to its distinction. Some nonspecific tissue inflammatory reactions may also simulate JXG [140].

Solitary JXG may also mimic Spitz nevus [141] and occasional positivity of JXG cells for S100 protein may further complicate their telling apart. Immunohistochemical expression of histiocytic markers and the absence of melanocytic markers such as Melan A or Sox 10 may be very helpful.

Clues and Pitfalls

- Expression of CD31 (usually considered a vascular marker) in histiocytic disorders [129] may be the cause of JXG misdiagnosis, especially in multiple, disseminated, or giant lesions [142].
- Xanthogranulomas developed at irradiation sites may be clinically misinterpreted as tumor relapse, or even as angiosarcoma, due to their CD31 positivity [143, 144].

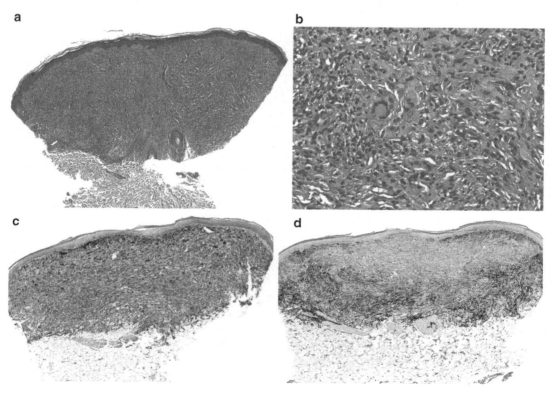

Fig. 11.30 Microscopical appearance of a cutaneous lesion from an Erdheim-Chester disease patient. The discrete histiocytic proliferation (**a**), with mild xanthomization (**b**), and the inmmunohistochemical profile, with expression of CD68 (**c**) and factor XIIIa (**d**), do not differ significantly from a typical juvenile xanthogranuloma

Hemophagocytic Lymphohistiocytosis

Hemophagocytic lymphohistiocytosis (HLH) is a rare life-threatening disorder of the immune regulatory system that may arise in any age group in relation to many different conditions. HLH is considered to be a hyperinflammatory syndrome more than a single disease [145–148].

HLH may occur in two forms: primary or familiar and secondary or sporadic. Primary HLH usually develops in infancy, although reports in adults and adolescents are becoming increasingly frequent [149]. Primary HLH is associated with gene defects in the familial hemophagocytic lymphohistiocytosis (FHL) locus, which codifies molecules involved in perforin-dependent cytotoxicity. Some congenital immunodeficiency syndromes with multisystemic disorders (frequently associated with albinism) present an increased incidence of HLH, which can be the first manifestation of the disease [148, 150]. In secondary HLH the usual triggering factor is an infection that is usually viral [146], herpes viruses and particularly EBV being the most frequent causes [145]. Rheumatologic diseases, immunodeficiency syndromes, and neoplasms, mainly T-cell lymphomas, are other conditions commonly related to secondary HLH. The term macrophage-activation syndrome (MAS) is used for a hemophagocytic syndrome associated with an inflammatory or autoimmune disease [145, 151]. Some patients with secondary HLH present mild genetic defects resulting in limited expression of the same proteins involved in primary cases [145].

In HLH pathogenesis a disproportionate cytokine production is responsible for excessive activation of macrophages [152, 153]. An infection is often the initiating factor and activation of toll-like receptors may contribute to the development of the condition [146, 148]. A defect of perforin-dependent cytotoxic function reduces the activity of natural killer and cytotoxic lymphocytes, which normally eliminate the infected antigen-presenting cells. As a result, uncontrolled expansion of cytotoxic T- cells and activated macrophages replaces physiological homeostatic mechanisms [146, 148].

The most frequent presenting symptoms are prolonged fever, lymphadenopathies, hepatosplenomegaly, and seizures or confusion. At the time of presentation, 80 % of patients present cytopenias that later on may evolve to pancytopenia. Hypertriglyceridemia, high serum ferritin levels, and coagulopathy are also common. Many patients develop hepatitis, renal failure, respiratory failure, encephalitis, and hypotension. Skin rashes occur in 25 % of patients and range from erythroderma with edema to purpuric or petequial rash [145–148]. Cases presenting multisystem failure, neurological deterioration, and superinfection secondary to cytopenia are usually fatal [145].

The diagnosis of HLH relies more on clinical and laboratory findings than on the histopathological study. Hemophagocytosis, the hallmark of the disease, is not a requisite symptom to make the diagnosis, and may well be absent in the early stages of the disease [145]. Microscopically, hemophagocytosis consists of the presence of macrophages containing phagozized erythrocytes, leukocytes, megakaryocytes and platelets or their cellular debris (Fig. 11.31a). Bone marrow, spleen, lymph node, and liver are the best sites to look for images of hemophagocytosis [145–148].

Cutaneous hemophagocytosis in the context of HLH is extremely rare, but erythrophagocytosis, a form of hemophagocytosis, has been reported in the skin of one MAS patient (Fig. 11.32) and in two patients with rheumatological diseases that could be considered incomplete forms of MAS [154].

Immunohistochemistry

Macrophages in hemophagocytosis express CD68 (KP1 and PG-M1) (Fig. 11.33) and CD163. The soluble form of the latter is also a useful marker for the diagnosis of MAS [155]. A significantly high population of CD8-positive T lymphocytes in the infiltrate, accompanied by a decrease in the number of CD5-expressing cells, is both a frequent finding and a useful diagnostic clue in Epstein-Barr virus-associated HLH [156].

Fig. 11.31 (a) Hemophagocytosis with engulfed inflammatory cells in the cytoplasm of a macrophage showing different grades of degeneration should be distinguished from (b) emperipolesis, which is characterized by the presence of intact inflammatory cells in the cytoplasm of a macrophage, sometimes surrounded by a retraction halo

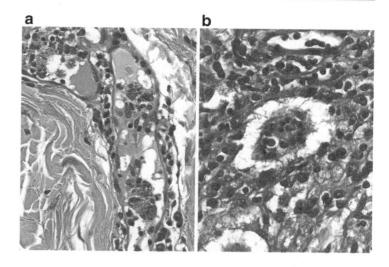

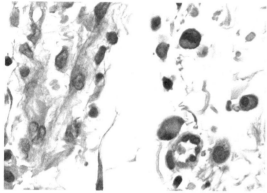

Fig. 11.32 Cutaneous erythrophagocytosis in a case of macrophage activation syndrome (courtesy of Prof. Dr. H. Kerl, Medical University of Graz, Graz, Austria)

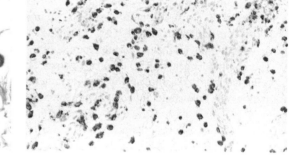

Fig. 11.33 Diffuse CD68 expression in macrophages from a case of cutaneous erythrophagocytosis in a case of macrophage activation syndrome (courtesy of Prof. Dr. H. Kerl, Medical University of Graz, Graz, Austria)

In addition, macrophages and activated T cells express high levels of cytokines (Fig. 11.34). When a virus is the triggering factor, immunohistochemical staining may contribute to its identification [157]. In the case of EBV, a type II latency-gene expression pattern has been demonstrated [158].

Molecular Biology

Many HLH cases contain clonal B-cell or T-cell populations, especially in cases related to EBV [159], but the demonstration of clonality does not carry a worse prognosis. Conversely, an abnormal karyotype would point towards a systemic EBV-driven T-cell lymphoproliferative disorder with clinical and histopathological overlap with EBV-related HLH and a high mortality rate [160].

Differential Diagnosis

Residual lesions of leucocytoclastic vasculitis may present perivascular hemophagocytosis [161, 162]. This finding, in the adequate clinical context, may raise the possibility of HLH. Although its presence makes further investigations advisable, the diagnosis of HLH should be based on the established criteria [163]. Hemophagocytosis should be distinguished from emperipolesis, in which intracytoplasmic cells are intact (Fig. 11.31b).

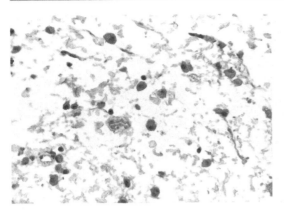

Fig. 11.34 Strong interferon γ expression in macrophages from a case of macrophage activation syndrome (courtesy of Prof. Dr. H. Kerl, Medical University of Graz, Graz, Austria)

Clues and Pitfalls

- If HLH is suspected, performance of immunohistochemical or in situ hybridization tests for detection of viruses (mainly members of the herpes virus family such as EBV and CMV) may help to unveil the triggering factor.
- The common phenomenon of phagocytosis of cellular debris in macrophages at areas of inflammation may be misinterpreted as hemophagocytosis. A background of long-standing inflammation with residual acute inflammatory infiltrates, necrosis, or fibrosis is an uncommon feature in HLH and favors inflammatory resolution with macrophagic infiltration.

Multicentric Reticulohistiocytosis

Multicentric reticulohistiocytosis (MRH) is a rare form of idiopathic non-Langerhans cell histiocytosis that manifests itself in the skin as papulonodular mucocutaneous lesions [164]. Destructive polyarthritis is present in almost half the cases, in which it causes a severe form of joint destruction known as arthritis mutilans. These cutaneous and rheumatological manifestations may coexist, appear in isolation, or follow one after the other [164, 165]. The dermatological features may range from tiny papules to nodules that may coalesce forming clusters or furrowing and coarsening the skin [164–167]. Skin lesions grow slowly, are often asymptomatic, show a skin-colored, translucent, reddish or yellowish surface and rarely ulcerate [164, 165]. Any skin site and occasionally the external mucosa may be affected, the hands and face being the most common locations [164, 165]. Clustering of papulonodules overlying the periungual areas may result in the characteristic "coral-bead" appearance [166]. Diffuse facial infiltration is less common, but it was the cause of a leonine facies in one case [167]. Patients may complain of malaise and systemic symptoms and rare instances of pulmonary, myocardic, and liver histiocytic infiltration have been reported [168, 169]. In other patients lung involvement consists of nonspecific fibrosis only [170]. Some lesions may be induced by ultraviolet light [171] and photodistribution is sometimes present [172]. The pathogenesis of MRH is not known but there are many evidences in favor of an immunological basis. Elevated cytokine serum levels seem to play a role in bone destruction [173]. In addition, TNF-alpha increase in both serum and lesional epidermis [174, 175] might trigger monocyte chemoattractant protein-1 (MCP-1) overexpression [176] leading to histiocyte attraction. Furthermore, MRH histiocytes show osteoclast-like characteristics that contribute to bone destruction [177]. Near a quarter of MFH cases are associated with neoplasia, but the two diseases do not necessarily follow a parallel course [178]. Autoimmune diseases have also been reported in association with MRH [179]. Spontaneous resolution occurs after an average of 8 years, but the diagnosis must be quickly established and aggressive therapy promptly initiated to prevent irreversible articular damage [180].

Microscopically, skin lesions are nodular and dermal-based but may spread to the subcutaneous tissue. The infiltrate is made up of large histiocytes, many of them multinucleated, with abundant pale or eosinophilic ground-glass cytoplasm and occasional fibrosis and xanthomization (Fig. 11.35) [181, 182]. T lymphocytes and neutrophils may also be present. An abundant accompanying population of dermal dendrocytes is identified in some cases. Additionally, an identical histological appearance is present in polyarthritis-related synovial membranes and in rarely involved internal organs [168, 169].

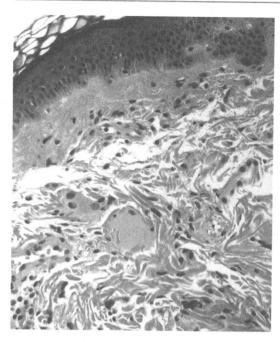

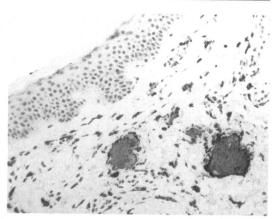

Fig. 11.36 Multicentric reticulohistiocytosis with CD68 KP1 positive cells

Fig. 11.35 Large multinucleated histiocytes with eosinophilic cytoplasm are scattered in the dermis in a case of multicentric reticulohistiocytosis

Immunohistochemistry

Immunohistohemically, cells express CD68 (KP1 and PGM1) (Fig. 11.36), CD163 and other histiocytic markers, as well as vimentin. Rare cases are S100-protein positive [183] or show light Factor XIIIa expression [184]. More often, positivity for these markers is due to a population of Langerhans cells and dermal dendrocytes, respectively. CD10 has been found to be positive in one case [185] and p53 in two cases associated with urological neoplasms [186]. MRH is consistently negative for both CD1a and CD34.

Molecular Biology

MRH is a non-neoplastic histiocytic proliferation caused by immunological dysregulation that may heal spontaneously. Cytogenetic alterations or clonality have never been described in the infiltrate [173–179].

Differential Diagnosis

At the initial stages, MRH shows clinical resemblance to rheumatic diseases such as rheumatoid arthritis [187], fibroblastic rheumatism [188] or dermatomyositis [189, 190]. MRH intense and

rapid articular damage, much more aggressive than in other rheumatological diseases, is a clue to the diagnosis. Nevertheless, an etiopathogenic pathway common to other rheumatological diseases cannot be excluded [179]. Cytological study of the synovial fluid is a quick and easy method [191] for obtaining the correct diagnosis, thus avoiding treatment delays. Nevertheless, in some cases a biopsy of the cutaneous or synovial lesions will be necessary.

Clues and Pitfalls

- MRH is a multisystemic disorder in which the presence of extracutaneous symptoms is the best clue to recognize the disease, since cutaneous lesions may be rather inconspicuous.
- A biopsy of an extracutaneous location demonstrating a histiocytic infiltrate that shares the immunophenotype and microscopical appearance of the cutaneous infiltrate is a highly specific method to confirm the diagnosis.
- S100-protein positive MRH cases could be unawarely misdiagnosed as LCH but their CD1a negativity allows to rule out LCH.

Solitary Reticulohistiocytoma (Solitary Epithelioid Histiocytoma)

Solitary lesions with a microscopic and immunohistochemical appearance similar to MRH lesions have been denominated solitary reticulohistiocytoma (SRH) [181, 182, 192] or solitary epithelioid histiocytoma [182]. In spite of these immunophenotypical similarities, there are many differences that have led to the conclusion that they are distinct entities. Whereas SRH occurs more frequent in young adults with a slight predominance in males, MRH is more common in middle-aged females. In addition, SRH does not usually involve the face or digits, which are the most typical locations of MRH [181, 182].

Ganglion-like histiocytes with finely granular and eosinophilic cytoplasm are the hallmark of SRH and MRH, but whereas in SRH they are the main component of the infiltrate, in MRH there is more fibrosis and xanthomization (Fig. 11.37). Besides, some cases of SRH with granular cell change have been described [192, 193].

Immunohistochemistry

The immunohistochemical profile of SRH does not differ from that of MRH. The large epithelioid histiocytes are positive for vimentin and histiocytic markers such as CD68 KP1 and PGM1 (Fig. 11.38) and CD163. Factor XIIIa and S-100 protein (Fig. 11.39) may be focally expressed, but widespread expression of these markers militates against the diagnosis of SRH. Expression of CD45 is also variable, whereas CD1a, CD3, CD20, CD30, and CD34 are consistently negative.

T lymphocytes and neutrophils may be abundant [181, 182, 193, 194].

Molecular Biology

Clonal rearrangement of the anaplastic lymphoma kinase (*ALK*) gene resulting in VCL-ALK and SQSTM1-ALK gene fusions has been reported in a case of SRH [195]. This finding has been interpreted as an additional argument in favor of considering this lesion as a neoplastic process.

Differential Diagnosis

Juvenile xanthogranuloma (JXG) and Rosai-Dorfman disease (RDD) may cause problems in

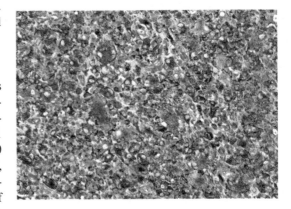

Fig. 11.38 CD68 PGM1 immunoreactivity decorates both the large histiocytes typical of solitary reticulohistiocytoma and the mononucleated cells

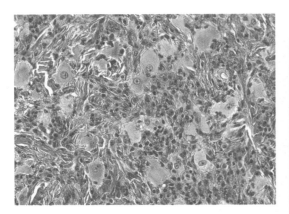

Fig. 11.37 Solitary reticulohistiocytoma with large multinucleated cells exhibiting ganglion-like features, in a background of lymphocytes, mononucleated histiocytes and dense collagen

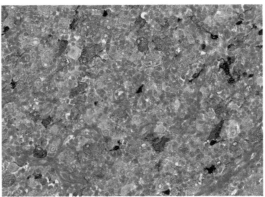

Fig. 11.39 Large histiocytes in solitary reticulohistiocytoma may show some positivity for S100 protein

SRH differential diagnosis. Nevertheless, the associated inflammatory infiltrate, microscopical characteristics of histiocytes and their immunophenotype provide definite clues for their distinction. Unlike what happens in SRH, JXG frequently contains eosinophils but neutrophils are rare. JXG may show histiocytes with large cytoplasms, but they tend to show xanthomization and factor XIIIa positivity. As for RDD, the infiltrate usually contains many plasma cells and large histiocytes, but they show emperipolesis and strong positivity for S100 protein. The latter, if present in SRH, is only focal.

SRH may also resemble melanoma and Spitz tumor. The presence of focal positivity for S100 protein and microphthalmia transcription factor (MITF) in some SRH instances [196] makes these two markers inadequate for this differential diagnosis, that should rely on a panel of antibodies including histiocytic markers such as CD68 and melanocytic markers such as Melan A.

SRH cases, especially those with a polypoid silhouette and granular cytoplasm, may simulate granular cell tumors. Their distinction from primitive polypoid granular-cell tumor is particularly difficult [193, 194].

Clues and Pitfalls

- When considering the diagnosis of SRH, pay attention to the associated inflammatory infiltrate. Consider the possibility of JXG if eosinophils are predominant or RDD whenever the plasma cell infiltrate in abundant. Look at the cytoplasm of large histiocytes, whose xanthomization points to JXG, whereas the presence of intact inflammatory cells (emperipolesis) makes RDD the first option.
- SRH may present focal and/or weak S100 protein positivity, a finding potentially leading to the wrong diagnosis of RDD or melanocytic lesion.
- Since SRH may focally express S100 protein and MITF, Use of a panel of histiocytic and melanocytic markers (other than those mentioned) is advisable when confronted with any supposed melanocytic lesion showing predominance of large cells with eosinophilic cytoplasm.

Rosai-Dorfman Disease

Rosai-Dorfman disease (RDD) is a non-neoplastic proliferative histiocytic disorder of unknown etiology. RDD was originally described in lymph nodes with the name of sinus histiocytosis with massive lymphadenopathy [197] due to the large-sized adenopathies shown by these patients, particularly in the cervical and submandibular regions. For many years extranodal involvement has been considered a rare event [198], but quite probably its real incidence has been underestimated due to unawareness. The number of extranodal cases, most of them cutaneous, has increased notably as diagnostic accuracy has improved, to the point that extranodal cases outnumbered nodal forms in a recent series [199].

Cutaneous RDD may occur in any age group, but whereas nodal cases are more common in young males of African origin, cutaneous RDD tends to appear in middle-aged white women [198, 200]. There are reports of RDD cases associated with lymphoproliferative disorders and histiocytosis [201, 203], viral infections (Epstein-Barr virus, human herpes virus 6, parvovirus B19, and polyomavirus) [204, 205] and Crohn's disease [206].

The relationship between RDD with IgG4-related disease (IgG4-RD) is not well established. Both entities share microscopical features and many cases of RDD show increased numbers of IgG4-positive cells (>40% IgG4/IgG-positive cells after averaging three high-power fields) [207–209]. Nevertheless, it is not clear whether IgG4 antibodies have a truly significant role in the pathogenesis of these diseases. Conversely, the T helper cells present in the infiltrate seem to be better candidates as key agents of tissue damage [207, 209].

Clinically, RDD cutaneous lesions often are papules or nodules with orange or erythematous discoloration that may involve any location but seem to be more common on the upper part of the body [200, 210].

The microscopic appearance of nodal and extranodal RDD is quite similar [200] and consists of a nonclonal proliferation of large histiocytes with abundant pale cytoplasm. Typically,

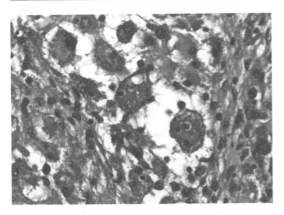

Fig. 11.40 The presence of large histiocytes with intact lymphocytes and neutrophils, a phenomenon known as emperipolesis, is a typical feature of Rosai Dorfman disease

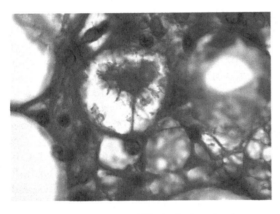

Fig. 11.41 Small eosinophilic inclusions in the cytoplasm of histiocytes from Rosai-Dorfman disease, simulating a viral infection

the cytoplasms of many histiocytes contain intact lymphocytes or neutrophils, a phenomenon known as emperipolesis (Fig. 11.40) [211]. Small granular pink cytoplasmic inclusions and nuclear viral-like changes can also be observed (Fig. 11.41) [206]. An inflammatory background of mature lymphocytes, plasma cells, and occasional eosinophils accompanies the histiocytic proliferation, often forming aggregates that provide RDD extranodal lesions an appearance reminiscent of a lymph node with sinus histiocytosis (Fig. 11.42a). A variable degree of stromal fibro-

sis with a storiform or lobulated pattern is often present [210].

The clinical course of RDD is unpredictable. Although the evolution in most cases is indolent and self-limited, fatal cases do exist [212]. Patients with severe and widespread forms, refractory to the usual therapeutic approaches, may require potent treatments [213].

Immunohistochemistry

Immunohistochemically, the proliferating histiocytes typically show intense S100-protein expression (Figs. 11.42b and 11.43). CD68 (KP1 and PGM1), (Figs. 11.42c and 11.44), CD163 and vimentin are also positive, although their intensity is more variable [200]. Some mesenchymal markers associated with the epithelial mesenchymal transition, such as β-catenin, N-cadherin, fibronectin, and Slig, have also been found to be positive [214]. Coexpression of histiocytic and mesenchymal markers in proliferating cells has led to speculate whether RDD might be considered a histiocytic mesenchymal transition disorder [214]. In one case, expression of p53, p16, and PTEN was also found [214], whereas CD1is consistently negative [200, 214].

The histiocytic proliferation is usually accompanied by a prominent lymphoplasmacytic infiltrate containing a mixed population of CD20-positive B lymphocytes and CD3-positive T lymphocytes.

Molecular Pathology

Genomic analysis have failed to demonstrate any significant mutation in the serum or the tissues involved [137, 214].

Differential Diagnosis

Lymphoproliferative disorders, histiocytosis, and autoimmune diseases (including IgG4-RD) constitute the main differential diagnosis. Actually, RDD may coexist, follow or precede various lymphoma types [201, 202]. A complete immunohistochemical profiling of the infiltrates allows to tell them apart.

S100 protein expression in RDD giant cells permits ruling out JXG, whereas RDD negativity

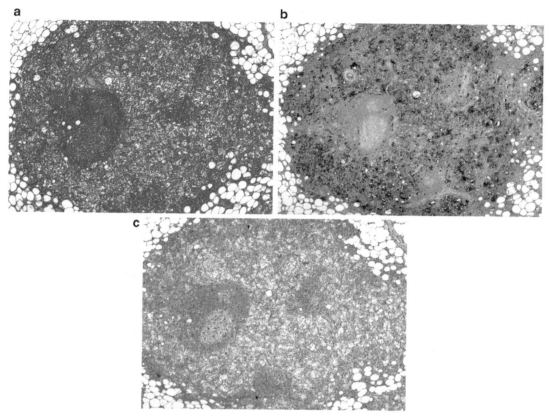

Fig. 11.42 (**a**) Nodular aggregate of histiocytes surrounding aggregates of lymphocytes containing germinal centers. The whole image of the infiltrate in this case of Rosai-Dorfman disease is reminiscent of a lymph node with massive sinus histiocytosis. Nevertheless, the infiltrate is located in the subcutaneous tissue, far from any lymph node. (**b**) Intense positivity for S100 in the histiocytic proliferation (**c**) Moderate CD68 PGM1 expression in the histiocytic proliferation

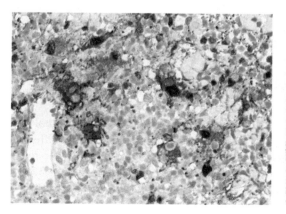

Fig. 11.43 Immunostaining for S100 highlights the phenomenon of emperipolesis, typical of Rosai-Dorfman disease, which appears in the form of nonstained cytoplasmic dots

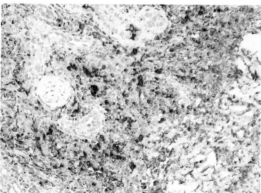

Fig. 11.44 Rosai-Dorfman disease with CD68 (PGM1)-positive histiocytic infiltrate among sweat glands

for CD1a and langerin contributes to the distinction from Langerhans cell histiocytosis (LCH). Nevertheless, there are exceptional reports of the coexistence of both histiocytosis [202].

Autoimmune disorders such as lupus erythematosus may produce dense inflammatory infiltrates, usually with lymphocytic predominance, but they rarely contain a prominent histiocytic infiltrate. IgG4-RD may exhibit an inflammatory infiltrate similar to RDD, but lacks the characteristic S100 protein-positive histiocytes with emperipolesis. Only the nodal and dermal infiltrates of H syndrome may display a microscopic and immunophenotypic appearance identical to RDD [20–22]. H syndrome is an autosomal recessive disorder with marked clinical variability. Patients with H syndrome often show low height, phalangeal flexion contractures, hearing loss, and hyperpigmented hypertrichotic cutaneous plaques [215–217]. Other systemic manifestations are hepatosplenomegaly, heart anomalies, hypogonadism, and hyperglycemia.

H syndrome is caused by the *SLC29A3* gene mutation, which results in alterations of hENT3, a member of the human equilibrative nucleoside transporter family [216]. The same mutation has been described in Faisalabad histiocytosis, also known as familial RDD, but has never been identified in sporadic cases of RDD [214].

Clues and Pitfalls

- The presence of emperipolesis with well-preserved granulocytes and some lymphocytes in the cytoplasm of proliferating histiocytes may be difficult to recognize using hematoxylin-eosin stainings, but it can be highlighted using S100 protein immunostaining, that shows nonstained dots corresponding to the internalized cells (Fig. 11.43).
- Conversely, the inflammatory cells internalized in the cytoplasm of histiocytes may be underlined with the aid of CD20, CD3, or myeloperoxidase antibodies.
- The deeply eosinophilic inclusions present in the cytoplasm of some histiocytes (Fig. 11.41)

may be misinterpreted as viral infections. Immunostaining with antibodies specific for CMV and other herpes viruses may help to rule out this possibility.

Cutaneous Kikuchi-Fujimoto Disease

Kikuchi-Fujimoto Disease (KFD), first described in 1972 and also known as histiocytic necrotizing lymphadenitis, is a rare lymphohistiocytic disorder of unknown pathogenesis [218]. It affects predominantly young adults, especially females of Asian descent. Patients often present with cervical lymphadenopathy, fever, and leukopenia, usually with spontaneous resolution in 1–4 months [219]. Several viruses, including HHV6, HHV8, Epstein-Barr virus, HTLV-1, and cytomegalovirus, have been incriminated in the pathogenesis of KFD, but the results of different studies have been contradictory [220].

Cutaneous involvement occurs in 4–14% of KFD patients [219, 221, 222]. Cutaneous lesions are nonspecific, most frequently in the form of rash or erythematous macules or papules, although atypical presentations have also been described [223].

Histologically, there are superficial and deep perivascular infiltrates of lymphocytes and histiocytes with lichenoid reaction, basal vacuolar change, and necrotic keratinocytes. Extension to the subcutis is common. Non-neutrophilic karyorrhectic debris, often phagocytosed by histiocytic cells, are frequent. Scattered plasma cells and eosinophils must be seen, but neutrophils are not present [223, 224]. KFD diagnostic criteria have been proposed on the basis of these microscopic findings [224].

Lymph nodes may show three histopathological images, probably representing different stages of disease progression [225]. In the most frequent necrotizing type, there is karyorrhectic necrosis in the paracortex with hystiocytes, plasmacytoid dendritic cells, and T lymphocytes, while neutrophils are absent (Figs. 11.45, 11.46, 11.47, and 11.48).

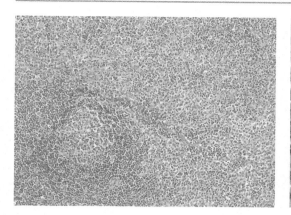

Fig. 11.45 Lymph node with Kikuchi-Fujimoto, disease showing parafollicular expansion with karyorrhectic necrosis (*upper-right* corner) and a reactive germinal center (Hematoxilin-eosin; 100×)

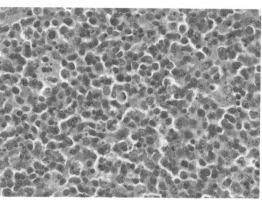

Fig. 11.47 Kikuchi-Fujimoto disease. High-power view showing karyorrhectic debris admixed with histiocytes, plasmacytoid dendritic cells and T lymphocytes, without neutrophils (Hematoxilin-eosin; 400×)

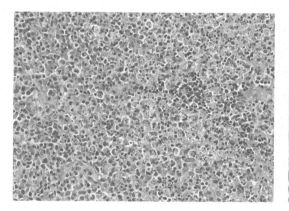

Fig. 11.46 Kikuchi-Fujimoto disease. Panoramic view of a Karyorrhectic necrotic focus (Hematoxilin-eosin; 200×)

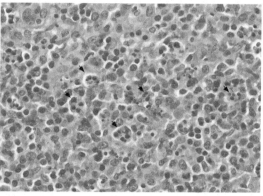

Fig. 11.48 Kikuchi-Fujimoto disease. Macrophages with phagosized karyorrhectic debris can be seen (Hematoxilin-eosin; 400×)

Immunohistochemistry

The infiltrate is composed of a mixture of hystiocityc cells (CD68+, CD4+,CD163+, myeloperoxidase+), plasmacytoid dendritic cells (CD68+, CD4+, CD123+, BDCA2+), and T lymphocytes (CD3+, with CD8+ cells outnumbering CD4+ cells) [224, 226, 227].

Molecular Biology

The molecular mechanisms that underlie KFD are largely unknown. A study based on gene-expression profiling (GEP) found upregulation of apoptosis-associated genes and downregulation of apoptosis-inhibitory genes compared to non-specific lymphadenitis [228]. Another GEP-based study found upregulation of interferon-induced genes both in lymph node and peripheral blood mononuclear cells of KFD [229]. A t(2:16) has been reported in a single case [230].

Differential Diagnosis

KFD must be differentiated from systemic lupus erythematosus (SLE), since both conditions may present with fever, lymphadenopathy, and cutaneous lesions. From a pathological point of view, in both KFD and SLE there is interface dermatitis with basal vacuolar change and apoptotic keratinocytes. The presence of abundant plasma cells and granular deposition of IgG, IgM, and IgA at the dermoepidermal junction favors SLE, whereas the observation of non-neutrophilic karyorrhectic debris favors KFD. Clinicopathological correlation, ANA screening, and long-term follow-up is encouraged to exclude SLE [222–224].

In some cases, differential diagnosis may also include panniculitis-like T-cell lymphoma (PTL), pityriasis lichenoides et varioliformis acuta (PLEVA) or erythema multiforme [224].

Clues and Pitfalls

- Always consider KFD in a cutaneous lymphohistiocytic infiltrate with interface damage, basal vacuolar change, and non-neutrophilic karyorrhectic debris.
- Clinical evaluation, ANA screening, and follow-up are mandatory in order to exclude SLE.

Cutaneous Intralymphatic Histiocytosis

Cutaneous intralymphatic histiocytosis (ILH) is a rare benign disorder characterized by dilated lymphatic vessels containing aggregates of mononuclear histiocytes (Fig. 11.49) [231, 232]. In most cases only the reticular dermis is involved. The inflammatory response in the adjacent dermis is usually scarce. Occasionally, granulomatous [233] or dense lymphocytic infiltrates forming follicles, abundant plasma cells or intense edema may be present [232]. ILH was initially described in relation to rheumatoid arthritis [234] and this seems to be the most common association, but ILH may also overly surgical scars [231] or orthopedic metal implants [235] or may be associated with neoplasia (breast cancer [231], Merkel cell carcinoma [231] and colon carcinoma) [236]. Cases of primary ILH, without any recognizable association, may also occur [232]. A single ILH case of the oral mucosa in a patient with multiple dental gold crowns simulating a lymphangioma circumscriptum has also been described [237].

Clinically, non-tender, poorly demarcated, erythematous lesions form patches, plaques, or nodules, sometimes with pseudovesicles or

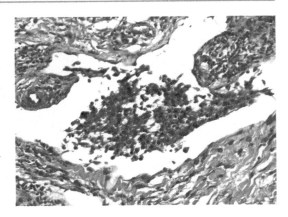

Fig. 11.49 Lymphatic vessel containing compact aggregate of histiocytes (courtesy of Dr. L. Requena, Dept. of Dermatology, Fundación Jiménez Díaz, Madrid, Spain)

livedo reticularis-like features. These lesions are usually located in the extremities and tend to overlie the inflamed joints in patients with rheumatoid arthritis. Lesions associated with joint prosthesis are also close to the articulation [231].

IJH is a benign reactive condition, but its exact pathogenesis is unknown. For some authors this could be considered the early stage of intravascular reactive angioendotheliomatosis [231, 238] or the consequence of local lymphatic damage or obstruction [231]. A recent hypothesis links ILH to the concept of the immunocompromised district [239], according to which a lesion develops at a cutaneous site that has been immune-marked by a previous clinical event. The local immune response would make this area especially susceptible to subsequent episodes of opportunistic infections, tumors, and immune disorders [240].

Immunohistochemistry

The immunohistochemical profile of ILH reflects, on the one hand, the histiocytic nature of the intravascular cells, which are positive for CD68 KP1 and PGM1 (Fig. 11.50), CD163 and CD31 and show variable positivity for myeloperoxidase, CD31, and podoplanin [231, 232]. On the other hand, vascular structures express markers characteristic of lymphatic endothelial cells such as podoplanin (Fig. 11.51), CD31, CD34, D2-40, Lyve-1, and Prox-1 [231, 232].

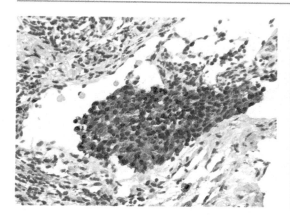

Fig. 11.50 Histiocytes present in the lumen of lymphatic vessels showing intense expression of CD68 PGM1 (courtesy of Dr. L. Requena, Dept. of Dermatology, Fundación Jiménez Díaz, Madrid, Spain)

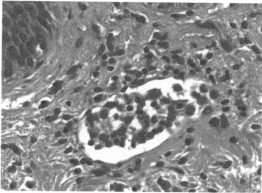

Fig. 11.52 Accumulation of histiocytes inside a lymphatic vessel at the base of an area of contact dermatitis (courtesy of Dr. L. Requena, Dept. of Dermatology, Fundación Jiménez Díaz, Madrid, Spain)

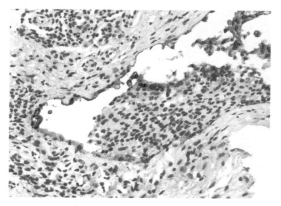

Fig. 11.51 Vessels walls in intralymphatic histiocytosis are typically positive for podoplanin. This antibody is also expressed in the cytoplasm of some histiocytic cells (courtesy of Dr. L. Requena, Dept. of Dermatology, Fundación Jiménez Díaz, Madrid, Spain)

Differential Diagnosis

The sole presence of dilated lymphatic vessels containing histiocytes in a focal area cannot be considered bona fide ILH, since it may be observed in many common dermatoses [241]. For instance, this finding may be present in contact dermatitis (Fig. 11.52), cheilitis granulomatosa, or RDD [241].

Two cases of necrotic genital lesions with intravascular histiocytosis (IVH) have been reported, but the changes involved blood vessels in which lymphatic markers were shown to be negative. One of these cases involved the scrotum of a young man with associated tonsillitis [242] and the other the vulva of an elderly woman [243] with lupus anticoagulant and elevated anticardiolipin antibodies. In both instances, the phenomenon was probably secondary to thrombogenic diathesis associated with a hypercoagulability state.

Reactive endotheliomatosis [244] and intravascular lymphomas [245] may also simulate IVH but in the first case the intravascular proliferation consist of endothelial cells and in the second case of lymphocytes, usually B-cells. Benign atypical intravascular CD30+ T-cell proliferation, a mimicker of intravascular lymphoma [246], may also be included in this differential diagnosis. An immunohistochemical study may easily demonstrate the absence of histiocytic markers in the intravascular cells of these lesions and the expression of the endothelial or lymphoid markers characteristic of each of them.

Clues and Pitfalls

- Not all intravascular accumulations of histiocytoid cells correspond to cutaneous ILH. Clinicopathological correlation may provide some clues to the nature of the lesion. A location overlying an orthopedic metal implant favors ILH.
- Conversely, the presence of large cells within hemangioma vessels is more probably a

benign intravascular CD30-positive proliferation or an intravascular lymphoma [247].

- The coexistence of intravascular histiocytosis and intravascular reactive angioendotheliomatosis has been reported. To confirm this rare association it is necessary to characterize endothelial cells with immunohistochemical markers other than CD31. The latter's positivity in histiocytic cells does not allow discrimination between the two differentiation lineages [248].

- In contrast to intralymphatic histiocytosis, the incidental accumulation of histiocytes inside a lymphatic vessel in the setting of inflammatory dermatosis is limited to one or very few vessels and shows the presence of an inflammatory infiltrate in the adjacent dermis.

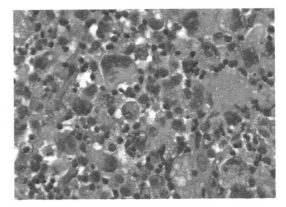

Fig. 11.53 Histiocytic sarcoma. Multinucleated neoplastic cells with abundant cytoplasm and nuclear atypia

Histiocytic Sarcoma

Histiocytic sarcoma (HS) is an aggressive and extremely rare neoplasm that may present at any age, although cases tend to cluster in two groups (0–29 and 50–69 years) [249, 250]. Lymph node involvement is frequent but extranodal involvement (gastrointestinal tract, spleen, soft tissue, or skin) is even more common. Tumor cells show morphologic and immunophenotypic features characteristic of histiocytes. In the skin, HS presents as either solitary or multiple tumors of the trunk and limbs. In cases suspicious for HS, it is mandatory to rule out other aggressive neoplasms with the aid of a broad immunohistochemical panel [249, 251, 252]. In fact, the diagnosis of HS requires exclusion of other conditions that are much more common [249].

Histologically, HS shows a diffuse, noncohesive growth of large round or oval cells that focally may adopt a sarcomatoid appearance. Cytoplasms usually are wide and eosinophilic and tend to be vacuolated. Images of hemophagocytosis may be present. Tumor cell nuclei are round or oval, often large, atypical and eccentric, with vesicular chromatin and variably sized nucleoli. Binucleation or multinucleation is common and high mitotic activity is frequently seen (Fig. 11.53) [51, 249, 253].

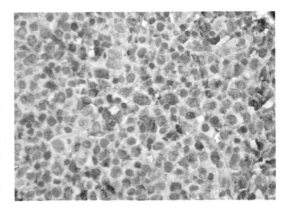

Fig. 11.54 Histiocytic sarcoma. Granular cytoplasmic immunoreactivity for CD68 in neoplastic cells

Immunohistochemistry

It is mandatory that neoplastic cells express some histiocytic markers in conjunction with their negativity for other tumor markers. The histiocytic markers more commonly used are CD163, CD68 (KP1 and PG-M1), and lysozyme. CD163 (Fig. 11.54), which shows plasma membrane and cytoplasmic positivity, is considered more specific than CD68 [254–256]. Granular cytoplasmic expression of CD68 is very reproducible, but may be found in melanoma, carcinoma, lymphoma, and dendritic cell tumor as well.

The immunohistochemical study should demonstrate negativity for Langerhans cells (CD1a and langerin), follicular dendritic cells (CD21 and CD35), myeloid cells (CD33, CD13, and myeloperoxidase), melanoma (HMB-45 and

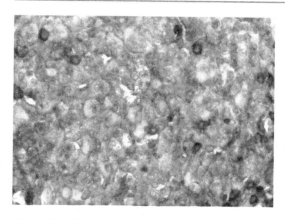

Fig. 11.55 Histiocytic sarcoma. Tumor cells are weakly positive for CD4. Follicular dendritic cell sarcoma and interdigitating dendritic cell sarcoma

Melan A) and epithelial cell (cytokeratins and EMA). Specific markers for B-cell and T-cell lymphomas should be negative. CD30 immuno-reactivity has to be equally negative. In contrast, S-100 protein, CD15, and CD1a may show some positivity, while CD4, CD45, CD45RO, and HLA-DR are commonly positive (Fig. 11.55) [51, 249, 250].

Molecular Biology

IgH or *TCR* rearrangements have been detected in some HS cases. These findings have been interpreted as transdifferentiation phenomena taking place in a previous or simultaneous B-cell or T-cell lymphoma. Indeed, several HS instances associated with previous or synchronic B-cell or T-cell lymphoblastic lymphoma or low grade B-cell lymphoma have been reported. Interestingly, in these cases HS and lymphoma share a clonality feature such as a *IgH, IGK* or *TCR* rearrangement, or a t(14:18) or t(11:14) translocation. This genetic connection with a well-characterized lymphoprolifera-tive disease does not preclude the diagnosis of HS [257–263].

Recently, BRAF(V600E) mutations have been reported in over 60 % of HS cases [5]. Nevertheless, it should be kept in mind that these mutations have also been described in Langerhans cell tumors and dendritic cell sarcomas. Additional studies are necessary to evaluate the diagnostic role of these alterations and their

potential to serve as predictors of therapeutic response to specific inhibitors [264].

Differential Diagnosis

HS differential diagnosis should be carried out with aggressive hematologic conditions such as diffuse large B-cell lymphoma, peripheral T-cell lymphoma, and anaplastic large cell lymphoma. Therefore, the immunohistochemical assessment should include B-cell and T-cell markers, CD30, and ALK-1 [249, 250, 265].

Equally important is to rule out poorly differen-tiated carcinoma and melanoma. In this regard, it should be remembered that CD68 expression may be present in both melanoma and carcinoma and, on the other hand, keratin expression may be absent in poorly differentiated carcinoma. In some cases, a generous sampling of the lesion is sufficient to identify with certainty focal histologic features characteristic of carcinoma [51, 249, 250, 253].

Langerhans cell histiocytosis has to be ruled out by demonstrating negativity for CD1a and, particularly, for langerin. Follicular dendritic cell sarcoma is easier to rule out, since follicular den-dritic cell markers are negative in HS. In contrast, interdigitating dendritic cell sarcoma poses more differential diagnostic difficulties due to the fact that, as HS, it may be positive for both S-100 pro-tein and CD68 [51, 249, 250, 253].

Clues and Pitfalls

- Positivity for histiocytic markers such as CD68 is not sufficient to establish the diagno-sis of HS. It is mandatory to rule out the diag-nosis of other aggressive neoplasms such as lymphoma, carcinoma, and melanoma.
- Although they are not diagnostically useful, CD15 and S100 protein may be focally posi-tive in HS.
- Detection of *IgH* or *TCR* rearrangements does not preclude the diagnosis of HS. Nonetheless, the presence of an aggressive lymphoma should always be ruled out by using the appro-priate immunohistochemical panel.
- In HS cases associated with lymphoma, the demonstration of shared clonality with the aid of molecular techniques is of interest.
- HS may show BRAF(V600E) mutations.

Follicular Dendritic Cell Sarcoma and Interdigitating Dendritic Cell Sarcoma

Introduction

Follicular dendritic cells (FDCs), whose origin is mesenchymal, are found in normal lymph node germinal centers, where they play an important role in the development of the immune response. Normal interdigitating dendritic cells (IDCs) are antigen-processing cells located in the paracortical T-cell zone of lymph nodes. Unlike FDCs, and similarly to Langerhans cells and histiocytes, IDCs arise from bone marrow precursor cells. Therefore, FDCs and IDCs are characterized by different immunophenotypes [266–268].

Follicular dendritic cell sarcoma (FDCS)is a rare tumor resulting from the transformation of FDCs. FDCS usually presents in adults as slowly growing tumor lesions involving cervical or abdominal lymph nodes, although extranodal sites such as the oral cavity, gastrointestinal tract, skin, mediastinum, liver, and spleen have also been described. Castleman disease may precede o coincide with FDCS. Paraneoplastic associations of FDCS with myasthenia gravis and pemphigus have been observed [269–273].

Histologically, FDCS shows moderately atypical cells that form fascicles, diffuse sheets, storiform arrays, or ill-defined nodules. Tumor cells reveal oval or elongated nuclei, vesicular or finely dispersed chromatin, and thin nuclear membranes (Fig. 11.56). Binucleated or multinucleated cells may be seen. Significant cytologic atypia, a high mitotic index, and necrosis are occasionally identified as well. Some cases show lymphoid infiltrates arranged in perivascular nests [269, 272, 274].

Interdigitating dendritic cell sarcoma (IDCS) is even rarer than FDCS. IDCS is usually seen in adults but may also arise in children. Commonly, it is a solitary lesion confined to lymph nodes, although disseminated cases have been described. Extranodal locations of IDCS include the skin, kidney, breast, lung, urinary bladder, and genitalia. Some IDCS instances associated with lymphoma have been reported [106, 274].

Histologically, IDCS may be very similar in appearance to FDCS. IDCS form fascicles and may exhibit a storiform pattern. Tumor cells

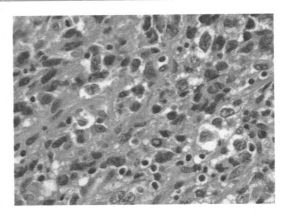

Fig. 11.56 Follicular dendritic cell sarcoma. Atypical spindle cell proliferation with some nuclear pseudoinclusions

show fusiform or ovoid indented nuclei, slightly eosinophilic abundant cytoplasm, and ill-defined cell borders. Multinucleated cells may be present and associated lymphoid infiltrates are commonly observed. Images of emperipolesis may also be present [106, 274].

Immunohistochemistry

FDCS usually shows immunopositivity for .several FDC markers (CD21, CD23, CD35, KIM4p, and CNA.42) (Figs. 11.57 and 11.58). Clusterin. is positive, often strongly so, whereas plasma membrane positivity for D2-40 is also very helpful. Additionally, positive immunoreactivity for CD4, CD20, CD45, CD68, EMA, S-100 protein, epithelial membrane antigen, fascin, and vimentin has been described in FDCS. In contrast, CD1a, langerin, CD3, CD34, CD79a, and HMB45 are negative [269, 272, 275–277].

As for IDCS, it is negative for FDC markers (CD21, CD23, and CD35), while S-100 protein, vimentin, and fascin are positive. With few exceptions CD1a and langerin are negative in IDCS. On the other hand, there is positivity for markers such as CD4, CD45, CD68, CD11c, CD14, and epithelial membrane antigen. The associated lymphoid infiltrate is mostly composed of T cells [106, 275, 277].

Molecular Biology

There is no IGH or TCR rearrangement in FDCS. Some IDCS cases associated with lymphoma have shown cytogenetic alterations characteristic

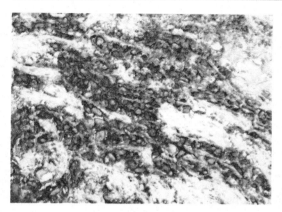

Fig. 11.57 Follicular dendritic cell sarcoma. CD23 cytoplasmic immunostaining of tumor cells

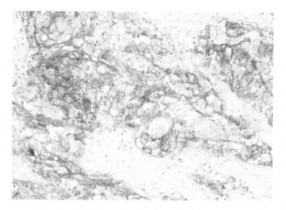

Fig. 11.58 Follicular dendritic cell sarcoma. .CD21 immunostaining showing predominantly membrane positivity in tumor cells

of the latter [106, 269, 278–280]. Recently, *BRAF* V600E mutations have been detected by direct Sanger sequencing in five of 27 FDCS instances. In contrast, this mutation was absent in an IDCS case included in the study [281]. Assessment of the diagnostic and therapeutic usefulness of these findings needs further study.

Differential Diagnosis

Morphologically, FDCS and IDCS may be very similar. Therefore, their distinction requires accurate immunophenotyping. Specifically, it is important to evaluate the expression of FDC markers (CD21, CD23, and CD35), as well as that of clusterin and D2-40 [282]. As already men-

tioned, clusterin usually is very strongly positive in FDCS [264, 269, 276, 277]. Although clusterin may be weakly positive in IDCS, its negativity for D2-40 and the FDC marker profile allows its distinction from FDCS [264, 269, 276, 277].

Langerhans cell histiocytosis (LCH) usually shows a more heterogeneous histologic appearance, with accompanying inflammatory infiltrates and a distinctive immunohistochemical profile. Although IDCS may express CD1a and S-100 protein, it is negative for langerin.

Immunohistochemical findings in histiocytic sarcoma (HS) may be similar to those of IDCS (positivity for S-100 protein and CD68 and negativity for FDC markers and langerin) [106, 269, 276].

Clues and Pitfalls

- FDCS shows characteristically strong positivity for clusterin and plasma membrane immunoreactivity for D2-40.
- Langerin immunostaining allows the distinction between LCH and IDCS.
- The T-cell immunophenotype is predominant in IDCS the lymphocytes of.
- Positivity for FDC markers distinguishes FDCS from IDCS, LCH, and histiocytic conditions.

References

1. Cho-Vega JH, Medeiros LJ, Prieto VG, Vega F. Leukemia cutis. Am J Clin Pathol. 2008;129(1):130–42.
2. Pileri SA, Orazi A, Falini B. Myeloid sarcoma. In: Swerdlow SH, Campo E, Harris NL, Jaffe ES, Pileri SA, Stein H, Thiele J, Vardiman JW, editors. WHO classification of tumours of haematopoietic and lymphoid tissues. 4th ed. Lyon, France: IARC Press; 2008. p. 140–1.
3. Hsi AC, Robirds DH, Luo J, Kreisel FH, Frater JL, Nguyen TT. T-cell prolymphocytic leukemia frequently shows cutaneous involvement and is associated with gains of MYC, loss of ATM, and TCL1A rearrangement. Am J Surg Pathol. 2014;38(11):1468–83.
4. Tokura Y, Sawada Y, Shimauchi T. Skin manifestations of adult T-cell leukemia/lymphoma: clinical, cytological and immunological features. J Dermatol. 2014;41(1):19–25.
5. Robak E, Robak T. Skin lesions in chronic lymphocytic leukemia. Leuk Lymphoma. 2007;48(5):855–65.

6. Cerroni L, Zenahlik P, Höfler G, Kaddu S, Smolle J, Kerl H. Specific cutaneous infiltrates of B-cell chronic lymphocytic leukemia: a clinicopathologic and prognostic study of 42 patients. Am J Surg Pathol. 1996;20(8):1000–10.

7. Tapia G, Mate JL, Fuente MJ, Navarro JT, Fernández-Figueras MT, Juncà J, et al. Cutaneous presentation of chronic lymphocytic leukemia as unique extramedullar involvement in a patient with normal peripheral blood lymphocyte count (monoclonal B-cell lymphocytosis). J Cutan Pathol. 2013;40(8):740–4.

8. Bénet C, Gomez A, Aguilar C, Delattre C, Vergier B, Beylot-Barry M, et al. Histologic and immunohistologic characterization of skin localization of myeloid disorders: a study of 173 cases. Am J Clin Pathol. 2011;135(2):278–90.

9. Hurley MY, Ghahramani GK, Frisch S, Armbrecht ES, Lind AC, Nguyen TT, et al. Cutaneous myeloid sarcoma: natural history and biology of an uncommon manifestation of acute myeloid leukemia. Acta Derm Venereol. 2013;93(3):319–24.

10. Amador-Ortiz C, Hurley MY, Ghahramani GK, Frisch S, Klco JM, Lind AC, et al. Use of classic and novel immunohistochemical markers in the diagnosis of cutaneous myeloid sarcoma. J Cutan Pathol. 2011;38(12):945–53.

11. Mathew RA, Bennett JM, Liu JJ, Komrokji RS, Lancet JE, Naghashpour M, et al. Cutaneous manifestations in CMML: indication of disease acceleration or transformation to AML and review of the literature. Leuk Res. 2012;36(1):72–80.

12. Patel LM, Maghari A, Schwartz RA, Kapila R, Morgan AJ, Lambert WC. Myeloid leukemia cutis in the setting of myelodysplastic syndrome: a crucial dermatological diagnosis. Int J Dermatol. 2012; 51(4):383–8.

13. Klco JM, Welch JS, Nguyen TT, Hurley MY, Kreisel FH, Hassan A, et al. State of the art in myeloid sarcoma. Int J Lab Hematol. 2011;33(6):555–65.

14. Aboutalebi A, Korman JB, Sohani AR, Hasserjian RP, Louissaint Jr A, Le L, et al. Aleukemic cutaneous myeloid sarcoma. J Cutan Pathol. 2013;40(12): 996–1005.

15. Angulo J, Haro R, González-Guerra E, Fariña MC, Martín L, Requena L. Leukemia cutis presenting as localized cutaneous hyperpigmentation. J Cutan Pathol. 2008;35(7):662–5.

16. Freiman A, Muhn CY, Trudel M, Billick RC. Leukemia cutis presenting with fingertip hypertrophy. J Cutan Med Surg. 2003;7(1):57–60.

17. Hattori T, Amano H, Nagai Y, Ishikawa O. Leukemia cutis in a patient with acute monocytic leukemia presenting as unique facial erythema. J Dermatol. 2008;35(10):671–4.

18. Cañueto J, Meseguer-Yebra C, Román-Curto C, Santos-Briz A, Fernández-López E, Fraile C, et al. Leukemic vasculitis: a rare pattern of leukemia cutis. J Cutan Pathol. 2011;38(4):360–4.

19. Martínez-Escanamé M, Zuriel D, Tee SI, Fried I, Massone C, Cerroni L. Cutaneous infiltrates of acute myelogenous leukemia simulating inflammatory dermatoses. Am J Dermatopathol. 2013;35(4): 419–24.

20. Baksh FK, Nathan D, Richardson W, Kestenbaum T, Woodroof J. Leukemia cutis with prominent giant cell reaction. Am J Dermatopathol. 1998;20(1): 48–52.

21. Chavan RN, Cappel MA, Ketterling RP, Wada DA, Rochet NM, Knudson R, et al. Histiocytoid Sweet syndrome may indicate leukemia cutis: a novel application of fluorescence in situ hybridization. J Am Acad Dermatol. 2014;70(6):1021–7.

22. Cibull TL, Thomas AB, O'Malley DP, Billings SD. Myeloid leukemia cutis: a histologic and immunohistochemical review. J Cutan Pathol. 2008;35(2): 180–5.

23. Cronin DM, George TI, Sundram UN. An updated approach to the diagnosis of myeloid leukemia cutis. Am J Clin Pathol. 2009;132(1):101–10.

24. Sangle NA, Schmidt RL, Patel JL, Medeiros LJ, Agarwal AM, Perkins SL. Optimized immunohistochemical panel to differentiate myeloid sarcoma from blastic plasmacytoid dendritic cell neoplasm. Mod Pathol. 2014;27(8):1137–43.

25. Cronin DM, George TI, Reichard KK, Sundram UN. Immunophenotypic analysis of myeloperoxidase-negative leukemia cutis and blastic plasmacytoid dendritic cell neoplasm. Am J Clin Pathol. 2012; 137(3):367–76.

26. Murphy MJ. Molecular testing of leukemia cutis. J Cutan Pathol. 2013;40(2):286–8.

27. Pileri SA, Ascani S, Cox MC, Campidelli C, Bacci F, Piccioli M, et al. Myeloid sarcoma: clinicopathologic, phenotypic and cytogenetic analysis of 92 adult patients. Leukemia. 2007;21(2):340–50.

28. Falini B, Lenze D, Hasserjian R, Coupland S, Jaehne D, Soupir C, et al. Cytoplasmic mutated nucleophosmin (NPM) defines the molecular status of a significant fraction of myeloid sarcomas. Leukemia. 2007;21(7):1566–70.

29. Sen F, Zhang XX, Prieto VG, Shea CR, Qumsiyeh MB. Increased incidence of trisomy 8 in acute myeloid leukemia with skin infiltration (leukemia cutis). Diagn Mol Pathol. 2000;9(4):190–4.

30. Agis H, Weltermann A, Fonatsch C, Haas O, Mitterbauer G, Müllauer L, et al. A comparative study on demographic, hematological, and cytogenetic findings and prognosis in acute myeloid leukemia with and without leukemia cutis. Ann Hematol. 2002;81(2):90–5.

31. Requena L, Kutzner H, Palmedo G, Pascual M, Fernández-Herrera J, Fraga J, et al. Histiocytoid Sweet syndrome: a dermal infiltration of immature neutrophilic granulocytes. Arch Dermatol. 2005; 141(7):834–42.

32. Facchetti F, Jones DM, Petrella T. Blastic plasmacytoid dendritic cells neoplasm. In: Swerdlow SH,

Campo E, Harris NL, Jaffe ES, Pileri SA, Stein H, Thiele J, Vardiman JW, editors. WHO classification of tumours of haematopoietic and lymphoid tissues. 4th ed. Lyon, France: IARC Press; 2008. p. 146–7.

33. Brody JP, Allen S, Schulman P, Sun T, Chan WC, Friedman HD, et al. Acute agranular CD4-positive natural killer cell leukemia. Comprehensive clinico-pathologic studies including virologic and in vitro culture with inducing agents. Cancer. 1995;75(10): 2474–83.

34. DiGiuseppe JA, Louie DC, Williams JE, Miller DT, Griffin CA, Mann RB, et al. Blastic natural killer cell leukemia/lymphoma: a clinicopathologic study. Am J Surg Pathol. 1997;21(10):1223–30.

35. Petrella T, Comeau MR, Maynadié M, Couillault G, De Muret A, Maliszewski CR, et al. "Agranular CD4+ CD56+ hematodermic neoplasm" (blastic NK-cell lymphoma) originates from a population of CD56+ precursor cells related to plasmacytoid monocytes. Am J Surg Pathol. 2002;26(7):852–62.

36. Julia F, Dalle S, Duru G, Balme B, Vergier B, Ortonne N, et al. Blastic plasmacytoid dendritic cell neoplasms: clinico-immunohistochemical correlations in a series of 91 patients. Am J Surg Pathol. 2014;38(5):673–80.

37. Petrella T, Bagot M, Willemze R, Beylot-Barry M, Vergier B, Delaunay M, et al. Blastic NK-cell lymphomas (agranular CD4+CD56+ hematodermic neoplasms): a review. Am J Clin Pathol. 2005;123(5): 662–75.

38. Khoury JD, Medeiros LJ, Manning JT, Sulak LE, Bueso-Ramos C, Jones D. CD56(+) TdT(+) blastic natural killer cell tumor of the skin: a primitive systemic malignancy related to myelomonocytic leukemia. Cancer. 2002;94(9):2401–8.

39. Herling M, Jones D. CD4+/CD56+ hematodermic tumor: the features of an evolving entity and its relationship to dendritic cells. Am J Clin Pathol. 2007;127(5):687–700.

40. Herling M, Teitell MA, Shen RR, Medeiros LJ, Jones D. TCL1 expression in plasmacytoid dendritic cells (DC2s) and the related CD4+ CD56+ blastic tumors of skin. Blood. 2003;101(12):5007–9.

41. Petrella T, Meijer CJ, Dalac S, Willemze R, Maynadié M, Machet L, et al. TCL1 and CLA expression in agranular CD4/CD56 hematodermic neoplasms (blastic NK-cell lymphomas) and leukemia cutis. Am J Clin Pathol. 2004;122(2):307–13.

42. Pilichowska ME, Fleming MD, Pinkus JL, Pinkus GS. CD4+/CD56+ hematodermic neoplasm ("blastic natural killer cell lymphoma"): neoplastic cells express the immature dendritic cell marker BDCA-2 and produce interferon. Am J Clin Pathol. 2007; 128(3):445–53.

43. Montes-Moreno S, Ramos-Medina R, Martínez-López A, Barrionuevo Cornejo C, Parra Cubillos A, Quintana-Truyenque S, et al. SPIB, a novel immunohistochemical marker for human blastic plasmacytoid dendritic cell neoplasms: characterization of its expression in major hematolymphoid neoplasms. Blood. 2013;121(4):643–7.

44. Marafioti T, Paterson JC, Ballabio E, Reichard KK, Tedoldi S, Hollowood K, et al. Novel markers of normal and neoplastic human plasmacytoid dendritic cells. Blood. 2008;111(7):3778–92.

45. Leroux D, Mugneret F, Callanan M, Radford-Weiss I, Dastugue N, Feuillard J, et al. CD4(+), CD56(+) DC2 acute leukemia is characterized by recurrent clonal chromosomal changes affecting 6 major targets: a study of 21 cases by the Groupe Français de Cytogénétique Hématologique. Blood. 2002;99(11): 4154–9.

46. Lucioni M, Novara F, Fiandrino G, Riboni R, Fanoni D, Arra M, et al. Twenty-one cases of blastic plasmacytoid dendritic cell neoplasm: focus on biallelic locus 9p21.3 deletion. Blood. 2011;118(17): 4591–4.

47. Sapienza MR, Fuligni F, Agostinelli C, Tripodo C, Righi S, Laginestra MA, et al. Molecular profiling of blastic plasmacytoid dendritic cell neoplasm reveals a unique pattern and suggests selective sensitivity to NF-kB pathway inhibition. Leukemia. 2014;28(8): 1606–16.

48. Alayed K, Patel KP, Konoplev S, Singh RR, Routbort MJ, Reddy N, et al. TET2 mutations, myelodysplastic features, and a distinct immunoprofile characterize blastic plasmacytoid dendritic cell neoplasm in the bone marrow. Am J Hematol. 2013; 88(12):1055–61.

49. Menezes J, Acquadro F, Wiseman M, Gómez-López G, Salgado RN, Talavera-Casañas JG, et al. Exome sequencing reveals novel and recurrent mutations with clinical impact in blastic plasmacytoid dendritic cell neoplasm. Leukemia. 2014;28(4):823–9.

50. Assaf C, Gellrich S, Whittaker S, Robson A, Cerroni L, Massone C, et al. CD56-positive haematological neoplasms of the skin: a multicentre study of the Cutaneous Lymphoma Project Group of the European Organisation for Research and Treatment of Cancer. J Clin Pathol. 2007;60(9):981–9.

51. Pileri SA, Grogan TM, Harris NL, Banks P, Campo E, Chan JK, et al. Tumours of histiocytes and accessory dendritic cells: an immunohistochemical approach to classification from the International Lymphoma Study Group based on 61 cases. Histopathology. 2002;41(1):1–29.

52. Vermi W, Facchetti F, Rosati S, Vergoni F, Rossi E, Festa S, et al. Nodal and extranodal tumor-forming accumulation of plasmacytoid monocytes/interferon-producing cells associated with myeloid disorders. Am J Surg Pathol. 2004;28(5):585–95.

53. Borowitz MJ, Chan JKC. T lymphoblastic leukemia/lymphoma. In: Swerdlow SHCE, Harris NL, Jaffe ES, et al., editors. WHO classification of tumours of haematopoietic and lymphoid tissues. Lyon: IARC; 2008. p. 176–8.

54. Borowitz MJ, Croker BP, Metzgar RS. Lymphoblastic lymphoma with the phenotype of common acute

lymphoblastic leukemia. Am J Clin Pathol. 1983; 79(3):387–91.

55. Nabhan C, Tolentino A, Meyer A, Tallman MS. Cutaneous involvement with B-lineage acute lymphoblastic leukemia. Leuk Lymphoma. 2012;53(5): 987–9.

56. Boccara O, Laloum-Grynberg E, Jeudy G, Aubriot-Lorton MH, Vabres P, de Prost Y, et al. Cutaneous B-cell lymphoblastic lymphoma in children: a rare diagnosis. J Am Acad Dermatol. 2012;66(1):51–7.

57. Lin P, Jones D, Dorfman DM, Medeiros LJ. Precursor B-cell lymphoblastic lymphoma: a predominantly extranodal tumor with low propensity for leukemic involvement. Am J Surg Pathol. 2000; 24:1480–90.

58. Gallagher G, Chhanabhai M, Song KW, Barnett MJ. Unusual presentation of precursor T-cell lymphoblastic lymphoma: involvement limited to breasts and skin. Leuk Lymphoma. 2007;48: 428–30.

59. Shafer D, Wu H, Al-Saleem T, Reddy K, Borghaei H, Lessin S, et al. Cutaneous precursor B-cell lymphoblastic lymphoma in 2 adult patients: clinicopathologic and molecular cytogenetic studies with a review of the literature. Arch Dermatol. 2008;144(9):1155–62.

60. Lee WJ, Moon HR, Won CH, Chang SE, Choi JH, Moon KC, et al. Precursor B- or T-lymphoblastic lymphoma presenting with cutaneous involvement: a series of 13 cases including 7 cases of cutaneous T-lymphoblastic lymphoma. J Am Acad Dermatol. 2014;70(2):318–25.

61. Suzumiya J, Ohshima K, Kikuchi M, Takeshita M, Akamatsu M, Tashiro K. Terminal deoxynucleotidyl transferase staining of malignant lymphomas in paraffin sections: a useful method for the diagnosis of lymphoblastic lymphoma. J Pathol. 1997;182:86–91.

62. Savage NM, Johnson RC, Natkunam Y. The spectrum of lymphoblastic, nodal and extranodal T-cell lymphomas: characteristic features and diagnostic dilemmas. Hum Pathol. 2013;44(4):451–71.

63. Chimenti S, Fink-Puches R, Peris K, Pescarmona E, Pütz B, Kerl H, et al. Cutaneous involvement in lymphoblastic lymphoma. J Cutan Pathol. 1999;26(8): 379–85.

64. Ishibashi M, Yamamoto K, Kudo S, Chen KR. Mantle cell lymphoma with skin invasion characterized by the common variant in the subcutis and blastoid transformation in the overlying dermis. Am J Dermatopathol. 2010;32(2):180–2.

65. Cao Q, Li Y, Lin H, Ke Z, Liu Y, Ye Z. Mantle cell lymphoma of blastoid variant with skin lesion and rapid progression: a case report and literature review. Am J Dermatopathol. 2013;35(8):851–5.

66. Motegi S, Okada E, Nagai Y, Tamura A, Ishikawa O. Skin manifestation of mantle cell lymphoma. Eur J Dermatol. 2006;16(4):435–8.

67. Shi Y, Wang E. Blastic plasmacytoid dendritic cell neoplasm: a clinicopathologic review. Arch Pathol Lab Med. 2014;138(4):564–9.

68. Machado I, Traves V, Cruz J, Llombart B, Navarro S, Llombart-Bosch A. Superficial small round-cell tumors with special reference to the Ewing's sarcoma family of tumors and the spectrum of differential diagnosis. Semin Diagn Pathol. 2013;30(1): 85–94.

69. Kolhe R, Reid MD, Lee JR, Cohen C, Ramalingam P. Immunohistochemical expression of PAX5 and TdT by Merkel cell carcinoma and pulmonary small cell carcinoma: a potential diagnostic pitfall but useful discriminatory marker. Int J Clin Exp Pathol. 2013;6(2):142–7.

70. Buresh CJ, Oliai BR, Miller RT. Reactivity with TdT in Merkel cell carcinoma: a potential diagnostic pitfall. Am J Clin Pathol. 2008;129(6):894–8.

71. Horny HP, Metcalfe DD, Bennett JM, Bain BJ. Mastocytosis. In: Swerdlow SH, Campo E, Harris NL, Jaffe ES, Pileri SA, Stein H, et al., editors. WHO classification of tumours of haematopoietic and lymphoid tissues. 4th ed. Lyon France: IARC Press; 2008. p. 54–63.

72. Berezowska S, Flaig MJ, Ruëff F, Walz C, Haferlach T, Krokowski M, et al. Adult-onset mastocytosis in the skin is highly suggestive of systemic mastocytosis. Mod Pathol. 2014;27(1):19–29.

73. Valent P, Escribano L, Broesby-Olsen S, Hartmann K, Grattan C, Brockow K, et al. Proposed diagnostic algorithm for patients with suspected mastocytosis: a proposal of the European Competence Network on Mastocytosis. Allergy. 2014;69(10):1267–74.

74. Valent P, Akin C, Escribano L, Födinger M, Hartmann K, Brockow K, et al. Standards and standardization in mastocytosis: consensus statements on diagnostics, treatment recommendations and response criteria. Eur J Clin Invest. 2007;37(6): 435–53.

75. Kiszewski AE, Durán-Mckinster C, Orozco-Covarrubias L, Gutiérrez-Castellón P, Ruiz-Maldonado R. Cutaneous mastocytosis in children: a clinical analysis of 71 cases. J Eur Acad Dermatol Venereol. 2004;18(3):285–90.

76. Wolff K, Komar M, Petzelbauer P. Clinical and histopathological aspects of cutaneous mastocytosis. Leuk Res. 2001;25(7):519–28.

77. Chiu A, Orazi A. Mastocytosis and related disorders. Semin Diagn Pathol. 2012;29(1):19–30.

78. Hollmann TJ, Brenn T, Hornick JL. CD25 expression on cutaneous mast cells from adult patients presenting with urticaria pigmentosa is predictive of systemic mastocytosis. Am J Surg Pathol. 2008; 32(1):139–45.

79. Morgado JM, Sánchez-Muñoz L, Teodósio CG, Jara-Acevedo M, Alvarez-Twose I, Matito A, et al. Immunophenotyping in systemic mastocytosis diagnosis: "CD25 positive" alone is more informative than the "CD25 and/or CD2" WHO criterion. Mod Pathol. 2012;25(4):516–21.

80. Valent P, Cerny-Reiterer S, Herrmann H, Mirkina I, George TI, Sotlar K, et al. Phenotypic heterogeneity, novel diagnostic markers, and target expression

profiles in normal and neoplastic human mast cells. Best Pract Res Clin Haematol. 2010;23(3):369–78.

81. Morgado JM, Perbellini O, Johnson RC, Teodósio C, Matito A, Álvarez-Twose I, et al. CD30 expression by bone marrow mast cells from different diagnostic variants of systemic mastocytosis. Histopathology. 2013;63(6):780–7.

82. Sotlar K, Cerny-Reiterer S, Petat-Dutter K, Hessel H, Berezowska S, Müllauer L, et al. Aberrant expression of CD30 in neoplastic mast cells in high-grade mastocytosis. Mod Pathol. 2011;24(4):585–95.

83. Baek JO, Kang HK, Na SY, Lee JR, Roh JY, Lee JH, et al. N822K c-kit mutation in CD30-positive cutaneous pleomorphic mastocytosis after germ cell tumour of the ovary. Br J Dermatol. 2012;166(6):1370–3.

84. Yanagihori H, Oyama N, Nakamura K, Kaneko F. c-kit Mutations in patients with childhood-onset mastocytosis and genotype-phenotype correlation. J Mol Diagn. 2005;7(2):252–7.

85. Bodemer C, Hermine O, Palmérini F, Yang Y, Grandpeix-Guyodo C, Leventhal PS, et al. Pediatric mastocytosis is a clonal disease associated with D816V and other activating c-KIT mutations. J Invest Dermatol. 2010;130(3):804–15.

86. Ma D, Stence AA, Bossler AB, Hackman JR, Bellizzi AM. Identification of KIT activating mutations in paediatric solitary mastocytoma. Histopathology. 2014;64(2):218–25.

87. Badalian-Very G, Vergilio JA, Fleming M, Rollins BJ. Pathogenesis of Langerhans cell histiocytosis. Annu Rev Pathol. 2013;8:1–20.

88. Jaffe R, Weis LM, Facchetti F. Tumours derived from Langerhans cells. In: Swerdlow SH, Campo E, Harris NL, Jaffe ES, et al., editors. WHO classification of tumours of haematopoietic and lymphoid tissues. 4th ed. Lyon: International Agency for Research on Cancer (IARC); 2008. p. 358–630.

89. Favara BE, Feller AC, Pauli M, Jaffe ES, Weiss LM, Arico M, et al. Contemporary classification of histiocytic disorders. The WHO Committee On Histiocytic/Reticulum Cell Proliferations. Reclassification Working Group of the Histiocyte Society. Med Pediatr Oncol. 1997;29(3):157–66.

90. Valentín-Nogueras SM, Seijo-Montes R, Montalván-Miró E, Sánchez JL. Langerhans cell sarcoma: a case report. J Cutan Pathol. 2013;40(7):670–5.

91. Valladeau J, Duvert-Frances V, Pin JJ, Dezutter-Dambuyant C, Vincent C, Massacrier C, et al. The monoclonal antibody DCGM4 recognizes Langerin, a protein specific of Langerhans cells, and is rapidly internalized from the cell surface. Eur J Immunol. 1999;29(9):2695–704.

92. Kim HK, Park CJ, Jang S, Cho YU, Park SH, Koh KN, et al. Bone marrow involvement of Langerhans cell histiocytosis: immunohistochemical evaluation of bone marrow for CD1a, Langerin, and S100 expression. Histopathology. 2014;65(6):742–8.

93. Lau SK, Chu PG, Weiss LM. Immunohistochemical expression of Langerin in Langerhans cell histiocytosis and non-Langerhans cell histiocytic disorders. Am J Surg Pathol. 2008;32(4):615–9.

94. Roden AC, Hu X, Kip S, Parrilla Castellar ER, Rumilla KM, Vrana JA, et al. BRAF V600E expression in Langerhans cell histiocytosis: clinical and mmunohistochemical study on 25 pulmonary and 54 extrapulmonary cases. Am J Surg Pathol. 2014;38(4):548–51.

95. Méhes G, Irsai G, Bedekovics J, Beke L, Fazakas F, Rózsa T, et al. Activating BRAF V600E mutation in aggressive pediatric Langerhans cell histiocytosis: demonstration by allele-specific PCR/direct sequencing and immunohistochemistry. Am J Surg Pathol. 2014;38(12):1644–8.

96. Sagransky MJ, Deng AC, Magro CM. Primary cutaneous langerhans cell sarcoma: a report of four cases and review of the literature. Am J Dermatopathol. 2013;35(2):196–204.

97. Badalian-Very G, Virgilio J, Degar BA, MacConaill LE, Brandner B, Calicchio ML, et al. Recurrent BRAF mutations in Langerhans cell histiocytosis. Blood. 2010;116(11):1919–23.

98. Brown NA, Furtado LV, Betz BL, Kiel MJ, Weigelin HC, Lim MS, et al. High prevalence of somatic MAP2K1 mutations in BRAF V600E-negative Langerhans cell histiocytosis. Blood. 2014;124(10):1655–8.

99. Hicks MJ, Bonilla DL, Dwyer KC, Berres ML, Poulikakos PI, Merad M, et al. Mutually exclusive recurrent somatic mutations in MAP2K1 and BRAF support a central role for ERK activation in LCH pathogenesis. Blood. 2014;124(19):3007–15.

100. Nelson DS, Quispel W, Badalian-Very G, van Halteren AG, van den Bos C, Bovée JV, et al. Somatic activating ARAF mutations in Langerhans cell histiocytosis. Blood. 2014;123(20):3152–5.

101. Kansal R, Quintanilla-Martinez L, Datta V, Lopategui J, Garshfield G, Nathwani BN. Identification of the V600D mutation in Exon 15 of the BRAF oncogene in congenital, benign langerhans cell histiocytosis. Genes Chromosomes Cancer. 2013;52(1):99–106.

102. Haroche J, Cohen-Aubart F, Emile JF, Arnaud L, Maksud P, Charlotte F, et al. Dramatic efficacy of vemurafenib in both multisystemic and refractory Erdheim-Chester disease and Langerhans cell histiocytosis harboring the BRAF V600E mutation. Blood. 2013;121(9):1495–500.

103. Baiocchi RA. Driving toward targeted therapy for LCH. Blood. 2014;124(10):1546–8.

104. Weitzman S, Jaffe R. Uncommon histiocytic disorders: the non-Langerhans cell histiocytoses. Pediatr Blood Cancer. 2005;45(3):256–64.

105. Rezk SA, Spagnolo DV, Brynes RK, Weiss LM. Indeterminate cell tumor: a rare dendritic neoplasm. Am J Surg Pathol. 2008;32(12):1868–76.

106. Weis LM, Chan JKC, Fletcher CDM. Other rare dendritic cell tumors. In: Swerdlow SH, Campo E, Harris NL, Jaffe ES, et al., editors. WHO classification of tumours of haematopoietic and lymphoid tissues. 4th ed. Lyon: International Agency for Research on Cancer (IARC); 2008. p. 365.

107. Ferran M, Toll A, Gilaberte M, Barranco C, Lloreta J, Pujol RM. Acquired mucosal indeterminate cell histiocytoma. Pediatr Dermatol. 2007;24(3):253–6.

108. Tardío JC, Aguado M, Borbujo J. Self-regressing S100-negative CD1a-positive cutaneous histiocytosis. Am J Dermatopathol. 2013;35(4):57–9.

109. Calatayud M, Güell JL, Gris O, Puig J, Arrondo E, Huguet P. Ocular involvement in a case of systemic indeterminate cell histiocytosis: a case report. Cornea. 2001;20(7):769–71.

110. Ratzinger G, Burgdorf WH, Metze D, Zelger BG, Zelger B. Indeterminate cell histiocytosis: fact or fiction? J Cutan Pathol. 2005;32(8):552–60.

111. Ventura F, Pereira T, da Luz DM, Marques H, Pardal F, Brito C. Indeterminate cell histiocytosis in association with acute myeloid leukemia. Dermatol Res Pract. 2010;2010:569345.

112. Buser L, Bihl M, Rufle A, Mickys U, Tavoriene I, Griskevicius L, et al. Unique composite hematolymphoid tumor consisting of a pro-T lymphoblastic lymphoma and an indeterminate dendritic cell tumor: evidence for divergent common progenitor cell differentiation. Pathobiology. 2014;81(4):199–205.

113. Dehner LP. Juvenile xanthogranulomas in the first two decades of life: a clinicopathologic study of 174 cases with cutaneous and extracutaneous manifestations. Am J Surg Pathol. 2003;27(5):579–93.

114. Zelger BG, Zelger B, Steiner H, Mikuz G. Solitary giant xanthogranuloma and benign cephalic histiocytosis—variants of juvenile xanthogranuloma. Br J Dermatol. 1995;133(4):598–604. 40.

115. Torrelo A, Juarez A, Hernández A, Colmenero I. Multiple lichenoid juvenile xanthogranuloma. Pediatr Dermatol. 2009;26(2):238.

116. Koren J, Matecek L, Zamecnik M. Mitotically active deep juvenile xanthogranuloma. Ann Diagn Pathol. 2010;14(1):36–40.

117. Newman CC, Raimer SS, Sánchez RL. Nonlipidized juvenile xanthogranuloma: a histologic and immunohistochemical study. Pediatr Dermatol. 1997;14(2):98–102.

118. Ngendahayo P, de Saint Aubain N. Mitotically active xanthogranuloma: a case report with review of the literature. Am J Dermatopathol. 2012;34(3):e27–30.

119. Fenot M, Stalder JF, Barbarot S. Juvenile xanthogranulomas are highly prevalent but transient in young children with neurofibromatosis type 1. J Am Acad Dermatol. 2014;71(2):389–90.

120. Iyengar V, Golomb CA, Schachner L. Neurilemmomatosis, NF2, and juvenile xanthogranuloma. J Am Acad Dermatol. 1998;39(5 Pt 2):831–4.

121. Zvulunov A, Barak Y, Metzker A. Juvenile xanthogranuloma, neurofibromatosis, and juvenile chronic myelogenous leukemia. World statistical analysis. Arch Dermatol. 1995;131(8):904–8.

122. Shin HT, Harris MB, Orlow SJ. Juvenile myelomonocytic leukemia presenting with features of hemophagocytic lymphohistiocytosis in association with neurofibromatosis and juvenile xanthogranulomas. J Pediatr Hematol Oncol. 2004;26(9):591–5.

123. Tran DT, Wolgamot GM, Olerud J, Hurst S, Argenyi Z. An "eruptive" variant of juvenile xanthogranuloma associated with langerhans cell histiocytosis. J Cutan Pathol. 2008;35 Suppl 1:50–4.

124. Gonzalez Ruíz A, Bernal Ruíz AI, Aragoneses Fraile H, Peral Martinez I, García MM. Progressive nodular histiocytosis accompanied by systemic disorders. Br J Dermatol. 2000;143(3):628–31.

125. Lüftl M, Seybold H, Simon Jr M, Burgdorf W. Progressive nodular histiocytosis—rare variant of cutaneous non-Langerhans cell histiocytosis. J Dtsch Dermatol Ges. 2006;4(3):236–8.

126. Veyssier-Belot C, Cacoub P, Caparros-Lefebvre D, Wechsler J, Brun B, Remy M, et al. Erdheim-Chester disease. Clinical and radiologic characteristics of 59 cases. Medicine. 1996;75(3):157–69.

127. Mazor RD, Manervich-Mazor M, Shoenfeld Y. Erdheim Chester Disease: A comprehensive review of the literature. Orphanet J Rare Dis. 2013;8:137.

128. Kraus MD, Haley JC, Ruiz R, Essary L, Moran CA, Fletcher CD. "Juvenile" xanthogranuloma: an immunophenotypic study with a reappraisal of histogenesis. Am J Dermatopathol. 2001;23(2):104–11.

129. Tidwell WJ, Googe PB. Tissue histiocyte reactivity with CD31 is comparable to CD68 and CD163 in common skin lesions. J Cutan Pathol. 2014; 41(6):489–93.

130. Pouryazdanparast P, Yu L, Cutlan JE, Olsen SH, Fullen DR, Ma L. Diagnostic value of CD163 in cutaneous spindle cell lesions. J Cutan Pathol. 2009;36(8):859–64.

131. Tomaszewski MM, Lupton GP. Unusual expression of S-100 protein in histiocytic neoplasms. J Cutan Pathol. 1998;25(3):129–35.

132. Amouri M, Gouiaa N, Chaaben H, Masmoudi A, Zahaf A, Boudawara T, et al. Disseminated juvenile xanthogranuloma expressing protein S100. Ann Dermatol Venereol. 2012;139(2):128–31.

133. Yamamoto Y, Kadota M, Nishimura Y. A case of S-100-positive juvenile xanthogranuloma: a longitudinal observation. Pediatr Dermatol. 2009;26(4): 475–6.

134. Perez-Becker R, Szczepanowski M, Leuschner I, Janka G, Gokel M, Imschweiler T, et al. An aggressive systemic juvenile xanthogranuloma clonally related to a preceding T-cell acute lymphoblastic leukemia. Pediatr Blood Cancer. 2011;56(5): 859–62.

135. Emile JF, Diamond EL, Hélias-Rodzewicz Z, Charlotte F, Hyman DM, Kim E, et al. Recurent RAS and PIK3CA mutations in Erdheim-Chester disease. Blood. 2014;124(19):3016–09.

136. Haroche J, Charlotte F, Arnaud L, von Deimling A, Hélias-Rodzewicz Z, et al. High prevalence of BRAF V600E mutations in Erdheim-Chester disease but not in other non-Langerhans cell histiocytoses. Blood. 2012;120(13):2700–3.

137. Bubolz AM, Weissinger SE, Stenzinger A, Arndt A, Steinestel K, Brüderlein S, et al. Potential clinical implications of BRAF mutations in histiocytic proliferations. Oncotarget. 2014;5(12):4060–70.

138. Janku F, Vibat CR, Kosco K, Holley VR, Cabrilo G, Meric-Bernstam F, et al. BRAF V600E mutations in urine and plasma cell-free DNA from patients with Erdheim-Chester disease. Oncotarget. 2014;5(11): 3607–10.

139. Cavalli G, Biavasco R, Borgiani B, Dagna L. Oncogene-induced senescence as a new mechanism of disease: the paradigm of Erdheim-Chester disease. Front Immunol. 2014;5:281. doi:10.3389/fimmu.2014.00281.eCollection2014.

140. Aldabagh B, Ly MN, Hessel AB, Usmani AS. Molluscum contagiosum involving an epidermoid cyst with xanthogranuloma-like reaction in an HIV-infected patient. J Cutan Pathol. 2010;37(2): 282–6.

141. Nakamura Y, Nakamura A, Muto M. Solitary spindle cell xanthogranuloma mimicking a spitz nevus. Am J Dermatopathol. 2013;35(8):865–7.

142. Berti S, Coronella G, Galeone M, Balestri R, Patrizi A, Neri I. Giant congenital juvenile xanthogranuloma. Arch Dis Child. 2013;98(4):317.

143. Cohen PR, Prieto VG. Radiation port xanthogranuloma: solitary xanthogranuloma occurring within the irradiated skin of a breast cancer patient-report and review of cutaneous neoplasms developing at the site of radiotherapy. J Cutan Pathol. 2010;37(8): 891–4.

144. Shimada R, Fujimura T, Kambayashi Y, Ohtani T, Nasu M, Numata Y, et al. CD163+ adult xanthogranuloma arising from Merkel cell carcinoma treated with local radiotherapy. Acta Derm Venereol. 2012;92(6):631–2.

145. Janka GE, Lehmberg K. Hemophagocytic syndromes—an update. Blood Rev. 2014;28(4): 135–42.

146. Ramos-Casals M, Brito-Zerón P, López-Guillermo A, Khamashta MA, Bosch X. Adult haemophagocytic syndrome. Lancet. 2014;383(9927):1503.

147. Li J, Wang Q, Zheng W, Ma J, Zhang W, Wang W, et al. Hemophagocytic lymphohistiocytosis: clinical analysis of 103 adult patients. Medicine. 2014; 93(2):100–5.

148. Janka GE, Lehmberg K. Hemophagocytic lymphohistiocytosis: pathogenesis and treatment. Hematology Am Soc Hematol Educ Program. 2013; 2013:605–11.

149. Zhang K, Jordan MB, Marsh RA, Johnson JA, Kissell D, Meller J, et al. Hypomorphic mutations in PRF1, MUNC13-4, and STXBP2 are associated with adult onset familial HLH. Blood. 2011;118(22):5794–8.

150. Jessen B, Bode SF, Ammann S, Chakravorty S, Davies G, Diestelhorst J, et al. The risk of hemophagocytic lymphohistiocytosis in Hermansky-Pudlak syndrome type 2. Blood. 2013;121(15): 2943–51.

151. Lin CI, Yu HH, Lee JH, Wang LC, Lin YT, Yang YH, et al. Clinical analysis of macrophage activation syndrome in pediatric patients with autoimmune diseases. Clin Rheumatol. 2012;31(8):1223–30.

152. Risma K, Jordan MB. Hemophagocytic lymphohistiocytosis: updates and evolving concepts. Curr Opin Pediatr. 2012;24(1):9–15.

153. Brisse E, Wouters CH, Matthys P. Hemophagocytic lymphohistiocytosis (HLH): a heterogeneous spectrum of cytokine-driven immune disorders. Cytokine Growth Factor Rev. 2014. doi:10.1016/j.cytogfr.2014.10.001.

154. Kerl K, Wolf IH, Cerroni L, Wolf P, French LE, Kerl H. Hemophagocytosis in cutaneous autoimmune disease. Am J Dermatopathol. 2015;37(7): 539–43.

155. Schaer DJ, Schleiffenbaum B, Kurrer M, Imhof A, Bächli E, Fehr J, et al. Soluble hemoglobin-haptoglobin scavenger receptor CD163 as a lineage-specific marker in the reactive hemophagocytic syndrome. Eur J Haematol. 2005;74:6–10.

156. Wada T, Sakakibara Y, Nishimura R, Toma T, Ueno Y, Horita S, et al. Down-regulation of CD5 expression on activated CD8+ T cells in familial hemophagocytic lymphohistiocytosis with perforin gene mutations. Hum Immunol. 2013;74(12):1579–85.

157. Ohkuma K, Saraya T, Sada M, Kawai S. Evidence for cytomegalovirus-induced haemophagocytic syndrome in a young patient with AIDS. BMJ Case Rep. 2013; 2013.

158. Ito Y, Kawamura Y, Iwata S, Kawada J, Yoshikawa T, Kimura H. Demonstration of type II latency in T lymphocytes of Epstein-Barr virus-associated hemophagocytic lymphohistiocytosis. Pediatr Blood Cancer. 2013;60(2):326–8.

159. Ahn JS, Rew SY, Shin MG, Kim HR, Kim HR, Yang DH, et al. Clinical significance of clonality and Epstein-Barr virus infection in adult patients with hemophagocytic lymphohistiocytosis. Am J Hematol. 2010;85:719–22.

160. Smith MC, Cohen DN, Greig B, Yenamandra A, Vnencak-Jones C, Thompson MA, et al. The ambiguous boundary between EBV-related hemophagocytic lymphohistiocytosis and systemic EBV-driven T cell lymphoproliferative disorder. Int J Clin Exp Pathol. 2014;7(9):5738–49.

161. Draper NL, Morgan MB. Dermatologic perivascular hemophagocytosis: a report of two cases. Am J Dermatopathol. 2007;29(5):467–9.

162. Valentín SM, Montalván E, Sánchez JL. Perivascular hemophagocytosis: report of 2 cases and review of the literature. Am J Dermatopathol. 2010;32(7): 716–9.

163. Henter JI, Horne A, Arico M, Egeler RM, Filipovich AH, Imashuku S, et al. HLH-2004: diagnostic and

therapeutic guidelines for hemophagocytic lympho-histiocytosis. Pediatr Blood Cancer. 2007;48(2):124–31.

164. Sroa N, Zirwas MJ, Bechtel M. Multicentric reticu-lohistiocytosis: a case report and review of the litera-ture. Cutis. 2010;85(3):153–5.

165. Baek IW, Yoo SH, Yang H, Park J, Kim KJ, Cho CS. A case of multicentric reticulohistiocytosis. Mod Rheumatol. 2014;1–4. [Epub ahead of print] PMID: 25211404.

166. Kandiah DA. Multicentric reticulohistiocytosis. Mayo Clin Proc. 2014;89(8):e73. doi:10.1016/j.mayocp.2013.10.036.

167. Lu YY, Lu CC, Wu CH. Leonine facies in the cuta-neous form of multicentric reticulohistiocytosis. Intern Med. 2012;51(15):2069–70.

168. West KL, Sporn T, Puri PK. Multicentric reticulo-histiocytosis: a unique case with pulmonary fibrosis. Arch Dermatol. 2012;148(2):228–32.

169. Yang HJ, Ding YQ, Deng YJ. Multicentric reticulo-histiocytosis with lungs and liver involved. Clin Exp Dermatol. 2009;34(2):183–5.

170. Webb-Detiege T, Sasken H, Kaur P. Infiltration of histiocytes and multinucleated giant cells in the myocardium of a patient with multicentric reticulo-histiocytosis. J Clin Rheumatol. 2009;15(1):25–6.

171. Taniguchi T, Asano Y, Okada A, Sugaya M, Sato S. Ultraviolet light-induced Köbner phenomenon contributes to the development of skin eruptions in multicentric reticulohistiocytosis. Acta Derm Venereol. 2011;91(2):160–3.

172. Arai S, Katsuoka K, Ishikawa A. Multicentric reticu-lohistiocytosis presenting with the cutaneous fea-tures of photosensitivity dermatitis. J Dermatol. 2012;39(2):180–1.

173. Bennàssar A, Mas A, Guilabert A, Julià M, Mascaró-Galy JM, Herrero C. Multicentric reticulohistiocyto-sis with elevated cytokine serum levels. J Dermatol. 2011;38(9):905–10.

174. Kovach BT, Calamia KT, Walsh JS, Ginsburg WW. Treatment of multicentric reticulohistiocytosis with etanercept. Arch Dermatol. 2004;140(8):919–21.

175. Lovelace K, Loyd A, Adelson D, Crowson N, Taylor JR, Cornelison R. Etanercept and the treatment of multicentric reticulohistiocytosis. Arch Dermatol. 2005;141(9):1167–8.

176. Iwata H, Okumura Y, Seishima M, Aoyama Y. Overexpression of monocyte chemoattractant protein-1 in the overlying epidermis of multicentric reticulohistiocytosis lesions: a case report. Int J Dermatol. 2012;51(4):492–4.

177. Codriansky KA, Rünger TM, Bhawan J, Kantarci A, Kissin EY. Multicentric reticulohistiocytosis: a sys-temic osteoclastic disease? Arthritis Rheum. 2008;59(3):444–8. doi:10.1002/art.23320.

178. Nicol C, Quereux G, Renaut JJ, Renac F, Dreno B. Paraneoplastic multicentric reticulohistiocytosis. Ann Dermatol Venereol. 2011;138(5):405–8.

179. Ben Abdelghani K, Mahmoud I, Chatelus E, Sordet C, Gottenberg JE, Sibilia J. Multicentric reticulohis-tiocytosis: an autoimmune systemic disease? Case report of an association with erosive rheumatoid arthritis and systemic Sjogren syndrome. Joint Bone Spine. 2010;77(3):274–6.

180. Macía-Villa CC, Zea-Mendoza A. Multicentric reticulohistiocytosis: case report with response to infliximab and review of treatment options. Clin Rheumatol. 2016;35(2):527–34.

181. Zelger B, Cerio R, Soyer HP, Misch K, Orchard G, Wilson-Jones E. Reticulohistiocytoma and multi-centric reticulohistiocytosis. Histopathologic and immunophenotypic distinct entities. Am J Dermatopathol. 1994;16(6):577–84.

182. Miettinen M, Fetsch JF. Reticulohistiocytoma (soli-tary epithelioid histiocytoma): a clinicopathologic and immunohistochemical study of 44 cases. Am J Surg Pathol. 2006;30(4):521–8.

183. Bialynicki-Birula R, Sebastian-Rusin A, Maj J, Wozniak Z, Baran E, Dziegiel P. Multicentric reticu-lohistiocytosis with S100 protein positive staining: a case report. Acta Dermatovenerol Croat. 2010;18(1):35–7.

184. Perrin C, Lacour JP, Michiels JF, Flory P, Ziegler G, Ortonne JP. Multicentric reticulohistiocytosis. Immunohistological and ultrastructural study: a pathology of dendritic cell lineage. Am J Dermatopathol. 1992;14(5):418–25.

185. Tashiro A, Takeuchi S, Nakahara T, Oba J, Tsujita J, Fukushi J, et al. Aberrant expression of CD10 in ground-glass-like multinucleated giant cells of mul-ticentric reticulohistiocytosis. J Dermatol. 2010;37(11):995–7.

186. Tan BH, Barry CI, Wick MR, White KP, Brown JG, Lee A, et al. Multicentric reticulohistiocytosis and urologic carcinomas: a possible paraneoplastic asso-ciation. J Cutan Pathol. 2011;38(1):43–8.

187. Krause ML, Lehman JS, Warrington KJ. Multicentric reticulohistiocytosis can mimic rheumatoid arthritis. J Rheumatol. 2014;41(4):780–1.

188. Trotta F, Colina M. Multicentric reticulohistiocyto-sis and fibroblastic rheumatism. Best Pract Res Clin Rheumatol. 2012;26(4):543–57.

189. Mun JH, Ko HC, Kim MB. Multicentric reticulohis-tiocytosis masquerading as dermatomyositis: similar and different features. J Dermatol. 2012;39(1):104–7.

190. Fett N, Liu RH. Multicentric reticulohistiocytosis with dermatomyositis-like features: a more common disease presentation than previously thought. Dermatology. 2011;222(2):102–8.

191. Spadaro A, Riccieri V, Sili-Scavalli A, Innocenzi D, Pranteda G, Taccari E. Value of cytological analysis of the synovial fluid in multicentric reticulohistiocy-tosis. A case. Rev Rhum Ed Fr. 1994;61(7–8):554–7.

192. Zak FG. Reticulohistiocytoma ("ganglioneuroma") of the skin. Br J Dermatol Syph. 1950;62(9):351–5.

193. Rabkin MS, Vukmer T. Granular cell variant of epi-thelioid cell histiocytoma. Am J Dermatopathol. 2012;34(7):766–9.

194. Caltabiano R, Magro G, Vecchio GM, Lanzafame S. Solitary cutaneous histiocytosis with granular cell changes: a morphological variant of reticulohistiocytoma? J Cutan Pathol. 2010;37(2):287–91.

195. Jedrych J, Nikiforova M, Kennedy TF, Ho J. Epithelioid cell histiocytoma of the skin with clonal ALK gene rearrangement resulting in VCL-ALK and SQSTM1-ALK gene fusions. Br J Dermatol. 2015;37(7):539–43.

196. Miettinen M, Fernandez M, Franssila K, Gatalica Z, Lasota J, Sarlomo-Rikala M. Microphthalmia transcription factor in the immunohistochemical diagnosis of metastatic melanoma: comparison with four other melanoma markers. Am J Surg Pathol. 2001; 25(2):205–11.

197. Rosai J, Dorfman RF. Sinus histiocytosis with massive lymphadenopathy. A newly recognized benign clinicopathological entity. Arch Pathol. 1969;87: 63–70.

198. Brenn T, Calonje E, Granter SR, Leonard N, Grayson W, Fletcher CD, et al. Cutaneous rosaidorfman disease is a distinct clinical entity. Am J Dermatopathol. 2002;24(5):385–91.

199. Zhu F, Zhang JT, Xing XW, Wang DJ, Zhu RY, Zhang Q, et al. Rosai-Dorfman disease: a retrospective analysis of 13 cases. Am J Med Sci. 2013; 345:200–10.

200. Frater JL, Maddox JS, Obadiah JM, Hurley MY. Cutaneous Rosai-Dorfman disease: comprehensive review of cases reported in the medical literature since 1990 and presentation of an illustrative case. J Cutan Med Surg. 2006;10(6):281–90.

201. Fernandez-Vega I, Santos-Juanes J, Ramsay A. Rosai-Dorfman disease following a classical Hodgkin lymphoma, nodular sclerosis subtype. Am J Dermatopathol. 2014;36(3):280–1.

202. Llamas-Velasco M, Cannata J, Dominguez I, García-Noblejas A, Aragües M, Fraga J, et al. Coexistence of Langerhans cell histiocytosis, Rosai-Dorfman disease and splenic lymphoma with fatal outcome after rapid development of histiocytic sarcoma of the liver. J Cutan Pathol. 2012;39(12):1125–30.

203. Venkataraman G, McClain KL, Pittaluga S, Rao VK, Jaffe ES. Development of disseminated histiocytic sarcoma in a patient with autoimmune lymphoproliferative syndrome and associated Rosai-Dorfman disease. Am J Surg Pathol. 2010;34(4):589–94.

204. Arakaki N, Gallo G, Majluf R, Diez B, Arias E, Riudavets MA, et al. Extranodal Rosai-Dorfman disease presenting as a solitary mass with human herpesvirus 6 detection in a pediatric patient. Pediatr Dev Pathol. 2012;15(4):324–8.

205. Al-Daraji W, Anandan A, Klassen-Fischer M, Auerbach A, Marwaha JS, Fanburg-Smith JC. Soft tissue Rosai-Dorfman disease: 29 new lesions in 18 patients, with detection of polyomavirus antigen in 3 abdominal cases. Ann Diagn Pathol. 2010;14(5): 309–16.

206. Salva KA, Stenstrom M, Breadon JY, Odland PB, Bennett D, Longley J, et al. Possible association of cutaneous Rosai-Dorfman disease and chronic Crohn disease: a case series report. JAMA Dermatol. 2014;150(2):177–81.

207. Zhang X, Hyjek E, Vardiman J. A subset of Rosai-Dorfman disease exhibits features of IgG4-related disease. Am J Clin Pathol. 2013;139(5):622–32.

208. Menon MP, Evbuomwan MO, Rosai J, Jaffe ES, Pittaluga S. A subset of Rosai-Dorfman disease cases show increased IgG4-positive plasma cells: another red herring or a true association with IgG4-related disease? Histopathology. 2014;64(3):455–9.

209. Liu L, Perry AM, Cao W, Smith LM, Hsi ED, Liu X, et al. Relationship between Rosai-Dorfman disease and IgG4-related disease: study of 32 cases. Am J Clin Pathol. 2013;140(3):395–402.

210. Vuong V, Moulonguet I, Cordoliani F, Crickx B, Bezier M, Vignon-Pennamen MD, et al. Cutaneous revelation of Rosai-Dorfman disease: 7 cases. Ann Dermatol Venereol. 2013;140(2):83–90.

211. Cangelosi JJ, Prieto VG, Ivan D. Cutaneous Rosai-Dorfman disease with increased number of eosinophils: coincidence or histologic variant? Arch Pathol Lab Med. 2011;135(12):1597–600.

212. Foucar E, Rosai J, Dorfman RF. Sinus histiocytosis with massive lymphadenopathy. An analysis of 14 deaths occurring in a patient registry. Cancer. 1984;54:1834–40.

213. Sasaki K, Pemmaraju N, Westin JR, Wang WL, Khoury JD, Podoloff DA, et al. A single case of Rosai-Dorfman disease marked by pathologic fractures, kidney failure, and liver cirrhosis treated with single-agent cladribine. Front Oncol. 2014;4:297.

214. Zheng M, Bi R, Li W, Landeck L, Chen JQ, Lao LM, et al. Generalized pure cutaneous Rosai-Dorfman disease: a link between inflammation and cancer not associated with mitochondrial DNA and SLC29A3 gene mutation? Discov Med. 2013;16(89): 193–200.

215. Avitan-Hersh E, Mandel H, Indelman M, Bar-Joseph G, Zlotogorski A, Bergman R. A case of H syndrome showing immunophenotye similarities to Rosai-Dorfman disease. Am J Dermatopathol. 2011;33(1):47–51.

216. Colmenero I, Molho-Pessach V, Torrelo A, Zlotogorski A, Requena L. Emperipolesis: an additional common histopathologic finding in H syndrome and Rosai-Dorfman disease. Am J Dermatopathol. 2012;34(3):315–20.

217. Molho-Pessach V, Ramot Y, Camille F, Doviner V, Babay S, Luis SJ, et al. H syndrome: the first 79 patients. J Am Acad Dermatol. 2014;70(1):80–8.

218. Kikuchi M. Lymphadenitis showing focal reticulum cell hyperplasia with nuclear debris and phagocytes. Acta Hematol Jpn. 1972;35:379–80.

219. Kim TY, Ha KS, Kim Y, Lee J, Lee K, Lee J. Characteristics of Kikuchi-Fujimoto disease in children compared with adults. Eur J Pediatr. 2014; 173(1):111–6.

220. Bosch X, Guilabert A, Miquel R, Campo E. Enigmatic Kikuchi-Fujimoto disease: a comprehensive

review. Am J Clin Pathol. 2004;122(1): 141–52.

221. Kucukardali Y, Solmazgul E, Kunter E, Oncul O, Yildirim S, Kaplan M. Kikuchi-Fujimoto disease: analysis of 244 cases. Clin Rheumatol. 2007; 26(1):50–4.

222. Cheng CY, Sheng WH, Lo YC, Chung CS, Chen YC, Chang SC. Clinical presentations, laboratory results and outcomes of patients with Kikuchi's disease: emphasis on the association between recurrent Kikuchi's disease and autoimmune diseases. J Microbiol Immunol Infect. 2010;43(5):366–71.

223. Atwater AR, Longley BJ, Aughenbaugh WD. Kikuchi's disease: case report and systematic review of cutaneous and histopathologic presentations. J Am Acad Dermatol. 2008;59(1):130–6.

224. Kim JH, Kim YB, In SI, Kim YC, Han JH. The cutaneous lesions of Kikuchi's disease: a comprehensive analysis of 16 cases based on the clinicopathologic, immunohistochemical, and immunofluorescence studies with an emphasis on the differential diagnosis. Hum Pathol. 2010;41(9):1245–54.

225. Kuo TT. Kikuchi's disease (histiocytic necrotizing lymphadenitis). A clinicopathologic study of 79 cases with an analysis of histologic subtypes, immunohistology, and DNA ploidy. Am J Surg Pathol. 1995;19(7):798–809.

226. Nomura Y, Takeuchi M, Yoshida S, Sugita Y, Niino D, Kimura Y, et al. Phenotype for activated tissue macrophages in histiocytic necrotizing lymphadenitis. Pathol Int. 2009;59(9):631–5.

227. Pilichowska ME, Pinkus JL, Pinkus GS. Histiocytic necrotizing lymphadenitis (Kikuchi-Fujimoto disease): lesional cells exhibit an immature dendritic cell phenotype. Am J Clin Pathol. 2009;131(2):174–82.

228. Ohshima K, Karube K, Hamasaki M, Makimoto Y, Fujii A, Kawano R, et al. Apoptosis- and cell cycle-associated gene expression profiling of histiocytic necrotising lymphadenitis. Eur J Haematol. 2004;72(5):322–9.

229. Ishimura M, Yamamoto H, Mizuno Y, Takada H, Goto M, Doi T, et al. A non-invasive diagnosis of histiocytic necrotizing lymphadenitis by means of gene expression profile analysis of peripheral blood mononuclear cells. J Clin Immunol. 2013;33(5): 1018–26.

230. Robertson KE, Forsyth PD, Batstone PJ, Levison DA, Goodlad JR. Kikuchi's disease displaying a t(2:16) chromosomal translocation. J Clin Pathol. 2007;60(4):433–5.

231. Requena L, El-Shabrawi-Caelen L, Walsh SN, Segura S, Ziemer M, Hurt MA, et al. Intralymphatic histiocytosis: a clinicopathologic study of 16 cases. Am J Dermatopathol. 2009;31:140–51.

232. Bakr F, Webber N, Fassihi H, Swale V, Lewis F, Rytina E, et al. Primary and secondary intralymphatic histiocytosis. J Am Acad Dermatol. 2014;70(5):927–33.

233. Watanabe T, Yamada N, Yoshida Y, Yamamoto O. Intralymphatic histiocytosis with granuloma formation associated with orthopedic metal implants. Br J Dermatol. 2008;158:402–4.

234. O'Grady JT, Shahidullah H, Doherty VR, Al-Nafussi A. Intravascular histiocytosis. Histopathology. 1994;24:265–8.

235. Rossari S, Scatena C, Gori A, Grazzini M, Corciova S, Scarfì F, et al. Intralymphatic histiocytosis: cutaneous nodules and metal implants. J Cutan Pathol. 2011;38(6):534–5.

236. Echeverría-García B, Botella-Estrada R, Requena C, Guillen C. Intralymphatic histiocytosis and cancer of the colon. Actas Dermosifiliogr. 2010;101:257–62.

237. Park YJ, Kwon JE, Han JH, Kim CH, Kang HY. Intralymphatic histiocytosis mimicking oral lymphangioma circumscriptum. Am J Dermatopathol. 2014;36(9):759–61.

238. Rieger E, Soyer HP, Leboit PE, Metze D, Slovak R, Kerl H. Reactive angioendotheliomatosis or intravascular histiocytosis? An immunohistochemical and ultrastructural study in two cases of intravascular histiocytic cell proliferation. Br J Dermatol. 1999;140(3):497–504.

239. Piccolo V, Ruocco E, Russo T, Baroni A. A possible relationship between metal implant-induced intralymphatic histiocytosis and the concept of the immunocompromised district. Int J Dermatol. 2014;53(7), e365.

240. Ruocco V, Brunetti G, Puca RV, Ruocco E. The immunocompromised district: a unifying concept for lymphoedematous, herpes-infected and otherwise damaged sites. J Eur Acad Dermatol Venereol. 2009;23(12):1364–73.

241. Franz R, Andres C. Cheilitis granulomatosa and Melkersson-Rosenthal syndrome. Intralymphatic histiocytosis as valuable diagnostic indication. Pathologe. 2014;35(2):177–81.

242. Asagoe K, Torigoe R, Ofuji R, Iwatsuki K. Reactive intravascular histiocytosis associated with tonsillitis. Br J Dermatol. 2006;154:560–2.

243. Pouryazdanparast P, Yu L, Dalton VK, Haefner HK, Brincat C, Mandell SH, et al. Intravascular histiocytosis presenting with extensive vulvar necrosis. J Cutan Pathol. 2009;36 Suppl 1:1–7.

244. Rongioletti F, Rebora A. Cutaneous reactive angiomatoses: patterns and classification of reactive vascular proliferation. J Am Acad Dermatol. 2003; 49(5):887–96.

245. Cathébras P, Laurent H, Guichard I. Generalized telangiectasia revealing intravascular large B-cell lymphoma. Br J Haematol. 2013;161(2):155.

246. Riveiro-Falkenbach E, Fernández-Figueras MT, Rodríguez-Peralto JL. Benign atypical intravascular CD30(+) T-cell proliferation: a reactive condition mimicking intravascular lymphoma. Am J Dermatopathol. 2013;35(2):143–50.

247. Adachi Y, Kosami K, Mizuta N, Ito M, Matsuoka Y, Kanata M, et al. Benefits of skin biopsy of senile hemangioma in intravascular large B-cell lymphoma: a case report and review of the literature. Oncol Lett. 2014;7(6):2003–6.

248. Aung PP, Ballester LY, Goldberg LJ, Bhawan J. Incidental simultaneous finding of intravascular histiocytosis and reactive angioendotheliomatosis: a case report. Am J Dermatopathol. 2015;37(5): 401–4.

249. Grogan TM, Pileri SA, Chan JKC, Weiss LM, Fletcher CDM. Histiocytic sarcoma. In: Swerdlow SH, Campo E, Harris NL, Jaffe ES, Pileri SA, et al., editors. World Health Organization Classification of Tumours, WHO classification of tumours of haematopoietic and lymphoid tissues. 4th ed. Lyon: International Agency for Research on Cancer (IARC); 2008. p. 356–7.

250. Takahashi E, Nakamura S. Histiocytic sarcoma :an updated literature review based on the 2008 WHO classification. J Clin Exp Hematop. 2013;53(1):1–8.

251. Ralfkiaer E, Delsol G, O'Connor NT, Brandtzaeg P, Brousset P, Vejlsgaard GL, et al. Malignant lymphomas of true histiocytic origin. A clinical, histological, immunophenotypic and genotypic study. J Pathol. 1990;160(1):9–17.

252. Kamel OW, Gocke CD, Kell DL, Cleary ML, Warnke RA. True histiocytic lymphoma: a study of 12 cases based on current definition. Leuk Lymphoma. 1995;18(1–2):81–6.

253. Hornick JL, Jaffe ES, Fletcher CD. Extranodal histiocytic sarcoma: clinicopathologic analysis of 14 cases of a rare epithelioid malignancy. Am J Surg Pathol. 2004;28(9):1133–44.

254. Nguyen TT, Schwartz EJ, West RB, Warnke RA, Arber DA, Natkunam Y. Expression of CD163 (hemoglobin scavenger receptor) in normal tissues, lymphomas, carcinomas, and sarcomas is largely restricted to the monocyte/macrophage lineage. Am J Surg Pathol. 2005;29(5):617–24.

255. Lau SK, Chu PG, Weiss LM. CD163: a specific marker of macrophages in paraffin-embedded tissue samples. Am J Clin Pathol. 2004;122(5):794–801.

256. Vos JA, Abbondanzo SL, Barekman CL, Andriko JW, Miettinen M, Aguilera NS. Histiocytic sarcoma: a study of five cases including the histiocyte marker CD163. Mod Pathol. 2005;18(5):693–704.

257. Soslow RA, Davis RE, Warnke RA, Cleary ML, Kamel OW. True histiocytic lymphoma following therapy for lymphoblastic neoplasms. Blood. 1996;87(12):5207–12.

258. Feldman AL, Minniti C, Santi M, Downing JR, Raffeld M, Jaffe ES. Histiocytic sarcoma after acute lymphoblastic leukaemia: a common clonal origin. Lancet Oncol. 2004;5(4):248–50.

259. Chen W, Lau SK, Fong D, Wang J, Wang E, Arber DA, et al. High frequency of clonal immunoglobulin receptor gene rearrangements in sporadic histiocytic/dendritic cell sarcomas. Am J Surg Pathol. 2009;33(6):863–73.

260. McClure R, Khoury J, Feldman A, Ketterling R. Clonal relationship between precursor B-cell acute lymphoblastic leukemia and histiocytic sarcoma: a case report and discussion in the context of similar cases. Leuk Res. 2010;34(2):71–3.

261. Bouabdallah R, Abéna P, Chetaille B, Aurran-Schleinitz T, Sainty D, Dubus P, et al. True histiocytic lymphoma following B-acute lymphoblastic leukaemia: case report with evidence for a common clonal origin in both neoplasms. Br J Haematol. 2001;113(4):1047–50.

262. Kumar R, Khan SP, Joshi DD, Shaw GR, Ketterling RP, Feldman AL. Pediatric histiocytic sarcoma clonally related to precursor B-cell acute lymphoblastic leukemia with homozygous deletion of CDKN2A encoding p16INK4A. Pediatr Blood Cancer. 2011;56(2):307–10.

263. Hure MC, Elco CP, Ward D, Hutchinson L, Meng X, Dorfman DM, et al. Histiocytic sarcoma arising from clonally related mantle cell lymphoma. J Clin Oncol. 2012;30(5):49–53.

264. Go H, Jeon YK, Huh J, Choi SJ, Choi YD, Cha HJ, et al. Frequent detection of BRAF(V600E) mutations in histiocytic and dendritic cell neoplasms. Histopathology. 2014;65(2):261–72.

265. Pletneva MA, Smith LB. Anaplastic large cell lymphoma: features presenting diagnostic challenges. Arch Pathol Lab Med. 2014;138(10):1290–4.

266. Wu J, Qin D, Burton GF, Szakal AK, Tew JG. Follicular dendritic cell-derived antigen and accessory activity in initiation of memory IgG responses in vitro. J Immunol. 1996;157(8): 3404–11.

267. Yamada K, Yamakawa M, Imai Y, Tsukamoto M. Expression of cytokine receptors on follicular dendritic cells. Blood. 1997;90(12):4832–41.

268. Steinman RM, Pack M, Inaba K. Dendritic cells in the T-cell areas of lymphoid organs. Immunol Rev. 1997;156:25–37.

269. Chan JKC, Pileri SA, Delsol G, Fletcher CDM, Weis LM, Grogg KL. Follicular dendritic cell sarcoma. In: Swerdlow SH, Campo E, Harris NL, Jaffe ES, et al., editors. WHO classification of tumours of haematopoietic and lymphoid tissues. 4th ed. Lyon: International Agency for Research on Cancer (IARC); 2008. p. 363–4.

270. Meijs M, Mekkes J, van Noesel C, Nijhuis E, Leeksma O, Jonkman M, et al. Paraneoplastic pemphigus associated with follicular dendritic cell sarcoma without Castleman's disease; treatment with rituximab. Int J Dermatol. 2008;47(6):632–4.

271. Lee IJ, Kim SC, Kim HS, Bang D, Yang WI, Jung WH, et al. Paraneoplastic pemphigus associated with follicular dendritic cell sarcoma arising from Castleman's tumor. J Am Acad Dermatol. 1999; 40:294–7.

272. Chan JK, Fletcher CD, Nayler SJ, Cooper K. Follicular dendritic cell sarcoma. Clinicopathologic analysis of 17 cases suggesting a malignant potential higher than currently recognized. Cancer. 1997; 79(2):294–313.

273. Cokelaere K, Debiec-Rychter M, De Wolf-Peeters C, Hagemeijer A, Sciot R. Hyaline vascular Castleman's disease with HMGIC rearrangement in follicular dendritic cells: molecular evidence of mesenchymal tumorigenesis. Am J Surg Pathol. 2002; 26(5):662–9.

274. Saygin C, Uzunaslan D, Ozguroglu M, Senocak M, Tuzuner N. Dendritic cell sarcoma: a pooled analysis including 462 cases with presentation of our case series. Crit Rev Oncol Hematol. 2013;88(2): 253–71.

275. Weiss LM, Grogan TM, Chan JKC. Interdigitating dendritic cell sarcoma. In: Swerdlow SH, Campo E, Harris NL, Jaffe ES, et al., editors. WHO classification of tumours of haematopoietic and lymphoid tissues. 4th ed. Lyon: International Agency for Research on Cancer (IARC); 2008. p. 361–2.

276. Fonseca R, Yamakawa M, Nakamura S, van Heerde P, Miettinen M, Shek TW, et al. Follicular dendritic cell sarcoma and interdigitating reticulum cell sarcoma: a review. Am J Hematol. 1998;59(2):161–7.

277. Grogg KL, Macon WR, Kurtin PJ, Nascimento AG. A survey of clusterin and fascin expression in sarcomas and spindle cell neoplasms: strong clusterin immunostaining is highly specific for follicular dendritic cell tumor. Mod Pathol. 2005;18(2):260–6.

278. Grogg KL, Lae ME, Kurtin PJ, Macon WR. Clusterin expression distinguishes follicular dendritic cell

tumors from other dendritic cell neoplasms: report of a novel follicular dendritic cell marker and clinicopathologic data on 12 additional follicular dendritic cell tumors and 6 additional interdigitating dendritic cell tumors. Am J Surg Pathol. 2004; 28(8):988–98.

279. Shao H, Xi L, Raffeld M, Feldman AL, Feldman AL, Ketterling RP, et al. Clonally related histiocytic/dendritic cell sarcoma and chronic lymphocytic leukemia/small lymphocytic lymphoma: a study of seven cases. Mod Pathol. 2011;24(11):1421–32.

280. Feldman AL, Arber DA, Pittaluga S, Martinez A, Burke JS, Raffeld M, et al. Clonally related follicular lymphomas and histiocytic/dendritic cell sarcomas: evidence for transdifferentiation of the follicular lymphoma clone. Blood. 2008;111(12): 5433–9.

281. Fraser CR, Wang W, Gomez M, Zhang T, Mathew S, Furman RR, et al. Transformation of chronic lymphocytic leukemia/small lymphocytic lymphoma to interdigitating dendritic cell sarcoma: evidence for transdifferentiation of the lymphoma clone. Am J Clin Pathol. 2009;132(6):928–39.

282. Xie Q, Chen L, Fu K, Harter J, Young KH, Sunkara J, et al. Podoplanin (d2-40): a new immunohistochemical marker for reactive follicular dendritic cells and follicular dendritic cell sarcomas. Int J Clin Exp Pathol. 2008;1(3):276–84.

Part VI

Immunohistology of Melanocytic Lesions

Immunohistology of Melanocytic Lesions

12

Jonathan L. Curry, Michael T. Tetzlaff,
Priyadharsini Nagarajan,
and Carlos A. Torres-Cabala

Introduction

Melanoma is a deadly skin disease, and accurate diagnosis and evaluation of melanocytic lesions are critical for optimal patient care. The majority of melanocytic lesions can be evaluated with routine hematoxylin and eosin (H&E) stained sections. However, a subset of these lesions require additional ancillary studies (e.g., immunohistochemical [IHC] studies), either to confirm the diagnosis or to provide insight into the mutation status (e.g., BRAFV600E, BAP-1). IHC studies aid in distinguishing melanoma from melanocytic nevi and its imitators. Furthermore, the use of IHC will provide prognostic information and identify biologically aggressive tumors.

In the following section, we will examine the utility of IHC markers for (a) melanocytic differentiation, (b) cell proliferation, (c) vascular invasion, and (d) mutation status; we will also examine the application of (e) dual IHC markers and how to integrate the IHC findings in the diagnosis and prognosis of melanoma. Table 12.1 highlights selected IHC markers used in evaluating melanocytic lesions.

J.L. Curry, M.D. (✉) • M.T. Tetzlaff, M.D., Ph.D. •
P. Nagarajan, M.D., Ph.D. • C.A. Torres-Cabala, M.D.
Department of Pathology, Section of
Dermatopathology, The University of Texas MD
Anderson Cancer Center,
Holcombe Blvd., Unit 445, Houston, TX 77030, USA
e-mail: jlcurry@mdanderson.org

IHC Markers Used in the Evaluation of Melanocytic Lesions

Markers of Melanocytic Differentiation

HMB45

HMB45 is a monoclonal antibody targeted against glycoprotein 100 (gp 100) localized to the inner cytoplasmic membranes of types I, II, and III pre-melanosomes [1, 2]. HMB45 is a highly specific marker of melanocytic differentiation with a specificity of ~95–100 % [1, 3, 4]. HMB45 is expressed in melanocytic nevi, melanomas, and nonmelanocytic tumors that demonstrate pre-melanosome synthesis such as perivascular epithelioid cell tumors (PEComas, angiomyolipomas, or clear cell sugar tumors) [5]. HMB45 expression may be seen in rare renal cell carcinomas characterized by chromosomal translocation t(6:11)(p21:q12) [6] and in uncommon steroid-producing tumors of the ovary [7]. The sensitivity of HMB45 ranges from ~70 to 100 % in primary melanomas and up to ~80 % in metastasis [8, 9].

HMB45 is expressed in fetal and neonatal melanocytes, activated melanocytes, nevus cells in the junction and papillary dermis, and in the dermal component in certain types of nevi (e.g., blue and Spitz nevi) [1, 10–13]. The pattern of HMB45 reactivity is helpful in distinguishing benign from malignant melanocytic processes and is discussed later in the chapter.

© Springer International Publishing Switzerland 2016
J.A. Plaza, V.G. Prieto (eds.), *Applied Immunohistochemistry in the Evaluation
of Skin Neoplasms*, DOI 10.1007/978-3-319-30590-5_12

Table 12.1 Clinical use of selected tissue biomarkers in evaluating melanocytic lesions

Category	Marker	Property	Clone (vender)	Concentration	IHC pattern	Internal control	Clinical application	Potential pitfalls
Melanocytic differentiation	HMB45	Melanosome glycoprotein-100 (GP-100)	HMB45 (Dako)	1:50	C	Skin melanocytes	Confirmation of melanocytic differentiation. Evaluate for "maturation" of dermal melanocytes	Spitz nevi may be diffusely positive
	Mart-1/Melan-A	Melanoma antigen recognized by T cells 1	M27C10 and M29E3 (Thermo Scientific)	1:500	C	Skin melanocytes	Confirmation of melanocytic differentiation	Reactive in macrophages, keratinocytes, activated melanocytes in the epidermis
	MiTF	Nuclear transcription factor	D5 (Thermo Scientific)	1:40	N	Skin melanocytes, macrophages, and fibroblasts	Distinction from melanocytic hyperplasia and LM. Confirmation of melanocytic differentiation	Reactive in macrophages, fibroblasts
	Sox10	Nuclear transcription factor	Polyclonal (Cell Marque)	1:50	N	Skin melanocytes, adnexae, nerve	Distinction from melanocytic hyperplasia and LM. Confirmation of melanocytic differentiation	Positive in salivary and breast carcinomas
	S100	Calcium-binding protein soluble in 100 % saturated ammonium sulfate solution	15E2E2 (Biogenex)	1:900	C and N	Nerve, Langerhans cells, skin melanocytes	Confirmation of melanocytic differentiation.	Not reactive in tissue previously frozen, or poorly fixed
	Panmelanocytic cocktail	Contains antibodies to HMB45, Mart-1/Melan-A, and tyrosinase	HMB45 (Dako) AB-3 (Labvision) T311 (Novocastra)	1:100 1:100 1:50	C	Skin melanocytes	Confirmation of melanocytic differentiation	Contains Mart-1/Melan-A that can react with macrophages
	Panmelanocytic cocktail 2	Contains antibodies to HMB45 and tyrosinase	HMB45 (Dako) T311 (Novocastra)	1:100 1:50	C	Skin melanocytes	Confirmation of melanocytic differentiation	Subset of melanomas may be negative

Category	Marker	Description	Clone (Source)	Dilution	Localization	Internal control	Purpose	Comments
Vascular invasion	D2-40	O-linked sialoglycoprotein on lymphatic endothelium	D2-40 (Signet)	1:50	C	Adnexae, basal keratinocytes	Evaluate for vascular invasion	Reactive in adnexae
Proliferation	Ki-67	Cell marker of proliferation present in all phases (G1, S, G2, and M) of the cell cycle	MIB1 (Dako)	1:100	N	Lymphocytes, basal keratinocytes	Evaluate proliferative index	Positive in lymphocytes, any proliferating cells
	PHH3	Mitotic associated histone involved in regulation of chromatin structure	Histone H3 (Ser10) (Millipore)	1:400	N	Mitotic figures in epidermis, adnexal, inflammatory cells	Evaluate or confirm mitotic figure	Positive in any mitotically active cell, some mitotic figures may fail to label with PHH3
Mutation status	BRAFV600E	Serine/threonine protein kinase	VE1 (Spring Bioscience)	1:50	C	Smooth muscle	Detect the presence of *BRAF V600E* mutation	Melanin pigment may obscure interpretation and correlation with molecular studies is critical
	BAP-1	Ubiquitin hydrolase and enhance BRCA-1 tumor suppression	C-4 (Santa Cruz)	1:150	N	Skin keratinocytes	Detect the presence of *BAP1* mutation	Nonspecific cytoplasmic reactivity
Double markers	Mart-1/Ki-67	See above	MIB1 (Dako)	1:100	Mart-1=C Ki-67=N	Junctional melanocytes	Evaluate proliferative index of dermal melanocytes	Melanocytic nevi may have increased proliferative rate
	Mart-1/PHH3	See above	Histone H3 (Ser10) (Millipore)	1:400	Mart-1=C PHH3=N	Junctional melanocytes	Detect mitotic figures in melanocytes	Mitotic figures may fail to label with PHH3
	MiTF/D2-40	See above	D5 (Thermo Scientific) D2-40 (Signet)	1:40 1:50	MiTF=N D2-40=C	Junctional melanocytes	Detect and confirm vascular invasion of melanoma	Labeling of epithelium with melanoma as positive for LVI

C cytoplasmic, *N* nuclear, *LVI* lymphovascular invasion

Mart-1/Melan-A

*M*elanoma *A*ntigen *R*ecognized by *T* cells-*1* (Mart-1) is an antigen expressed in normal melanocytes, nevus cells, and melanoma cells. There are two antibody clones, Mart-1 (clone M2-7C10) and Melan-A (clone A-103), that target the same antigen and are used as markers of melanocytic differentiation [14]. Both clones share similar sensitivity (~75–92%) and specificity (~95–100%) for melanoma and, as with HMB45, are reactive in PEComas [5, 8, 15]. Melan-A (clone A-103) is also used to label adrenal cortical tumors and steroid-producing tumors, which is not seen with Mart-1 (clone M2-7C10) [14]. Mart-1/Melan-A is expressed in junctional melanocytes, nevus cells in the epidermis and dermis in all types of nevi, and in melanoma cells [16]. Some pitfalls in interpretation of Mart-1/Melan-A staining are discussed later.

Tyrosinase

Tyrosinase is a critical enzyme in melanogenesis and functions in the conversion of L-tyrosine to L-3,4-dihydroxyphenylalanine (L-DOPA), a key regulatory step in the synthesis of melanin [17]. There are several antibody clones commercially available (including T311 and MAT-1) that demonstrate a sensitivity of 84–94% as melanocytic markers of differentiation [18–22]. As seen with HMB45, tyrosinase also has excellent specificity (>97%) for melanocytic differentiation and shares a similar expression pattern in junctional and dermal nevus cells and different types of nevi [8, 21].

MiTF

Microphthalmia-associated transcription factor (MiTF) is a basic-helix-loop-helix leucine zipper transcription factor that regulates genes in melanin synthesis and is critical for melanocyte differentiation [23, 24]. The monoclonal antibody clone D5 targets human MiTF expressed in the nucleus and is thus a clinically useful nuclear marker of melanocytic differentiation. The sensitivity of anti-MiTF (clone D5) is ~80–100% and similar to that of HMB45, tyrosinase, and Melan-A [25, 26]. MiTF is expressed in junctional melanocytes and nevus cells in the epidermis and dermis and in melanoma cells. However,

MiTF is also expressed in nonmelanocytic cells including mast cells, fibroblasts, and macrophages; thus, it has a lower specificity (<88%) compared with that of HMB45, tyrosinase, and Melan-A [25]. Despite the lower specificity of anti-MiTF, its nuclear expression is a valuable quality utilized in certain clinical settings.

S100

S100 is a family of calcium-binding proteins that are soluble in 100% saturated ammonium sulfate solution [27]. S100 is composed of two related protein fractions, S100B and S100A, and includes several protein subtypes (e.g., S100A1 and S100A6). Polyclonal and monoclonal antibodies are available to, and primarily detect, S100B antigen. Some polyclonal antibodies may also be reactive with some S100A protein subtypes, and anti-S100A6 is a useful marker in the detection of neurothekeoma, a tumor in the histologic differential diagnosis of melanocytic lesions [28].

The S100 marker is routinely used for neural and melanocytic differentiation. The sensitivity of S100 for melanocytic lesions is 97–100% [9, 29–31]. However, S100 antigen is soluble in acetone and alcohol; thus, S100 expression may be affected by the type of fixative, fixation time, or in previously frozen tissue, and caution is warranted to avoid false-negative interpretation [30, 32]. Since S100 is also reactive in myoepithelial cells, nerve sheath cells, Langerhans cells, adipocytes, and chondrocytes, its specificity for melanoma is less than 90% [3, 33, 34]. Schwann cell precursors may be positive for S100 in skin excision specimens for melanoma and erroneously interpreted as residual melanoma, particularly if the melanoma had a desmoplastic/spindle cell morphology [9, 35].

Sox10

Sox10, which belongs to the *Sox* (*Sry-related box*) family of genes involved in neural crest cell development, regulates expression of genes (e.g., *MiTF*) involved in melanin synthesis [36–38]. Sox10 is expressed in melanocytes, skin adnexal structures, oligodendrocytes, Schwann cells, and myoepithelial cells [39]. As with S100, Sox10 is a highly sensitive (~97–100%) marker of melanocytic proliferation [39–43]. Furthermore, since Sox10 expression is absent in fibroblasts and macrophages in skin excision specimens (in contrast to MiTF) and in follicular dendritic cells in the lymph nodes (as opposed to S100), Sox10 has a greater specificity (>90 %) for primary and metastatic melanomas when compared to MiTF and S100 [42–45]. Awareness of Sox10 expression in cutaneous adnexal structures, a subset of salivary gland and breast carcinomas, will help to avoid pitfalls in interpretation of the tissue biomarker in melanocytic lesions.

Sox10 protein is localized to the nucleus; therefore, anti-Sox10 is a nuclear marker similar to MiTF and has some advantages in certain clinical contexts. Several polyclonal and monoclonal anti-Sox10 antibodies are commercially available and appear to have comparable sensitivity and specificity, when nuclear expression is required for positive labeling [45, 46].

Melanocytic Cocktails

The clinical necessity to improve overall sensitivity and specificity of melanocytic markers in order to best evaluate the sentinel lymph node (SLN), which may contain only a microscopic cluster of tumor cells (at times fewer than five tumor cells or even a single isolated tumor cell), has led to the development of pan-melanocytic markers [47]. We developed and currently use two types of melanocytic cocktails at our institution. The first, panmelanocytic cocktail 1, contains a mixture of HMB45, anti-tyrosinase, anti-Mart-1 (clone M2-7C10), and anti-Melan-A (clone A-103). The second panmelanocytic cocktail, includes HMB45 and anti-tyrosinase (anti-Mart-1 and anti-Melan-A are not included). Both melanocytic cocktail markers are used in certain clinical contexts, ultimately to enhance overall sensitivity and specificity in the detection of melanocytic differentiation.

In our clinical practice, we routinely use panmelanocytic cocktail-1 stain (includes HMB45, anti-Mart-1/Melan-A, anti-tyrosinase) in the evaluation of SLNs or to demonstrate melanocytic differentiation in poorly differentiated neoplasms. We use panmelanocytic cocktail-2 stain (includes HMB45, anti-tyrosinase) when a greater degree

of specificity is required in the IHC analysis (e.g., to avoid labeling of macrophages and keratinocytes). There are now commercially available anti-melanoma cocktails that contain a mixture of melanocytic markers that can be used to evaluate for melanocytic differentiation in a single assay using one section of tissue.

Markers of Cellular Proliferation

MIB-1 (anti-Ki-67)

Ki-67 is a cell cycle–associated protein expressed in G1, M, G2, and S phases of the cell cycle in proliferating cells [48]. MIB-1 is a monoclonal antibody used to detect Ki-67–positive cells. When proportions of Ki-67–positive cells were compared in banal melanocytic nevi, dysplastic nevi, and primary and metastatic melanomas, expression levels of Ki-67 were significantly higher in the melanoma cells (11–48 % positive cells) than in the nevus cells (0–2 % positive cells) [49]. Furthermore, in a quantitative analysis, metastatic melanoma cells included higher numbers of MIB-1–positive cells than did nevus cells $(47.0–95.2 \times 10^3/mm^3$ vs. $6.3–6.4 \times 10^3/mm^3$, respectively) [50, 51]. Examination of the proliferative index (PI), as measured by the percentage of MIB-1–positive cells in Spitz nevi, showed that melanomas tend to have a PI greater than 10 %, in contrast to Spitz nevi, which yield a PI of 2–10 % [52]. At times, other cell types (e.g., lymphocytes) may affect accurate evaluation of melanocyte-specific PI; thus, to better interpret and quantitate MIB-1–positive cells, a Ki-67/Mart-1 dual IHC cocktail could be used. This marker has the advantage of highlighting Mart-1–positive cells that are proliferating [53, 54]. The use of digital image analysis with automated quantification of Mart-1/Ki-67–positive cells in melanocytic lesions further increases the certainty in distinguishing between melanocytic nevi and melanoma [55].

PHH3

Antibody to PHH3 specifically detects *p*hosphorylated *h*istone *H3* (at serine residue 10)–associated cell division and chromatin condensation at

G2 and M phases of the cell cycle [56]. PHH3 is a sensitive and specific cell division-associated histone marker that may be used for detecting mitotic figures in melanoma that may aid in diagnosis and provide prognostic information [57–60]. PHH3 has been shown to facilitate mitotic count and correlate with worse survival [59, 60]. PHH3 may be used in certain clinical scenarios to confirm the presence of mitotic figures in melanoma [61]. Similar to the dual Mart-1/Ki-67 IHC stain, a dual Mart-1/PHH3 IHC stain is available and improves test specificity in the identification of mitotic figures in melanocytes.

H3KT

Dual modified histones have been shown to be critical for chromatin condensation and proper cell division. Histone modification of H3K79me3T80ph (H3KT) and more recently H3K9me3S10ph (H3KS) has been associated with G2 and M phases of the cell cycle [62, 63]. Antibodies targeted against these modified histones detected mitotic figures in melanoma and in Merkel cell carcinomas and the levels of H3KT positive cells were associated with more aggressive clinical behavior and worse survival [62, 64].

Markers of Vascular Invasion

D2-40

D2-40 (podoplanin) is a highly specific antibody of lymphatic endothelium that facilitates detection of vascular invasion in cutaneous melanoma [65, 66]. The presence of vascular invasion identified using D2-40 has been associated with positive SLN and poor survival [66]. To enhance the specificity of lymphatic invasion by melanoma cells, we have developed a dual MiTF/D2-40 stain; this marker can confirm cells with melanocytic differentiation in a highlighted lymphatic vessel [61].

CD31

CD31, or platelet-endothelial cell adhesion molecule type 1 (PECAM-1), is located on endothelial cells, platelets, and macrophages [67]. CD31 detects both lymphatic and blood vessel endothelium [68] and aids in the evaluation of microvessel density and blood vascular invasion [69]. In sinonasal melanomas, detection of vascular invasion with S100/CD31 dual stain was associated with worse prognosis [70].

CD34

CD34 is a cell surface glycoprotein detected on immature hematopoietic cells, endothelial cells, and dermal dendritic cells [68, 71, 72]. As seen with D2-40, CD34 facilitated identification of vascular invasion in melanoma and was associated with worse disease-free survival and overall survival rates [73]. Since CD34 labels other structures in the skin that may interfere with interpretation, we prefer D2-40 for evaluating vascular invasion in cutaneous melanoma [66].

Markers of Mutation Status

BRAF V600E

Mutations in the *BRAF* gene, the most commonly seen somatic mutations in cutaneous melanoma, are detected in ~50–60 % of melanoma patients [74]. IHC detection of BRAF V600E protein with monoclonal anti-BRAF V600E (clone VE1) has been a highly sensitive (97–100 %) and specific (97–100 %) surrogate marker of the *BRAF* mutation status in patients with melanoma, particularly when there is strong homogeneous labeling of tumor cells [75–80]. A subset of tumors demonstrates heterogeneous BRAF V600E expression; molecular analysis by next-generation sequencing in fact shows that these tumors harbor the *BRAF V600E* mutation. However, in our experience, this heterogeneous BRAF V600E IHC group also had a higher rate of false-positive IHC test results compared with NGS results and thus decreased overall BRAF V600E IHC test specificity [80].

At times, melanoma samples that are heavily pigmented with melanin may interfere with interpretation of BRAF V600E IHC test results, especially if the detection system is with brown chromogen DAB (3,3'-diaminobenzidine). In cases with tumor samples with prominent melanin pigment, pretreatment with a mild H_2O_2

(bleach) and heat to remove endogenous melanin or the use of red chromogen detection agent AEC (3-amino-9-ethylcarbazole) may be beneficial [61, 81]. Alternatively, staining sections with Giemsa, in contrast to labeling with DAB, may facilitate detecting the presence of melanin. Ultimately, interpretation of heterogeneous BRAF IHC test results or staining of heavily pigmented melanin tumor samples requires correlation with sequencing information before initiation of BRAF inhibitor therapy.

BAP-1

BAP-1 (BRCA1-associated protein 1) is a tumor suppressor involved in G1/S cell cycle transition [82]. Germline mutations in BAP-1 predispose family members with uveal and cutaneous melanomas to the development of multiple melanocytic nevi (so-called Bap-omas) with distinct clinical and histologic features [83, 84]. These nevi demonstrate histomorphologic features of Spitz nevi, yet characteristically harbor BRAF V600E and BAP-1 mutations, in contrast to typical Spitz nevi that have increased copy numbers in chromosome 11p and HRAS mutations [85, 86]. Melanocytic nevi with acquired somatic mutations in BAP-1 have similar morphologic features, and evaluation with an anti-BAP-1 IHC study is a useful surrogate marker of BAP-1 mutation. Nevi that harbor the BAP-1 mutation demonstrate loss of BAP-1 expression in the nucleus [85, 87].

KIT

A subset of melanomas that occur on acral or chronically sun-damaged skin and at mucosal sites are known to harbor oncogenic KIT mutations and/or amplifications that have been associated with melanoma tumorigenesis [88–90]. Activation of c-KIT (CD117), a transmembrane receptor tyrosine kinase for stem cell factor, promotes melanocyte proliferation, migration, and survival via signaling of MAP kinase and PI3K-AKT pathways [91–93].

IHC expression of KIT protein in some melanomas has been shown to correlate with KIT protein expression and the presence of KIT mutation or gene amplification [94, 95]. Furthermore, the intensity of KIT IHC expression was associated

with particular mutations in exon 11 KIT mutations (e.g., L576P) [90, 96]. However, other studies failed to demonstrate significant correlation with KIT protein expression and the presence of KIT mutation or gene amplification [89, 97–99]. KIT mutations were also identified in KIT-negative cells isolated by laser capture microdissection [100]. Thus, KIT IHC expression does not appear to share the same positive predictive value as a surrogate marker for KIT mutations as seen with BRAF V600E IHC expression. The variability of results may be from differences in staining protocols, antibodies, subtypes of melanomas, type of genetic alteration in KIT, as well as geographic or ethnic diversity of patients examined in these various studies.

p16^{INK4a}

The cyclin dependent kinase 2a (CDKN2a) gene is located on chromosome 9p21 and encodes for two major tumor suppressor proteins, p16^{INK4a} and p14^{ARF} [101]. Mutations in CDKN2a account for the majority of genetic alterations in familial melanoma, and loss of nuclear p16INK4a protein function in melanoma has been associated with worse survival [102, 103]. Homozygous deletion of the 9p21 probe by fluorescence in situ hybridization has been shown to be associated with sporadic melanomas with spitzoid morphology [104]. IHC staining for p16^{INK4a} may provide insight into diagnosis and prognosis in a subset of melanomas, particularly those with spitzoid morphology.

Dual IHC Markers

Dual IHC markers allow for specific evaluation of proliferative rate (with Mart-1/Ki-67 and Mart-1/PHH3) and vascular invasion (Sox10/D2-40 and MiTF/D2-40) in cells with melanocytic differentiation. In particular, examination of Mart-1/Ki-67 in melanocytic lesions with dense lymphocytic infiltrate (e.g., halo reaction) helps discern reactive Ki-67 lymphocytes from Mart-1/Ki-67 melanocytes. The use of D2-40 combined with MiTF or Sox10 (both nuclear markers of melanocytic differentiation) confirms the presence of vascular invasion.

Clinical Applications of IHC Markers in Melanocytic Lesions

Confirm Melanocytic Differentiation

Distinguish Lentigo Maligna from Lentigo

Biopsy examination of pigmented lesions on chronically sun-damaged skin may pose a diagnostic challenge. These lesions may appear atypical clinically and are often submitted by the clinician to rule out melanoma. Histologically, these lesions may appear with atrophic epidermis, prominent solar elastosis, and an attenuated rete ridge pattern (Fig. 12.1). The presence of melanocytes is typically not apparent on initial review of H&E-stained sections, and often lesions may be interpreted as "lentigo." This is the classic scenario in which a lentigo maligna may be overlooked. In such cases, the utility of melanocytic markers such as HMB45, anti-tyrosinase, MiTF, and Sox10 may aid in enumerating the melanocytes along the dermal-epidermal junction and reveal the appropriate diagnosis. Lentigo, by strict histologic criteria, is a keratinocytic process with elongation of rete ridges and pigmented basal keratinocytes (Fig. 12.1). Diagnosis of lentigo in the setting of chronically sun-damaged skin with attenuated rete ridges is a potential diagnostic pitfall for lentigo maligna.

The use of Melan-A to enumerate melanocytes along the dermal-epidermal junction on chroni-

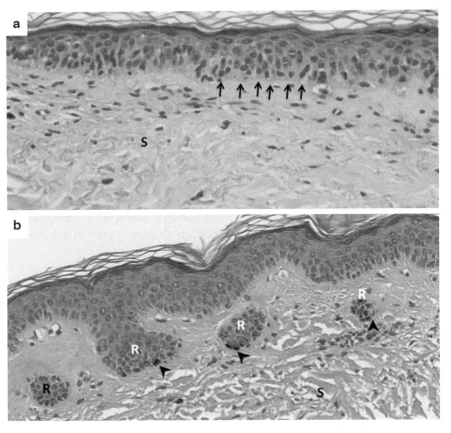

Fig. 12.1 Melanoma in situ, lentigo maligna type. (**a**) Atrophic sun-damaged skin with dermal solar elastosis (S) and attenuated (flattened) rete ridge pattern. Confluent proliferation of atypical melanocytes (*arrows*) are present along the dermal-epidermal junction (Hematoxylin and Eosin (H&E), 200× magnification). (**b**) Solar lentigo. Skin with elongated rete ridges (R) with notable pigmentation of basal keratinocytes (*arrows*) in the setting of sun damage with dermal solar elastosis (S) (H&E, 200× magnification)

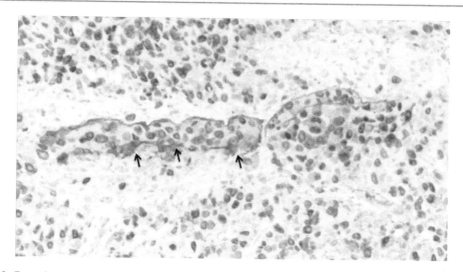

Fig. 12.2 Detection of vascular invasion by melanoma cells with dual stain MiTF/D2-40. MiTF labels nucleus of melanocytes (*brown color*). D2-40 highlights vascular channel (*arrows*, *red color*) (IHC, 400× magnification)

cally sun-damaged skin may cause overestimation of melanocytes and the appearance of melanoma in situ since Melan-A labels dendritic processes and may also label keratinocytes [105]. The use of HMB45 and anti-tyrosinase IHC may be more specific. Alternatively, MiTF and Sox10 have been utilized recently in this setting. These are nuclear markers that help identify melanocytes, avoiding labeling of melanocytic dendritic processes and thus the appearance of increased numbers of intraepidermal melanocytes [106, 107].

Confirm the Presence of Vascular Invasion in Melanoma

Identification of vascular invasion in melanoma has prognostic significance. The presence of vascular invasion has been associated with increased rates in SLN positivity and worse survival [66]. IHC stain with anti-D2-40 facilitates detection of vascular channels and may highlight tumor cells within the vascular lumen. However, at times the vascular lumen may contain cells that may be morphologically difficult to discern between melanoma cells and inflammatory cells on H&E (e.g., lymphocytes and macrophages). The use of MiTF or Sox10 (both nuclear markers) combined with D2-40, which highlights the lymphatic endothelium, allows confirmation of vascular invasion by melanoma cells (Fig. 12.2).

Confirm Proliferating and/or Mitotic Figures in Melanocytes

Ki-67 and PHH3 are markers of proliferation. Ki-67 labels proliferating cells throughout all phases of the cell cycle (G1, S, G2, and M) [48]. PHH3 more specifically labels mitotic figures and labels cells in the G2 and M phases of the cell cycle [64]. Although Ki-67 and PHH3 are proliferative markers, they are not specific to melanocytes; thus, evaluation of the proliferative rate in melanocytic lesions with inflammatory infiltrate (e.g., halo nevus) may be difficult since Ki-67 and PHH3 are also reactive in lymphocytes. The use of double IHC stain with anti-Mart-1 with either Ki-67 (Mart-1/Ki-67) or PHH3 (Mart-1/PPH3) will facilitate evaluation of the proliferative rate and/or confirm the presence of mitotic figures in melanocytes (Fig. 12.3).

Distinguish Melanocytic Nevi from Melanoma

Common Compound Melanocytic Nevi and Dysplastic Nevi

The pattern of HMB45 expression in the dermal nests of compound melanocytic nevi (either common or dysplastic) aids in distinguishing melanocytic nevi from melanoma. In melanocytic nevi,

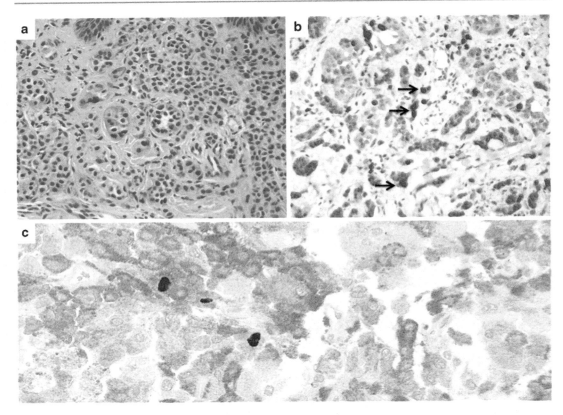

Fig. 12.3 Invasive melanoma. (**a**) Melanoma cells in dermis with patchy melanin pigment (H&E, 200× magnification). (**b**) Increased proliferative rate of the dermal nests of melanocytes measured by Mart-1 (*red*)/Ki-67 (*brown*) (*arrows*). (**c**) Detection of mitotic figure (*brown*, nuclear) with PHH3 in melanoma cells (*red* cytoplasmic). Note the patchy labeling of Mart-1 by the melanoma cells

HMB45 expression tends to "mature" with progressive descent into the deeper dermis (positive in melanocytes in the papillary dermis and negative in melanocytes situated in the deeper dermis) (Fig. 12.4). Exceptions include nevus cells beneath an area of trauma and around hair follicles that may be positive for HMB45 [108]. Blue nevi and variants (see below) should be diffusely positive for HMB45. In contrast, melanoma tends to have patchy labeling with HMB45 or may entirely lose HMB45 expression (Fig. 12.5).

Anti-Mart-1 in melanocytic nevi should be positive throughout the lesion. Melanomas may show patchy labeling with anti-Mart-1, or as with HMB45, may be negative. Anti-Mart-1 is not as specific a marker of melanocytic differentiation as HMB45 is and may also label macrophages in excision specimens (Fig. 12.6) and lymph nodes.

Awareness that anti-Mart-1 may label cells besides melanocytes is important to avoid misinterpretation of this marker.

S100 and Sox10 are reactive in melanocytic nevi and melanoma. S100 and Sox10 are sensitive markers of melanocytic differentiation and are particularly useful in evaluating melanomas that have lost expression of other markers of melanocytic differentiation (e.g., HMB45, anti-tyrosinase, anti-Mart-1). However, S100 and Sox10 may also be reactive in neural tumors, myoepithelial tumors, and some breast carcinomas, so interpretation of these markers requires appropriate clinical context.

Examination of the proliferative rate with Mart-1/Ki-67 has greatly enhanced our interpretation of borderline melanocytic lesions. The use of Mart-1/Ki-67 stain allows specific identifica-

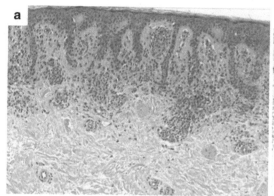

Fig. 12.4 Compound melanocytic nevus. (**a**) Dermal nests of melanocytes disperse with progressive descent into the reticular dermis. (**b**) HMB45 demonstrates "mat- uration" of dermal melanocytes or absence of labeling of melanocytes with progressive descent into the dermis (H&E, 100×; IHC, 100×)

tion of proliferating melanocytes that is particu- larly useful when a lesion is accompanied by lymphocytes. A proliferative rate of less than ~5 % of dermal melanocytes (positive Mart-1/ Ki-67 cells) is supportive of the diagnosis of melanocytic nevi; in contrast, a proliferative rate of greater than ~10 % of dermal melanocytes aids in the diagnosis of melanoma [52, 54, 109]. The pattern of Ki-67 labeling in dermal melanocytes also aids in distinguishing melanocytic nevi from melanoma. Melanocytic nevi typically show mat- uration or loss of Ki-67 labeling with progressive descent into the deeper reticular dermis (similar to the maturation pattern with HMB45 seen in melanocytic nevi). Melanomas, in contrast, often have patchy labeling with Ki-67 including mela- nocytes at the deep aspect of the lesion. Recently, automated quantification with anti-Mart-1/Ki-67 was shown to aid in distinguishing melanocytic nevi from melanoma [55]. At times, an increased proliferative rate may occur in melanocytic nevi, as well as in nevi associated with hormonal changes and congenital nevi with proliferative nodules; thus, clinical pathologic correlation is essential [110, 111].

Desmoplastic Melanocytic Nevi

Desmoplastic or sclerotic melanocytic nevi are mor- phologically composed of spindle cells in a fibrotic or keloidal collagen and may have histologic fea- tures reminiscent of blue or Spitz nevi. However,

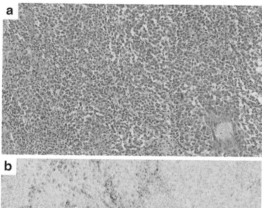

Fig 12.5 Invasive melanoma. (**a**) Sheets of invasive mel- anoma cells with (**b**) patchy labeling with HMB45 (H&E 200×, IHC 200×)

desmoplastic nevi are considered a distinct type of melanocytic nevi [112]. Immunohistochemically, desmoplastic melanocytic nevi are positive for S100 and demonstrate "maturation" (similar to HMB45 labeling in compound melanocytic nevi) with pro- gressive dermal descent of melanocytes with respect

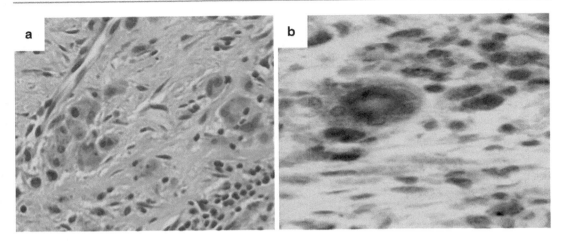

Fig. 12.6 Healing surgical wound/scar in a melanoma excision. (**a**) Multinucleated giant cells in excision scar (H&E, 400×) (**b**) reactive for Melan-A (IHC, 400×)

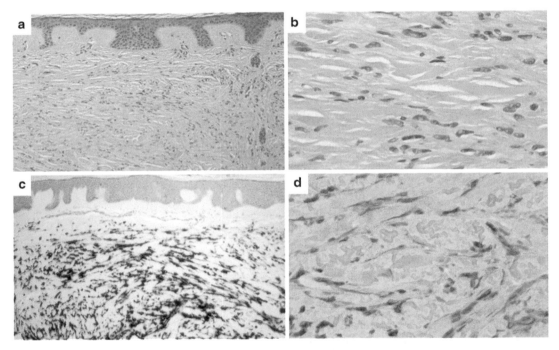

Fig. 12.7 Desmoplastic nevi. (**a, b**) Spindle-shaped melanocytes disperse between fibrotic collagen bundles in the dermis without prominent melanin pigment (H&E, 100×; 400×). (**c**) Melanocytes are uniformly reactive with

HMB45 (IHC, 100×) (**d**) and double stain with Mart-1/Ki-67 highlights melanocytes (*red* cytoplasmic color) without reactivity for Ki-67 (*brown* nuclear color) indicating a low proliferative rate (IHC, 400×)

to HMB45 [113]. This pattern of labeling differs from that of blue nevi, which demonstrates diffuse reactivity to HMB45 [30]. Desmoplastic melanocytic nevi are uniformly positive for Melan-A and demonstrate a low proliferative rate measured by Ki-67 (Fig. 12.7) [113, 114].

Blue Nevi and Cellular Blue Nevi

Blue nevi or cellular blue nevi are dermal-based melanocytic proliferations typically associated with prominent melanin pigment, melanophages, and fibrotic stroma. Lesions with areas of increased cellularity are designated as cellular blue nevi. Blue nevi demonstrate uniform labeling with both anti-Mart-1 and HMB45 (in the hypocellular and cellular areas) and a low proliferative rate with Ki-67 [9, 11]. Cellular blue nevi must be distinguished from pigmented epithelioid melanocytoma (PEM), epithelioid blue nevus associated with Carney complex, and melanomas arising in association with a blue nevus since cellular blue nevi are considered benign lesions whereas the others are malignant. Increased mitotic activity, associated tumor necrosis, and cytologic atypia are more associated with PEM and melanomas arising in association with a blue nevus [115, 116]. Examination of proliferative markers (e.g., Mart-1/Ki-67 and Mart-1/PHH3) may be useful in evaluating these lesions.

Spitz Nevi and Variants

Spitz nevi are melanocytic proliferations that typically occur in children. When Spitz nevi present with classic morphologic features, these lesions may be distinguished from other melanocytic nevi and melanoma. Some variants of Spitz nevi include pigmented spindle cell nevus of Reed, angiomatoid Spitz nevus, and intradermal Spitz nevus [117–119]. Spitz nevi demonstrate marked cytologic atypia of melanocytes that may be misinterpreted as malignant tumor cells. The use of IHC analysis is helpful, particularly in Spitz lesions that demonstrate morphologic features of atypia that include asymmetry, poor circumscription, prominent pagetoid migration, increased dermal mitotic figures, absence of maturation of cells with descent into the dermis, and necrosis. Spitz nevi tend to demonstrate either maturation with HMB45 with descent into the dermis or uniform labeling with HMB45. Both HMB45 and anti-Mart-1 allow examination of the extent of pagetoid migration. As with other nevi, Spitz nevi should have a low proliferative rate measured with Ki-67 (Fig. 12.8); in contrast, melanomas with Spitz features (spitzoid melanomas) often have patchy labeling with HMB45 and an increased proliferative rate measured by Ki-67 stain [120]. Homozygous deletion of 9p21 has been shown to be a feature of spitzoid melanomas, and a subset of spitzoid melanomas have

loss of p16 protein expression [104, 121]. However, loss of p16 protein expression may also be seen in Spitz nevi [122]. Thus, retained expression of p16 protein detected by IHC appears to better correlate with the absence of homozygous deletion of 9p21 [104, 123].

BAP-omas

A distinct melanocytic proliferation associated with inactivating mutations of the *BAP1* tumor suppressor gene and the risk of developing uveal melanomas have been described by Wiesner et al. [83]. These "BAP-omas" demonstrate cytologic atypia seen in Spitz nevi and may sporadically and characteristically harbor the *BRAF V600E* mutation [85, 124]. Loss of nuclear BAP1 protein expression in melanocytes by IHC analysis may provide insight into the *BAP1* mutation status in these lesions. Furthermore, the combined presence of *BRAF V600E* mutation allows further distinction from Spitz nevi.

Melanoma

IHC markers have been a valuable ancillary test in the examination of melanocytic lesions that do meet the criteria for diagnosis of melanoma on initial histologic evaluation. These borderline melanocytic lesions require incorporation of all the clinical, histologic, IHC, and molecular studies (discussed elsewhere in this book) to arrive at a final pathologic diagnosis. Abnormal IHC features seen in melanoma include patchy labeling with HMB45 (absence of "maturation") (Fig. 12.9) and with anti-Mart-1 and increase in the proliferative rate of the dermal melanocytes with anti-Mart-1/Ki-67 double stain. A subset of melanomas may also show variable reactivity for S100 and Sox10. S100 is a labile antigen and may be damaged if the tissue is improperly fixed, previously frozen, or enzymatically treated [11]. The use of other markers of melanocytic differentiation such as Sox10 or MiTF may be helpful in these cases.

Melanomas may also demonstrate keratin and myogenic differentiation and be reactive with cytokeratin cocktail and desmin [125]. At times, when keratin or desmin appears to be the only reactive marker (loss of melanocytic markers), the lesion may be misinterpreted as

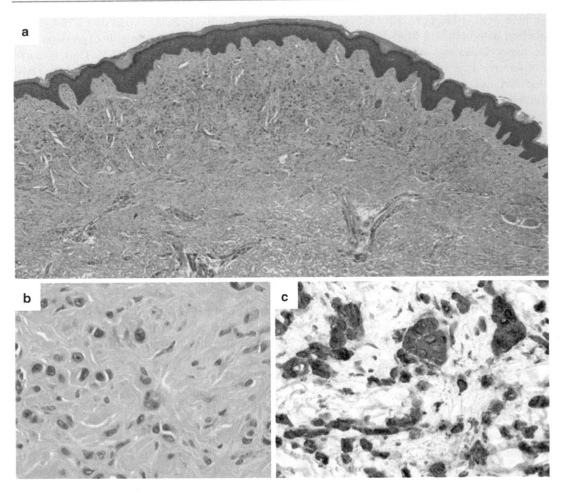

Fig. 12.8 Spitz nevi. (**a**) Wedge-shaped dermal proliferation of atypical epithelioid melanocytes with maturation of cell size and dispersion with progressive descent into the deeper dermis (H&E, 40×). (**b**) Melanocytes demonstrate severe cytologic atypia with enlarged nuclei and prominent nucleoli (H&E, 400×). (**c**) Mart-1/Ki-67 demonstrates a low proliferative rate with labeling of melanocytes (*red*, cytoplasmic color) and absence of Ki-67 reactivity (*brown*, nuclear color) (IHC, 400×)

poorly differentiated carcinoma or sarcoma (Fig. 12.10). It is important to correlate the IHC expression profile with the clinical history and, if available, with any molecular data since the known mutations that occur in melanoma (e.g., BRAF and NRAS) would be rare in sarcoma.

Desmoplastic Melanoma

S100 and Sox10 are highly sensitive markers of desmoplastic melanomas compared with HMB45 and Melan-A, which typically show poor positive staining [8, 126]. However, in

excision specimens it is critical not to misinterpret S100- or Sox10-positive cells as residual tumors since scars may have labeling of scattered regenerative nerve fibers [35, 127]. Desmoplastic melanoma should be considered only when most of the lesional cells are positive for S100 or Sox10 (Fig. 12.11) [11]. It is important to recognize "pure" desmoplastic melanomas from melanomas with spindle cell morphology and/or mixed desmoplastic features since risk of regional nodal metastasis is lower in pure desmoplastic melanomas and SLN biopsy may not be indicated [128]. At our

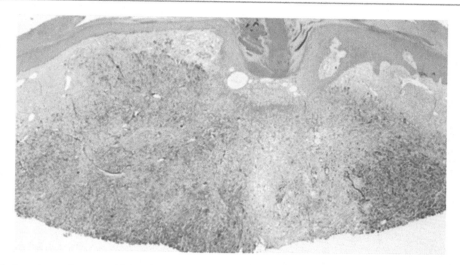

Fig. 12.9 Invasive melanoma with labeling of HMB45 in melanoma cells in the superficial and deep dermis, thus absence of "maturation" with respect to HMB45 labeling (IHC, 20×)

institution if greater than 90 % of the invasive component contains hypocellular areas of spindle-shaped melanoma cells in a fibrotic stroma, then the lesion is classified as a "pure" desmoplastic melanoma and surgically treated by complete excision (Fig. 12.12).

Evaluation of SLNs

IHC evaluations of SLNs for melanomas require sensitive and specific markers of melanocytic differentiation. Although S100 is a sensitive marker, its utility in SLNs is limited due to its labeling of follicular dendritic cells. In our experience, a pan-melanocytic cocktail marker (that includes HMB45, anti-Mart-1, and anti-tyrosinase) is a sensitive and specific marker that allows for the detection of micrometastasis (Fig. 12.13) [11]. Since anti-Mart-1 may be expressed in macrophages [35], at times we may use HMB45 or Sox10 by itself to help differentiate between macrophages and melanoma cells (HMB45 usually does not label macrophages). Sox10 was recently shown to be a sensitive and specific marker in the detection of melanoma micrometastasis in SLNs and may also be useful in spindle/desmoplastic melanomas whose tumor cells are negative for HMB45 or anti-

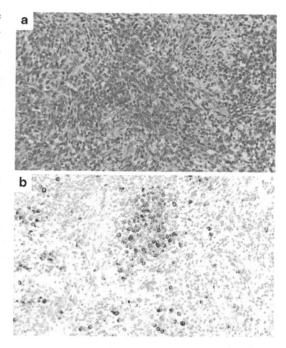

Fig. 12.10 Invasive melanoma. (**a**) Tumor cells with epithelioid and spindle-shaped morphology (H&E, 200×) and (**b**) focal reactivity to desmin (IHC, 200×)

Mart-1 [129]. Comparison of the morphology of the primary tumor to a few isolated cells in the SLN is often beneficial in the final IHC interpretation of SLN biopsies.

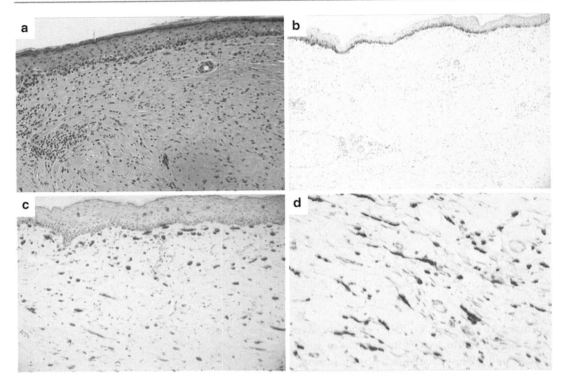

Fig. 12.11 Desmoplastic melanoma. (**a**) Epidermis with confluent proliferation of atypical melanocytes and dermis with invasive spindle-shaped tumor cells in fibrotic stroma with associated lymphocytic inflammation (H&E, 200×). (**b**) Melan-A highlights in situ component with confluent proliferation of atypical melanocytes in the epidermis and absence of labeling of invasive tumor cells in the dermis (IHC, 100×). (**c**) S100 (IHC, 200×) and Sox10 (IHC, 400×) label increased numbers of atypical spindle cells in the dermis

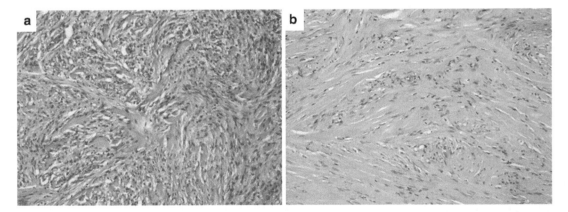

Fig. 12.12 The cellularity of the lesion separates classification of melanoma as mixed melanoma with desmoplastic features from "pure" desmoplastic melanoma. (**a**) Hypercellular invasive melanoma with spindle cells and desmoplastic features that does not meet criteria at our institution for pure desmoplastic melanoma (H&E, 400×). (**b**) Hypocellular invasive melanoma. Tumor cells separated by notable fibrotic dermis. When 90% of the tumor demonstrates with this morphology, the lesion will meet our criteria for a "pure" desmoplastic melanoma (H&E, 400×)

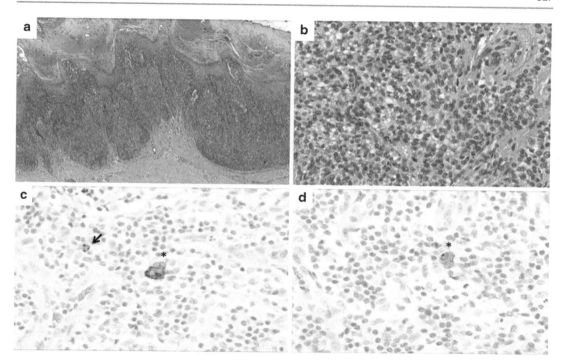

Fig. 12.13 Invasive acral lentiginous melanoma. (**a, b**) Tumor cells appear atypical with epithelioid and nevoid morphology (H&E, 20× and 400×, respectively). (**c**) Sentinel lymph node biopsy with cluster of cells (*) positive for pan-melanocytic cocktail (HMB45, anti-Mart-1, anti-Tyrosinase) in contrast to labeling of adjacent macrophage (*arrow*) (IHC, 400×). (**d**) Cluster of tumor cells positive for HMB45 and demonstrates similar morphologic features to invasive primary melanoma seen in image **b**. (IHC, 400×)

The degree of cytologic atypia, pattern of HMB45 labeling, location, and proliferative rate in melanocytes in the SLN aid in distinguishing nodal nevi from metastatic melanoma [11]. Nodal nevi frequently occur in the capsule, are negative for HMB45 (Fig. 12.14), and demonstrate a low proliferative rate with Mart-1/Ki-67. However, nevus cells may be detected in the lymph node parenchyma, and melanoma cells may be detected in the vascular lumen of the capsule. Thus, when available, comparison with the morphology of the primary tumor is recommended.

Provide Mutation Status

The identification of the targetable *BRAF* mutation in melanoma has fundamentally changed treatment in patients with advanced-stage dis-ease. Patients whose tumor contain the BRAF V600E protein may benefit from BRAF inhibitor therapy (vemurafenib or dabrafenib); therefore, identification of BRAF V600E mutant melanomas is critical [130, 131]. IHC detection of BRAF V600E (with anti-VE1 antibody) in melanoma cells highly correlates with the presence of *BRAF V600E* mutation and is a useful surrogate marker of *BRAF* mutation status [80]. Since IHC BRAF detection is a rapid and reliable marker of mutation status, some patients may benefit from initiation of therapy before completion of molecular testing (Fig. 12.15). Thus, accurate interpretation of BRAF IHC is necessary. Some pitfalls in BRAF IHC interpretation include tumor samples that are heavily pigmented with melanin and tumor samples with focal or patchy labeling with BRAF stain. Samples with prominent melanin pigment may benefit from counterstain with Giemsa.

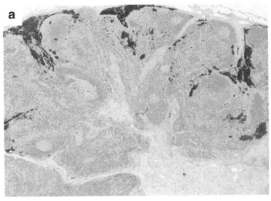

Fig. 12.14 Sentinel lymph node with nodal nevi. (**a**) Nevus cells are positive for pan-melanocytic cocktail stain (HMB45, anti-Mart-1, anti-Tyrosinase) (IHC, 20×).

(**b**) Nodal nevus cells with notable diminished labeling with HMB-45 (IHC, 20×)

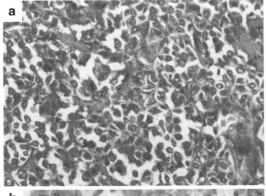

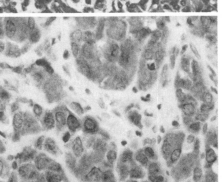

Fig. 12.15 BRAF V600E mutant melanoma (**a**) with epithelioid morphology (H&E, 400×) with (**b**) diffuse cytoplasmic expression of BRAF V600E (IHC, 400×)

However, in these settings, discussion with the clinical team and correlation with molecular tests are necessary before making treatment decisions with BRAFi (Fig. 12.16).

The loss of BAP1 nuclear expression by IHC analysis with anti-BAP1 is a reliable surrogate marker in the *BAP1* mutation status. Bap-omas are nevi that typically have combined mutations in *BAP1* and *BRAF* that correlate to melanocytes with nuclear loss of BAP1 expression and BRAF V600E positivity [85, 124].

Conclusions

The diagnosis and treatment of melanoma continue to be a challenge; however, improved understanding of the molecular pathogenesis of melanoma and the development of targeted therapy have resulted in personalized therapy. The use of IHC markers facilitates the examination of challenging melanocytic lesions and provides prognostic information and insight into the mutation status in patients with melanoma, which will ultimately guide clinical teams in the treatment of this deadly disease.

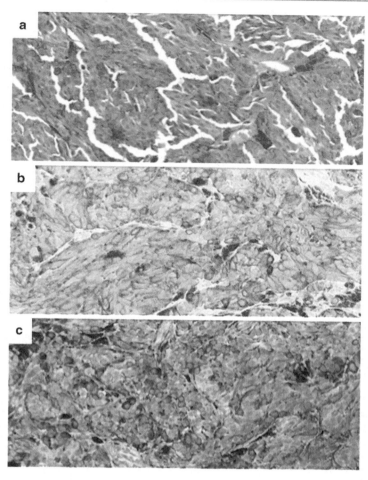

Fig. 12.16 BRAF V600E wild-type melanoma with (**a**) prominent melanin pigment in the tumor cells (H&E, 400×). (**b**) Melanin pigment may obscure interpretation of BRAF V600E immunohistochemical stain with DAB (*brown* color) detection system (IHC, 400×). (**c**) Counterstain with giemsa demonstrates presence of melanin pigment (*dark green* color) and absence of reactivity with anti-BRAF V600E (*brown color*) (giemsa, 400×)

References

1. Gown AM, Vogel AM, Hoak D, Gough F, McNutt MA. Monoclonal antibodies specific for melanocytic tumors distinguish subpopulations of melanocytes. Am J Pathol. 1986;123(2):195–203.
2. Adema GJ, de Boer AJ, Vogel AM, Loenen WA, Figdor CG. Molecular characterization of the melanocyte lineage-specific antigen gp100. J Biol Chem. 1994;269(31):20126–33.
3. Ordonez NG, Ji XL, Hickey RC. Comparison of HMB-45 monoclonal antibody and S-100 protein in the immunohistochemical diagnosis of melanoma. Am J Clin Pathol. 1988;90(4):385–90.
4. Wick MR, Swanson PE, Rocamora A. Recognition of malignant melanoma by monoclonal antibody HMB-45. An immunohistochemical study of 200 paraffin-embedded cutaneous tumors. J Cutan Pathol. 1988;15(4):201–7.
5. Fetsch PA, Fetsch JF, Marincola FM, Travis W, Batts KP, Abati A. Comparison of melanoma antigen recognized by T cells (MART-1) to HMB-45: additional evidence to support a common lineage for angiomyolipoma, lymphangiomyomatosis, and clear cell sugar tumor. Mod Pathol. 1998;11(8):699–703.
6. Argani P, Hawkins A, Griffin CA, Goldstein JD, Haas M, Beckwith JB, et al. A distinctive pediatric renal neoplasm characterized by epithelioid morphology, basement membrane production, focal HMB45 immunoreactivity, and t(6;11)(p21.1;q12) chromosome translocation. Am J Pathol. 2001;158(6):2089–96.
7. Deavers MT, Malpica A, Ordonez NG, Silva EG. Ovarian steroid cell tumors: an immunohistochemical study including a comparison of calretinin

with inhibin. Int J Gynecol Pathol. 2003;22(2):162–7.

8. Ohsie SJ, Sarantopoulos GP, Cochran AJ, Binder SW. Immunohistochemical characteristics of melanoma. J Cutan Pathol. 2008;35(5):433–44.

9. Ivan D, Prieto VG. Use of immunohistochemistry in the diagnosis of melanocytic lesions: applications and pitfalls. Future Oncol. 2010;6(7):1163–75.

10. Smoller BR, McNutt NS, Hsu A. HMB-45 recognizes stimulated melanocytes. J Cutan Pathol. 1989;16(2):49–53.

11. Prieto VG, Shea CR. Use of immunohistochemistry in melanocytic lesions. J Cutan Pathol. 2008;35 Suppl 2:1–10.

12. Bergman R, Dromi R, Trau H, Cohen I, Lichtig C. The pattern of HMB-45 antibody staining in compound Spitz nevi. Am J Dermatopathol. 1995;17(6):542–6.

13. Skelton 3rd HG, Smith KJ, Barrett TL, Lupton GP, Graham JH. HMB-45 staining in benign and malignant melanocytic lesions. A reflection of cellular activation. Am J Dermatopathol. 1991;13(6):543–50.

14. Fetsch PA, Marincola FM, Abati A. The new melanoma markers: MART-1 and Melan-A (the NIH experience). Am J Surg Pathol. 1999;23(5):607–10.

15. Orchard GE. Comparison of immunohistochemical labelling of melanocyte differentiation antibodies melan-A, tyrosinase and HMB 45 with NKIC3 and S100 protein in the evaluation of benign naevi and malignant melanoma. Histochem J. 2000;32(8):475–81.

16. Busam KJ, Chen YT, Old LJ, Stockert E, Iversen K, Coplan KA, et al. Expression of melan-A (MART1) in benign melanocytic nevi and primary cutaneous malignant melanoma. Am J Surg Pathol. 1998;22(8):976–82.

17. Slominski A, Tobin DJ, Shibahara S, Wortsman J. Melanin pigmentation in mammalian skin and its hormonal regulation. Physiol Rev. 2004;84(4):1155–228.

18. Jungbluth AA, Iversen K, Coplan K, Kolb D, Stockert E, Chen YT, et al. T311 – an anti-tyrosinase monoclonal antibody for the detection of melanocytic lesions in paraffin embedded tissues. Pathol Res Pract. 2000;196(4):235–42.

19. Sato N, Suzuki S, Takimoto H, Masui S, Shibata K, Nakano H, et al. Monoclonal antibody MAT-1 against human tyrosinase can detect melanogenic cells on formalin-fixed paraffin-embedded sections. Pigment Cell Res. 1996;9(2):72–6.

20. Hofbauer GF, Kamarashev J, Geertsen R, Boni R, Dummer R. Tyrosinase immunoreactivity in formalin-fixed, paraffin-embedded primary and metastatic melanoma: frequency and distribution. J Cutan Pathol. 1998;25(4):204–9.

21. Clarkson KS, Sturdgess IC, Molyneux AJ. The usefulness of tyrosinase in the immunohistochemical assessment of melanocytic lesions: a comparison of

the novel T311 antibody (anti-tyrosinase) with S-100, HMB45, and A103 (anti-melan-A). J Clin Pathol. 2001;54(3):196–200.

22. Ordonez NG. Value of melanocytic-associated immunohistochemical markers in the diagnosis of malignant melanoma: a review and update. Hum Pathol. 2014;45(2):191–205.

23. Hemesath TJ, Steingrimsson E, McGill G, Hansen MJ, Vaught J, Hodgkinson CA, et al. Fisher DE: microphthalmia, a critical factor in melanocyte development, defines a discrete transcription factor family. Genes Dev. 1994;8(22):2770–80.

24. Yasumoto K, Yokoyama K, Shibata K, Tomita Y, Shibahara S. Microphthalmia-associated transcription factor as a regulator for melanocyte-specific transcription of the human tyrosinase gene. Mol Cell Biol. 1994;14(12):8058–70.

25. Busam KJ, Iversen K, Coplan KC, Jungbluth AA. Analysis of microphthalmia transcription factor expression in normal tissues and tumors, and comparison of its expression with S-100 protein, gp100, and tyrosinase in desmoplastic malignant melanoma. Am J Surg Pathol. 2001;25(2):197–204.

26. Miettinen M, Fernandez M, Franssila K, Gatalica Z, Lasota J, Sarlomo-Rikala M. Microphthalmia transcription factor in the immunohistochemical diagnosis of metastatic melanoma: comparison with four other melanoma markers. Am J Surg Pathol. 2001;25(2):205–11.

27. Moore BW. A soluble protein characteristic of the nervous system. Biochem Biophys Res Commun. 1965;19(6):739–44.

28. Fullen DR, Lowe L, Su LD. Antibody to S100a6 protein is a sensitive immunohistochemical marker for neurothekeoma. J Cutan Pathol. 2003;30(2):118–22.

29. Fernando SS, Johnson S, Bate J. Immunohistochemical analysis of cutaneous malignant melanoma: comparison of S-100 protein, HMB-45 monoclonal antibody and NKI/C3 monoclonal antibody. Pathology. 1994;26(1):16–9.

30. Prieto VG, Shea CR. Immunohistochemistry of melanocytic proliferations. Arch Pathol Lab Med. 2011;135(7):853–9.

31. Cochran AJ, Wen DR. S-100 protein as a marker for melanocytic and other tumours. Pathology. 1985;17(2):340–5.

32. Edgerton ME, Roberts SA, Montone KT. Immunohistochemical performance of antibodies on previously frozen tissue. Appl Immunohistochem Mol Morphol. 2000;8(3):244–8.

33. Takahashi K, Isobe T, Ohtsuki Y, Akagi T, Sonobe H, Okuyama T. Immunohistochemical study on the distribution of alpha and beta subunits of S-100 protein in human neoplasm and normal tissues. Virchows Arch B Cell Pathol Incl Mol Pathol. 1984;45(4):385–96.

34. Blessing K, Sanders DS, Grant JJ. Comparison of immunohistochemical staining of the novel antibody

melan-A with S100 protein and HMB-45 in malignant melanoma and melanoma variants. Histopathology. 1998;32(2):139–46.

35. Trejo O, Reed JA, Prieto VG. Atypical cells in human cutaneous re-excision scars for melanoma express p75NGFR, C56/N-CAM and GAP-43: evidence of early Schwann cell differentiation. J Cutan Pathol. 2002;29(7):397–406.

36. Ludwig A, Rehberg S, Wegner M. Melanocyte-specific expression of dopachrome tautomerase is dependent on synergistic gene activation by the Sox10 and Mitf transcription factors. FEBS Lett. 2004;556(1–3):236–44.

37. Kiefer JC. Back to basics: Sox genes. Dev Dyn. 2007;236(8):2356–66.

38. Bondurand N, Pingault V, Goerich DE, Lemort N, Sock E, Le Caignec C, et al. Interaction among SOX10, PAX3 and MITF, three genes altered in Waardenburg syndrome. Hum Mol Genet. 2000;9(13):1907–17.

39. Nonaka D, Chiriboga L, Rubin BP. Sox10: a pan-schwannian and melanocytic marker. Am J Surg Pathol. 2008;32(9):1291–8.

40. Agnarsdottir M, Sooman L, Bolander A, Stromberg S, Rexhepaj E, Bergqvist M, et al. SOX10 expression in superficial spreading and nodular malignant melanomas. Melanoma Res. 2010;20(6):468–78.

41. Karamchandani JR, Nielsen TO, van de Rijn M, West RB. Sox10 and S100 in the diagnosis of soft-tissue neoplasms. Appl Immunochem Mol Morphol. 2012;20(5):445–50.

42. Ramos-Herberth FI, Karamchandani J, Kim J, Dadras SS. SOX10 immunostaining distinguishes desmoplastic melanoma from excision scar. J Cutan Pathol. 2010;37(9):944–52.

43. Mohamed A, Gonzalez RS, Lawson D, Wang J, Cohen C. SOX10 expression in malignant melanoma, carcinoma, and normal tissues. Appl Immunochem Mol Morphol. 2013;21(6):506–10.

44. Jennings C, Kim J. Identification of nodal metastases in melanoma using sox-10. Am J Dermatopathol. 2011;33(5):474–82.

45. Tacha D, Qi W, Ra S, Bremer R, Yu C, Chu J, et al. A newly developed mouse monoclonal SOX10 antibody is a highly sensitive and specific marker for malignant melanoma, including spindle cell and desmoplastic melanomas. Arch Pathol Lab Med. 2015;139(4):530–6.

46. Ordonez NG. Value of SOX10 immunostaining in tumor diagnosis. Adv Anat Pathol. 2013;20(4):275–83.

47. Orchard G. Evaluation of melanocytic neoplasms: application of a pan-melanoma antibody cocktail. Br J Biomed Sci. 2002;59(4):196–202.

48. Gerdes J, Lemke H, Baisch H, Wacker HH, Schwab U, Stein H. Cell cycle analysis of a cell proliferation-associated human nuclear antigen defined by the monoclonal antibody Ki-67. J Immunol. 1984;133(4):1710–5.

49. Kanter L, Blegen H, Wejde J, Lagerlof B, Larsson O. Utility of a proliferation marker in distinguishing between benign naevocellular naevi and naevocellular naevus-like lesions with malignant properties. Melanoma Res. 1995;5(5):345–50.

50. Smolle J, Soyer HP, Kerl H. Proliferative activity of cutaneous melanocytic tumors defined by Ki-67 monoclonal antibody. A quantitative immunohistochemical study. Am J Dermatopathol. 1989;11(4):301–7.

51. Rieger E, Hofmann-Wellenhof R, Soyer HP, Kofler R, Cerroni L, Smolle J, et al. Comparison of proliferative activity as assessed by proliferating cell nuclear antigen (PCNA) and Ki-67 monoclonal antibodies in melanocytic skin lesions. A quantitative immunohistochemical study. J Cutan Pathol. 1993;20(3):229–36.

52. Vollmer RT. Use of Bayes rule and MIB-1 proliferation index to discriminate Spitz nevus from malignant melanoma. Am J Clin Pathol. 2004;122(4):499–505.

53. Puri PK, Valdes CL, Burchette JL, Grichnik JM, Turner JW, Selim MA. Accurate identification of proliferative index in melanocytic neoplasms with Melan-A/Ki-67 double stain. J Cutan Pathol. 2010;37(9):1010–2.

54. Nielsen PS, Riber-Hansen R, Steiniche T. Immuno-histochemical double stains against Ki67/MART1 and HMB45/MITF: promising diagnostic tools in melanocytic lesions. Am J Dermatopathol. 2011;33(4):361–70.

55. Nielsen PS, Spaun E, Riber-Hansen R, Torben S. Automated quantification of MART1-verified Ki-67 indices: useful diagnostic aid in melanocytic lesions. Hum Pathol. 2014;45(6):1153–61.

56. Juan G, Traganos F, James WM, Ray JM, Roberge M, Sauve DM, et al. Histone H3 phosphorylation and expression of cyclins A and B1 measured in individual cells during their progression through G2 and mitosis. Cytometry. 1998;32(2):71–7.

57. Balch CM, Gershenwald JE, Soong SJ, Thompson JF, Atkins MB, Byrd DR, et al. Final version of 2009 AJCC melanoma staging and classification. J Clin Oncol. 2009;27(36):6199–206.

58. Schimming TT, Grabellus F, Roner M, Pechlivanis S, Sucker A, Bielefeld N, et al. pHH3 immunostaining improves interobserver agreement of mitotic index in thin melanomas. Am J Dermatopathol. 2012;34(3):266–9.

59. Tetzlaff MT, Curry JL, Ivan D, Wang WL, Torres-Cabala CA, Bassett RL, et al. Immunodetection of phosphohistone H3 as a surrogate of mitotic figure count and clinical outcome in cutaneous melanoma. Mod Pathol. 2013;26(9):1153–60.

60. Ladstein RG, Bachmann IM, Straume O, Akslen LA. Prognostic importance of the mitotic marker phosphohistone H3 in cutaneous nodular melanoma. J Invest Dermatol. 2012;132(4):1247–52.

61. Tetzlaff MT, Torres-Cabala CA, Pattanaprichakul P, Rapini RP, Prieto VG, Curry JL. Emerging clinical applications of selected biomarkers in melanoma. Clin Cosmet Investig Dermatol. 2015;8:35–46.

62. Martinez DR, Richards HW, Lin Q, Torres-Cabala CA, Prieto VG, Curry JL, et al. H3K79me3T80ph is

a novel histone dual modification and a mitotic indicator in melanoma. J Skin Cancer. 2012;2012:823534.

63. Hammond SL, Byrum SD, Namjoshi S, Graves HK, Dennehey BK, Tackett AJ, et al. Mitotic phosphorylation of histone H3 threonine 80. Cell Cycle. 2014;13(3):440–52.

64. Henderson SA, Tetzlaff MT, Pattanaprichakul P, Fox P, Torres-Cabala CA, Bassett RL, et al. Detection of mitotic figures and G2+ tumor nuclei with histone markers correlates with worse overall survival in patients with Merkel cell carcinoma. J Cutan Pathol. 2014;41(11):846–52.

65. Niakosari F, Kahn HJ, Marks A, From L. Detection of lymphatic invasion in primary melanoma with monoclonal antibody D2-40: a new selective immunohistochemical marker of lymphatic endothelium. Arch Dermatol. 2005;141(4):440–4.

66. Petersson F, Diwan AH, Ivan D, Gershenwald JE, Johnson MM, Harrell R, et al. Immunohistochemical detection of lymphovascular invasion with D2-40 in melanoma correlates with sentinel lymph node status, metastasis and survival. J Cutan Pathol. 2009;36(11):1157–63.

67. Newman PJ, Berndt MC, Gorski J, White 2nd GC, Lyman S, Paddock C, et al. PECAM-1 (CD31) cloning and relation to adhesion molecules of the immunoglobulin gene superfamily. Science. 1990;247(4947):1219–22.

68. Sauter B, Foedinger D, Sterniczky B, Wolff K, Rappersberger K. Immunoelectron microscopic characterization of human dermal lymphatic microvascular endothelial cells. Differential expression of CD31, CD34, and type IV collagen with lymphatic endothelial cells vs blood capillary endothelial cells in normal human skin, lymphangioma, and hemangioma in situ. J Histochem Cytochem. 1998;46(2):165–76.

69. Massi D, Franchi A, Borgognoni L, Paglierani M, Reali UM, Santucci M. Tumor angiogenesis as a prognostic factor in thick cutaneous malignant melanoma. A quantitative morphologic analysis. Virchows Arch. 2002;440(1):22–8.

70. Wermker K, Brauckmann T, Klein M, Hassfeld S, Schulze HJ, Hallermann C. Prognostic value of S100/CD31 and S100/podoplanin double immunostaining in mucosal malignant melanoma of the head and neck. Head Neck. 2015;37(9):1368–74.

71. Nickoloff BJ. The human progenitor cell antigen (CD34) is localized on endothelial cells, dermal dendritic cells, and perifollicular cells in formalin-fixed normal skin, and on proliferating endothelial cells and stromal spindle-shaped cells in Kaposi's sarcoma. Arch Dermatol. 1991;127(4):523–9.

72. Greaves MF, Brown J, Molgaard HV, Spurr NK, Robertson D, Delia D, et al. Molecular features of CD34: a hemopoietic progenitor cell-associated molecule. Leukemia. 1992;6 Suppl 1:31–6.

73. Rose AE, Christos PJ, Lackaye D, Shapiro RL, Berman R, Mazumdar M, et al. Clinical relevance of detection of lymphovascular invasion in primary

74. Davies H, Bignell GR, Cox C, Stephens P, Edkins S, Clegg S, et al. Mutations of the BRAF gene in human cancer. Nature. 2002;417(6892):949–54.

75. Capper D, Berghoff AS, Magerle M, Ilhan A, Wöhrer A, Hackl M, et al. Immunohistochemical testing of BRAF V600E status in 1,120 tumor tissue samples of patients with brain metastases. Acta Neuropathol. 2012;123(2):223–33.

76. Long GV, Wilmott JS, Capper D, Preusser M, Zhang YE, Thompson JF, et al. Immunohistochemistry is highly sensitive and specific for the detection of V600E BRAF mutation in melanoma. Am J Surg Pathol. 2013;37(1):61–5.

77. Busam KJ, Hedvat C, Pulitzer M, von Deimling A, Jungbluth AA. Immunohistochemical analysis of BRAF(V600E) expression of primary and metastatic melanoma and comparison with mutation status and melanocyte differentiation antigens of metastatic lesions. Am J Surg Pathol. 2013;37(3):413–20.

78. Marin C, Beauchet A, Capper D, Zimmermann U, Julie C, Ilie M, et al. Detection of BRAF p.V600E mutations in melanoma by immunohistochemistry has a good interobserver reproducibility. Arch Pathol Lab Med. 2014;138(1):71–5.

79. Feller JK, Yang S, Mahalingam M. Immunohistochemistry with a mutation-specific monoclonal antibody as a screening tool for the BRAFV600E mutational status in primary cutaneous malignant melanoma. Mod Pathol. 2013;26(3):414–20.

80. Tetzlaff MT, Pattanaprichakul P, Wargo J, Fox PP, Patel KP, Estrella JS, Broaddus RR, Williams MD, Davies MA, Routbort MJ et al. Utility of BRAF V600E immunohistochemical expression pattern as a surrogate of BRAF mutation status in 154 patients with advanced melanoma. Hum Pathol. 2015;46(8):1101–10.

81. Chen Q, Xia C, Deng Y, Wang M, Luo P, Wu C, et al. Immunohistochemistry as a quick screening method for clinical detection of BRAF(V600E) mutation in melanoma patients. Tumour Biol. 2014;35(6):5727–33.

82. Jensen DE, Rauscher 3rd FJ. BAP1, a candidate tumor suppressor protein that interacts with BRCA1. Ann N Y Acad Sci. 1999;886:191–4.

83. Wiesner T, Obenauf AC, Murali R, Fried I, Griewank KG, Ulz P, et al. Germline mutations in BAP1 predispose to melanocytic tumors. Nat Genet. 2011;43(10):1018–21.

84. Aoude LG, Wadt K, Bojesen A, Cruger D, Borg A, Trent JM, et al. A BAP1 mutation in a Danish family predisposes to uveal melanoma and other cancers. PLoS One. 2013;8(8):e72144.

85. Wiesner T, Murali R, Fried I, Cerroni L, Busam K, Kutzner H, et al. A distinct subset of atypical Spitz tumors is characterized by BRAF mutation and loss of BAP1 expression. Am J Surg Pathol. 2012;36(6):818–30.

86. Bastian BC, LeBoit PE, Pinkel D. Mutations and copy number increase of HRAS in Spitz nevi with

distinctive histopathological features. Am J Pathol. 2000;157(3):967–72.

87. Llamas-Velasco M, Perez-Gonzalez YC, Requena L, Kutzner H. Histopathologic clues for the diagnosis of Wiesner nevus. J Am Acad Dermatol. 2014;70(3):549–54.

88. Curtin JA, Fridlyand J, Kageshita T, Patel HN, Busam KJ, Kutzner H, et al. Distinct sets of genetic alterations in melanoma. N Engl J Med. 2005;353(20):2135–47.

89. Beadling C, Jacobson-Dunlop E, Hodi FS, Le C, Warrick A, Patterson J, et al. KIT gene mutations and copy number in melanoma subtypes. Clin Cancer Res. 2008;14(21):6821–8.

90. Satzger I, Schaefer T, Kuettler U, Broecker V, Voelker B, Ostertag H, et al. Analysis of c-KIT expression and KIT gene mutation in human mucosal melanomas. Br J Cancer. 2008;99(12):2065–9.

91. Carlson JA, Linette GP, Aplin A, Ng B, Slominski A. Melanocyte receptors: clinical implications and therapeutic relevance. Dermatol Clin. 2007;25(4):541–57. viii-ix.

92. Alexeev V, Yoon K. Distinctive role of the cKit receptor tyrosine kinase signaling in mammalian melanocytes. J Invest Dermatol. 2006;126(5):1102–10.

93. Grichnik JM, Burch JA, Burchette J, Shea CR. The SCF/KIT pathway plays a critical role in the control of normal human melanocyte homeostasis. J Invest Dermatol. 1998;111(2):233–8.

94. Curtin JA, Busam K, Pinkel D, Bastian BC. Somatic activation of KIT in distinct subtypes of melanoma. J Clin Oncol. 2006;24(26):4340–6.

95. Torres-Cabala CA, Wang WL, Trent J, Yang D, Chen S, Galbincea J, et al. Correlation between KIT expression and KIT mutation in melanoma: a study of 173 cases with emphasis on the acral-lentiginous/mucosal type. Mod Pathol. 2009;22(11):1446–56.

96. Antonescu CR, Busam KJ, Francone TD, Wong GC, Guo T, Agaram NP, et al. L576P KIT mutation in anal melanomas correlates with KIT protein expression and is sensitive to specific kinase inhibition. Int J Cancer. 2007;121(2):257–64.

97. Kong Y, Si L, Zhu Y, Xu X, Corless CL, Flaherty KT, et al. Large-scale analysis of KIT aberrations in Chinese patients with melanoma. Clin Cancer Res. 2011;17(7):1684–91.

98. Alessandrini L, Parrozzani R, Bertorelle R, Valentini E, Candiotto C, Giacomelli L, et al. C-Kit SCF receptor (CD117) expression and KIT gene mutation in conjunctival pigmented lesions. Acta Ophthalmol. 2013;91(8):e641–5.

99. Santi R, Simi L, Fucci R, Paglierani M, Pepi M, Pinzani P, et al. KIT genetic alterations in anorectal melanomas. J Clin Pathol. 2014;68(2):130–4.

100. Schoenewolf NL, Bull C, Belloni B, Holzmann D, Tonolla S, Lang R, et al. Sinonasal, genital and acrolentiginous melanomas show distinct characteristics of KIT expression and mutations. Eur J Cancer. 2012;48(12):1842–52.

101. Chin L, Garraway LA, Fisher DE. Malignant melanoma: genetics and therapeutics in the genomic era. Genes Dev. 2006;20(16):2149–82.

102. Goldstein AM, Chan M, Harland M, Gillanders EM, Hayward NK, Avril MF, et al. High-risk melanoma susceptibility genes and pancreatic cancer, neural system tumors, and uveal melanoma across GenoMEL. Cancer Res. 2006;66(20):9818–28.

103. Lade-Keller J, Riber-Hansen R, Guldberg P, Schmidt H, Hamilton-Dutoit SJ, Steiniche T. Immunohistochemical analysis of molecular drivers in melanoma identifies p16 as an independent prognostic biomarker. J Clin Pathol. 2014;67(6):520–8.

104. Gammon B, Beilfuss B, Guitart J, Gerami P. Enhanced detection of spitzoid melanomas using fluorescence in situ hybridization with 9p21 as an adjunctive probe. Am J Surg Pathol. 2012;36(1):81–8.

105. Beltraminelli H, Shabrawi-Caelen LE, Kerl H, Cerroni L. Melan-a-positive "pseudomelanocytic nests": a pitfall in the histopathologic and immunohistochemical diagnosis of pigmented lesions on sun-damaged skin. Am J Dermatopathol. 2009;31(3):305–8.

106. Buonaccorsi JN, Prieto VG, Torres-Cabala C, Suster S, Plaza JA. Diagnostic utility and comparative immunohistochemical analysis of MITF-1 and SOX10 to distinguish melanoma in situ and actinic keratosis: a clinicopathological and immunohistochemical study of 70 cases. Am J Dermatopathol. 2014;36(2):124–30.

107. Nybakken GE, Sargen M, Abraham R, Zhang PJ, Ming M, Xu X. MITF accurately highlights epidermal melanocytes in atypical intraepidermal melanocytic proliferations. Am J Dermatopathol. 2013;35(1):25–9.

108. Leleux TM, Prieto VG, Diwan AH. Aberrant expression of HMB-45 in traumatized melanocytic nevi. J Am Acad Dermatol. 2012;67(3):446–50.

109. Rudolph P, Schubert C, Schubert B, Parwaresch R. Proliferation marker Ki-S5 as a diagnostic tool in melanocytic lesions. J Am Acad Dermatol. 1997;37(2 Pt 1):169–78.

110. Chan MP, Chan MM, Tahan SR. Melanocytic nevi in pregnancy: histologic features and Ki-67 proliferation index. J Cutan Pathol. 2010;37(8):843–51.

111. Nguyen TL, Theos A, Kelly DR, Busam K, Andea AA. Mitotically active proliferative nodule arising in a giant congenital melanocytic nevus: a diagnostic pitfall. Am J Dermatopathol. 2013;35(1):e16–21.

112. Sherrill AM, Crespo G, Prakash AV, Messina JL. Desmoplastic nevus: an entity distinct from spitz nevus and blue nevus. Am J Dermatopathol. 2011;33(1):35–9.

113. Harris GR, Shea CR, Horenstein MG, Reed JA, Burchette Jr JL, Prieto VG. Desmoplastic (sclerotic) nevus: an underrecognized entity that resembles dermatofibroma and desmoplastic melanoma. Am J Surg Pathol. 1999;23(7):786–94.

114. Kucher C, Zhang PJ, Pasha T, Elenitsas R, Wu H, Ming ME, et al. Expression of Melan-A and Ki-67 in desmoplastic melanoma and desmoplastic nevi. Am J Dermatopathol. 2004;26(6):452–7.

115. Loghavi S, Curry JL, Torres-Cabala CA, Ivan D, Patel KP, Mehrotra M, et al. Melanoma arising in association with blue nevus: a clinical and pathologic study of 24 cases and comprehensive review of the literature. Mod Pathol. 2014;27(11):1468–78.

116. Zembowicz A, Carney JA, Mihm MC. Pigmented epithelioid melanocytoma: a low-grade melanocytic tumor with metastatic potential indistinguishable from animal-type melanoma and epithelioid blue nevus. Am J Surg Pathol. 2004;28(1):31–40.

117. Sau P, Graham JH, Helwig EB. Pigmented spindle cell nevus: a clinicopathologic analysis of ninety-five cases. J Am Acad Dermatol. 1993;28(4):565–71.

118. Tetzlaff MT, Xu X, Elder DE, Elenitsas R. Angiomatoid spitz nevus: a clinicopathological study of six cases and a review of the literature. J Cutan Pathol. 2009;36(4):471–6.

119. Plaza JA, De Stefano D, Suster S, Prieto VG, Kacerovska D, Michal M, et al. Intradermal spitz nevi: a rare subtype of spitz nevi analyzed in a clinicopathologic study of 74 cases. Am J Dermatopathol. 2014;36(4):283–94. quiz 295-287.

120. Paradela S, Fonseca E, Pita S, Kantrow SM, Goncharuk VN, Diwan H, et al. Spitzoid melanoma in children: clinicopathological study and application of immunohistochemistry as an adjunct diagnostic tool. J Cutan Pathol. 2009;36(7):740–52.

121. Al Dhaybi R, Agoumi M, Gagne I, McCuaig C, Powell J, Kokta V. p16 expression: a marker of differentiation between childhood malignant melanomas and Spitz nevi. J Am Acad Dermatol. 2011;65(2):357–63.

122. Mason A, Wititsuwannakul J, Klump VR, Lott J, Lazova R. Expression of p16 alone does not differentiate between Spitz nevi and Spitzoid melanoma. J Cutan Pathol. 2012;39(12):1062–74.

123. Horst BA, Terrano D, Fang Y, Silvers DN, Busam KJ. 9p21 gene locus in Spitz nevi of older individu-

als: absence of cytogenetic and immunohistochemical findings associated with malignancy. Hum Pathol. 2013;44(12):2822–8.

124. Busam KJ, Sung J, Wiesner T, von Deimling A, Jungbluth A. Combined BRAF(V600E)-positive melanocytic lesions with large epithelioid cells lacking BAP1 expression and conventional nevomelanocytes. Am J Surg Pathol. 2013;37(2):193–9.

125. Romano RA, Ortt K, Birkaya B, Smalley K, Sinha S. An active role of the DeltaN isoform of p63 in regulating basal keratin genes K5 and K14 and directing epidermal cell fate. PLoS One. 2009;4(5):e5623.

126. Romano RC, Carter JM, Folpe AL. Aberrant intermediate filament and synaptophysin expression is a frequent event in malignant melanoma: an immunohistochemical study of 73 cases. Mod Pathol. 2015;28(8):1033–42.

127. Robson A, Allen P, Hollowood K. S100 expression in cutaneous scars: a potential diagnostic pitfall in the diagnosis of desmoplastic melanoma. Histopathology. 2001;38(2):135–40.

128. Pawlik TM, Ross MI, Prieto VG, Ballo MT, Johnson MM, Mansfield PF, et al. Assessment of the role of sentinel lymph node biopsy for primary cutaneous desmoplastic melanoma. Cancer. 2006;106(4):900–6.

129. Chapman PB, Hauschild A, Robert C, Haanen JB, Ascierto P, Larkin J, et al. Improved survival with vemurafenib in melanoma with BRAF V600E mutation. N Engl J Med. 2011;364(26):2507–16.

130. Chapman PB, Hauschild A, Robert C, Haanen JB, Ascierto P, Larkin J, Dummer R, Garbe C, Testori A, Maio M et al. Improved survival with vemurafenib in melanoma with BRAF V600E mutation. N Engl J Med 364(26):2507–16.

131. Long GV, Stroyakovskiy D, Gogas H, Levchenko E, de Braud F, Larkin J, et al. Dabrafenib and trametinib versus dabrafenib and placebo for Val600 BRAF-mutant melanoma: a multicentre, double-blind, phase 3 randomised controlled trial. Lancet. 2015;386(9992):444–51.

Part VII
Molecular Studies of Melanocytic Lesions

Molecular Studies Informing the Diagnosis of Melanocytic Lesions

Rami Al-Rohil, Priyadharsini Nagarajan, and Michael T. Tetzlaff

Introduction

Primary cutaneous melanoma remains the deadliest among most common types of skin cancer and accounts for the majority of skin cancer related mortality. The incidence of cutaneous melanoma continues to rise, and the percentage of people with this disease has more than doubled in the past 30 years [1]. The estimated lifetime risk of an American developing invasive melanoma is 1 in 59 and is projected to be 1 in 50 by the year 2015 [2]. As a consequence, the number of biopsies procured to exclude melanoma continues to increase, and histopathologic evaluation of biopsies of pigmented lesions comprises a significant component of the practice of dermatopathology, accounting for approximately one fifth of all biopsies in a general dermatopathology practice [3, 4].

Further, the significance of correctly distinguishing between benign and malignant melanocytic proliferations carries tremendous clinical implications. A benign (albeit atypical) lesion is considered to be cured with conservative re-excision, while the diagnosis of melanoma requires significantly greater medical intervention, subsequent lifetime surveillance and consequent morbidity in the form of wide local excision (WLE) and in some cases, sentinel lymph node biopsy (SLNB) in addition to the attendant psychiatric burden borne by the patient who carries a malignant diagnosis with well-known lethal potential for the remainder of his or her life.

The diagnosis of pigmented lesions has historically relied on a systematic appraisal of the light microscopic features of a lesion, and the morphologic distinction between benign and malignant melanocytic lesions is achieved without the aid of ancillary tests in most cases. However, studies report considerable inter-observer variability among certain lesions with this approach [5–7]. Thus, a subset of melanocytic lesions requires additional studies to characterize the lesional cells, including immunohistochemical studies [8–10]. Advances in immunohistochemistry have provided refinement to light microscopy, including an assessment of markers of melanocytic differentiation, like gp100 (with HMB-45) [11], together with markers

R. Al-Rohil, M.D. • P. Nagarajan, M.D., Ph.D.
Department of Pathology, Section of Dermatopathology, The University of Texas MD Anderson Cancer Center, 1515 Holcombe Blvd, Unit 85, Houston, TX 77005, USA
e-mail: pnagarajan@mdanderson.org

M.T. Tetzlaff, M.D., Ph.D. (✉)
Department of Pathology, Section of Dermatopathology, The University of Texas MD Anderson Cancer Center, 1515 Holcombe Blvd, Unit 85, Houston, TX 77005, USA

Department of Translational and Molecular Pathology, The University of Texas MD Anderson Cancer Center, Houston, TX, USA
e-mail: mtetzlaff@mdanderson.org

© Springer International Publishing Switzerland 2016
J.A. Plaza, V.G. Prieto (eds.), *Applied Immunohistochemistry in the Evaluation of Skin Neoplasms*, DOI 10.1007/978-3-319-30590-5_13

of proliferation, like Ki-67 [12]. Nevertheless, despite a rigorous diagnostic algorithm integrating light microscopy and immunohistochemistry, there continues to be a subset of ambiguous melanocytic lesions that demonstrate features of benignity together with additional worrisome histopathologic and/or immunophenotypic features of melanoma. In our practice, such histopathologically challenging lesions exhibit at least one but typically more of the following atypical light microscopic/immunohistochemical features: (1) asymmetric pattern of growth or inflammatory infiltrate, (2) confluent or expansile pattern of growth, (3) dermal inflammation and/or fibrosis, (4) upward pagetoid migration within the intraepidermal component, (5) severe cytologic atypia (including enlarged and irregular nuclei with prominent nucleoli), (6) dermal mitotic figures, (7) abnormal dermal maturation pattern (morphologically and/or as determined by HMB-45 immunohistochemistry), and (8) increased dermal proliferative rate, particularly at the base of the lesion (at least >5 % as measured by Ki-67 immunohistochemistry). For these lesions, there is a critical need for additional diagnostic tests to further refine our appraisal of these lesions.

The past decade has witnessed a transformative expansion of our understanding of the molecular characteristics distinguishing melanocytic nevi from melanoma, which has been leveraged into diagnostically relevant tests. One of the most important advances to date in our understanding of the biology of melanocytic tumors was derived from the application of comparative genomic hybridization (CGH) to a series of benign and malignant melanocytic proliferations [13, 14]. These early CGH studies demonstrated a reproducible pattern of chromosomal aberrations typical of melanoma (~96 % of the lesions studied exhibited gains and losses in portions of chromosomes) that was entirely distinct from melanocytic nevi (which either lacked chromosomal changes altogether or carried alterations of whole chromosomes) [14–16]. From this work, it became quickly apparent that this fundamental genomic disparity could be exploited in a diagnostic setting to differentiate malignant melanocytic tumors from benign ones. However, for a variety of reasons (ranging from cost to technical), it is often not feasible to apply CGH in a routine diagnostic setting [17]. Thus, fluorescence in situ hybridization (FISH) evolved as a surrogate of the genomic instability captured by CGH to identify those melanocytic proliferations which carried chromosomal aberrations most typical of melanoma [18, 19]. The earliest study assessing the utility of first generation FISH in a diagnostic setting demonstrated a sensitivity of 86.7 % and a specificity of 95.4 % in the distinction of melanoma from nevus [18]. Since this pioneering effort, a number of confirmatory "proof of principle" studies have validated the diagnostic utility of FISH in a variety of different diagnostic settings and reported a comparably high sensitivity and specificity of the assay [20–28]. Most of the earliest proof of principle studies utilized histopathologically unambiguous nevi and melanomas to demonstrate the utility of FISH as an ancillary diagnostic test. However, FISH is not typically deployed in the setting of morphologically unambiguous melanocytic tumors. Instead, the ideal setting to utilize an ancillary test like FISH would be for histopathologically ambiguous lesions, where additional ancillary testing has the potential to most usefully inform the diagnosis. Despite early reports that FISH might prove helpful in distinguishing among ambiguous melanocytic proliferations, it has become clear from larger series that the diagnostic utility of FISH is controversial in the setting of such ambiguous melanocytic lesions, where the overall reported sensitivity lies between 43 and 60 % and the specificity between 50 and 80 % using clinical behavior as the gold standard [29, 30]. Furthermore, more recent studies have identified newer probe combinations to improve the sensitivity and specificity of FISH and to overcome technical issues that engender false positive results [31]. FISH has not only demonstrated suitability as an informative diagnostic assay, but also FISH results have been shown to correlate with clinical outcome, since FISH-positive melanomas exhibit a more aggressive clinical course than FISH-negative melanomas. Specific FISH probes appear to have greater prognostic relevance than others [32–34].

This chapter examines the application of molecular pathology to the diagnosis of melanocytic lesions of the skin. In particular, the application of molecular techniques (e.g., FISH and CGH) to facilitate the distinction between benign and malignant melanocytic neoplasms and potential pitfalls in interpretation of some ancillary diagnostic techniques are discussed in detail.

Comparative Genomic Hybridization: The Beginning

Since the initial description of the technique, comparative genomic hybridization (CGH) has systematically revolutionized our understanding of the core genomic landscape of solid and hematopoietic tumors [35]. Up to that point, a systematic description of tumor-specific genomic alterations in melanocytic lesions relied on either conventional cytogenetic approaches and/or molecular genetic studies of isolated tumor DNA (restriction fragment length polymorphisms: RFLP; loss of heterozygosity: LOH). However, cytogenetics provides a relatively low-resolution image of the genomic changes typical of a tumor, relies on tumor cells with high quality metaphase nuclei and requires a considerable amount of fresh tumor cells for effective analysis. Similarly, molecular-genetic studies of tumor DNA (RFLP and LOH) typically only focus on a specific genomic/chromosomal region, are limited by the relative informativeness of a given RFLP marker and further, require a significant amount of relatively pure tumor DNA for successful analysis.

In contrast, CGH utilizes a straightforward approach: DNA from a tumor cell of interest is amplified and labeled with a fluorescent probe and is simultaneously hybridized together with reference DNA from a normal cell (labeled with a different fluorescent probe) to a substrate of complete genomic DNA. The fundamental premise of CGH is that regions of relative gain or loss in the tumor cells will be directly reflected in the relative differences in the intensity of the different fluorophores. Namely, regions of gain in the tumor cell genome will preferentially hybridize to the substrate platform due to their relative

greater numbers (tumor fluorophore predominant signal) compared to the control, whereas regions of deletion in the tumor cell will hybridize less frequently to the substrate platform in fewer numbers than the control (control fluorophore predominant signal), while all other regions will contain the same relative number of fluorescent signals between tumor and control (Fig. 13.1). The advantage of CGH is its ability to simultaneously survey the entire genome of a tumor for relative DNA copy number changes (gains and losses) in a relatively high-throughput setting. CGH facilitates the identification of previously unknown tumor suppressors (correspond to regions of loss in a tumor) or oncogene (region of gain in a tumor) in a single experiment. Conventional CGH utilized a normal chromosome spread as the target [35] and provided a resolution of ~10–20 Mb [36]. Subsequent implementations of CGH employed a microarray containing the entire genome in small sequential fragments of the genome contained within bacterial artificial chromosomes (BAC) [37, 38]. In contrast to conventional CGH, array CGH (aCGH) facilitates a much more precise resolution to the extent of genomic alterations: the resolution is limited only by the spacing/length of the BAC clones (Fig. 13.1).

In one of the first studies to apply CGH to cutaneous melanomas, Wiltshire et al. coupled microdissection techniques with CGH to define the complex genomic heterogeneity within lesions of cutaneous melanomas and described a genomic progression from radial growth phase (RGP) melanomas to vertical growth phase melanoma (VGP) from the same patient. They showed for example that portions of chromosome 17 and the short arm of chromosome 1 (1p) were lost in the RGP and VGP of melanomas from two of the three samples tested. In contrast, there were important disparities between RGP and VGP, including gains at 6p in one case and variable gains in chromosome 7 in two of the three cases tested [39].

In the first comprehensive application of conventional CGH to cutaneous melanoma, Bastian and colleagues described the genomic content of 32 primary melanomas [13]. Their findings confirmed and expanded on earlier cytogenetic

Fig. 13.1 Schematic of
Comparative Genomic
Hybridization. Regions
of gain in the tumor
cell genome will
preferentially hybridize
to the substrate platform
due to their relative
greater numbers (tumor
fluorophore predominant
signal) compared to the
control, whereas regions
of deletion in the tumor
cell will hybridize less
frequently to the
substrate platform in
fewer numbers than the
control (control
fluorophore predominant
signal), while all other
regions will contain the
same relative number of
fluorescent signals
between tumor and
control

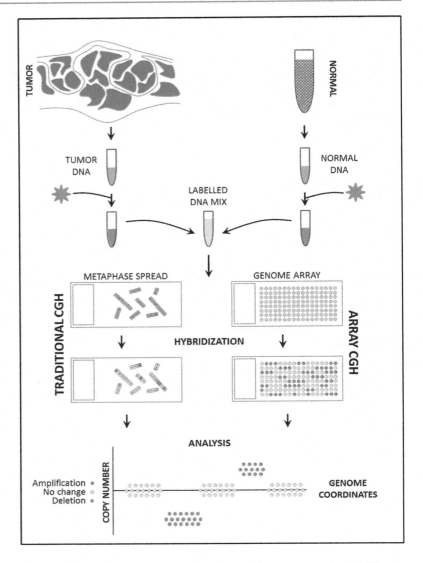

studies and RFLP/LOH studies in melanoma. In
particular, they identified the short arm of chromosome 9 (9p) as the most commonly deleted
locus in melanoma: identified in 26/32 cases
(81 %) they analyzed in their series. Additional
commonly deleted genomic regions in melanoma
included: chromosome 10 (63 %), the long arm of
chromosome 6 (6q; 28 %), and the short arm of
chromosome 8 (8p; 22 %). Additional commonly
amplified genomic regions in melanoma included
areas on chromosome 7 (50 %), the long arm of
chromosome 8 (8q; 34 %), the short arm of chromosome 6 (6p; 28 %), the long arm of chromosome 1 (1q; 25 %), the long arm of chromosome
20 (20q; 13 %), the long arm of chromosome 17

(17q; 13 %), and chromosome 2 (13 %). In
addition, the authors identified important correlations between the absolute number of chromosomal changes and parameters predictive of
outcome in cutaneous melanoma. First, there was
a strong correlation between the number of aberrations and increasing patient age ($p = 0.007$), and
there was apparent clustering of discrete changes
in specific age groups: gains of chromosomes 5
and 17 and losses of chromosome 18 occurring
almost exclusively in patients older than 70 years.
Although there was no statistically significant
correlation between the absolute number of aberrations and increasing tumor thickness ($p = 0.34$),
other important histopathologic correlations were

identified: when tumors of <3.0 mm were compared to tumors ≥3.0 mm, although losses of chromosomes 9 and 10 were comparable in both groups, losses of chromosome 7 were significantly more common among thicker tumors ($p=0.05$). In addition to identifying potentially important tumor suppressors and oncogenes in melanoma, their findings also implicated specific chromosomal loci (in particular the loss of chromosome 9p) as an important and early contributor to melanomagenesis: (1) it was the most frequently altered locus in their series and (2) its alteration occurred at an equal frequency among thin and thick lesions [13].

In a subsequent landmark study, Bastian and colleagues applied conventional CGH to a series of 186 melanocytic lesions comprised of 132 melanomas and 54 nevi, and demonstrated a striking difference in the genomic composition of melanomas compared to melanocytic nevi [14]. In particular, 127/132 (96.2 %) of the melanomas harbored some chromosomal copy aberration, and similar to the previous study, to the extent that they were frequently altered in melanoma, several discrete genomic loci were implicated as critical to melanomagenesis. These included gains in 6p (37.1 %), 1q (32.6 %), 7p (31.8 %), 7q (31.8 %), 8q (25.0 %), 17q (24.2 %) and 20q (22.0 %), while the most frequent chromosomal losses included 9p (64.4 %), 9q (36.4 %), 10q (36.4 %), 10p (29.5 %), 6q (25.8 %), and 11q (21.2 %). Furthermore, they interrogated melanomas according to the anatomic site on which they arose. They identified more frequent amplifications among acral melanomas (AM; 100 % contained at least one amplification) compared to melanomas arising on cutaneous sites (non-AM; only 22.2 % carried one amplification). AMs further contained discretely amplified loci at a significantly higher frequency that non-AMs, including 5p (36.4 % compared 4.6 %, $p=0.00015$), 12q (22.2 % compared to 0 %; $p=0.000092$), 4q (18.2 % compared to 0.9 %; $p=0.0076$), and 11q (36.4 % compared to 9.3 %; $p=0.0028$). In addition, AM were also typified by specific chromosomal deletions compared to non-AMs: 6q (50 % compared to

9.4 %; $p=0.0052$), 15q (22.7 % compared to 0.9 %; $p=0.00049$), and 16q (36.4 % compared to 10.2 %; $p=0.0044$). Similarly, when cutaneous melanomas were grouped according to histopathologic pattern (superficial spreading melanoma (SSM) type versus lentigo maligna (LM) type), there were also differences in their genomic composition: LM had gains at 15q and 17q more frequently than in SSM (20.0 % compared to 0 %; $p=0.0027$ and 40 % compared to 11.5 %; $p=0.0066$, respectively) and losses at 13q and 17p (32 % compared to 5.8 %; $p=0.0040$ and 36.0 % compared to 3.8 %; $p=0.00043$, respectively) [14].

When cutaneous melanomas were grouped according to the degree of solar elastosis and thus according to whether the melanoma arose in a background of chronic sun damage (CSD) versus non-chronically sun damaged (non-CSD) skin, analogous genomic differences emerged: namely, in CSD compared to non-CSD there were more frequent amplifications overall (43.8 % compared to 13.2 %; $p=0.00046$) and specifically, gains at 15q (12.5 % compared to 0 %; $p=0.0067$) and losses at 17p (28.1 % compared to 6.6 %; $p=0.0044$). Similarly, there were more frequent losses at chromosome 10p (36.8 % compared to 9.4 %; $p=0.0046$) and 10q (40.8 % compared to 12.5 %; $p=0.0037$) in non-CSD compared to CSD [14]. These latter results were expanded upon in a subsequent benchmark study from Bastian and colleagues in which they characterized the genomic profile of an additional 126 melanomas arising on different body sites [40]. The authors again grouped the melanomas according to body site and degree of antecedent sun exposure and generated four categories that they interrogated and compared: mucosal melanomas, acral melanomas, cutaneous melanomas with evidence of chronic sun damage (CSD), and cutaneous melanomas without evidence of chronic sun damage (non-CSD), and using these broad categories several fundamental principles emerged. First, melanomas from non-sun-exposed sites (acral and mucosal) had a higher overall number of chromosomal aberrations: there were more total gains and losses of chromosomal DNA ($p=0.004$), a greater number of copy-number transitions ($p<0.001$) within chromosomes and a higher number of overall contiguous amplifications ($p<0.001$). Whereas amplifications were found in 89 % of acral and 85 % of mucosal melanomas, they were relatively rare among CSD and non-CSD (cutaneous) melanomas. Although there were changes common to all the groups of melanomas, there were also changes that occurred with differing frequency among the groups. The latter was best reflected by the ~70 % of lesions in the total cohort that were correctly classified according to anatomic location/degree of sun exposure based on their DNA copy aberrations alone. The identification of statistically significant differences in the genomic composition of melanomas according to both anatomic site as well as the relative degree of sun exposure provided a critical mechanistic correlation for the relative contribution of sun exposure (and other factors) to melanomagenesis: namely, there are distinct pathways driving this process derived in part from different environmental agents (sun) [40].

Similar results were described by Balazs et al. [41] who applied CGH to characterize the genomic profile of 16 primary and 12 metastatic melanomas (including paired primary and metastatic melanoma samples from the same patients). All 16 primary tumors showed some form of chromosomal copy aberration, with an average number of 6.3 alterations/primary tumor (range 1–14). The most frequent changes among the primary melanomas in their series included gains of 6p (10/16; 63 %), gains of 8q (8/16; 50 %) and gains at 1q (6/16; 38 %) and losses at 10q (10/16; 63 %) and losses at 9p (7/16; 44 %). Similarly all 12 of the metastatic melanomas showed some form of chromosomal copy aberration in their series with an average number of 7.8 alterations/metastatic tumor. The most frequent changes among the metastatic melanomas in their series included gains of 6p (6/12; 50 %) and 8q (5/12; 42 %) and losses at 10q (6/12; 50 %) and 9p (7/12; 58 %). Although there was considerable overlap in the genomic profile of the four paired primary and metastatic lesions analyzed in their series, there were also important differences and

implicated specific regions, including gains in chromosome 13q, chromosome 3, and chromosome 7 and losses at chromosome 16q, 2p21, and 9p21 as important loci in the evolution of melanoma metastases. To further analyze their CGH findings, they assessed several of the more commonly altered loci by fluorescence in situ hybridization (FISH). FISH studies confirmed alterations in chromosome 1 in all four primary tumors tested; FISH studies confirmed the status of 8q (the c-MYC locus) for three of the four primary and three of the four metastatic tumors tested; and FISH confirmed deletion of the 9p21 locus in four of eight primary tumors tested (FISH identified an additional two lesions with 9p21 deletion not identified by CGH, which was attributed to improved sensitivity of FISH compared to CGH).

They also correlated changes detected by CGH with conventional parameters of clinical outcome in melanoma, including tumor thickness, age, and the propensity to form metastases. Similar to the findings of Bastian et al. they found that there although there was a trend towards an increasing number of chromosomal copy number aberrations with increasing tumor thickness (4.4 ± 4.5 alterations in tumors ≤4 mm versus 7.4 ± 3.7 alterations in tumors >4 mm), this failed to achieve statistical significance ($p=0.161$). Of note, the authors noted a more frequent gain on chromosome 7 among thicker tumors. Finally, when they compared the primary tumors that developed metastases within 1 year of the primary surgery ($n=12$ versus $n=4$), the number of chromosomal copy aberrations was higher in this group (7.8 ± 4.1) compared to those who did not develop metastases during this time period (2.0 ± 1.4) ($p=0.017$). Among those who developed metastases, six patients died within 2 years of surgery, and the primary tumors in these patients carried more alterations (9.8 ± 4.2) than those who survived this time period (4.2 ± 3.0), and this, too, was statistically significant ($p=0.007$) [41].

Virtually all of the studies applying CGH to melanocytic tumors proved important indicators of the critical chromosomal imbalances contributing to melanomagenesis to the extent that specifically altered loci were either held in common or distinctly different across multiple different studies and multiple different lesions. What was more striking was the absolutely fundamental difference observed between melanomas and nevi. In their original study [14], whereas most of the melanomas (96.2 %) carried some form of chromosomal copy alteration, only 13 % of the nevi tested showed any chromosomal changes, and these were limited to Spitz nevi with isolated gains in the entire short arm of 11p. Only a single case of melanoma showed changes in 11p, and this involved only *a portion of 11p* as opposed to the *entire chromosomal arm* as seen in Spitz nevi. These findings argued that gross chromosomal abnormalities (in the form of gains/losses in discrete regions of the chromosome) are a central feature of melanomas and for the first time, implicated CGH as a potentially informative diagnostic tool, particularly in histopathologically challenging melanocytic lesions. This utility of CGH as a diagnostic adjunct was explored in a series of subsequent studies. Two cases with challenging differential diagnoses according to histopathologic parameters (essentially melanoma versus atypical nevus) were investigated by CGH and diagnosed as nevus and melanoma based upon the absence and presence, respectively, of chromosomal copy aberrations [16].

The latter paradigm was further tested in a study applying CGH to define the genomic composition of large congenital melanocytic nevi (CMN) and congenital melanocytic nevi containing different patterns of secondary melanocytic proliferations worrisome for melanoma [15]. In this study, the authors applied CGH to a series of 29 CMN with differing attributes, ranging from conventional CMN to melanomas arising in CMN. They showed that lesions with a mostly benign morphology contained no abnormalities by CGH (*n* = 13), whereas 100 % of the melanomas tested (*n* = 6) manifested chromosomal abnormalities typical of melanoma (changes in copy number of portions of chromosomes). In contrast, those lesions consisting of CMN with expansile nodular proliferations with "…high

cellularity, nuclear atypia and markedly increased proliferation rate…" (Group IV) contained chromosomal copy number alterations in 7 of 9 cases. However, this was a distinctive pattern and included changes in the number of *whole chromosomes* (rather than *portions of chromosomes* as is typical of melanomas) seen in 86 % (6/7) of the cases. Only rare cases of melanomas (5 % in their study) also contained copy number alterations involving whole chromosomes. Together, these findings suggested distinctive patterns of genomic instability in different melanocytic lesions that correlate with the observed differences in biological behavior, and further, exploiting these could provide a useful tool to inform their diagnosis. Indeed, even when melanomas showed whole chromosomal copy number alterations, the pattern of chromosomes involved was distinctive: losses of chromosome 9 and 10 occurred in melanomas, whereas these changes were less frequently seen in the benign category. Furthermore, in the cases of melanoma arising in association with a benign melanocytic nevus in this study with sufficient material to analyze the benign and malignant components separately either by FISH or CGH (*n* = 3), the nevus component showed none of the chromosomal changes observed in the melanomas [15].

Because lesions with features of blue nevus occasionally pose diagnostic challenges, a series of melanocytic lesions with varying features of blue nevi were also studied by CGH. Among 11 lesions with features of conventional cellular blue nevus or deep penetrating nevus, none showed any chromosomal abnormalities. Among 11 lesions with an intermediate histopathology (defined by variable presence of nuclear atypia/pleomorphism, >1 mitotic figure/10 high power fields (hpf), focal necrosis, and sheet-like growth or a focus of increased cellularity), three contained chromosomal changes. One of these three cases exhibited three chromosomal abnormalities and given the reported presence of cytologic atypia, 3 mitotic figures/10 hpf, and focal necrosis, might also be better classified as melanoma, blue nevus type [42]. Finally, among the group of lesions classified as melanomas with features of or an associated blue nevus, all seven lesions (100 %) exhibited multiple chromosomal abnormalities (mean=8 abnormalities/case) typical of melanoma. The most common changes seen were losses in portions of chromosome 9 and gains of portions of chromosome 20. Among the histopathologic features that most strongly correlated with the presence of chromosomal abnormalities, all cases with necrosis ($n=4$) had chromosomal abnormalities; in addition, both cytologic atypia (odds ratio=9.4; $p=0.0004$); and a mitotic rate>2/10hpf (odds ratio=8.5; $p=0.017$) correlated with genomic alterations [42].

Given their typically challenging morphology, the genomic profile of Spitz nevi was further explored in a series of subsequent studies [43–45]. In a confirmation of their prior findings, 17 Spitz nevi were assessed by CGH and FISH and ~20 % of Spitz nevi (4/17 cases analyzed) were typified by gains in the entire short arm of chromosome 11 (11p) [44]. A smaller study utilized array CGH to study 3 Spitz nevi and showed 1/3 cases with 11p amplification [45]. In a larger cohort of lesions ($n=102$, amenable to direct FISH testing of the 11p locus), Bastian and colleagues showed that ~12 % of Spitz nevi carried copy number increases in 11p, and this change correlated with increased tumor thickness (mean=1.1 mm for cases with increased copy numbers of 11p versus 0.6 mm for those cases with two copies of 11p; $p=0.01$). Within 11p, the authors identified the HRAS gene locus as a candidate oncogene and showed further that 5/9 cases (56 %) with 11p amplification by FISH also carried activating HRAS mutations. Additional sequencing of 3 of the Spitz nevi with 11p amplification identified by CGH in their previous study [44] demonstrated that these lesions also carried activating mutations in HRAS. Thus, between their two studies [43, 44], a total of 8/12 Spitz nevi with amplification of 11p also carried activating mutations in HRAS. In contrast, only 1/13 cases (~8 %) with diploid copy numbers of 11p by FISH carried HRAS mutations, while all seven of the cases with diploid copy numbers of 11p by CGH were wild type for HRAS (total of 1/20 diploid

11p cases with activating mutations in HRAS). This predilection of HRAS mutation for lesions with amplified 11p was statistically significant ($p<0.0001$) [43, 44]. In addition, cases with increased copy numbers of 11p demonstrated a typical morphology: increased desmoplasia and single cell infiltration of the deep dermis towards the deeper aspects of the lesion, and these single cells had a characteristic eosinophilic, reticulin-positive membrane surrounding them. The tumor cell nuclei in cases with gains in 11p exhibited greater pleomorphism than Spitz nevi diploid for 11p. There was, however, no statistically significant difference in the proliferative index (assessed by Ki-67 immunohistochemistry) between Spitz nevi with 11p copy number increases compared to those cases diploid for 11p [43].

Although CGH has transformed our understanding of and ability to more thoroughly quantify the genomic composition of melanocytic lesions, there are important limitations to a broader application of the technique in routine diagnosis. From a practical perspective, CGH is expensive and time-consuming, and CGH requires considerable technical expertise. More importantly, the results of CGH analysis reflect the average DNA content contributed by the total admixture of cells analyzed. As such, CGH requires a considerable amount of relatively pure population of tumor cells containing a particular chromosomal copy aberration in order to detect that change, and different types of changes will be detected more easily than others (for example, amplifications more readily detected than simple chromosomal gains and losses). Thus, because copy number alterations must be present in at least ~30–50 % of the tumor cells in order to be detected by CGH [16], genomic changes occurring in only a minority of cells analyzed might go undetected by CGH. This would thus complicate the application of CGH to melanocytic lesions with a small dermal component, lesions with a significant associated benign nevus or lesions with a significant associated lymphohistiocytic/adnexal component, as the tumor cells of interest might contribute only a minority of DNA to the overall analysis [16].

Fluorescence In Situ Hybridization (FISH): A Surrogate of the Genomic Instability Described by CGH

Because CGH provides an image of the entire genomic landscape of a given melanocytic proliferation, it still represents the gold standard for ancillary testing in melanocytic tumor diagnosis. However, given its aforementioned limitations, it was rapidly realized that there was a critical need to develop a test with capacity for higher throughput, a more feasible utility in laboratories of all sizes and capabilities to further inform melanocytic tumor diagnosis. Similar approaches had been previously applied to develop fluorescence in situ hybridization (FISH) tests as surrogates of genomic instability in other cancer types, including bladder and lung cancer [46, 47]. Gerami and colleagues thus developed the initial conventional melanoma FISH assay [18]. Using an exhaustive statistical approach, they performed a combinatorial analysis of Bastian's existing CGH data to delineate the most frequently altered genomic loci in melanoma. This identified 13 chromosomal loci from eight different chromosomes. FISH probes corresponding to each of these loci were generated, and given the known frequency of *KIT* amplifications and the potential implications for *KIT* alterations in directing targeted therapy [48] an additional probe for this locus was generated. Different combinations of these fluorescently labeled probes were applied to a series of 97 melanomas and 95 nevi, comprising the "discovery cohort." This approach identified 6p25 (*RREB1*), centromere 6, 6q23 (*MYB*), 7q34 (*BRAF*), 11q13 (*CCND1*), 17q25 (*TK1*), and 20q13 (*ZNF217*) as informative probes to distinguish between melanomas and nevi. A subsequent systematic analysis identified 6p25 (*RREB1*), centromere 6, 6q23 (*MYB*), and 11q13 (*CCND1*) as the most sensitive and specific combination to distinguish melanomas from nevi, and this probe set was selected for application to a new cohort of 58 melanomas and nevi to define the best diagnostic cutoffs for the FISH assay. This analysis yielded the following algorithm: (1) >38 % of tumor nuclei contain more than two signals for 11q13 (*CCND1*); (2) >55 % of the tumor nuclei contain more 6p25 (*RREB1*) signals than centromere 6 signals; (3) >40 % of the tumor nuclei contain fewer 6q23 (*MYB*) signals than centromere six signals; (4) >29 % of the tumor nuclei contain more than two signals for 6p25 (*RREB1*) (Fig. 13.2). Any one of these changes indicated a positive FISH result. The application of these diagnostic criteria to a 3rd cohort of 83 melanomas and 86 melanocytic nevi resulted in the correct classification of 72 melanomas and 82 nevi for sensitivity of 86.7 % and a specificity of 95.4 %, respectively. They also applied the set of probes to a series of 27 histopathologically ambiguous tumors. A total of 12 of these 27 tumors were positive by FISH— including all of the lesions (*n* = 6) that eventually metastasized, further supporting the concept that this FISH assay was a diagnostically informative one (to the extent that it correctly identified all the histopathologically ambiguous melanocytic tumors that produced metastases) [18].

In comparison to CGH, there are important advantages offered by FISH, albeit with new limitations. Whereas CGH scanned the entire genome, FISH only interrogates the composition of specific genomic loci; however, FISH enables the interrogation of the discrete tumor cells and does not require a pure population of tumor cells for this. An important caveat to that, however, is that FISH relies on the ability of the 4-"6"-diamidino-2-phenylindole dihydrochloride hydrate (DAPI) counterstain to identify the tumor cells. This presents an important limitation when considering the applicability of FISH to assess single cell predominant intraepidermal proliferations or dermal based lesions with a nevoid morphology in the background of an associated lymphohistiocytic inflammatory infiltrate—to the extent that the tumor cells would be difficult to precisely distinguish in the absence of obvious morphologic features, which are not always readily evident under fluorescence microscopic visualization of tumor nuclei. An additional shortcoming (already realized in the initial FISH study) was the presence of polyploidy among the benign melanocytic nevi yielding a false positive result (apparent gains in both chromosomes 6 and 11 without concomitant

Fig. 13.2 Schematic of First Generation FISH assay. (1) >38 % of tumor nuclei contain more than two signals for 11q13 (CCND1); (2) >55 % of the tumor nuclei contain more 6p25 (RREB1) signals than centromere 6 signals; (3) >40 % of the tumor nuclei contain fewer 6q23 (MYB) signals than centromere 6 signals; (4) >29 % of the tumor nuclei contain more than two signals for 6p25 (RREB1)

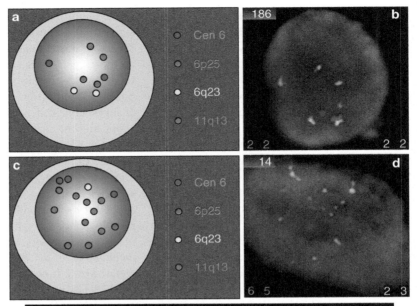

Probe Set	UCSF/Northwestern	Neogenomics
RREB (6p25)>2	>29%	>16%
RREB (6p25)>CEN6	>55%	>53%
MYB (6q23)<CEN6	>40%	>42%
CCND1 (11q13)>2	>38%	>19%

alterations in the ratio of chromosome 6 probes and centromere 6) in three of the four cases [18]. (This important limitation is described in more detail below.) In an independent validation study, Morey et al. applied FISH to a series of 20 unambiguous melanomas (including 10 primaries and 10 metastases) and 20 nevi and demonstrated a sensitivity of 90 % and a specificity of 95 % [19]. Of note, among the false negative cases were two melanoma metastases.

The applicability of the FISH assay as defined above was subsequently exhaustively explored in a variety of different diagnostic contexts—including both distinctive subtypes of unambiguous melanoma in comparison to their unequivocally benign counterparts (i.e., blue nevus-like melanomas compared to blue nevi) as well as ambiguous melanocytic tumors. When considering the utility of FISH in the literature, among unambiguous melanomas [$n=583$) compared to unambiguous nevi [$n=720$), the overall sensitivity described is ~82.2 % [479/583; range: 40–100 %) and the

overall specificity is ~95.3 % [686/720; range: 93–100 %) [18, 19, 21–28, 30, 49–57] (Table 13.1). In particular, FISH enjoys high sensitivity (84–88 %) and specificity (100 %) in the distinction of lentiginous nevus of the elderly from melanoma in situ [26, 56]; FISH also enjoys a comparably high sensitivity (90–100 %) and specificity (100 %) in the distinction of blue nevus-like melanoma from benign blue nevus mimickers [22, 28]; FISH reliably distinguishes nevoid melanoma from benign nevi [24] and conjunctival melanomas from conjunctival nevi [20] with 100 % sensitivity and specificity. However, there are specific differential diagnostic contexts in which FISH has a reduced utility—even when considering unambiguous lesions. One of the first studies to demonstrate this showed a markedly reduced sensitivity for the distinction of desmoplastic melanoma from desmoplastic nevus [52]. Only 7 of 15 desmoplastic melanomas tested by FISH yielded positive results (Sensitivity = 47 %); not surprisingly, however, the specificity for the

Table 13.1 Studies examining the application and utility of FISH assays in the diagnosis of melanocytic lesions

Reference	Melanomas tested	Melanomas positive	Sensitivity (%)	Nevi tested	Nevi negative	Specificity (%)	Type of case tested
[53]	123	102	83	110	103	94	Unambiguous MM versus nevus
[19]	20	18	90	20	19	95	Unambiguous MM versus nevus
[25]	36	28	78	36	36	100	Unambiguous MM versus nevus
[29]	7	3	43	3	3	100	Unambiguous MM versus nevus
[55]	167	140	83	333	314	94	Unambiguous MM versus nevus
[30]	20	17	85	19	17	90	Unambiguous MM versus nevus
[51]	50	41	82	50	47	98	Unambiguous MM versus nevus
	15	13	85				Metastases from these lesions
[26]	19	16	84	19	19	100	Lentiginous nevus of the elderly = MM
[56]	8	7	88	5	5	100	Lentiginous nevus of the elderly = MM
[28]	10	9	90	10	10	100	Blue nevus-like MM versus epithelioid blue nevus
[22]	5	5	100	12	12	100	Blue nevus-like MM versus epithelioid blue nevus
[52]	15	7	47	15	15	100	Desmoplastic melanoma versus desmoplastic nevus
[23]	7	5	71	6	6	100	Superficial melanocytic neoplasms with pagetoid melanocytosis = MM
[24]	10	10	100	10	10	100	Nevoid melanoma versus nevus
[20]	6	6	100	4	4	100	Conjunctival melanoma versus nevus
[21]	18	14	78				Metastatic melanoma versus nodal nevus; primary MM
	24	20	83	17	16	94	
[57]	12 (8)	7	88	6 (5)	5	100	Spitzoid MM versus Spitzoid nevus
[54]				3	3	100	Sclerosing melanocytic nevus
[50]	15	11	73	15	14	93	Spindle cell MM versus pigmented spindle cell nevus of Reed
[27]				28	28	100	Nevus with atypical epithelioid cell component (NAECC)

diagnosis was 100 % (all 15 desmoplastic nevi were FISH-negative). An additional differential diagnostic context where FISH has limited diagnostic utility is the distinction of spindle cell melanoma from its mimic, the pigmented spindle cell nevus of Reed; although the specificity of FISH remained high at 93 % (14 of 15 Reed nevi were FISH negative), only 11 of 15 spindle cell melanomas were FISH-positive (Sensitivity=73 %) [50]. Finally, FISH has modest sensitivity in the distinction of nodal nevi from microscopic lymph node metastases: among 24 metastases tested, only 20 were FISH positive (Sensitivity=83 %), whereas 16 of 17 nodal nevi were FISH negative (Specificity=94 %) [21]. It is unclear the extent to which the small size and spindled morphology of nodal nevus cells contribute to this reduced sensitivity. Furthermore, this study did not correlate the FISH status of the metastasis with its primary melanoma, as a FISH-negative primary melanoma might likely produce a FISH-negative metastasis and thus, an apparent false-negative result.

The work of Bastian and colleagues demonstrated many nonoverlapping genomic changes in melanomas arising on different anatomic sites. At some level, this is presumably a function of the degree of antecedent sun exposure [40]. This raised the question whether FISH might have similarly different sensitivity across the various subtypes of melanoma and more specifically, whether different FISH probes would show a different frequency of altered copy numbers among different subtypes of primary melanoma. Gerami and colleagues addressed this question directly in a large scale study describing FISH results across 123 melanomas of different subtypes [53]. Several important principles emerged from this important study: (1) the overall sensitivity and specificity of FISH in this group of lesions was similar to the findings in their original study and the literature overall at 83.0 and 94.0 %, respectively; (2) FISH was most sensitive in detecting nodular (90.9 % sensitive, $n=22$) and acral lentiginous melanomas (100 %, $n=3$) compared to lentigo maligna (82.1 %, $n=28$) and superficial spreading types (81.4 %, $n=70$); (3) gains at 6p25 were the most frequent alteration across all melanoma subtypes; and (4) gains at 11q13 were

enriched in melanomas arising on chronically sun damaged skin—confirming the finding of the original CGH studies showing an identical relative frequency of 11q13 amplifications among CSD melanomas compared to non-CSD lesions [53].

One of the most important limitations to the early studies to assess the applicability of FISH to melanocytic tumor diagnosis was that most of these were proof of principle studies utilizing histopathologically unambiguous nevi in comparison to histopathologically unambiguous melanomas. In contrast, the utility of FISH to distinguish among histopathologically ambiguous lesions—where additional ancillary testing would most usefully inform the diagnosis—remains a challenging and controversial topic. Despite the initial reports that FISH might prove helpful in distinguishing among ambiguous melanocytic proliferations [18], larger series with histopathologically challenging melanocytic lesions have shown the diagnostic utility of FISH in this setting to be less definitive, with an overall lower sensitivity (between 43 and 60 %) and lower specificity (between 50 and 80 %) using clinical behavior as the gold standard [29, 30]. In one of the largest studies addressing the utility of FISH in ambiguous melanocytic tumors, Vergier et al. assessed a series of 113 morphologically ambiguous melanocytic proliferations [30]. Assuming clinical outcome to be the gold standard, they demonstrated that histopathologic review by expert dermatopathologists had a sensitivity of 95 % but a specificity of only 52 % for the distinction of benign from malignant. For the same question, FISH demonstrated a sensitivity of only 43 %, but a specificity of 80 %. Their results were significant to the extent that among histopathologically ambiguous lesions, FISH negativity could be observed among lesions with a malignant behavior (i.e., false negatives) at a rate of ~8 % overall. These included both lesions with an overall malignant histopathologic impression ($n=8$) as well as an isolated lesion with an overall benign morphology ($n=1$). Each of these lesions showed negativity by FISH, but ultimately produced metastases. Similarly, among lesions with an overall benign morphology and benign follow-up, there were occasional false positives ($n = 3$). Given the relatively high specificity of FISH in their study, the findings of Vergier et al. were significant to the extent that they systematically defined how best to incorporate FISH into the diagnosis of morphologically ambiguous melanocytic tumors. Namely, adding FISH to histopathologic assessment improved the specificity of the diagnosis, and they concluded that the application of conventional FISH is most effective in those cases in which the FISH result reinforced the conclusions of expert histopathologic review: namely, a negative FISH assay in a "favor benign" lesion or a positive FISH in a "favor malignant" lesion. Furthermore, the FISH result ought not supplant the time tested principles of a careful histopathologic assessment by seasoned dermatopathologists [30]. Gaiser et al. similarly applied FISH (albeit using slightly different criteria for FISH positivity) to a series of 22 melanocytic lesions, including 12 ambiguous cases, to provide an even less favorable appraisal of the utility of the FISH assay: demonstrating a sensitivity of 60 % and a specificity of only 50 % to detect those lesions that produced subsequent metastasis [29].

Zembowicz et al. also reported their experience with the conventional FISH assay in a large series of 140 challenging melanocytic lesions encountered in their consultation practice [58]. Among 66 "favor benign" lesions, 59 demonstrated a negative FISH result, while the remaining 7 "favor benign" lesions exhibited abnormal FISH results that the authors attributed to "false positivity" either due to tetraploidy (5 cases; see discussion below) or poor hybridization (2 cases). All 66 of these cases were ultimately diagnosed as atypical nevus. Among 27 "favor malignant cases," 14 exhibited FISH positivity (one of these attributable to tetraploidy) and 13 were FISH negative. All 27 of these cases were ultimately diagnosed as melanoma. Finally, among 47 borderline lesions, 29 cases were FISH negative; these were ultimately diagnosed as "borderline lesions." In contrast, 18 cases exhibited a positive FISH result. Among the latter, 4 were interpreted as secondary to tetraploidy. Among the

remaining 14, 10 cases were finally diagnosed as melanoma, while 4 cases were designated as "borderline melanocytic tumors of uncertain malignant potential with abnormal FISH test results." Overall, the authors reported a high rate of false positives dues to tetraploidy (26 %) and thus (similar to that of Vergier and colleagues) concluded that in the context of the morphologic findings of an atypical nevus, a negative FISH test is reassuring. Furthermore, in the context of a morphologically worrisome lesion, they argued that a positive FISH test "clinches" the diagnosis of "outright melanoma." They argued that when there is discordance ("favor benign" and positive FISH or "favor malignant" and negative FISH), the FISH result should not supplant the more rigorously "time-tested" criteria of morphology and proposed that perhaps FISH results should be considered *prognostic* rather than *diagnostic* [58]. This notion ultimately found concrete support in a landmark study by Bastian and colleagues who demonstrated that FISH-positive melanomas carried a significantly higher risk of developing future metastases than FISH-negative melanomas (Hazard Ratio = 5.9; $p = 0.04$) [34].

We performed FISH on a series of 34 ambiguous melanocytic tumors encountered in our consultation service. Eight of these cases exhibited FISH positivity (three in which the morphologic features favored a benign diagnosis and five in which the morphologic features favored a diagnosis of melanoma). In all cases, the final diagnosis mirrored the initial consensus impression rendered prior to FISH testing. Namely, we ultimately diagnosed 24 lesions in which we "favored benign" as melanocytic nevus (albeit with atypical features); among the three cases in this category that were positive for FISH, we believed the combined morphologic and immunophenotypic features of these lesions ultimately did not merit a malignant diagnosis. Two of these cases exhibited gains of 6p25 together with gains of 11q13 while one case revealed an altered ratio of 6q23/cen6 [59]. It is possible that the FISH positivity in the former two cases could be attributable to tetraploidy/polyploidy [22, 31, 58, 60–62], although this was not formally demonstrated in these cases.

Similarly, for the ten lesions in which we favored an overall malignant histopathologic impression, we diagnosed these as malignant, whereas only five were FISH positive. Our conclusions are supported by the follow-up in our cases (range 7–25 months at the time of publication) which showed only a single metastasis to a lymph node in a FISH-negative melanoma in a 4 year old boy, and they are in agreement with the opinions of similar studies in the literature [30, 58]. Namely, the results of a FISH test (positive or negative) did not necessarily alter the overall morphologic impression. The sensitivity of FISH in our study for the diagnosis of melanoma was 50%, while the specificity is 87.5%—findings similar to that described by Vergier et al. [30] Similar to previous studies which also show a high specificity and high negative predictive value [30, 58, 63], we found further support for the idea that a negative FISH assay in a lesion whose histopathologic and immunophenotypic parameters confer an overall benign diagnostic impression is a reassuring finding to further reinforce a benign diagnosis. Similarly, a positive FISH assay in a lesion with mostly atypical histopathologic and/or immunophenotypic findings provides additional confirmation for a malignant diagnosis.

A critical consideration in assessing the utility of the FISH assay is the variability in the thresholds employed by different centers performing it for the designation of a positive FISH result. In fact, the empirically derived cutoffs utilized by the centers at the University of California, San Francisco (UCSF) and Northwestern University (NW) are slightly different than that of the commercially available test at Neogenomics as follows: (1) >2 signals for RREB1 [6p25] in >29% of the nuclei at UCSF and NW versus >16% of the nuclei at Neogenomics (2) >2 signals for CCND1 [11q13] in >38% of the nuclei at UCSF and NW versus >19% of the nuclei at Neogenomics (3) ratio of RREB [6p25]:centromere 6 [cen6] >1 in >55% of the nuclei at UCSF and NW versus >53% of the nuclei at Neogenomics or (4) ratio of MYB [6q23]:centromere 6 [cen6] signal <1 in >40% of the nuclei at UCSF and NW versus in >42% of the nuclei at Neogenomics [17, 18] (Fig. 13.2).

The generally higher thresholds used by UCSF and NW compared to Neogenomics reflect an amalgamation of differing methodologies, but result in a different test sensitivity and specificity [17]. Moreover, these differences underscore an important caveat in assessing the impact of a FISH test result on diagnosis: FISH results for the same lesion might differ according to the laboratory in which the test was performed. Therefore, since Neogenomics applies a lower threshold to some criteria to designate a positive result, the likelihood of a false positive might be greater; for the same reasons, the possibility of a false negative might be greater at UCSF or NW. Of note, Vergier et al. [30] applied the thresholds proposed by UCSF and NW, whereas our study and Zembowicz et al. [58] relied on the thresholds derived at Neogenomics. The variability used to define FISH positivity and negativity (inherent when different methodologies are used) is an important consideration requiring further study—particularly with the introduction of "second generation" FISH assays (see below). In addition, since the cutoffs are themselves derived using unambiguous cases, the applicability of these FISH parameters to ambiguous cases (the scenario in which a diagnostic assay would most often be deployed) warrants ongoing and rigorous reassessment.

In the largest single study to date to interrogate the impact of FISH testing on morphologically challenging melanocytic lesions, North et al. described the impact of FISH testing on the diagnosis of 804 melanocytic lesions encountered in the consultation practice at UCSF [64]. Among these 804 cases, 754 were amenable to analysis by FISH (94%), and of these, a total of 124 (~16.4%) were FISH-positive by at least one criterion, whereas 630 (83.6%) were FISH-negative. Several critically important themes were underscored in this study. First, and not surprisingly, the most frequently tested differential diagnosis was among lesions with Spitzoid morphology, comprising 378 cases (~47% of the total cohort). Of these, however, only 46 were FISH-positive—constituting 38% of the FISH-positive cases overall and only 12% of the Spitzoid cases tested. The lesional subtype that exhibited the greatest frequency of FISH positivity included the group of lesions where the histopathologic differential diagnosis included dysplastic nevus versus melanoma. Whereas only 53 of these cases were submitted for FISH analysis (~6.6% of the total), 14 of these were positive. This constituted 11.3% of the total FISH-positive cases overall, but showed that 26.4% of the cases of dysplastic nevus versus melanoma were FISH positive (the highest frequency among the differential diagnostic considerations) [64]. Finally, and in contrast to the previous findings of Gerami et al. [53], the most frequently altered locus among the ambiguous lesions tested in the UCSF study was relative loss of 6q23, which occurred in 78 cases (62.9% of all the FISH positive cases). Gain of 6p25 (the most frequently encountered alteration in Gerami's study) occurred in 42 FISH positive cases (33.9% of all the FISH positive cases). The latter suggests that ambiguous lesions may be characterized by distinctive patterns of FISH abnormalities in comparison to conventional, unambiguous melanomas. When they considered the impact of a FISH result on their final diagnosis, the findings were largely in keeping with that observed in previous studies. Namely, among the 630 FISH-negative cases, 489 (78%) received a final diagnosis of benign melanocytic nevus, 91 (14%) received an equivocal/indeterminate diagnosis that included both melanoma and nevus, and 50 (8%) received a final diagnosis of melanoma (despite FISH negativity). Of note, a subset of the latter cases ($n=6$) was subjected to CGH studies, and all six exhibited chromosomal abnormalities by CGH other than that assessed by FISH (i.e., loci not at 6p25, 6q23, and 11q13). Similarly, among the 124 FISH-positive cases, 117 (94%) were given a diagnosis of melanoma, one (1%) was given an equivocal/indeterminate diagnosis and six (5%) were given a benign diagnosis. Among the latter six cases, (1) there was an isolated relative 6q23 loss in three cases, and two of these only "…marginally exceeded the threshold…" for positivity; (2) a fourth case exhibited isolated gain of 6p25—again, only marginally exceeding the threshold for positivity; (3) one case exhibited polysomy for chromosome 6; and (4) only one case exhibited both loss of 6q23 and gain of 6p25 [64].

Overall, the emerging consensus in the literature is that in the context of ambiguous lesions, FISH by itself has a lower sensitivity and specificity for the diagnosis of benign versus malignant [58]. Furthermore, the consensus from the above studies of FISH in ambiguous melanocytic tumors underscored important potential pitfalls in the utility of FISH among lesions difficult to classify by conventional light microscopic and/or immunophenotypic features: (1) FISH may be negative in lesions (ambiguous and unambiguous) with malignant behavior, (2) FISH may be positive in lesions with benign morphology and behavior—a common explanation being tetraploidy/polyploidy and (3) there are specific subtypes of melanocytic lesions where FISH might have limited utility because such lesions are typified by their own specific subset of genomic alterations not necessarily interrogated by the conventional probe set of 6p25, 6q23, and 11q13.

One important example of this include melanomas with copy number gains at 8q24, which are typically nodular melanomas arising on non-chronically sun damaged skin, lacking obvious clinical or histopathologic pigmentation (amelanotic) and infrequently associated with a precursor nevus (i.e., "primary dermal melanoma") [65, 66]. In addition, melanomas with gains at 8q24 actually showed frequent alterations of 6p25, 6q23, and 11q13: among 40 melanomas with 8q24 gains, 37 were also typified by gains of chromosome 6p25 (92.5%), 21 exhibited gains in 11q13 (52.5%), 12 showed relative loss at 6q23 (30%), and 6 of 40 showed homozygous deletions in 9p21 (15%). The coexistence of multiple chromosomal alterations among melanomas with 8q24 loss is consistent with a high level of chromosomal instability among these unique melanomas. It was therefore not surprising that melanoma metastases occurred in 19 of 33 cases with 8q24 gains, including 11 deaths from melanoma. In contrast, only 1 of 30 cases without 8q24 gains developed metastasis, with only a single death occurring in this group due to melanoma [66].

One obvious conclusion of the UCSF study [64] is that the most commonly encountered and vexing challenging problems in diagnosing melanocytic tumors includes differentiating Spitzoid melanomas from Spitz nevi—a dilemma for which conventional FISH probes demonstrated low sensitivity and specificity [67]. Some studies have suggested a relatively high sensitivity and specificity for conventional FISH in differentiating Spitzoid melanomas from Spitz nevi: Requena et al. assessed 12 Spitzoid melanomas and 6 Spitz nevi by conventional FISH and showed a sensitivity of 87.5 % and a specificity of 100 % [57]. However, in a subsequent study assessing the utility of conventional FISH studies among Spitzoid melanomas, Gammon et al. demonstrated that conventional FISH probes (6p25, 6q23, cen6, and 11q13) showed a positive result in only 30 of 43 cases of Spitzoid melanoma (sensitivity = 70 %). In the search for additionally informative loci, however, they defined homozygous deletion of 9p21 as a relatively frequent occurrence in this subtype of melanoma: 11/27 cases (41 %) for which sufficient material was available for additional studies showed homozygous deletion of 9p21. Furthermore, adding the probe for homozygous deletion of 9p21 to their original FISH study set significantly improved the sensitivity of melanoma diagnosis among lesions with this morphology: in total, 37/43 Spitzoid melanomas were positive when homozygous deletion for 9p21 was combined with conventional FISH (Sensitivity = 86 %) [67].

Spitz Nevi with Tetraploidy: A Pitfall for FISH

One of the main limitations of the first generation FISH assay is the presence of polyploidy/tetraploidy (most often occurring in a subset of Spitz nevi—the lesion most commonly tested by FISH [64]). Tetraploidy is the balanced gain in copy numbers of *all of the chromosomes* from a 2 N status to a 4 N status that results after a melanocyte undergoes a cycle of DNA replication without subsequent cell division [60, 61]. In a study of 38 Spitz nevi, four lesions from two patients were identified with a significant number of

nuclei showing balanced gains in all four probes (6p25, 6q23, 11q13, and cen6); most cells had 3–4 copies of each chromosomal region. All four lesions were confirmed as polyploid using a probe for the X chromosome, which revealed four copies for women and two copies for men [61]. One of these two patients (a 17-year-old woman with multiple Spitz nevi exhibiting tetraploidy) was described in contrast to a 51 year old woman who also presented with multiple Spitz nevi which were diploid and without FISH abnormalities. From a diagnostic standpoint the presence of tetraploidy would favor a benign diagnosis. Although tetraploid melanomas have been described [68], they are rare. From a genomic standpoint, melanomas are more typically aneuploid, typified by amplifications or deletions in *discrete regions of chromosomes*. However, the FISH assay does not discriminate between gains in all of the chromosomes from gains in discrete regions of chromosomes; it detects changes in copy numbers at specific loci without the context of the content of the remainder of that chromosome. Thus, tetraploidy is the most common source of false positivity among histopathologically benign lesions, since to the untrained observer, tetraploidy would result in balanced gains in both 6p25 and 11q13 (usually in a significant number of cells) without altering the ratio between 6p25 or 6q23 and cen6. In one series [58], tetraploidy was the overwhelming source of false positive results in a series of histopathologically benign lesions.

Second Generation FISH: Improved Sensitivity for Spitzoid Lesions

Together, the relatively low sensitivity of conventional FISH for ambiguous lesions—in particular, lesions with a Spitzoid morphology—and the compromised specificity due to the relatively high frequency of tetraploidy (resulting in a relatively high number of false positive results) prompted a search for new FISH probes that would improve diagnostic sensitivity and specificity [31]. To achieve this, the authors interrogated a series of histopathologically unambiguous melanomas—negative by conventional/first generation FISH—with probes targeting other loci known to be frequently altered in melanoma: 9p21, cen9, 8q24, 7q34, cen17, cen10, 20q13, and 1q25 (essentially comprising the remainder of the 14 loci originally tested by Gerami et al. [18]). This analysis identified 9p21, cen9, 20q13, and 8q24 as the most complementary set of probes to conventional FISH, and they applied these together with conventional FISH probes to a second cohort of 49 melanomas and 51 nevi (not previously analyzed by FISH) and showed that five probes yielded the highest discriminatory capacity between melanoma and nevus: 6p25, 8q24, 9p21, 11q13, and 20q13. Given the extensive experience with 6p25 and the previous studies showing prognostic importance of 8q24 and 11q13 (see below), the final probe set selected for so-called "second generation FISH" included:

6p25, 8q24, 9p21, and 11q13. The cutoffs determined for these probes to indicate a positive result was >29 % of tumor cells with either gains at 6p25, 8q24, or 11q13 or homozygous deletion at 9p21 (Fig. 13.3). In their final validation set consisting of 51 melanomas and 51 nevi the new probe set demonstrated a sensitivity of 94 % and a specificity of 98 %, whereas conventional FISH showed a sensitivity of 75 % and a specificity of 96 % in the same set of lesions. Based upon their approach to enumeration, the problem of tetraploidy was largely eliminated: namely, they defined as tetraploid a cell with gains at 6p25, 8q24, *and* 11q13 and a value other than 0 for 9p21. Such a cell was counted in the denominator but excluded from the numerator in their tabulation, thus increasing the stringency for a true positive result and effectively buffering the impact of alterations in DNA ploidy on the FISH result [18, 67].

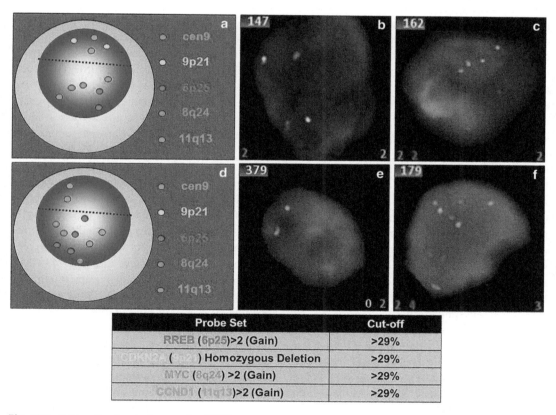

Probe Set	Cut-off
RREB (6p25)>2 (Gain)	>29%
CDKN2A (9p21) Homozygous Deletion	>29%
MYC (8q24) >2 (Gain)	>29%
CCND1 (11q13)>2 (Gain)	>29%

Fig. 13.3 Schematic of second generation FISH assay

Correlation Between CGH and FISH

An important question remains the degree to which CGH—the gold standard for assessing genomic content—correlates with FISH. In one of the first studies to address this question, Gaiser et al. studied a series of 22 melanocytic lesions by FISH and CGH (subset of cases), spanning the complete spectrum of lesions: three benign nevi with benign follow-up (all 3 FISH negative); seven cases with ambiguous morphology but benign follow-up (only 3 cases in this group amenable to FISH and 2 were FISH-positive); five cases with ambiguous morphology but malignant follow-up (3 of 5 FISH-positive); four cases of melanoma without metastases (2 of 4 FISH-positive) and three cases of melanoma with metastases (1 of 3 FISH-positive). Among these cases, nine had sufficient material for correlative CGH studies with the following results: in four cases, the FISH and CGH findings were in agreement (i.e., CGH identical or showed the same changes as FISH plus additional changes not detected by FISH), whereas there was discordance in the remaining five cases: CGH was negative in two FISH-positive lesions; CGH was positive in two FISH-negative lesions; and FISH detected a different change (6p25 gain) than CGH (11q13 gain) in one case. These findings suggested significant limitations to FISH in predicting behavior of challenging melanocytic lesions to the extent that there were FISH-negative lesions of varying morphologies (including bona fide melanomas as well as morphologically ambiguous tumors) that produced metastases. Of greater concern was the apparent significant incongruity between FISH and CGH: only 4/9 (44 %) cases were found to have overlapping results with both approaches, while 5/9 (56 %) were dissimilar [29].

However, different results were obtained by Wang et al. who showed a much stronger concordance between FISH and CGH [69]. They first applied array CGH to a series of 5 benign nevi and 25 melanomas. Similar to the original findings described by Bastian et al. [13, 14], they detected multiple DNA copy number aberrations in 23/25 (92 %) of melanomas but none of the 5 benign nevi. They then applied conventional FISH probes to 20 of the melanomas, and they obtained positive FISH results for 13/20 melanomas and a negative FISH result for 5/20 lesions. Two of the lesions were technically inadequate. In addition, they performed FISH on a subset of melanomas using probes not included in the standard four-panel FISH panel to confirm additional specific changes identified by aCGH. In contrast to Gaiser et al. [29], Wang et al. reported an overall concordance of 90 % between FISH and aCGH and noted that 85 % of the discrepancies resulted because the analytical sensitivity of FISH was greater than aCGH: the proportion of positive cells by FISH was below the analytical threshold determined for the aCGH assay conditions they devised [69].

FISH as a Surrogate of Clinical Outcome

In addition to informing the diagnosis, a pivotal question is whether melanocytic lesions with genomic instability detected by FISH have a different clinical outcome than those which are FISH negative—particularly for malignant lesions. This question was directly assessed by North et al. who studied 144 unambiguous melanomas by conventional FISH (6p25, 6q23, cen6, and 11q13) [34]. These melanomas represented a wide spectrum of histopathologic subtypes, including 51 superficial spreading, 26 lentigo maligna, 27 nodular, eight acral lentiginous, 32 unclassifiable, and six Spitzoid, and these corresponded to anatomic sites with varying degrees of antecedent sun exposure, including 43 CSD, 82 non-CSD, 14 acral, and five unclassifiable. Among the 144 cases, 118 (82 %) were FISH-positive by at least one of the four possible criteria. With the exception of patient age, there was no association between conventional prognostic indicators of outcome in cutaneous melanoma including gender, tumor thickness, ulceration, or sentinel lymph node status and a positive or negative FISH result. FISH-positive lesions tended to occur in older patients (mean=62 years, range: 28–97) compared to FISH-negative lesions (54 years, range: 17–82), and this was statistically significant ($p = 0.049$). With a median follow-up time of 32 months, a total of 43 patients had developed metastases, and 40 of these (93 %) were FISH-positive. Furthermore, 27 patients died of melanoma, and 26/27 (96.7 %) tested positive by FISH. These differences were statistically significant: $p = 0.02$ for disease-specific survival and $p = 0.04$ for disease-free survival. There was an increased risk for the development of metastatic disease (Odds ratio = 4.11; $p = 0.02$) and death from melanoma (Odds ratio = 7.0; $p = 0.04$) among FISH-positive compared to FISH-negative melanomas. Multivariate analysis which accounted for sentinel lymph node status, tumor thickness, ulceration and patient age demonstrated a positive FISH test to be independently associated with an increased risk for the development of metastasis (Hazard ratio = 5.9, $p = 0.04$). These results positioned FISH as both a diagnostically informative and prognostically relevant assay in the evaluation of melanocytic lesions and argue that FISH-negative melanomas are less likely to produce metastases and death compared to FISH-positive lesions [34].

In a study correlating outcome among primary cutaneous melanomas with copy number alterations [33], Gerami et al. analyzed 97 melanomas, including 55 with metastasis and 42 without metastasis, by FISH with probes for 6p25, 6q23, cen6, 11q13, 8q34, 9p21, cen9, and 20q13. Of note, these melanomas were derived from patients of a comparable mean age and gender distribution. The lesions themselves did not exhibit statistically significant differences in mean Breslow thickness or mitotic figure count, although there was a statistically significant increase in the number of cases with ulceration among the cases with metastases ($n = 26$ of 54) compared to those without metastases ($n = 3$ of 42; $p < 0.001$). In this study, copy number gains at 11q13 and 8q34 were shown to most significantly correlate with an increased risk for metastasis, and in multivariate analyses, copy number gains at 11q13 and 8q34 demonstrated a statistically significant association with the development of subsequent metastases. In fact, when compared to conventional prognostic indicators of outcome (according to the AJCC) the relative association between copy number gains at 8q34 and 11q13 and metastasis was second only to ulceration [33].

As highlighted by these studies, the utility of FISH is not only to inform the diagnosis but also to stratify risk among patients with histopathologically malignant lesions. Among atypical Spitzoid lesions, however, morphologic and immunophenotypic parameters are often inconclusive, and experts fail to reach a consensus on lesions that will or will not produce metastases [5]. There is, thus, a critical need to provide additional information to facilitate risk stratification in particular among this class of lesions, and a landmark multi-institutional study led by Gerami addressed this question directly. They applied both "first generation FISH" probes (6p25, cen6, 6q23, and 11q13) [18] as well as the "second generation FISH" probes (6p25, 8q24, 9p21, and 11q13) [31] to a series of 75 Atypical Spitz Tumors (AST) with long-term clinical follow-up using the previously published cutoffs [70]. Their series included 11 patients with evidence of tumor spread beyond the sentinel lymph node: four patients with both in-transit metastases and positive sentinel and/or non-sentinel nodes; four patients with positive sentinel and subsequent lymph node involvement of the nodal basin after completion lymphadenectomy; and three patients with distant metastases and death due to melanoma. Of note, all 11 patients comprising the group of "advanced locoregional disease, distant metastasis, and/or death" had a positive result by FISH, demonstrating copy number alterations in at least one of the loci analyzed. In contrast, only 15/64 patients with "benign follow-up" (no metastasis or disease spread confined to the sentinel lymph node only): $p < 0.001$ for "low risk" versus "high risk" patients. Furthermore, among the 11 patients with "advanced locoregional disease," nine patients (including all three who died of melanoma) showed homozygous deletion of 9p21, with an average of 80 % of the tumor nuclei showing this change. In contrast, only 3/64 patients with benign follow-up demonstrated homozygous deletion of 9p21 ($p<0.001$). When they applied multivariate logistic regression analysis to analyze the relative importance of both FISH abnormalities together with both conventional AJCC prognostic indicators (age, sex, Breslow thickness, mitotic rate, and ulceration) and other factors typically described in Spitz lesions (epidermal consumption, Kamino bodies, growth pattern, and cellular morphology), only mitotic rate ($p=0.03$) and homozygous loss of 9p21 ($p<0.0001$) emerged as statistically significant indicators of the likelihood of tumor spread beyond a regional lymph node, and only homozygous deletion of 9p21 correlated with an increased risk of death from disease ($p=0.01$). In contrast to the more aggressive phenotype associated with homozygous deletion of 9p21, ASTs with relative loss of 6q23 ($n=6$) enjoyed a less aggressive disease course: none reported advanced locoregional disease, distant metastasis, or death with follow-up of at least 5 years. To the extent that these specific genomic changes correlated with/predicted biological behavior, this study was among the first to demonstrate the utility of FISH studies in assessing risk among histopathologically challenging Spitzoid lesions. The authors therefore envisioned a revision to conventional melanoma nomenclature that would add significant value by incorporating the specific type of genomic alterations present as a more specific surrogate of biological behavior, including "Spitzoid melanoma with homozygous deletion of 9p21" to designate those lesions with a likely aggressive course versus "Atypical Spitz tumor with loss of 6q23" to designate those lesions more likely to behave in a less aggressive fashion [70].

To explore the significance of isolated loss of 6q23 in Spitzoid neoplasms further, Gerami and colleagues performed a retrospective review of 24 ASTs with isolated loss of 6q23 (but intact 6p25, 11q13, 8q23, and 9p21 by FISH). Although ~55 % of these patients (6/11 for whom sentinel lymph node was performed) had a positive sentinel lymph node biopsy, none developed metastatic disease beyond the sentinel node (follow-up: 2–60 months); in fact, the risk of developing disease beyond a sentinel node for these lesions was no different than Spitzoid tumors without chromosomal abnormalities assayed by FISH. Taken together, the findings in this study provided further support for the assertion that lesions with a Spitzoid morphology and an isolated loss of 6q23 likely have an overall benign prognosis [71].

In a subsequent study specifically interrogating the relative contribution of FISH to risk assessment among ASTs and conventional melanomas among children, Gerami and colleagues correlated FISH results with clinical outcomes for 37 FISH-positive ASTs and 21 conventional melanomas in children under the age of 18 [32]. Among the 37 FISH-positive ASTs, there were 15 cases with homozygous deletion of 9p21 (7 of which developed disease beyond a sentinel lymph node), five cases with gains of 11q13 and 6p25 (2 of which developed disease beyond the sentinel lymph node), two cases with gains of 6p25 only, 14 cases with loss of 6q23, and 1 case with gains of 8q24. In keeping with the findings in their previous study, among the nine pediatric ASTs with metastatic disease beyond the sentinel node, seven showed homozygous deletion of 9p21 (including 2 with brain metastases). Among the 21 conventional melanomas, conventional FISH (6p25, 6q23, cen6, and 11q13) was performed in 18 cases and was positive in 16. Additional FISH studies were performed with 9p21 in 16 cases and 8q24 in ten cases. Among these conventional melanomas in the pediatric population, there was no clinical, histopathologic or molecular (FISH) feature shown to correlate with outcome [32]. This study provided further justification to designate lesions with a Spitzoid histopathology and specific genomic alterations (in particular homozygous deletion of 9p21) as a distinct subtype of melanoma given their proclivity for aggressive behavior.

To further solidify this designation, Gerami and colleagues next characterized Spitzoid lesions with either heterozygous ($n=31$) or homozygous ($n=30$) deletion of 9p21 but without other chromosomal abnormalities (as detected by FISH) [72]. Spitzoid lesions with homozygous deletion of 9p21 showed a statistically significant increase in the mean mitotic rate ($p=0.042$), epithelioid morphology ($p=0.0004$), and severe cytologic atypia ($p=0.0003$). More importantly, in follow-up, ~41 % of the patients with Spitzoid lesions harboring homozygous deletion of 9p21 developed metastases beyond the sentinel node (9/22 for whom follow-up information was available), whereas none of the 16 patients with available follow-up and heterozygous deletion of 9p21 developed metastatic disease beyond the sentinel lymph node. Of note, p16 immunohistochemistry was shown to be an excellent surrogate of the integrity of the 9p21 gene locus: whereas 100 % of either the ASTs or conventional melanomas known to harbor homozygous deletion of 9p21 were negative with antibodies for p16, only ~33 % of the ASTs with heterozygous 9p21 were p16 negative (~67 % were p16 positive). Finally, in contrast to conventional melanomas with homozygous deletion of 9p21, BRAF^{V600E} mutations were rare among the Spitzoid lesions studied: only 1/42 (~2 %) were positive for BRAF^{V600E} immunohistochemistry, whereas conventional melanomas with homozygous deletion of 9p21 show BRAF V600E in ~53 % of cases (9/17) [72] — similar to that previously described [73]. Taken together, these findings (1) support the concept that homozygous deletion of 9p21 is a specific indicator of poor prognosis among Spitzoid neoplasms; (2) indicate that p16 immunohistochemistry is a suitable, first-pass surrogate of the status of 9p21: significant p16 positivity would imply an intact 9p21 locus; and (3) the generation of Spitzoid melanomas with homozygous loss of 9p21 is distinct from conventional melanomas with a similar genotype to the extent that activating mutations in BRAF (BRAF^{V600E}) are uncommon in the former but common in the latter [72]. Consistent with the above assertions, among 25 benign Spitz nevi from older individuals (>50 years old) there were no abnormalities by conventional FISH studies, there was retention of p16 expression by immunohistochemistry and normal diploid status of 9p21 by FISH [74, 75].

Other Genomic Changes: Loss of *BAP1*

In a multi-institutional study, Wiesner et al. described a discrete genomic alteration with autosomal dominant inheritance in a pair of families in which offspring harbored multiple similar distinctive melanocytic nevi [76]. Affected family members had ~5–50 dome-shaped, well-circumscribed papules that were usually pale brown to red in color. Histopathologically, the lesions were characterized by predominantly intradermal proliferations of markedly atypical epithelioid melanocytes with abundant amphophilic cytoplasm, large vesicular nuclei with prominent nucleoli—reminiscent of Spitz nevi. A subset of these lesions further exhibited atypical features, including increased cellularity, nuclear pleomorphism, and mitotic figures—features worrisome for melanoma. Finally, 88 % (37/42) of the lesions showed BRAF^{V600E} mutations, and each of the respective families had members with melanoma: there was a single uveal melanoma in each family and 3 additional cases of cutaneous melanoma in family #2. Further analysis of the tumor cells from affected individuals of both families by array CGH revealed variably sized deletions in chromosome 3 (ranging from the entire chromosome to discrete fragments of the short arm mapping to 3p21). To analyze the 3p21 region further, they performed haplotype analyses using single nucleotide polymorphism arrays on one affected family and showed that among the tumors with 3p loss, the paternal chromosome was consistently the one deleted, and each affected family member only carried the maternal chromosome. This led to the hypothesis that the maternal copy carried a specific inherited mutation, and that loss of the paternal 3p constituted a "second hit." This prediction was confirmed after sequencing of the minimally deleted region in both families revealed discrete mutations in the *BAP1* gene that segregated with the affected family members: in family #1, there was an inactivating frameshift mutation in *BAP1* (c.1305delG, pGln436AS-Nfs*135) and a *BAP1* mutation in family #2 affecting a splice site receptor (c.2057-2A>G, pMet687Glufs*). Mutations in *BAP1* were not identified when sequence data from 629 unrelated individuals were reviewed indicating a specific change that segregated with the phenotypes in the affected individuals. Furthermore, they confirmed by various other approaches that loss of the remaining *BAP1* allele in the affected family members must have occurred by either deletion, second mutation or other "...copy number neutral mechanisms..." of gene repression (transcriptional or translational). Finally, to assess the functional significance of *BAP1* in the pathogenesis of sporadically acquired melanocytic lesions, they sequenced *BAP1* in 156 melanocytic lesions from individuals without family history, including common banal nevi (*n*=28), Spitz nevi (*n*=17), so-called atypical spitz tumors (ASTs, *n*=18), and primary melanomas from (1) acral skin (*n*=15), (2) mucosa (*n*=15), (3) skin with or without CSD (*n*=15 for each) or uveal melanomas (*n*=33) and showed that 40% (13/33) of sporadic uveal melanomas, ~11% (2/18) of ASTs and ~5% (3/45) of the remaining cutaneous melanomas carried somatic *BAP1* mutations. Of interest, two of the melanomas with *BAP1* mutation arose in association with a preexisting nevus component; each of these showed *BAP1* mutation confined to the melanoma but not the nevus component, suggesting that inactivation of *BAP1* potentially contributes to melanomagenesis [76].

To further assess the role of *BAP1* in the evolution of sporadic melanocytic tumors, the authors then assessed the relative frequency of *BAP1* loss in a series of ASTs from patients without a family history of melanoma or melanocytic lesions [77]. They first confirmed the utility of BAP1 immunohistochemistry as a surrogate of *BAP1* loss by demonstrating that in a series of 42 melanocytic lesions from known *BAP1* germline carriers that BAP1 protein was not detectable by immunohistochemical studies: this included 33 cases with documented biallelic loss of *BAP1* and an additional nine cases without an identifiable "second hit" of the *BAP1* locus. In contrast, among 29 common nevi and 17 Spitz nevi without *BAP1* mutations, BAP1 protein expression was retained by immunohistochemistry. Among the 32 ASTs

chosen for study, they showed loss of BAP1 protein in 28% (9/32) cases. Sequencing *BAP1* in these 9 cases confirmed somatically acquired frameshift mutations in 5/9 cases, whereas the remaining 4 BAP-1 negative and 20/23 BAP-1 positive case amenable to sequencing did not reveal *BAP-1* mutations; these findings argued that somatic inactivation of *BAP1* may also occur through mechanisms other than deletions or mutations (i.e., epigenetic changes). Furthermore, sequencing of *BRAF* and *HRAS* in these lesions revealed *BRAF*^{V600E} in 8/9 BAP-1 negative tumors and 1/22 BAP-1 positive cases ($p<0.0001$); no *HRAS* mutations were found. Similar to the familial cases described previously, these sporadic ASTs exhibited a predominantly dermal location and were comprised of mostly large epithelioid cells with increased amphophilic cytoplasm with well-demarcated cytoplasmic borders, pleomorphic nuclei with vesicular chromatin and conspicuous nucleoli. Statistically significant parameters between the BAP1-positive and the BAP1-negative tumors included: (1) more frequent location on the trunk (50% of BAP1-negative versus 10% of BAP1-positive) and less often on the limbs (13% of BAP1-negative versus 62% of BAP1-positive; $p=0.04$); (2) predominantly dermal location versus compound (100% of BAP1-negative versus 52% of BAP1-positive; $p=0.01$); (3) well defined cytoplasmic borders (100% of BAP1-negative versus 22% of BAP1-positive; $p<0.001$); (4) binucleation or multinucleation (78% of BAP1- negative versus 9% of BAP1-positive; $p=0.0003$); and (5) moderate to marked tumor infiltrating lymphocytes (55% of BAP1-negative versus 22% of BAP1-positive; $p=0.02$). Together, the findings of these two studies identified a histopathologically distinct subset of Spitzoid neoplasms defined by loss of BAP-1 protein expression and the presence of *BRAF*^{V600E} mutations, which together with the Spitzoid lesions previously described with mutations in *HRAS* and gains at 11p establish the foundation for a genomic framework for the classification of benign melanocytic tumors with Spitzoid morphology: (1) lesions with BAP1 loss and *BRAF*^{V600E} (2) lesions with *HRAS* mutations and gains of 11p and (3) others [77].

The above findings were extended to an additional subset of Spitzoid tumors: namely, lesions with combined morphology comprised of conventional banal nevoid and Spitzoid melanocytes [78, 79]. In two studies, the authors described a series of eight sporadically acquired papulonodular lesions arising in six patients and an additional 8 lesions present since childhood in a single patient—all of which were compound melanocytic nevi consisting of an admixture of small and large epithelioid melanocytes in a stereotypical distribution: small nevoid melanocytes typically towards the peripheral aspects of the lesion, which blended together with the larger epithelioid melanocytes that were usually located centrally in the lesion. Immunohistochemical and molecular genetic studies were performed on the lesions. Namely, whereas the large epithelioid melanocytes exhibited loss of nuclear BAP-1 expression by immunohistochemistry, the smaller melanocytes retained BAP-1 expression, and both populations of melanocytes demonstrated positivity with antibodies for $BRAF^{V600E}$. DNA sequencing analysis showed a frameshift mutation in BAP-1 (c568_569delinsT, p.P190Sfs*41) and $BRAF^{V600E}$ [79] and in the patient with multiple lesions, a frameshift mutation in BAP-1 (c.214del, p172L*6) in both the lesional and non-lesional tissue and $BRAF^{V600E}$ confined to the lesional tissue [78]. In the latter case, germline mutation of BAP-1 mutation was confirmed. Their longstanding presence and overall indolent behavior supported their benignity.

To more precisely determine the relative frequency of BAP-1 loss in cutaneous melanoma and its relative distribution among the histopathologic/anatomic subtypes, Murali et al. performed BAP1 immunohistochemical studies on 158 primary cutaneous melanomas, including acral lentiginous ($n=24$), desmoplastic ($n=23$), lentigo maligna ($n=13$), nodular ($n=56$), superficial spreading ($n=39$) and unclassified types ($n=3$). They showed BAP-1 loss in ~6% (9/158) of cutaneous melanomas [80]. Interestingly, desmoplastic melanomas were more frequently BAP-1-negative (~22%; 5/23) than non-desmoplastic melanomas

(~3%; 4/135), and this was statistically significant ($p<0.001$). No other clinical or pathologic parameters were statistically significantly associated with BAP-1 loss. However, with a median follow-up of 17.6 months (range: 0–158.8 months), BAP-1 loss was among the factors (together with higher stage at initial diagnosis, mitotic figures, and lymphovascular invasion) that were independently associated with reduced disease-free and melanoma-specific survival, although there was some acknowledged selection bias built into the study to the extent that desmoplastic melanomas—which constituted a significant number of BAP-1-negative lesions— exhibited a greater comparative tumor thickness than other lesions in the study set. Furthermore, the lesions selected for analysis exhibited a greater frequency of ulceration, a greater number of mitotic figures, and increasing tumor thickness on average than melanomas typically encountered in the general population. Nevertheless, the finding of BAP-1 loss predominantly in desmoplastic melanomas (whereas its loss otherwise correlates with an epithelioid morphology in lesions with a benign course) was provocative and awaits further study [80].

The spectrum of melanocytic tumors with *BAP-1* loss was further characterized in a study from UCSF in which they described the relative frequency of isolated *BAP-1* loss among a series of 436 cases encountered in their consultation practice [81]. They performed array CGH to inform their diagnosis of histopathologically challenging lesions and identified 29 cases (~6%) which exhibited *isolated loss* of variable regions of chromosome 3 spanning the *BAP-1* locus. The *BAP-1* gene locus was sequenced in 11 cases, and 10 contained loss of function mutations in *BAP-1*. Overall, *BAP-1* loss was confirmed in all 17/29 cases for which sufficient material was available—either by sequencing or immunohistochemical approaches, and among these, 11/17 (~65%) were positive for $BRAF^{V600E}$, and a single case showed a mutation in $NRAS^{Q61R}$. The presence of an *NRAS* mutation suggested that the morphology typical of nevi previously only described in the context of *BAP1* loss and $BRAF^{V600E}$ might be better classified as "BAP-1 loss with MAPK pathway activation." Clinical follow-up was available for nine patients, and all nine were negative for recurrence. Histopathologic examination of the lesions revealed morphologic changes similar to that already described for familial and sporadic melanocytic tumors with *BAP-1* loss: namely, the lesions were characteristically dome shaped papules comprised of predominantly intradermal, not densely cellular proliferations of atypical epithelioid melanocytes with interspersed lymphocytes (Fig. 13.4). The melanocytes exhibited variable amounts of eosinophilic cytoplasm and oval nuclei (some eccentrically placed). The authors further described a unique interaction in these lesions between melanocytes and infiltrating lymphocytes: namely, the more inflamed tumors contained larger melanocytes with glassy eosinophilic cytoplasm and more prominent nuclear eccentricity, and these cells were surrounded by lymphocytes in what the authors termed a "kiss of

death" [81]. Similar to sporadic *BAP-1* negative lesions already described, five cases exhibited features of combined Spitz and conventional (banal nevi), and interestingly in these lesions, the lymphocytic infiltrate appeared to be confined to the epithelioid component. A single case was classified as a melanoma with features of a cellular blue nevus, suggesting a rare association between BAP-1 loss and malignancy among blue nevus-like melanomas [81].

Detecting Translocations in Morphologically Ambiguous Melanocytic Tumors

In a large scale sequencing effort, Wiesner and colleagues described for the first time the presence of kinase fusion events (translocations) in Spitzoid neoplasms [82]. They analyzed a total

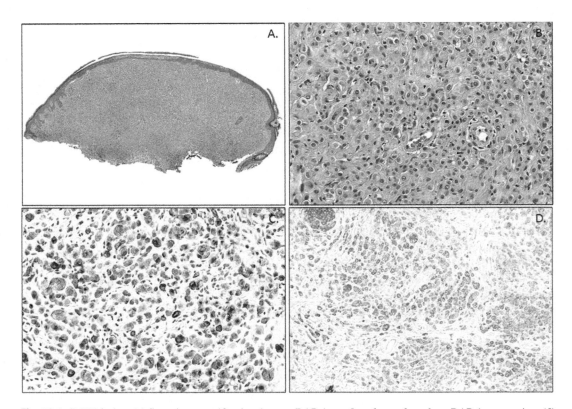

Fig. 13.4 BAP1 lesion. (**a**) Scanning magnification demonstrates papular architecture of the lesion (**b**) higher magnification of the lesion demonstrates well-spaced epithelioid melanocytes (**c**) immunohistochemical studies for BAP-1 confirm loss of nuclear BAP-1 expression (**d**) immunohistochemical studies for BRAF V600E confirm BRAF V600E expression in the tumor cells

of 140 Spitzoid melanocytic proliferations by targeted sequencing, including 75 Spitz nevi, 32 Atypical Spitz tumors, and 33 Spitzoid melanomas. In total, they identified rearrangements involving 72/140 lesions tested (51%), involving the following kinase gene loci: *ROS1* (24/140; 17%), *ALK* (14/140; 10%); *NTRK1* (23/140; 16%), *BRAF* (7/140; 5%) and *RET* (4/140; 3%). The fusions consisted of a portion of a gene encoding a coiled-coil domain at the 5′ fused to a kinase domain at the 3′ end; in a subset of cases, these were confirmed to generate a constitutively activated 3′ kinase domain, and these were amenable to known kinase inhibitors. In total, 41/75 (~55%) of Spitz nevi, 18/32 (56%) of Atypical Spitz tumors and 13/33 (39%) of Spitzoid melanomas harbored a kinase fusion, and the presence of one fusion event was mutually exclusive with another. Given the tendency of Spitzoid lesions to produce metastases, these findings were significant to the extent that they implied potential targets for systemic therapy in such cases. In particular, patients with advanced stage ROS1-rearranged non-small cell lung cancer, showed marked responses to crizotinib, a small-molecule tyrosine kinase inhibitor of anaplastic lymphoma kinase (ALK) [83, 84].

To determine whether any of the translocation associated Spitzoid neoplasms exhibited distinctive clinical and/or pathologic features, Busam et al. described these parameters in a series of 17 Spitzoid tumors with *ALK* fusions, which included 11 lesions fusing *TPM3* (the gene for tropomyosin 3) and six lesions fusing *DCTN1* (the gene for dynactin 1) to *ALK* [85]. They found that Spitzoid lesions with an *ALK* fusion tended to be polypoid and amelanotic. Furthermore, FISH break-apart probes confirmed an *ALK* rearrangement, and all cases were positive for ALK immunohistochemistry in a strong, diffuse pattern. Among eight cases that were tested by conventional melanoma FISH (using probes for 6p25, 6q23, cen6, 11q13, and 9p21), none of the lesions met conventional FISH criteria for malignancy.

Together, the above studies further expanded the genetic spectrum typical for Spitzoid lesions

and suggested a genetic classification system for this morphologically and biologically diverse set of lesions. Namely, there are benign Spitz nevi with (1) no genomic alterations; (2) mutations in HRAS and/or isolated gains in chromosome 11p; (3) loss of 3p21 and mutations in BRAF ($BRAF^{V600E}$); (4) homozygous deletion of 9p21 and a typically more aggressive phenotype; (5) loss of 6q23 and a typically less aggressive clinical behavior and (6) lesions with translocations resulting in the constitutive activation of various oncogenic kinases, including *ROS1, ALK, NTRK1, BRAF,* or *RET*. Additional studies are warranted to confirm the biological potential of these different genotypes.

References

1. Rigel DS. Epidemiology of melanoma. Semin Cutan Med Surg. 2010;29(4):204–9.
2. Jemal A, Siegel R, Ward E, Hao Y, Xu J, Thun MJ. Cancer statistics, 2009. Cancer J Clin. 2009;59(4):225–49.
3. Green AR, Elgart GW, Ma F, Federman DG, Kirsner RS. Documenting dermatology practice: ratio of cutaneous tumors biopsied that are malignant. Dermatol Surg. 2004;30(9):1208–9.
4. Hansen C, Wilkinson D, Hansen M, Argenziano G. How good are skin cancer clinics at melanoma detection? Number needed to treat variability across a national clinic group in Australia. J Am Acad Dermatol. 2009;61(4):599–604.
5. Barnhill RL, Argenyi ZB, From L, Glass LF, Maize JC, Mihm Jr MC, et al. Atypical Spitz nevi/tumors: lack of consensus for diagnosis, discrimination from melanoma, and prediction of outcome. Hum Pathol. 1999;30(5):513–20.
6. Brochez L, Verhaeghe E, Grosshans E, Haneke E, Pierard G, Ruiter D, et al. Inter-observer variation in the histopathological diagnosis of clinically suspicious pigmented skin lesions. J Pathol. 2002;196(4):459–66.
7. Gerami P, Busam K, Cochran A, Cook MG, Duncan LM, Elder DE, et al. Histomorphologic assessment and interobserver diagnostic reproducibility of atypical spitzoid melanocytic neoplasms with long-term follow-up. Am J Surg Pathol. 2014;38(7):934–40.
8. Zembowicz A, Prieto VG. Melanocytic lesions: current state of knowledge—part III. Arch Pathol Lab Med. 2011;135(7):824.
9. Zembowicz A, Prieto VG. Melanocytic lesions: current state of knowledge? Part II. Arch Pathol Lab Med. 2011;135(3):298–9.

10. Zembowicz A, Prieto VG. Melanocytic lesions: current state of knowledge. Arch Pathol Lab Med. 2010;134(12):1738–9.

11. Prieto VG, Shea CR. Immunohistochemistry of melanocytic proliferations. Arch Pathol Lab Med. 2011; 135(7):853–9.

12. Rudolph P, Lappe T, Schubert C, Schmidt D, Parwaresch RM, Christophers E. Diagnostic assessment of two novel proliferation-specific antigens in benign and malignant melanocytic lesions. Am J Pathol. 1995;147(6):1615–25. Pubmed Central PMCID: 1869947.

13. Bastian BC, LeBoit PE, Hamm H, Brocker EB, Pinkel D. Chromosomal gains and losses in primary cutaneous melanomas detected by comparative genomic hybridization. Cancer Res. 1998;58(10):2170–5.

14. Bastian BC, Olshen AB, LeBoit PE, Pinkel D. Classifying melanocytic tumors based on DNA copy number changes. Am J Pathol. 2003;163(5):1765–70. Pubmed Central PMCID: 1892437.

15. Bastian BC, Xiong J, Frieden IJ, Williams ML, Chou P, Busam K, et al. Genetic changes in neoplasms arising in congenital melanocytic nevi: differences between nodular proliferations and melanomas. Am J Pathol. 2002;161(4):1163–9. Pubmed Central PMCID: 1867277.

16. Bauer J, Bastian BC. Distinguishing melanocytic nevi from melanoma by DNA copy number changes: comparative genomic hybridization as a research and diagnostic tool. Dermatol Ther. 2006;19(1):40–9.

17. Gerami P, Zembowicz A. Update on fluorescence in situ hybridization in melanoma: state of the art. Arch Pathol Lab Med. 2011;135(7):830–7.

18. Gerami P, Jewell SS, Morrison LE, Blondin B, Schulz J, Ruffalo T, et al. Fluorescence in situ hybridization (FISH) as an ancillary diagnostic tool in the diagnosis of melanoma. Am J Surg Pathol. 2009;33(8):1146–56.

19. Morey AL, Murali R, McCarthy SW, Mann GJ, Scolyer RA. Diagnosis of cutaneous melanocytic tumours by four-colour fluorescence in situ hybridisation. Pathology. 2009;41(4):383–7.

20. Busam KJ, Fang Y, Jhanwar SC, Pulitzer MP, Marr B, Abramson DH. Distinction of conjunctival melanocytic nevi from melanomas by fluorescence in situ hybridization. J Cutan Pathol. 2010;37(2):196–203.

21. Dalton SR, Gerami P, Kolaitis NA, Charzan S, Werling R, LeBoit PE, et al. Use of fluorescence in situ hybridization (FISH) to distinguish intranodal nevus from metastatic melanoma. Am J Surg Pathol. 2010;34(2):231–7. Pubmed Central PMCID: 2831773.

22. Gammon B, Beilfuss B, Guitart J, Busam KJ, Gerami P. Fluorescence in situ hybridization for distinguishing cellular blue nevi from blue nevus-like melanoma. J Cutan Pathol. 2011;38(4):335–41.

23. Gerami P, Barnhill RL, Beilfuss BA, LeBoit P, Schneider P, Guitart J. Superficial melanocytic neoplasms with pagetoid melanocytosis: a study of interobserver concordance and correlation with FISH. Am J Surg Pathol. 2010;34(6):816–21.

24. Gerami P, Wass A, Mafee M, Fang Y, Pulitzer MP, Busam KJ. Fluorescence in situ hybridization for distinguishing nevoid melanomas from mitotically active nevi. Am J Surg Pathol. 2009;33(12):1783–8.

25. Newman MD, Lertsburapa T, Mirzabeigi M, Mafee M, Guitart J, Gerami P. Fluorescence in situ hybridization as a tool for microstaging in malignant melanoma. Mod Pathol. 2009;22(8):989–95.

26. Newman MD, Mirzabeigi M, Gerami P. Chromosomal copy number changes supporting the classification of lentiginous junctional melanoma of the elderly as a subtype of melanoma. Mod Pathol. 2009;22(9):1258–62.

27. Pouryazdanparast P, Haghighat Z, Beilfuss BA, Guitart J, Gerami P. Melanocytic nevi with an atypical epithelioid cell component: clinical, histopathologic, and fluorescence in situ hybridization findings. Am J Surg Pathol. 2011;35(9):1405–12.

28. Pouryazdanparast P, Newman M, Mafee M, Haghighat Z, Guitart J, Gerami P. Distinguishing epithelioid blue nevus from blue nevus-like cutaneous melanoma metastasis using fluorescence in situ hybridization. Am J Surg Pathol. 2009;33(9):1396–400.

29. Gaiser T, Kutzner H, Palmedo G, Siegelin MD, Wiesner T, Bruckner T, et al. Classifying ambiguous melanocytic lesions with FISH and correlation with clinical long-term follow up. Mod Pathol. 2010;23(3):413–9.

30. Vergier B, Prochazkova-Carlotti M, de la Fouchardiere A, Cerroni L, Massi D, De Giorgi V, et al. Fluorescence in situ hybridization, a diagnostic aid in ambiguous melanocytic tumors: European study of 113 cases. Mod Pathol. 2011;24(5):613–23.

31. Gerami P, Li G, Pouryazdanparast P, Blondin B, Beilfuss B, Slenk C, et al. A highly specific and discriminatory FISH assay for distinguishing between benign and malignant melanocytic neoplasms. Am J Surg Pathol. 2012;36(6):808–17.

32. Gerami P, Cooper C, Bajaj S, Wagner A, Fullen D, Busam K, et al. Outcomes of atypical spitz tumors with chromosomal copy number aberrations and conventional melanomas in children. Am J Surg Pathol. 2013;37(9):1387–94.

33. Gerami P, Jewell SS, Pouryazdanparast P, Wayne JD, Haghighat Z, Busam KJ, et al. Copy number gains in 11q13 and 8q24 [corrected] are highly linked to prognosis in cutaneous malignant melanoma. J Mol Diagn. 2011;13(3):352–8. Pubmed Central PMCID: 3077735.

34. North JP, Vetto JT, Murali R, White KP, White Jr CR, Bastian BC. Assessment of copy number status of chromosomes 6 and 11 by FISH provides independent prognostic information in primary melanoma. Am J Surg Pathol. 2011;35(8):1146–50. Pubmed Central PMCID: 4153784.

35. Kallioniemi A, Kallioniemi OP, Sudar D, Rutovitz D, Gray JW, Waldman F, et al. Comparative genomic hybridization for molecular cytogenetic analysis of solid tumors. Science. 1992;258(5083):818–21.

36. Bastian BC. Molecular cytogenetics as a diagnostic tool for typing melanocytic tumors. Recent Results Cancer Res. 2002;160:92–9.

37. Albertson DG, Ylstra B, Segraves R, Collins C, Dairkee SH, Kowbel D, et al. Quantitative mapping of amplicon structure by array CGH identifies CYP24 as a candidate oncogene. Nat Genet. 2000;25(2):144–6.
38. Pinkel D, Segraves R, Sudar D, Clark S, Poole I, Kowbel D, et al. High resolution analysis of DNA copy number variation using comparative genomic hybridization to microarrays. Nat Genet. 1998;20(2):207–11.
39. Wiltshire RN, Duray P, Bittner ML, Visakorpi T, Meltzer PS, Tuthill RJ, et al. Direct visualization of the clonal progression of primary cutaneous melanoma: application of tissue microdissection and comparative genomic hybridization. Cancer Res. 1995; 55(18):3954–7.
40. Curtin JA, Fridlyand J, Kageshita T, Patel HN, Busam KJ, Kutzner H, et al. Distinct sets of genetic alterations in melanoma. N Engl J Med. 2005;353(20):2135–47.
41. Balazs M, Adam Z, Treszl A, Begany A, Hunyadi J, Adany R. Chromosomal imbalances in primary and metastatic melanomas revealed by comparative genomic hybridization. Cytometry. 2001;46(4):222–32.
42. Maize Jr JC, McCalmont TH, Carlson JA, Busam KJ, Kutzner H, Bastian BC. Genomic analysis of blue nevi and related dermal melanocytic proliferations. Am J Surg Pathol. 2005;29(9):1214–20.
43. Bastian BC, LeBoit PE, Pinkel D. Mutations and copy number increase of HRAS in Spitz nevi with distinctive histopathological features. Am J Pathol. 2000;157(3):967–72. Pubmed Central PMCID: 1885704.
44. Bastian BC, Wesselmann U, Pinkel D, Leboit PE. Molecular cytogenetic analysis of Spitz nevi shows clear differences to melanoma. J Invest Dermatol. 1999;113(6):1065–9.
45. Harvell JD, Kohler S, Zhu S, Hernandez-Boussard T, Pollack JR, van de Rijn M. High-resolution array-based comparative genomic hybridization for distinguishing paraffin-embedded Spitz nevi and melanomas. Diagn Mol Pathol. 2004;13(1):22–5.
46. Sokolova IA, Bubendorf L, O'Hare A, Legator MS, Jacobson KK, Grilli BSB, et al. A fluorescence in situ hybridization-based assay for improved detection of lung cancer cells in bronchial washing specimens. Cancer. 2002;96(5):306–15.
47. Sokolova IA, Halling KC, Jenkins RB, Burkhardt HM, Meyer RG, Seelig SA, et al. The development of a multitarget, multicolor fluorescence in situ hybridization assay for the detection of urothelial carcinoma in urine. J Mol Diagn. 2000;2(3):116–23. Pubmed Central PMCID: 1906906.
48. Curtin JA, Busam K, Pinkel D, Bastian BC. Somatic activation of KIT in distinct subtypes of melanoma. J Clin Oncol. 2006;24(26):4340–6.
49. Busam KJ, Fang Y, Jhanwar S, Lacouture M. Diagnosis of blue nevus-like metastatic uveal melanoma confirmed by fluorescence in situ hybridization (FISH) for monosomy 3. J Cutan Pathol. 2012;39(6):621–5.
50. Diaz A, Valera A, Carrera C, Hakim S, Aguilera P, Garcia A, et al. Pigmented spindle cell nevus: clues for differentiating it from spindle cell malignant melanoma. A comprehensive survey including clinicopathologic, immunohistochemical, and FISH studies. Am J Surg Pathol. 2011;35(11):1733–42.
51. Fang Y, Dusza S, Jhanwar S, Busam KJ. Fluorescence in situ hybridization (FISH) analysis of melanocytic nevi and melanomas: sensitivity, specificity, and lack of association with sentinel node status. Int J Surg Pathol. 2012;20(5):434–40.
52. Gerami P, Beilfuss B, Haghighat Z, Fang Y, Jhanwar S, Busam KJ. Fluorescence in situ hybridization as an ancillary method for the distinction of desmoplastic melanomas from sclerosing melanocytic nevi. J Cutan Pathol. 2011;38(4):329–34.
53. Gerami P, Mafee M, Lurtsbarapa T, Guitart J, Haghighat Z, Newman M. Sensitivity of fluorescence in situ hybridization for melanoma diagnosis using RREB1, MYB, Cep6, and 11q13 probes in melanoma subtypes. Arch Dermatol. 2010;146(3):273–8.
54. Kiuru M, Patel RM, Busam KJ. Desmoplastic melanocytic nevi with lymphocytic aggregates. J Cutan Pathol. 2012;39(10):940–4.
55. Moore MW, Gasparini R. FISH as an effective diagnostic tool for the management of challenging melanocytic lesions. Diagn Pathol. 2011;6:76. Pubmed Central PMCID: 3162533.
56. Pennacchia I, Garcovich S, Gasbarra R, Leone A, Arena V, Massi G. Morphological and molecular characteristics of nested melanoma of the elderly (evolved lentiginous melanoma). Virchows Arch. 2012;461(4):433–9.
57. Requena C, Rubio L, Traves V, Sanmartin O, Nagore E, Llombart B, et al. Fluorescence in situ hybridization for the differential diagnosis between Spitz naevus and spitzoid melanoma. Histopathology. 2012;61(5):899–909.
58. Zembowicz A, Yang SE, Kafanas A, Lyle SR. Correlation between histologic assessment and fluorescence in situ hybridization using MelanoSITE in evaluation of histologically ambiguous melanocytic lesions. Arch Pathol Lab Med. 2012;136(12):1571–9.
59. Tetzlaff MT, Wang WL, Milless TL, Curry JL, Torres-Cabala CA, McLemore MS, et al. Ambiguous melanocytic tumors in a tertiary referral center: the contribution of fluorescence in situ hybridization (FISH) to conventional histopathologic and immunophenotypic analyses. Am J Surg Pathol. 2013;37(12):1783–96.
60. Boone SL, Busam KJ, Marghoob AA, Fang Y, Guitart J, Martini M, et al. Two cases of multiple spitz nevi: correlating clinical, histologic, and fluorescence in situ hybridization findings. Arch Dermatol. 2011;147(2):227–31.
61. Isaac AK, Lertsburapa T, Pathria Mundi J, Martini M, Guitart J, Gerami P. Polyploidy in spitz nevi: a not uncommon karyotypic abnormality identifiable by fluorescence in situ hybridization. Am J Dermatopathol. 2010;32(2):144–8.
62. Martin V, Banfi S, Bordoni A, Leoni-Parvex S, Mazzucchelli L. Presence of cytogenetic abnormalities in Spitz naevi: a diagnostic challenge for fluorescence in-situ hybridization analysis. Histopathology. 2012;60(2):336–46.

63. McCalmont TH. Fillet of FISH. J Cutan Pathol. 2011;38(4):327–8.

64. North JP, Garrido MC, Kolaitis NA, LeBoit PE, McCalmont TH, Bastian BC. Fluorescence in situ hybridization as an ancillary tool in the diagnosis of ambiguous melanocytic neoplasms: a review of 804 cases. Am J Surg Pathol. 2014;38(6):824–31.

65. Pouryazdanparast P, Brenner A, Haghighat Z, Guitart J, Rademaker A, Gerami P. The role of 8q24 copy number gains and c-MYC expression in amelanotic cutaneous melanoma. Mod Pathol. 2012;25(9):1221–6.

66. Pouryazdanparast P, Cowen DP, Beilfuss BA, Haghighat Z, Guitart J, Rademaker A, et al. Distinctive clinical and histologic features in cutaneous melanoma with copy number gains in 8q24. Am J Surg Pathol. 2012;36(2):253–64.

67. Gammon B, Beilfuss B, Guitart J, Gerami P. Enhanced detection of spitzoid melanomas using fluorescence in situ hybridization with 9p21 as an adjunctive probe. Am J Surg Pathol. 2012;36(1):81–8.

68. Satoh S, Hashimoto-Tamaoki T, Furuyama J, Mihara K, Namba M, Kitano Y. High frequency of tetraploidy detected in malignant melanoma of Japanese patients by fluorescence in situ hybridization. Int J Oncol. 2000;17(4):707–15.

69. Wang L, Rao M, Fang Y, Hameed M, Viale A, Busam K, et al. A genome-wide high-resolution array-CGH analysis of cutaneous melanoma and comparison of array-CGH to FISH in diagnostic evaluation. J Mol Diagn. 2013;15(5):581–91.

70. Gerami P, Scolyer RA, Xu X, Elder DE, Abraham RM, Fullen D, et al. Risk assessment for atypical spitzoid melanocytic neoplasms using FISH to identify chromosomal copy number aberrations. Am J Surg Pathol. 2013;37(5):676–84.

71. Shen L, Cooper C, Bajaj S, Liu P, Pestova E, Guitart J, et al. Atypical spitz tumors with 6q23 deletions: a clinical, histological, and molecular study. Am J Dermatopathol. 2013;35(8):804–12.

72. Yazdan P, Cooper C, Sholl LM, Busam K, Rademaker A, Weitner BB, et al. Comparative analysis of atypical spitz tumors with heterozygous versus homozygous 9p21 deletions for clinical outcomes, histomorphology, BRAF mutation, and p16 expression. Am J Surg Pathol. 2014;38(5):638–45.

73. Da Forno PD, Pringle JH, Fletcher A, Bamford M, Su L, Potter L, et al. BRAF, NRAS and HRAS mutations in spitzoid tumours and their possible pathogenetic significance. Br J Dermatol. 2009;161(2):364–72.

74. Horst BA, Terrano D, Fang Y, Silvers DN, Busam KJ. 9p21 gene locus in Spitz nevi of older individuals: absence of cytogenetic and immunohistochemical findings associated with malignancy. Hum Pathol. 2013;44(12):2822–8.

75. Horst BA, Fang Y, Silvers DN, Busam KJ. Chromosomal aberrations by 4-color fluorescence in situ hybridization not detected in Spitz nevi of older individuals. Arch Dermatol. 2012;148(10):1152–6.

76. Wiesner T, Obenauf AC, Murali R, Fried I, Griewank KG, Ulz P, et al. Germline mutations in BAP1 predispose to melanocytic tumors. Nat Genet. 2011;43(10):1018–21. Pubmed Central PMCID: 3328403.

77. Wiesner T, Murali R, Fried I, Cerroni L, Busam K, Kutzner H, et al. A distinct subset of atypical Spitz tumors is characterized by BRAF mutation and loss of BAP1 expression. Am J Surg Pathol. 2012;36(6):818–30. Pubmed Central PMCID: 3354018.

78. Busam KJ, Wanna M, Wiesner T. Multiple epithelioid Spitz nevi or tumors with loss of BAP1 expression: a clue to a hereditary tumor syndrome. JAMA Dermatol. 2013;149(3):335–9.

79. Busam KJ, Sung J, Wiesner T, von Deimling A, Jungbluth A. Combined BRAF(V600E)-positive melanocytic lesions with large epithelioid cells lacking BAP1 expression and conventional nevomelanocytes. Am J Surg Pathol. 2013;37(2):193–9.

80. Murali R, Wilmott JS, Jakrot V, Al-Ahmadie HA, Wiesner T, McCarthy SW, et al. BAP1 expression in cutaneous melanoma: a pilot study. Pathology. 2013;45(6):606–9.

81. Yeh I, Mully TW, Wiesner T, Vemula SS, Mirza SA, Sparatta AJ, et al. Ambiguous melanocytic tumors with loss of 3p21. Am J Surg Pathol. 2014;38(8):1088–95. Pubmed Central PMCID: 4101029.

82. Wiesner T, He J, Yelensky R, Esteve-Puig R, Botton T, Yeh I, et al. Kinase fusions are frequent in Spitz tumours and spitzoid melanomas. Nat Commun. 2014;5:3116. Pubmed Central PMCID: 4084638.

83. Shaw AT, Ou SH, Bang YJ, Camidge DR, Solomon BJ, Salgia R, et al. Crizotinib in ROS1-rearranged non-small-cell lung cancer. N Engl J Med. 2014;371(21):1963–71.

84. Solomon B, Wilner KD, Shaw AT. Current status of targeted therapy for anaplastic lymphoma kinase-rearranged non-small cell lung cancer. Clin Pharmacol Ther. 2014;95(1):15–23.

85. Busam KJ, Kutzner H, Cerroni L, Wiesner T. Clinical and pathologic findings of Spitz nevi and atypical Spitz tumors with ALK fusions. Am J Surg Pathol. 2014;38(7):925–33.

Part VIII

Immunohistology of Sentinel Lymph Node in Melanoma

Sentinel Lymph Node in Melanoma

14

Victor G. Prieto

Introduction

Cutaneous melanoma has become a significant health problem. Not only has its incidence risen strikingly over the past several decades, but it has a relatively high mortality and affects patients at a younger age than most cancers, thus resulting in a high social impact.

Although histologic examination of the primary lesion provides very important prognostic information included in the AJCC classification (i.e., Breslow thickness, ulceration, and mitotic figures), there are still some patients with relatively thin melanomas that progress to recur locally or metastasize to internal organs. Therefore, in melanoma, as well as in other solid tumors, clinical research has continued to try to detect features to further refine the prognosis of patients with these tumors. Among them, examination of sentinel lymph node (SLN) is probably one of the most important ones. SLN is defined as the first lymph node to receive lymphatic drainage from a particular anatomic area, and thus it is the lymph node most likely to contain any metastatic deposits. Evaluation of SLN is a popular method of staging of several malignancies, particularly breast

carcinoma and melanoma. The main advantages of SLN biopsy are the relatively low number/ degree of side effects (when compared with complete lymphadenectomy) and the restricted number of lymph nodes obtained, which can then be extensively analyzed by Pathology.

Criteria for Recommendation of Sentinel Lymphadenectomy

Most protocols recommend SLN examination in patients with melanomas with Breslow thickness ≥1 mm, or with ulceration. In addition, traditionally, lesions thinner than 1 mm and without ulceration, but with invasion to the reticular dermis (i.e., Clark level IV) were also considered to be at risk for metastatic disease and thus, patients with such lesions were recommended sentinel lymph node. This latter criterion changed in current AJCC classification in favor of mitotic count [1]. At our institution, other criteria also considered in such thin lesions are vascular invasion (particularly highlighted with anti-D2-40 [2, 3]) and satellitosis. At least one study has indicated that paucity of lymphocytic infiltrate is associated with higher positivity rate of SLN [4]. It is unclear if the presence of regression correlates with higher rate of positive SLN [5, 6], so most protocols do not consider regression as a criterion for SLN analysis. On the other hand, a melanoma subgroup that may not benefit of the examination of SLN regarding Breslow thickness is that of pure desmoplastic melanoma, since such lesions only rarely metastasize to the SLN [7, 8]. The

V.G. Prieto, M.D., Ph.D. (✉)
Department of Pathology, University of Texas MD Anderson Cancer Center, 1515 Holcombe Blvd, Unit 0085, Houston, TX 77545, USA
e-mail: vprieto@mdanderson.org

© Springer International Publishing Switzerland 2016
J.A. Plaza, V.G. Prieto (eds.), *Applied Immunohistochemistry in the Evaluation of Skin Neoplasms*, DOI 10.1007/978-3-319-30590-5_14

definition of "pure" desmoplastic melanoma is more than 90 % of their invasive component with spindle cells arranged in a dense, fibromyxoid stroma. Thus, a number of institutions recommend only wide local excision and not sentinel lymph node for those patients.

Procedure

Identification of the SLN is usually achieved by using both lymphoscintigraphy and a colored dye. Most institutions use lymphoscintigraphy some time before the surgery to determine the drainage pattern of that particular area. After injection in the skin, the radioactive dye is then transported by the lymphatic system to a lymphatic basin where it can be detected with a Geiger counter placed above the skin. As an example, a lesion on the forearm or lower leg may drain first to the epitrochlear or popliteal lymph nodes respectively. Other areas in which lymphoscintigraphy is useful are central back and abdomen (drainage can be directed to any of the two axillae or groins) and face (drainage to different areas in the neck). Early on the day of the surgery, the radioactive dye is again injected in the area of the lesion followed, during surgery, by a blue dye injected to the same area. With the Geiger counter, the surgeon determines the area in the basin(s) with the highest count and, after opening the skin, then locates the SLN (s) that are labeled with the blue dye. Both "hot" and blue lymph nodes are considered "sentinel" and are then submitted for pathology examination.

In order to provide the highest sensitivity and specificity, the entire lymph node should be examined.

Regarding histologic examination, in general, it is not recommended to perform frozen sections in the SLN since (a) the quality of the sections is not optimal, (b) there may be incomplete sectioning of the subcapsular region (the area most likely to contain small, microscopic metastases), and (c) there will be loss of tissue when the frozen tissue block is processed for permanent sections and the paraffin block is sectioned [9]. A possible alternative is touch

preparations/cytologic specimens [10, 11]; however, it is not a widespread technique since evaluation of such specimens requires expertise in cytologic smears, particularly to be able to distinguish between melanoma cells and pigmented macrophages.

For the reasons just described, most institutions process SLN in a routine manner, with fixation in formalin and embedding in paraffin [12]. The classical processing used in lymph nodes, i.e., bivalving of the node and examination of a single, routine hematoxylin and eosin (H&E) slide, misses a number of small metastases. In an early study from our institution with 243 patients with negative SLN initially examined with one H&E slide per block, ten (4.3 %) presented a recurrence in the same lymphatic basin. Of those ten patients, when the original SLN was re-examined using new serial sections or immunohistochemistry, eight (80 %) were found to contain metastatic melanoma [13]. In another study, three of seven patients with recurrent disease had metastatic MM in the originally negative SLN after re-examination with serial sections and immunohistochemistry [14]. Based upon these studies, most current protocols in SLN require examination of more than one hematoxylin and eosin section, usually with the addition of immunohistochemistry [12].

There are two main ways of processing these lymph nodes. The original method bisects the lymph node along the long axis, through the lymph node hilum [15]. A simpler, but equivalent way, is to breadloaf the lymph nodes (perpendicular to the long axis) to allow examination of a large surface of the lymph node (Fig. 14.1), avoiding the problem of finding the hilum in small lymph nodes [16] and requiring less technical work [17].

At our institution, if the first routine hematoxylin and eosin section is negative, we then cut three consecutive sections deeper in the paraffin block (after approximately 200 μm) and examine one routine section along with one immunohistochemical slide labeled with a cocktail containing anti-MART1, anti-tyrosinase, and HMB-45 (Fig. 14.2). The second unstained slide is preserved in case there is need to perform additional studies.

Microscopic Features

Approximately 20 % of patients with cutaneous melanoma show deposits of melanoma cells in the SLN. Metastatic melanoma cells may display a large variety of morphologies, epithelioid or spindled, pigmented or amelanotic. Most commonly metastatic melanoma cells resemble the cells in the primary lesion. Thus, when examining SLN, it

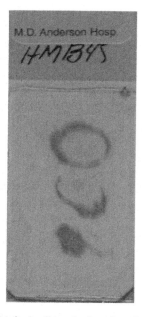

Fig. 14.1 Histologic slide of a lymph node breadloafed along the long axis

may be very important to study the original melanoma specimen, to compare the morphologic features, particularly to distinguish metastatic cells from macrophages or nevus cells (see also below). It may be difficult to distinguish pigmented melanoma cells from melanophages; however, pigment granules are usually coarser and larger in macrophages than in melanoma cells.

In general, melanoma cells in the SLN usually are located in the subcapsular sinus, as single cells, small nests, or large, expansile clusters (Fig. 14.3). Less frequently the metastasis is located within the parenchyma (Fig. 14.4). Very rarely do melanoma cells involve the fibrous capsule, and in such cases it is likely secondary to involvement of intracapsular lymphatic vessels. Similar to other solid tumors, there may be (<5 % of cases) extracapsular extension into the perinodal fibroadipose tissues.

Immunohistochemical studies are very helpful when trying to detect small metastatic deposits and also to differentiate metastasis from nodal (capsular) nevus. Of the approximately 20 % of patients that have positive SLN, 16 % are detected in the initial hematoxylin and eosin slide and the remaining 4 % are detected with the serial sections or immunoperoxidase [16]. Some authors propose the use of anti-S100 protein [18, 19]. However, since S100 labels lymph node dendritic cells in addition to melanocytes, in our opinion, it is difficult to distinguish single melanoma cells from a background

Fig. 14.2 Algorithm for diagnosis of sentinel lymph nodes. If the initial hematoxylin and eosin section is negative we cut three additional sections deeper in the block (approximately 200 μm in the block). The first one is stained with hematoxylin and eosin and the second is labeled with a pan-melanocytic cocktail (HMB45 and anti-MART1). The third slide is left in reserve in case examination of additional markers is needed (e.g., HMB45 alone, anti-S100 protein, anti-SOX10)

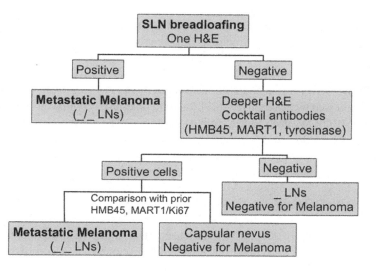

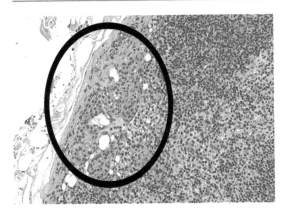

Fig. 14.3 Subcapsular metastasis. Note the epithelioid, large cells in the area immediately beneath the fibrous capsule, and thus likely involving the subcapsular sinus

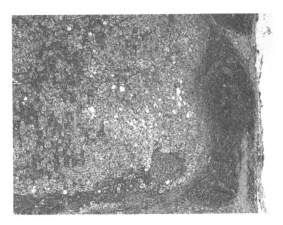

Fig. 14.4 Intraparenchymal metastasis. Cluster of melanoma cells located deep in the lymph node parenchyma

of dendritic cells. Therefore other markers may be more useful [20, 21]. Among the different options, we recommend a pan-melanocytic cocktail (HMB45, anti-MART1, and anti-tyrosinase) (Fig. 14.5) [22]. In addition, since MART1 can be expressed by macrophages [23], we sometimes use HMB45 by itself when trying to differentiate between macrophages and melanoma cells (HMB45 usually does not label macrophages). In cases of spindle cell melanoma in which the tumor cells do not express MART1 or gp100 (with HMB45) we may run anti-S100 and anti-SOX10.

The differential diagnosis also includes capsular nevi. Up to 20 % of lymphadenectomies from the axilla or groin contain such benign collections of melanocytes [24] (Fig. 14.6). The characteristic capsular location of these nevus deposits is different from the common subcapsular location of metastatic melanoma. Therefore, clusters of melanocytes in the capsule are usually benign (nodal nevus) while subcapsular/intraparenchymal clusters are malignant. However, a potential problem is the presence of vascular metastasis in the intracapsular lymphatic vessels of the node thus mimicking a capsular nevus (in our experience, it is extremely rare to detect nevus aggregates within the vessels of the SLN capsule) (Fig. 14.7). Immunohistochemistry against vascular markers (CD31, CD34, or D2-40) may be helpful in detecting the rim of endothelial cells, thus confirming the intravascular location of the melanoma cells.

Capsular nevi may rarely extend into the underlying node parenchyma. In general, those lymph nodes contain similar melanocytes in the capsular region, lack gp100 expression (with HMB45), and show very low Ki67 expression, thus consistent with benign melanocytes [25, 26]. In order to facilitate the identification of proliferating melanocytes, we have developed a homegrown cocktail that includes anti-MART1 and MIB1 (against Ki67). Since these two markers are expressed in different cellular components (Ki67 in the nucleus and MART1 in the cytoplasm) it is relatively easy to determine how many of the melanocytes (i.e., cells expressing MART1) are proliferating (i.e., expressing Ki67) [27].

Regarding metastasis, when examining lymph nodes, the report should contain the number of positive lymph nodes and the total number of lymph nodes examined, both spelled out and as numbers to avoid possible typographical errors (e.g., "two of three lymph nodes (2/3)"). The current AJCC/CAP recommendations for sentinel lymph node evaluation include tumor size and location among the required parameters to be included in the pathology report. Also important to remember is that identification of melanoma bells by immunohistochemistry is sufficient for a diagnosis of positive lymph node (and thus Stage III) even if the cells cannot be fully detected in the routine, hematoxylin and eosin sections.

Quantification of melanoma metastasis size in SLN correlates with subsequent involvement of

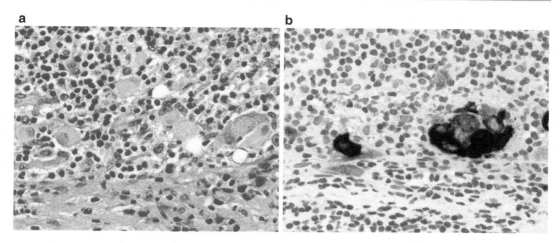

Fig. 14.5 Sentinel lymph node with micrometastatic melanoma. (**a**) Routine, hematoxylin and eosin stain shows only a few mononuclear cells, which may correspond to melanoma or lymphoid cells. (**b**) Anti-melanocytic cocktail labels these cells, therefore supporting the diagnosis of metastatic melanoma (**b**, anti-MART1, anti-MelanA, HMB45, and anti-tyrosinase with diaminobenzidine and light hematoxylin)

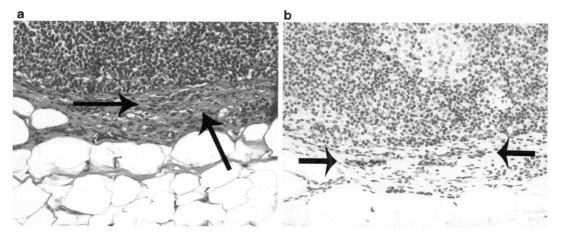

Fig. 14.6 Small capsular nevus in a sentinel lymph node. (**a**) Notice the small size of the cells, uniform nuclei, and location in the fibrous area of the lymph node capsule. (**b**) These melanocytes react against a panmelanocytic cocktail (**b**, anti-MART1, anti-MelanA, HMB45, and anti-tyrosinase with diaminobenzidine and light hematoxylin)

non-sentinel lymph nodes from the same anatomic region [28–34] and with prognosis [30, 35–40]. Some authors recommend a modification of Breslow thickness (i.e., measurement of the distance between the capsule and the most deeply located deposit) [12]. Based upon our results [40], we measure the tumor burden in the SLN as determined by the size of the largest tumor deposit (in two dimensions in mm), the location (subcapsular versus other), and presence or absence of extracapsular extension. Not all studies have detected an association between tumor location (subcapsular/intraparenchymal) and survival [28] but at any rate, a majority of responders to a European survey also report the size of the largest tumor deposit in the SLN [12].

Our preliminary data on 237 positive SLN out of 1417 patients [40], suggest a stratification in three groups with progressive worse prognosis: (1) involvement of one or two SLN *AND* metastasis

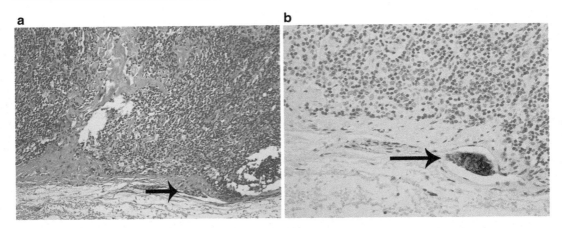

Fig. 14.7 Sentinel lymph node. (**a**) Metastatic melanoma involving a small vessel located in the fibrous capsule of the lymph node. (**b**) HMB45 confirms the presence of melanoma cells within a vascular space

size ≤2 mm (in the largest nest), *AND* lack of ulceration (in the primary lesion), (2) ulceration in the primary lesion OR any metastatic nest >2 mm, (3) involvement of three or more SLN *OR* ulceration in the primary lesion *AND* any metastatic nest >2 mm. Additional studies are necessary to determine if such stratification scheme provides clinically significant prognostic information. Regarding the relationship between tumor size and prognosis, an unexpected finding in our study was the lack of a definite cut-off. Unlike breast carcinomas, in which SLN with tumor deposits smaller than 0.2 mm are not considered positive by some authors, we have seen at least two cases in which only a single melanoma cell was identified in the SLN, and both lesions had recurred as multiple distant metastases within 4 years of diagnosis.

Regarding additional techniques, some studies have indicated that PCR detection of melanocytic mRNA in SLN correlates with decreased survival [41–43], a finding not shown by other authors [44, 45]. A possible explanation for these differences may be the presence of nodal nevi in some SLN that would result in positive PCR results. Therefore, unless mRNA specific for melanoma cells becomes available for PCR studies, it seems that histologic examination will remain the gold standard in SLN for melanoma.

In most institutions, after detection of a positive SLN, the surgeon recommends completion lymphadenectomy of the affected basin, in order to reduce the possibility of local recurrence. These lymphadenectomy specimens, due to the complexity of the method employed for the examination of sentinel lymph nodes, are examined histopathologically in a simpler manner, identical to that used for other lymph nodes in the body. Briefly, the entire lymph node is processed and examined in hematoxylin and eosin sections. Occasionally, if there are any cells suspicious to be metastatic melanoma, immunohistochemical studies may be used, but this is not performed in every single case.

Some studies have suggested improved survival after removal of positive SLN [46, 47] while other have failed to show such advantage [36]. Additional studies are necessary to determine such possible therapeutic value.

References

1. Balch CM, Gershenwald JE, Soong SJ, et al. Final version of 2009 AJCC melanoma staging and classification. J Clin Oncol. 2009;27(36):6199–206.
2. Petersson F, Diwan AH, Ivan D, et al. Immunohistochemical detection of lymphovascular invasion with D2-40 in melanoma correlates with sentinel lymph node status, metastasis and survival. J Cutan Pathol. 2009;36:1157–63.
3. Niakosari F, Kahn HJ, McCready D, et al. Lymphatic invasion identified by monoclonal antibody D2-40, younger age, and ulceration: predictors of sentinel

lymph node involvement in primary cutaneous melanoma. Arch Dermatol. 2008;144(4):462–7.

4. Taylor RC, Patel A, Panageas KS, Busam KJ, Brady MS. Tumor-infiltrating lymphocytes predict sentinel lymph node positivity in patients with cutaneous melanoma. J Clin Oncol. 2007;25(7):869–75.

5. Kaur C, Thomas RJ, Desai N, et al. The correlation of regression in primary melanoma with sentinel lymph node status. J Clin Pathol. 2008;61(3):297–300.

6. Morris KT, Busam KJ, Bero S, Patel A, Brady MS. Primary cutaneous melanoma with regression does not require a lower threshold for sentinel lymph node biopsy. Ann Surg Oncol. 2008;15(1):316–22.

7. Jung JY, Roh MR, Chung HJ, Chung KY. Desmoplastic malignant melanoma evaluated with 18F-fluorodeoxyglucose positron emission tomography-computed tomography and sentinel lymph node biopsy. J Eur Acad Dermatol Venereol. 2008;22(1):126–7.

8. Pawlik TM, Ross MI, Prieto VG, et al. Assessment of the role of sentinel lymph node biopsy for primary cutaneous desmoplastic melanoma. Cancer. 2006;106(4):900–6.

9. Prieto VG. Use of frozen sections in the examination of sentinel lymph nodes in patients with melanoma. Semin Diagn Pathol. 2008;25(2):112–5.

10. Messina JL, Glass LF, Cruse CW, Berman C, Ku NK, Reintgen DS. Pathologic examination of the sentinel lymph node in malignant melanoma. Am J Surg Pathol. 1999;23(6):686–90.

11. Creager AJ, Shiver SA, Shen P, Geisinger KR, Levine EA. Intraoperative evaluation of sentinel lymph nodes for metastatic melanoma by imprint cytology. Cancer. 2002;94(11):3016–22.

12. Batistatou A, Cook MG, Massi D, Group ESPDW. Histopathology report of cutaneous melanoma and sentinel lymph node in Europe: a web-based survey by the Dermatopathology Working Group of the European Society of Pathology. Virchows Arch. 2009;454(5):505–11.

13. Gershenwald JE, Colome MI, Lee JE, et al. Patterns of recurrence following a negative sentinel lymph node biopsy in 243 patients with stage I or II melanoma. J Clin Oncol. 1998;16(6):2253–60.

14. Clary BM, Brady MS, Lewis JJ, Coit DG. Sentinel lymph node biopsy in the management of patients with primary cutaneous melanoma: review of a large single-institutional experience with an emphasis on recurrence. Ann Surg. 2001;233(2):250–8.

15. Morton DL, Wen DR, Wong JH, et al. Technical details of intraoperative lymphatic mapping for early stage melanoma. Arch Surg. 1992;127(4):392–9.

16. Prieto VG, Clark SH. Processing of sentinel lymph nodes for detection of metastatic melanoma. Ann Diagn Pathol. 2002;6(4):257–64.

17. Mitteldorf C, Bertsch HP, Zapf A, Neumann C, Kretschmer L. Cutting a sentinel lymph node into slices is the optimal first step for examination of sentinel lymph nodes in melanoma patients. Mod Pathol. 2009;22(12):1622–7.

18. Gibbs JF, Huang PP, Zhang PJ, Kraybill WG, Cheney R. Accuracy of pathologic techniques for the diagnosis of metastatic melanoma in sentinel lymph nodes. Ann Surg Oncol. 1999;6(7):699–704.

19. Yu LL, Flotte TJ, Tanabe KK, et al. Detection of microscopic melanoma metastases in sentinel lymph nodes. Cancer. 1999;86(4):617–27.

20. Shidham VB, Qi DY, Acker S, et al. Evaluation of micrometastases in sentinel lymph nodes of cutaneous melanoma: higher diagnostic accuracy with Melan-A and MART-1 compared with S-100 protein and HMB-45. Am J Surg Pathol. 2001;25(8):1039–46.

21. Abrahamsen HN, Hamilton-Dutoit SJ, Larsen J, Steiniche T. Sentinel lymph nodes in malignant melanoma: extended histopathologic evaluation improves diagnostic precision. Cancer. 2004;100(8):1683–91.

22. Shidham VB, Qi D, Rao RN, et al. Improved immunohistochemical evaluation of micrometastases in sentinel lymph nodes of cutaneous melanoma with "MCW Melanoma Cocktail"—a mixture of monoclonal antibodies to MART-1, melan-A, and tyrosinase. BMC Cancer. 2003;3(1):15.

23. Trejo O, Reed JA, Prieto VG. Atypical cells in human cutaneous re-excision scars for melanoma express p75NGFR, C56/N-CAM and GAP-43: evidence of early Schwann cell differentiation. J Cutan Pathol. 2002;29(7):397–406.

24. Carson KF, Wen DR, Li PX, et al. Nodal nevi and cutaneous melanomas. Am J Surg Pathol. 1996;20(7):834–40.

25. Lohmann CM, Iversen K, Jungbluth AA, Berwick M, Busam KJ. Expression of melanocyte differentiation antigens and ki-67 in nodal nevi and comparison of ki-67 expression with metastatic melanoma. Am J Surg Pathol. 2002;26(10):1351–7.

26. Biddle DA, Evans HL, Kemp BL, et al. Intraparenchymal nevus cell aggregates in lymph nodes: a possible diagnostic pitfall with malignant melanoma and carcinoma. Am J Surg Pathol. 2003;27(5):673–81.

27. Prieto VG, Shea CR. Immunohistochemistry of melanocytic proliferations. Arch Pathol Lab Med. 2011;135(7):853–9.

28. Frankel TL, Griffith KA, Lowe L, et al. Do micromorphometric features of metastatic deposits within sentinel nodes predict nonsentinel lymph node involvement in melanoma? Ann Surg Oncol. 2008;15(9):2403–11.

29. Page AJ, Carlson GW, Delman KA, Murray D, Hestley A, Cohen C. Prediction of nonsentinel lymph node involvement in patients with a positive sentinel lymph node in malignant melanoma. Am Surg. 2007;73(7):674–8. discussion 678–679.

30. Debarbieux S, Duru G, Dalle S, Beatrix O, Balme B, Thomas L. Sentinel lymph node biopsy in melanoma: a micromorphometric study relating to prognosis and completion lymph node dissection. Br J Dermatol. 2007;157(1):58–67.

31. Sabel MS, Griffith K, Sondak VK, et al. Predictors of nonsentinel lymph node positivity in patients with a positive sentinel node for melanoma. J Am Coll Surg. 2005;201(1):37–47.

32. Gershenwald JE, Andtbacka RH, Prieto VG, et al. Microscopic tumor burden in sentinel lymph nodes predicts synchronous nonsentinel lymph node

involvement in patients with melanoma. J Clin Oncol. 2008;26(26):4296–303.

33. Guggenheim M, Dummer R, Jung FJ, et al. The influence of sentinel lymph node tumour burden on additional lymph node involvement and disease-free survival in cutaneous melanoma—a retrospective analysis of 392 cases. Br J Cancer. 2008;98(12):1922–8.

34. Dewar DJ, Newell B, Green MA, Topping AP, Powell BW, Cook MG. The microanatomic location of metastatic melanoma in sentinel lymph nodes predicts nonsentinel lymph node involvement. J Clin Oncol. 2004;22(16):3345–9.

35. Rossi CR, De Salvo GL, Bonandini E, et al. Factors predictive of nonsentinel lymph node involvement and clinical outcome in melanoma patients with metastatic sentinel lymph node. Ann Surg Oncol. 2008;15(4):1202–10.

36. van Akkooi AC, Bouwhuis MG, de Wilt JH, Kliffen M, Schmitz PI, Eggermont AM. Multivariable analysis comparing outcome after sentinel node biopsy or therapeutic lymph node dissection in patients with melanoma. Br J Surg. 2007;94(10):1293–9.

37. Wright BE, Scheri RP, Ye X, et al. Importance of sentinel lymph node biopsy in patients with thin melanoma. Arch Surg. 2008;143(9):892–9. discussion 899–900.

38. Guggenheim MM, Hug U, Jung FJ, et al. Morbidity and recurrence after completion lymph node dissection following sentinel lymph node biopsy in cutaneous malignant melanoma. Ann Surg. 2008;247(4):687–93.

39. Satzger I, Völker B, Al Ghazal M, Meier A, Kapp A, Gutzmer R. Prognostic significance of histopathological parameters in sentinel nodes of melanoma patients. Histopathology. 2007;50(6):764–72.

40. Prieto VG, Diwan AD, Lazar AFJ, Johnson MM, Shacherer C, Gershenwald J. Histologic quantification of tumor size in sentinel lymph node metastases correlates with prognosis in patients with cutaneous malignant melanoma. Mod Pathol. 2006;19:87A.

41. Romanini A, Manca G, Pellegrino D, et al. Molecular staging of the sentinel lymph node in melanoma patients: correlation with clinical outcome. Ann Oncol. 2005;16(11):1832–40.

42. Gradilone A, Ribuffo D, Silvestri I, et al. Detection of melanoma cells in sentinel lymph nodes by reverse transcriptase-polymerase chain reaction: prognostic significance. Ann Surg Oncol. 2004;11(11):983–7.

43. Mocellin S, Hoon DS, Pilati P, Rossi CR, Nitti D. Sentinel lymph node molecular ultrastaging in patients with melanoma: a systematic review and meta-analysis of prognosis. J Clin Oncol. 2007;25(12):1588–95.

44. Scoggins CR, Ross MI, Reintgen DS, et al. Prospective multi-institutional study of reverse transcriptase polymerase chain reaction for molecular staging of melanoma. J Clin Oncol. 2006;24(18):2849–57.

45. Hershko DD, Robb BW, Lowy AM, et al. Sentinel lymph node biopsy in thin melanoma patients. J Surg Oncol. 2006;93(4):279–85.

46. Nowecki ZI, Rutkowski P, Michej W. The survival benefit to patients with positive sentinel node melanoma after completion lymph node dissection may be limited to the subgroup with a primary lesion Breslow thickness greater than 1.0 and less than or equal to 4 mm (pT2-pT3). Ann Surg Oncol. 2008;15(8):2223–34.

47. Morton DL, Thompson JF, Cochran AJ, et al. Sentinel-node biopsy or nodal observation in melanoma. N Engl J Med. 2006;355(13):1307–17.

Index

© Springer International Publishing Switzerland 2016
J.A. Plaza, V.G. Prieto (eds.), *Applied Immunohistochemistry in the Evaluation
of Skin Neoplasms*, DOI 10.1007/978-3-319-30590-5